Clinical Aspects of Parasitology and Immunology

Clinical Aspects of Parasitology and Immunology

Editor: Arron Henderson

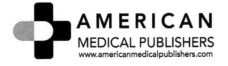

AMERICAN
MEDICAL PUBLISHERS
www.americanmedicalpublishers.com

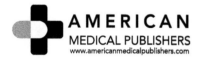
AMERICAN
MEDICAL PUBLISHERS
www.americanmedicalpublishers.com

Cataloging-in-Publication Data

Clinical aspects of parasitology and immunology / edited by Arron Henderson.
    p. cm.
Includes bibliographical references and index.
ISBN 978-1-63927-988-3
1. Medical parasitology. 2. Clinical immunology. 3. Diagnostic parasitology. 4. Medical microbiology.
5. Parasitology. 6. Immunology. I. Henderson, Arron.
QR251 .C55 2023
616.96--dc23

American Medical Publishers,
41 Flatbush Avenue,
1st Floor, New York,
NY 11217, USA

ISBN 978-1-63927-988-3 (Hardback)

Contents

Preface

This book aims to highlight the current researches and provides a platform to further the scope of innovations in this area. This book is a product of the combined efforts of many researchers and scientists, after going through thorough studies and analysis from different parts of the world. The objective of this book is to provide the readers with the latest information of the field.

Parasitology refers to the study of the biology of parasites and diseases caused by them. It is also concerned with their evolution, distribution, ecology, biochemistry, molecular biology and physiology along with the clinical aspects like host responses towards parasites. It studies various groups of parasites, including arthropods, protozoa and helminthes. Immunology involves the study of immune systems of the sapient species, animals, plants and humans. It has applications in various medical disciplines such as oncology, virology, parasitology and bacteriology. A parasite is a living organism that obtains its food from a host. The majority of parasites that reside inside and on the body of the host do not cause illness. This book elucidates the concepts and innovative models around prospective developments with respect to parasitology and immunology. It presents researches and studies performed by experts across the globe. This book will prove to be immensely beneficial to students and researchers in these fields.

I would like to express my sincere thanks to the authors for their dedicated efforts in the completion of this book. I acknowledge the efforts of the publisher for providing constant support. Lastly, I would like to thank my family for their support in all academic endeavors.

Editor

Genome-Wide Bimolecular Fluorescence Complementation-Based Proteomic Analysis of *Toxoplasma gondii* ROP18's Human Interactome Shows its Key Role in Regulation of Cell Immunity and Apoptosis

Jing Xia[1], Ling Kong[1†], Li-Juan Zhou[1†], Shui-Zhen Wu[1†], Li-Jie Yao[1†], Cheng He[1], Cynthia Y. He[2] and Hong-Juan Peng[1]*

[1] Department of Pathogen Biology, Guangdong Provincial Key Laboratory of Tropical Disease Research, School of Public Health, Southern Medical University, Guangzhou, China, [2] Department of Biological Sciences, National University of Singapore, Singapore, Singapore

Correspondence:
Hong-Juan Peng
hongjuan@smu.edu.cn

[†]These authors have contributed equally to this work.

Toxoplasma gondii rhoptry protein ROP18 (*Tg*ROP18) is a key virulence factor secreted into the host cell during invasion, where it modulates the host cell response by interacting with its host targets. However, only a few *Tg*ROP18 targets have been identified. In this study, we applied a high-throughput protein–protein interaction (PPI) screening in human cells using bimolecular fluorescence complementation (BiFC) to identify the targets of Type I strain ROP18 (ROP18$_I$) and Type II strain ROP18 (ROP18$_{II}$). From a pool of more than 18,000 human proteins, 492 and 141 proteins were identified as the targets of ROP18$_I$ and ROP18$_{II}$, respectively. Gene ontology, search tool for the retrieval of interacting genes/proteins PPI network, and Ingenuity pathway analyses revealed that the majority of these proteins were associated with immune response and apoptosis. This indicates a key role of *Tg*ROP18 in manipulating host's immunity and cell apoptosis, which might contribute to the immune escape and successful parasitism of the parasite. Among the proteins identified, the immunity-related proteins N-myc and STAT interactor, IL20RB, IL21, ubiquitin C, and vimentin and the apoptosis-related protein P2RX1 were further verified as ROP18$_I$ targets by sensitized emission-fluorescence resonance energy transfer (SE-FRET) and co-immunoprecipitation. Our study substantially contributes to the current limited knowledge on human targets of *Tg*ROP18 and provides a novel tool to investigate the function of parasite effectors in human cells.

Keywords: *Toxoplasma gondii*, ROP18, human interactome, bimolecular fluorescence complementation, genome-wide

INTRODUCTION

Toxoplasma gondii is an obligate intracellular protozoon that causes zoonotic toxoplasmosis. It is estimated that one third of the world's population is chronically infected with this parasite (1). *T. gondii* belongs to the phylum of Apicomplexa, characterized by the presence of an apical complex containing secretory organelles, including rhoptries, micronemes, and dense granules (2). Rhoptry discharges a family of proteins termed rhoptry proteins (ROPs) that are of importance for host cell invasion, intracellular survival, and interference with host functions (3, 4).

T. gondii isolates collected from North America and Europe primarily fall into one of the three distinct clonal lineages, types I, II, and III (5), which present a number of different phenotypes, such as growth, migration, and transmigration (6). The best characterized phenotype is their virulence in laboratory mice (7, 8): Type I strains exhibit acute lethal virulence [lethal dose (LD$_{100}$) $\approx$ 1], whereas types II and III strains are much less virulent [median LD$_{50}$ $\geq$ 10^5] (9, 10). According to previous forward genetic mapping studies, in which Types I, II, or III were intercrossed to identify the virulence determinant genes, the highly polymorphic *rop18* gene was identified as a key virulence determinant (11, 12). TgROP18 is a serine/threonine kinase secreted from the rhoptry into the parasitophorous vacuole membrane (PVM) and host cytosol during parasite invasion (13), of which the Type I strain (ROP18$_I$) (RH strain, GenBank accession NO: AFO54817.1) and the Type II strain (ROP18$_{II}$) (ME49, GenBank accession NO: XP_002367757.1) are different at 28 amino acid sites.

In murine cells, ROP18$_I$ can target and inactivate the immunity-related GTPases (IRGs) Irga6 and Irgb6 by phosphorylating a critical threonine residue in the switch loop 1 of the IRGs, thereby disrupting their accumulation on the PVM and protecting the parasites from destruction (14, 15). Although the precise molecular functions of TgROP18 in human cells remain obscure, it is known that it regulates parasite's multiplication in human cells and host cell apoptosis. It has been reported that a Type III strain (CEP) expressing ROP18$_I$ showed a dramatic increase in replication rate in human foreskin fibroblasts (HFFs) in comparison to the wild-type CEP strain without TgROP18 expression (13). It has also been shown that ROP18$_I$ inhibits cell apoptosis *via* the mitochondrial apoptosis pathway in human embryonic kidney 293 T cells (16). TgROP18 exerts its regulation on some important host cell signaling by interacting with its host targets. For instance, ROP18$_I$ phosphorylates and mediates the degradation of the host endoplasmic reticulum (c)-bound transcription factor ATF6β, which is expressed in both human and murine cells, resulting in compromised CD8$^+$ T cell-mediated host defense against T. gondii infection (17). ROP18$_I$ has also been shown to associate with p65, a member of the human NF-κB family of transcription factors, and targets this protein for ubiquitin-dependent degradation to suppress the human NF-κB pathway (18). Despite the important roles of the virulence factor TgROP18 in disrupting host cell functions and preserving survival of parasites in human cells, only a few binding partners of ROP18$_I$ have been determined, and the complex regulatory network of protein–protein interactions (PPIs) between ROP18$_I$ and host cell proteins remains to be elucidated. Moreover, very little is known regarding the host targets of ROP18$_{II}$, even though it is functionally expressed in Type II strains and is capable of conferring virulence to a Type III strain (11, 19).

A previous study has identified eight TgROP18-interacting proteins with a yeast two-hybrid (YTH) system (20). However, YTH generates a high occurrence of false positives and requires that the interacting proteins accumulate in the yeast nucleus (21). More recently, by using a protein array approach, Yang et al. have identified 68 substrates of the TgROP18 kinase, and four of them have been validated as the host targets (22). Although protein array is useful for comprehensive screens of protein functions, it requires pure functional proteins that are difficult to obtain because of the difficulties in expressing the proteins in a soluble form with correct folding (23). The bimolecular fluorescence complementation (BiFC) technique has been proven to be a useful and efficient tool to study PPIs. The BiFC assay is based on the principle that two non-fluorescent fragments [e.g., amino-yellow fluorescence protein, NYFP, or carboxyl-yellow fluorescence protein, C-terminal fragment of YFP (CYFP)] of a fluorescent reporter protein (e.g., yellow fluorescence protein, YFP) can refold together and reconstitute the functional fluorescent entity when they are in close proximity, for example by fusing to a pair of interacting proteins (**Figure 1A**) (24). Thus, the fluorescence intensity is proportional to the amount of formed dimer and can be detected by microscopy or flow cytometry (25). Here, we applied a high-throughput PPI screening based on BiFC (HT-BiFC) combined with a Gateway cloning system (26) to identify the potential TgROP18 (ROP18$_I$ and ROP18$_{II}$) interaction partners within a human ORFeome library containing more than 18,000 human cDNA clones (27). This screening helped us gain insights into the biological functions of TgROP18 in human cells.

MATERIALS AND METHODS

Parasites and Cell Lines

The RH and PRU strains of T. gondii were maintained by serial passage in HFFs, as described previously (28). The HFFs (#ATCC SCRC-1041), Phoenix (#ATCC CRL-3213), and COS-7 (#ATCC CRL-1651) cell lines were purchased from the American Type Culture Collection (Manassas, VA, USA). The HTC75 cell line was kindly provided by Professor Wenbin Ma (Sun Yat-Sen University, Guangzhou, China). Parasites and cells were cultured in Dulbecco's Modified Eagle Medium (DMEM, Gibco, #11995065) supplemented with 10% fetal bovine serum (Gibco, #16000044) and 1% penicillin/streptomycin (Gibco, #15070063) at 37°C in a 5% CO$_2$ incubator.

Antibodies

Anti-NMI rabbit monoclonal antibody (#183724) was obtained from Abcam (Cambridge, MA, USA). Anti-FLAG mouse monoclonal antibody (#AE005) was obtained from Abclonal (Woburn, MA, USA). Anti-HA rabbit monoclonal (#3724) and anti-β-Actin rabbit monoclonal (#4970) antibodies were obtained from Cell Signaling Technology (Danvers, MA, USA). Normal rabbit control IgG (#AB-105-C) was obtained from R&D Systems (Minneapolis, MN, USA). Anti-P2RX1 goat polyclonal (#sc-31491) and normal goat IgG (#sc-2028) antibodies were obtained from Santa Cruz Biotechnology (Dallas, TX, USA). Normal mouse IgG (#12-371) was obtained from Sigma-Aldrich (Billerica, MA, USA). Mono- and polyubiquitinylated conjugates monoclonal (FK2) antibody (#BML-PW8810) was obtained from Enzo Life Sciences (Farmingdale, NY, USA).

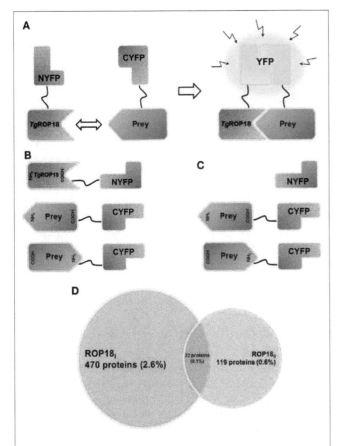

FIGURE 1 | Establishment of the HT-BiFC screening system and *Tg*ROP18-interacting proteins. **(A)** Principle of the bimolecular fluorescence complementation (BiFC) assay. The non-fluorescent fragments of a fluorescent reporter protein are fused with the proteins of interest and expressed in human cells. If the interaction between the proteins of interest takes place, the split fragments will be pulled close enough to refold together and reconstitute the functional fluorescent entity. **(B)** Schematic representation illustrating the *Tg*ROP18/prey BiFC constructs generated in the present study. *Tg*ROP18 is fused with the N-terminal fragment of YFP (NYFP) at the C-terminus, and the prey protein is tethered with the C-terminal fragment of YFP (CYFP) at either the N- or C-terminus. **(C)** Schematic representation illustrating the control screening. Non-fused NYFP is mated with each CYFP-prey/prey-CYFP constructs. **(D)** Venn diagram depicting the number (percentage) of ROP18$_I$-specific targets (blue), ROP18$_{II}$-specific targets (green), and ROP18$_I$/ROP18$_{II}$ targets (in the middle).

Plasmid Construction

Total RNA of *T. gondii* RH and PRU tachyzoites was extracted using the RNeasy Plus Mini Kit (#74034, Qiagen, Germantown, MD, USA) following manufacturer's instructions. The cDNA fragments of ROP18$_I$ (ToxoDB #TGGT1_205250) and ROP18$_{II}$ (ToxoDB #TGME49_205250) were amplified by RT-PCR from the total RNA of the RH and PRU tachyzoites with the forward primer 5'-ATAGCGGCCGCAATGTTTTCGGTACAGCG-3' and the reverse primer 5'-GGCGCGCCCTTCTGTGTGGAGATG-3'. The cDNAs of ROP18$_I$ and ROP18$_{II}$ were then fused with the N-terminal fragment (residues 1–155) of yellow fluorescent protein (NYFP) at the C-terminus to construct the bait vectors, pBabe-CMV-ROP18$_I$-NYFP-neo and pBabe-CMV-ROP18$_{II}$-NYFP-neo,

respectively (**Figure 1B**). The cDNAs of N-myc and STAT interactor (NMI), interleukin 20 receptor-β (IL20RB), purinergic receptor P2X1 (P2RX1), interleukin 21 (IL21), ubiquitin C (UBC), and vimentin were individually amplified by PCR from the human ORFeome v3.1 (Open Biosystems) and subcloned into pcDNA3.1 for eukaryotic expression, or into pEYFP-C1 for expression fused with enhanced yellow fluorescent protein. In addition, ROP18$_I$ and ROP18$_{II}$ cDNAs were, respectively, subcloned into pcDNA3.1 for eukaryotic expression, and into pECFP-N1 for expression fused with enhanced cyan fluorescent protein. All constructs were verified by DNA sequencing.

HT-BiFC Assay

The HT-BiFC screening was conducted by Longjie Biotechnology Co., Ltd. (Foshan, Guangdong, China). Bait vectors were transfected into the packaging cell lines, Phoenix cells, to generate the retrovirus, and the harvested retroviruses were used to infect HTC75 cells. Stable bait cell lines expressing ROP18$_I$-NYFP or ROP18$_{II}$-NYFP were obtained after 10 days of selection with 300 μg/mL G418. Meanwhile, a pool of prey vectors were constructed from the human ORFeome v7.1 library, containing 18,414 human open reading frames (ORFs), using the Gateway recombination system. At the end of the process, 17,076 colonies with a coverage of 93% of all human ORFs were successfully obtained (27). The prey collections were tethered to the C-terminal fragment (residues 156–239) of YFP (CYFP) at either the N- or C-terminus (pCL-CMV-prey-CYFP-puro and pCL-CMV-CYFP-prey-puro) (**Figure 1B**). CYFP-tagged prey retroviruses were produced as mentioned above and used to infect the stable NYFP tagged ROP18$_I$ (or ROP18$_{II}$) bait cells. Two days after infection, the infected cells were subjected to 5–10 days of selection with 1 μg/mL puromycin to obtain the stable cell lines co-expressing NYFP-tagged ROP18$_I$ (or ROP18$_{II}$) and CYFP-tagged prey. All procedures were performed in 96-well plates, using the Biomek 3000 Laboratory Automation Workstation (Beckman Coulter, Brea, CA, USA). The resulting diploid cells were then harvested, and the fluorescent cells were sorted out using the LSRII flow cytometer equipped with a high-throughput sampler (BD Biosciences, San Jose, CA, USA), along with the HTC75 cells infected with only CYFP-EV retroviruses as the negative control group. The positive fluorescent cells were harvested and subjected to another round of sorting until the desired positive rate (more than 90%) was reached (Figure S1 in Supplementary Material). mRNAs of the final positive cells were extracted and reverse-transcribed into cDNA by RT-PCR amplification and were then identified through Illumina/Solexa sequencing (29).

To determine the false-positive BiFC signals resulting from the self-assembly of the two YFP fragments, a control screening was performed, in which a stable bait cell line was generated to express NYFP without fusion to ROP18$_I$ or ROP18$_{II}$. The expressed NYFP was then mated with each CYFP-prey/prey-CYFP in the prey library (**Figure 1C**). The Original Total Reads of each prey was calculated through the high-throughput sequencing analysis of the whole prey library, and the NYFP Total Reads were calculated through the sequencing analysis of the positive cells obtained from the control screening. A Bias Ratio was then defined as the tendency of the NYFP fragment to associate with the CYFP-prey/prey-CYFP, by comparing the NYFP Total Reads to the Original Total Reads for each prey. The higher the Bias Ratio, the higher risk of identifying the prey as a positive signal. The preys with a Bias Ratio of more than 1% were regarded as false-positives and discarded.

SE-FRET Assay

The day before transfection, a total of 1×10^5 COS-7 cells were seeded in each well of a 12-well plate with 1 mL DMEM growth medium (no antibiotics). When the cells were about 60% to 80% confluent, 1 µg of pEYFPC1-NMI (pEYFPC1-IL20RB, pEYFPC1-P2RX1, pEYFPC1-IL21, pEYFPC1-UBC, or pEYFPC1-vimentin) and/or 1 µg of pECFPN1-ROP18$_I$ plasmids were transfected into COS-7 cells for the experimental groups, using Lipofectamine 2000 transfection reagent (#11668-019, Invitrogen, Waltham, MA, USA). For the negative control group, pECFPN1 and pEYFPC1 empty vectors were transfected into the cells, while for the positive control group, pECFPN1-EYFP was transfected into the cells. At 6 h post-transfection, the medium was replaced with fresh complete growth medium.

For the SE-FRET assay, prior to the testing of co-transfection samples, the images of the donor (CFP-ROP18$_I$ only) and acceptor (YFP-prey only) channels were collected to determine the spectral bleed-through. The images of the donor, acceptor, and FRET channels were simultaneously collected for selection of the region of interest during detection of the samples co-transfected with CFP-ROP18$_I$ and YFP-prey. The adjusted fluorescence density was obtained by subtraction of the background light density from the fluorescence density of the protein signal. The fluorescence signal, FRET efficiency, and distance between donor and acceptor were analyzed and calculated using the Olympus FluoView FV1000 viewer software (Olympus, Tokyo, Japan).

Co-immunoprecipitation (Co-IP) Assay

COS-7 cells overexpressing ROP18$_I$ and/or NMI (IL20RB, P2RX1, IL21, or vimentin) were prepared as mentioned previously in the FRET assay. Cell extracts were prepared by lysing the cells in cell lysis buffer (#P0013, Beyotime, Shanghai, China) with 1 mM phenylmethanesulfonyl fluoride (#WB-0181, Beijing Dingguo Changsheng Biotechnology, Beijing, China). Cell lysates were incubated with the primary antibody (anti-NMI rabbit monoclonal antibody anti-HA rabbit monoclonal antibody, anti-P2RX1 goat polyclonal antibody, or anti-FLAG mouse monoclonal antibody) with gentle rotation for 1 h at 4°C. Protein A-Agarose (#sc-2001, Santa Cruz Biotechnology, Santa Cruz, CA, USA) was then added to the immunoprecipitation reaction with incubation overnight at 4°C. The immunoprecipitates were washed four times with phosphate-buffered saline and then eluted by boiling with SDS-PAGE loading buffer (#9173, TAKARA, Kusatsu, Japan). The eluates were analyzed by western blotting with the indicated antibodies, as described previously (28). For the UBC experiment, cells were treated with 10 µM proteasome inhibitor MG132 (#S1748, Beyotime, Shanghai, China) for 12 h before harvesting.

Data Analysis

Each protein sequence and functional information was obtained from the UniProt Database (http://www.uniprot.org/). To further define the biological functions of the TgROP18 interactome, the TgROP18-interacting proteins were analyzed using DAVID Bioinformatics Resources 6.8 (30, 31) for gene ontology (GO) annotation and enrichment analysis. Pathway analyses were done using Ingenuity Pathway Analysis (IPA, Ingenuity® Systems, www.ingenuity.com) by importing the Entrez GeneID of the TgROP18-interacting proteins into online servers. Additionally, a combination of the search tool for the retrieval of interacting genes/proteins (STRING) version 10.0 database (32) and Cytoscape version 3.4.0 (33) was used to explore and build the PPI network. Statistical analysis data are presented as mean ± SD. Student's t-test was utilized for statistical analysis to evaluate the significant difference between different groups using IBM SPSS Statistics 20.0 (34). Statistical significance was accepted if $p < 0.05$.

RESULTS

Characterization of the TgROP18 Interactome

After multiple rounds of flow cytometric sorting, the final positive sorting rate of the HTC75 cells co-expressing ROP18$_I$-NYFP and CYFP-tagged prey and the HTC75 cells co-expressing ROP18$_{II}$-NYFP and CYFP-tagged prey were 93.2 and 98.6%, respectively (Figure S1 in Supplementary Material). After background noises in sequencing were filtered out using a cutoff value of five in total reads, 492 ROP18$_I$ (2.88%) and 141 ROP18$_{II}$ (0.83%) interacting proteins were identified, compared to control cells (**Figure 1D**). Tables S1 and S2 in Supplementary Material present the list of ROP18$_I$- and ROP18$_{II}$-interacting proteins with their total reads, respectively. Based on the specificity of the interaction, we classified the interacting proteins into three groups: A. 470 ROP18$_I$-specific targets; B. 119 ROP18$_{II}$-specific targets; and C. 22 targets for both ROP18$_I$ and ROP18$_{II}$ (**Figure 1D**). Regarding the ROP18$_I$ specific targets, many were ribosomal proteins (e.g., RPL23, RPL11, RPL37A, RPS14, and RPS6), GTPases (e.g., SAR1B, ARL17B, and RND2), and receptors (e.g., PTPRF, FPR1, IL9R, IL20RB, and KLRD1), whereas for the ROP18$_{II}$ specific targets, many were transmembrane proteins (e.g., TM4SF20, CMTM3, TMEM147, and TMBIM4) and zinc finger proteins (e.g., ZNF232, ZSCAN2, ZSCAN32, and ZNF273). Interestingly, we found that some humoral regulating factors (e.g., UTS2, CST2, and DEFB129) and some enzymes (e.g., DEGS1 and TPO) were targeted by both ROP18$_I$ and ROP18$_{II}$.

Among the ROP18$_I$-interacting proteins, CNBP, DCTD, NUP160, and PRAC, which had been previously confirmed as ROP18$_I$-interacting proteins by a previous human proteome array (22), were also identified in our HT-BiFC assay, indicating the reliability and quality of our results. In addition to these known interactions, 488 interactions of ROP18$_I$ with human proteins were newly defined in our study. Notably, to our knowledge, our findings provided the first report of ROP18$_{II}$-interacting proteins in human cells and specifically identified 141 ROP18$_{II}$-interacting human proteins.

Validation of the *Tg*ROP18-Interacting Proteins

To further validate the interactions identified by the HT-BiFC assay, six ROP18$_I$-interacting proteins (NMI, IL20RB, P2RX1, IL21, UBC, and vimentin) with a broad range of total reads (169793, 30861, 25144, 2214, 116, and 6, respectively) were selected for two independent assays, the SE-FRET assay and the Co-IP assay.

In the SE-FRET assay (**Figure 2A**), the donor and acceptor channels show the co-localizations of ROP18$_I$ with NMI, IL20RB, P2RX1, IL21, or UBC in the cytoplasm, suggesting the potential PPIs and their cytoplasmic localization. In addition, positive FRET signals were observed in the positive control cells and the COS-7 cells co-expressing ROP18$_I$ and NMI, IL20RB, P2RX1, IL21, or UBC (**Figure 2A**), yielding significantly higher FRET efficiency and less intermolecular distance than negative control cells ($p < 0.05$, see **Figure 2B**). The SE-FRET results of ROP18$_I$ and vimentin have been published recently in a study from our laboratory (35). These findings demonstrate the stable interactions

of ROP18$_I$ with NMI, IL20RB, P2RX1, IL21, UBC, and vimentin in the cytoplasm and are consistent with the HT-BiFC results, despite slight differences between the FRET efficiency values and total reads.

The interactions were also confirmed by our three replicates of Co-IP assays (**Figure 3**). The results show that in the dually transfected cells, ROP18$_I$ could be readily detected in the immunoprecipitates by using the specific antibodies anti-NMI, HA, P2RX1, and FLAG, but not with the control IgG. The Co-IP result of ROP18$_I$ and vimentin has been published recently in a study from our laboratory (35). These results confirmed the consistency between the two assays, suggesting the robustness and reliability of the HT-BiFC results.

Bioinformatic Analysis of the *Tg*ROP18-Interacting Proteins

To obtain a comprehensive view of the *Tg*ROP18 interactome, we performed a GO analysis to identify significantly enriched functional terms of *Tg*ROP18-interacting proteins. The top

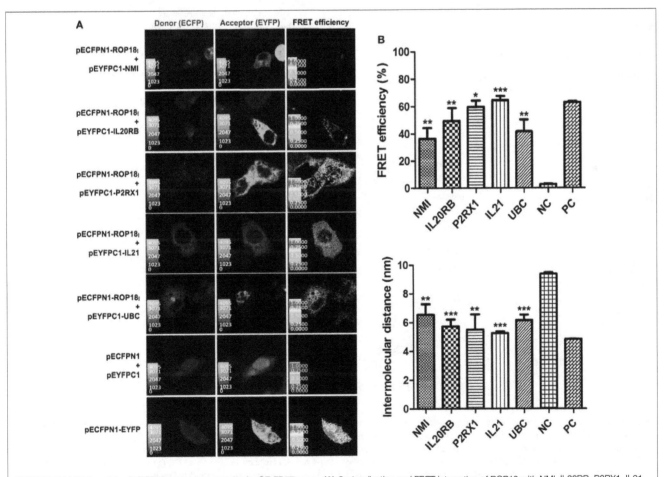

FIGURE 2 | Validation of the *Tg*ROP18-interacting proteins by SE-FRET assay. **(A)** Co-localization and FRET interaction of ROP18$_I$ with NMI, IL20RB, P2RX1, IL21, and UBC. Localization and co-localization of ROP18$_I$ and the five indicated candidates are shown in the donor channel (column 1) and the acceptor channel (column 2), respectively. The FRET efficiency is shown in column 3, in which a thermal pseudo color-matched FRET signal intensity scale is indicated for each image. **(B)** Quantitative analysis of FRET efficiency and intermolecular distance between ROP18$_I$ and the five indicated candidates. Error bars represent the means ± SD of triplicates. Student's *t*-tests results are between the six experimental groups and NC, *$p < 0.05$; **$p < 0.01$; ***$p < 0.001$. Abbreviations: NC, negative control; PC, positive control.

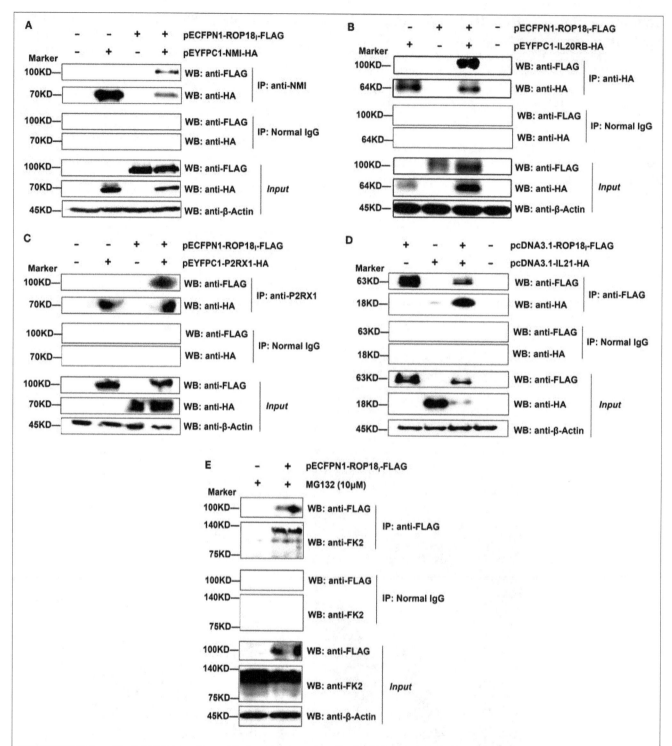

FIGURE 3 | Validation of the *Tg*ROP18-interacting proteins by co-immunoprecipitation (Co-IP) assay. **(A–D)** Lysates of COS-7 cells co-overexpressing ROP18ᵢ and the indicated interacting proteins were immunoprecipitated with the indicated antibodies. Rabbit, mouse, or goat normal control IgG were used as negative controls. The immunoprecipitates were detected by SDS-PAGE and western blotting using the antibodies indicated. **(E)** Lysates of COS-7 cells overexpressing ROP18ᵢ in the presence of MG132 (10 μM) for 12 h were immunoprecipitated with the anti-FLAG antibody. Endogenous UBC (a smear of bands) was detected in the immunoprecipitates through western blotting with anti-FK2 antibody, which recognizes mono- and polyubiquitinylated conjugates.

five enriched terms within the "Biological Process" ontology category, together with their protein counts and p-values, are shown in **Figure 4**. The results reveal that both ROP18ᵢ and

ROP18ᵢᵢ-interacting proteins were significantly enriched in a variety of biological processes ($p < 0.05$). As expected, ROP18ᵢ-interacting proteins were significantly overrepresented in the

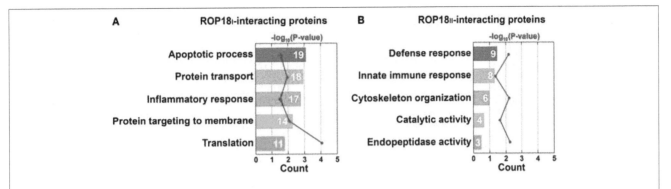

FIGURE 4 | Top five enriched biological processes for ROP18$_I$ **(A)** and ROP18$_{II}$-interacting proteins **(B)** identified by GO analysis. **(A)** ROP18$_I$-interacting proteins were significantly overrepresented in the biological processes of apoptotic process, protein transport, inflammatory response, protein targeting to membrane, and translation. **(B)** ROP18$_{II}$-interacting proteins were significantly overrepresented in the biological processes of defense response, innate immune response, cytoskeleton organization, catalytic activity, and endopeptidase activity.

biological processes of apoptotic process ($p = 2.7 \times 10^{-2}$), inflammatory response ($p = 1.1 \times 10^{-2}$), and protein targeting to membrane ($p = 8.7 \times 10^{-5}$), and for ROP18$_{II}$, we also added host targets to the expected biological processes, including defense response ($p = 7.8 \times 10^{-3}$) and innate immune response ($p = 4.0 \times 10^{-2}$). In addition to the roles of TgROP18 in the expected biological processes mentioned above, interesting roles of ROP18$_I$ in protein transport ($p = 3.0 \times 10^{-2}$) and translation ($p = 8.5 \times 10^{-5}$), and ROP18$_{II}$ in cytoskeleton organization ($p = 6.9 \times 10^{-3}$), catalytic activity ($p = 2.2 \times 10^{-2}$), and endopeptidase activity ($p = 6.1 \times 10^{-3}$) were also identified with great significance.

To elucidate whether the TgROP18-interacting proteins were functionally related, we conducted a deeper exploration of the PPI networks by using the STRING 10.0 database. By applying a medium confidence ($p > 0.4$), 353 (71.7%) of the ROP18$_I$-interacting proteins were tied to a single large network with a PPI enrichment p-value < 0.001; whereas for the ROP18$_{II}$-interacting proteins, 55 (39.0%) were enriched in a large PPI network, with a PPI enrichment p-value of 0.009 (**Figure 5**), which indicated that each one of the two sets of interacting proteins were biologically connected as a network with a significantly greater number of interactions, rather than as a random set of proteins. As shown in **Figure 5A**, 785 edges (PPIs) were observed among the 353 ROP18$_I$-interacting proteins, and seven protein–protein-interacting clusters were evident in the network, such as a cluster of ribosomal proteins containing RPS4X, RPL35, RPL23, RPL37A, and RPS6; a cluster of chemokines containing CXCL6, CXCL5, CCL19, CXCL11, and CXCL10; and a cluster of interleukins containing IL2, IL9, IL21, and IL24. Notably, UBC was observed as a main hub situated in the core of the network with 211 edges. Among the 55 ROP18$_{II}$-interacting proteins, 44 edges and four protein–protein-interacting clusters were determined by STRING analysis (**Figure 5B**). The cytoskeleton proteins ACTL7B, TUBB6, and TBCB were in close proximity and formed a cluster; TNS3 and UTS2 tensins were closely clustered with a tachykinin, TAC1; several functional regulators, such as TBRG4, PPIA, S100A1, and FKBP4 were tied together as a cluster; and several disease-related proteins, such as SNCG, STMN1, SSSCA1, and S100A16, were identified to be clustered.

By using the IPA database, we carried out an Ingenuity pathway analysis to further investigate the significant human signaling pathways influenced by ROP18$_I$/ROP18$_{II}$. Among the 492 ROP18$_I$-interacting proteins, 71 (14.4%) were mapped to 34 pathways, and 13 (9.2%) out of the 141 ROP18$_{II}$-interacting proteins were mapped to 16 pathways in total. All the involved significant pathways with their p-values and associated molecules are listed in Table S3 in Supplementary Material. The top five enriched pathways for the ROP18$_I$ and ROP18$_{II}$-interacting proteins shown in **Figure 6** were closely related to cell growth, cytokine signaling, and cellular immune response. For the ROP18$_I$-interacting proteins, MRAS was involved in the higher number of pathways, followed by ATM; whereas for the ROP18$_{II}$-interacting proteins, human leukocyte antigen (HLA)-DRB5 was involved in the higher number of pathways, followed by HLA-DQA1.

DISCUSSION

Protein–protein interaction plays indispensable roles in structuring and regulating biological processes in all biological systems. The "protein-protein interactome" refers to the whole union of all PPIs in a particular cell or organism (36). In addition to serving as a foundation for more detailed studies on the prediction of protein functions or disease associated genes (37, 38), interactome mapping has become a critical and powerful postgenomic research tool that facilitates a better understanding of genotype-to-phenotype relationship and biological systems (39). TgROP18, which is a key virulence determinant of T. gondii, modulates the host cell and mediates the parasite virulence by interacting with host proteins. However, only a few host targets of ROP18$_I$ have been identified, and knowledge about the host targets of ROP18$_{II}$ is still very limited.

The BiFC technique is an effective and robust tool for studying PPIs, as it enables not only the direct visualization of the occurrence and subcellular localization of PPIs in live cells (40, 41) but also the detection of weak or transient interactions due to the strong signal and high stability of the reconstituted fluorescent complex (25, 42). In the present study, we used a genome-wide BiFC-based proteomic approach to profile the TgROP18 (ROP18$_I$ and ROP18$_{II}$) interactome in human cells.

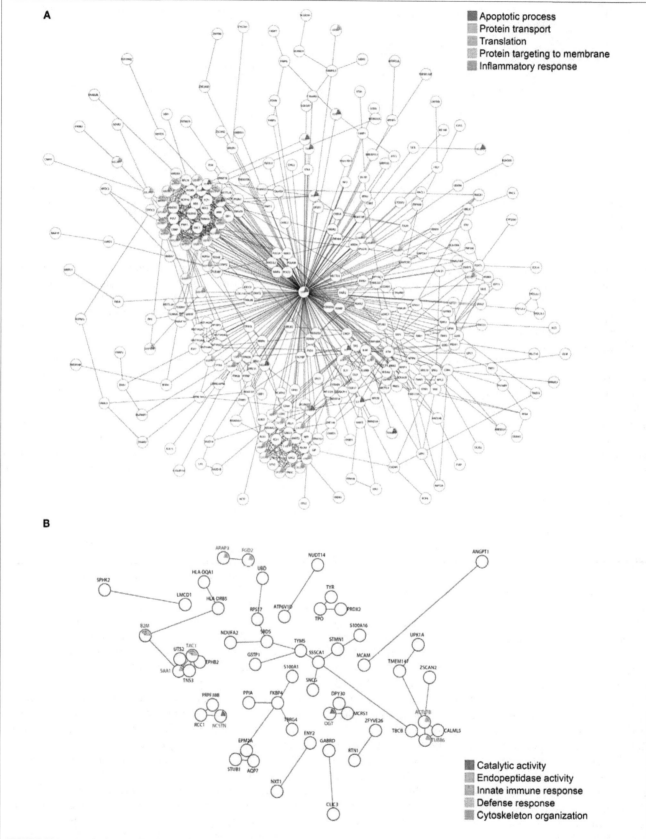

FIGURE 5 | Protein–protein interaction (PPI) networks of the *Tg*ROP18-interacting proteins. **(A)** Among the ROP18ᵢ-interacting proteins, 353 (71.7%) are tied to a single large network with 785 edges. **(B)** Among the ROP18ᵢᵢ-interacting proteins, 55 (39.0%) are enriched in a PPI network with 44 edges.

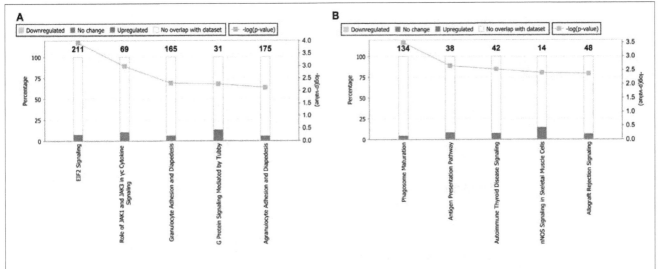

FIGURE 6 | Top five enriched pathways for ROP18$_I$ **(A)** and ROP18$_{II}$ **(B)** interacting proteins. The stacked bar chart indicates the number of proteins overlapped with the database, and the connected orange points represent the logarithm of the p-values.

Compared with control cells, a total of 492 ROP18$_I$ and 141 ROP18$_{II}$-interacting proteins were identified. Among these proteins, six of them, NMI, IL20RB, P2RX1, IL21, UBC, and vimentin, were further confirmed as authentic ROP18$_I$ targets by our SE-FRET and Co-IP assays and, furthermore, four of them, CNBP, DCTD, NUP160, and PRAC, had been previously reported as TgROP18 substrates by a human protein array (22). All of these results confirming the TgROP18 targets have strongly supported the power of our HT-BiFC assay. In this HT-BiFC assay, the NYFP- or CYFP-tagged prey collections covered 93% of all human ORFs, facilitating a much more complete and previously unavailable description of the TgROP18 interactome. We also newly identified 488 ROP18$_I$-interacting proteins when compared to the two previous screenings for ROP18$_I$ targets (20, 22). Such findings have demonstrated the significant advantages of the BiFC system to detect not only strong binding, but also transient or weak PPIs that would often be missed by using YTH and protein arrays (20, 22). The discovery of the novel TgROP18-interacting proteins have also shown the differences between the experimental methods used in the present study and in previous studies using YTH (20) and protein array methods (22), which analyzed the PPIs in yeast or *in vitro*. To our knowledge, ours is the first study to report the TgROP18 interactome in the natural cellular context. Our data appears to be highly complementary to the existing information about TgROP18, and the newly identified TgROP18-interacting proteins will be potential candidates for further investigations into the regulatory roles of TgROP18 in human cells.

TgROP18 and Immune Response

During *T. gondii* infection, immune defense against the parasite is strongly induced in its mammalian hosts, and T cell-mediated immune response plays a key role in this defense (43, 44). In our results, most TgROP18-interacting proteins were associated to the processes of immune response, including innate immune response, antigen presentation, activation and chemotaxis of

naïve T lymphocytes, and cytotoxic reaction of effector T lymphocytes (**Figure 7**).

Innate immune response provides a first line of defense against *T. gondii* infection and is essential for the activation of the adaptive immune response (45). Following the infection of *T. gondii*, innate cells, including macrophages, dendritic cells, and neutrophils, are recruited to the sites of infection, producing proinflammatory cytokines, phagocytizing the parasites, or generating reactive chemical substances in order to inhibit the replication and dissemination of the parasites (46–49). Human NPY, LGALS1, S100A12, SAA1, and TREM1 have been reported as regulators of innate immunity, modulating the innate immune functions by controlling the innate cells physiology and cytokines release (50–55). In this study, NPY, LGALS1, and TREM1 were found as targets of ROP18$_I$, and S100A12, SAA1, and TREM1 were targets of ROP18$_{II}$. These results indicate a potential role of TgROP18 in manipulating and disarming the host innate immune response, which may contribute to the increase in parasites' survival in infected cells.

Antigen presentation is the first step for induction of T cell-mediated response (56). Infection with *T. gondii* provides a strong stimulus for antigen-specific CD4$^+$ and CD8$^+$ T cells, which suggests that the parasite antigens are efficiently acquired by APCs and presented to antigen-specific T lymphocytes during infection. It has been reported that intermediate filament protein vimentin plays a key role in antigen presentation, and disruption of vimentin in Langerhans cells results in failed antigen presentation of these cells (57). HLA molecules have also been known to carry out an indispensable role in antigen processing and presentation, by binding the pathogen antigens and displaying them on the cell surface for recognition by T lymphocytes (56). In this study, we found an interaction between ROP18$_I$ and vimentin, and this interaction was confirmed by FRET and Co-IP assays (35). Moreover, HLA-DQA1 and HLA-DRB5 were identified as the targets of ROP18$_{II}$. These results suggest that TgROP18 may confer the virulence to the parasite and exert its influence on

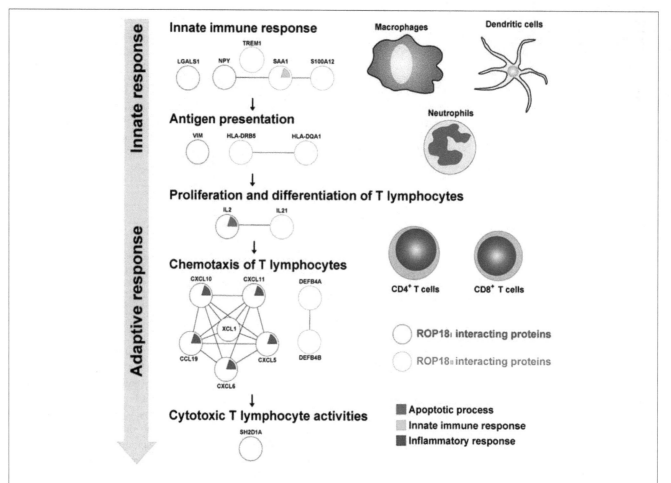

FIGURE 7 | *Tg*ROP18-interacting proteins involved in the immune response. Numerous ROP18ᵢ (red circles) and ROP18ᵢᵢ (blue circles) identified interacting proteins related to the processes of immune response. During *T. gondii* infection, innate immune response acts rapidly to provide the first line of defense and activate the adaptive immune response, with release of proinflammatory cytokines by macrophages, dendritic cells, and neutrophils. In the milieu of proinflammatory cytokines, T cell-mediated immune response is initiated when naïve CD4+ or CD8+ T cells encounter the parasite antigens presented by antigen presenting cells (APCs). Once the antigen-specific T lymphocytes are activated, they proliferate, differentiate, and traffic to the sites of infection, protecting the host by exhibiting cytotoxic T lymphocyte (CTL) activities toward infected cells.

human cellular immunity by forming PPIs with the key proteins involved in antigen processing and presentation.

Once the T lymphocytes are specifically sensitized by exposure to the parasite antigens, they undergo proliferation and differentiation, which is regulated by inflammatory cytokines (58). Proinflammatory cytokines, such as IL-2 and IL-21, are pivotal mediators in triggering development of T cell populations and effector functions against *T. gondii* infection mediated by T lymphocytes. Though the IL-2 response is not potently induced during *T. gondii* infection (59), IL-2⁻/⁻ mice have a defect in production of IFN-γ and exhibit poor CD8+ T cell responses against the parasite (60). In addition, Khan et al. have reported that in mice lacking functional IL-21, expression of co-stimulatory molecules on CD8+ T cells is strongly downregulated by *T. gondii* infection, and in the absence of IL-21 receptors, the functions of CD8+ T cells are significantly affected (61). In the present study, we identified IL-2 and IL-21 as the host targets of ROP18ᵢ. In particular, IL-21 was further confirmed as the ROP18ᵢ-interacting protein by FRET and Co-IP assays (**Figures 2** and **3**). These data

suggest that ROP18ᵢ may inhibit the activation and development of host T lymphocytes by targeting the key cytokines, resulting in the dysregulation of T cell-mediated immunity.

During *T. gondii* infection, multiple chemokines are upregulated, contributing to T cells entry into the sites of infection and targeting of parasites (62). In murine ocular and cerebral toxoplasmosis, there is a significant increase in the expression levels of CXCL10 and CXCL11 over the course of infection (63, 64). CCL19 is a vital chemokine in multiple immunological processes, including generation of thymocytes, promotion of regulatory T cells activity, and homing of leukocytes (65–67). The family of β-defensins (DEFB) consists of a number of cationic host defense peptides, such as DEFB4A and DEFB4B, which play a dual role in both innate and adaptive immune response (68). In this study, chemokines CXCL5, CXCL6, CXCL10, CXCL11, CCL19, and XCL1 were identified as the ROP18ᵢ-interacting proteins, and DEFB4A and DEFB4B were identified as the ROP18ᵢᵢ targets, which indicate a regulatory role of *Tg*ROP18 in human chemokines, enabling the parasite to interfere with the host immune responses and finally promote parasite's survival.

After being attracted to the sites of infection, the antigen-specific effector T lymphocytes display strong effector functions toward infected cells for host protection (69). SH2D1A (or signaling lymphocytic activation molecule-associated protein, SAP) is an adaptor protein that regulates signaling through signaling lymphocytic activation molecule family receptors expressed on T lymphocytes and NK cells (70). Mutations in the *sh2d1a* gene or lack of SH1D2A protein show a significant decrease in the production of IFN-γ, resulting in disruption of cytotoxic T lymphocyte (CTL) function and defective lytic activity against EBV-positive target cells (71). In our study, we identified SH2D1A as a host target of ROP18$_I$. Given the importance of SH2D1A in CTL activities, being targeted by ROP18$_I$ may lead to impaired function of SH2D1A, thereby decreasing cytotoxic activity against *T. gondii* infection.

*Tg*ROP18 and Apoptosis

Apoptosis is a programmed, regulated form of cell death that permits the active and safe self-destruction of the cell (72). It plays a major role in cell development, tissue homeostasis, immune defense, and protection against tumorigenesis (73). *T. gondii* appears to use various strategies to interfere with host cell apoptosis through both pro-apoptotic and anti-apoptotic activities. Such complex dual activities of the parasite may be crucial for stable host-parasite interaction and sustained toxoplasmosis (74, 75). After acute infection, increased apoptosis of immune cells induced by *T. gondii* may suppress the immune responses against the parasite, thereby leading to immune evasion. On the other hand, inhibition of host cell apoptosis may serve as a mechanism for preserving intracellular replication and long-term survival of the parasite (76).

*Tg*ROP18 has been shown to use a variety of mechanisms, including the mitochondrial pathway, to modulate the host cell apoptosis (16). As a mitochondrial inner membrane protein, HIGD1A inhibits cytochrome c release and reduces caspases activities, thus suppressing the mitochondrial pathway of apoptosis (77). IGF1R, which is a tyrosine kinase, acts as an anti-apoptotic agent by upregulating the expression of anti-apoptotic members of the BCL2 family. Inhibition of IGF1R not just leads to reduced anti-apoptotic BCL2 proteins, but also increases expression of proapoptotic Bax/Bak-like BCL2 proteins and cleavage of caspase 3 (78). In our research, we found that HIGD1A and IGFIR were targeted by ROP18$_I$, suggesting that these host proteins might be significant for ROP18$_I$ to manipulate human cell apoptosis through the mitochondrial pathway.

The death receptor pathway is another major pathway of apoptosis. Fas apoptotic inhibitory molecule (FAIM) is a death receptor antagonist that protects the cell from Fas-induced apoptosis by inhibiting auto-ubiquitinylation and proteasome-dependent degradation of the apoptotic suppressor protein XIAP (79). Cells overexpressing FAIM show increased resistance to apoptosis triggered by the death receptor, and suppression of FAIM expression protects the cell against death receptor-induced apoptotic cell death (80). We found an interaction between ROP18$_I$ and FAIM in this study, which suggested that

the parasite might interfere with the death receptor pathway of host cell apoptosis through targeting the key component in this pathway by *Tg*ROP18.

The ER is a central cellular organelle responsible for several crucial biological processes, and ER stress condition can trigger cell apoptosis when the stress is prolonged and severe (81). It has been reported that *T. gondii* can induce apoptosis of host cells *via* the ER stress pathway by upregulating the expression of C/EBP homologous protein, c-JUN NH2-terminal kinase, and activated caspase 12 (82, 83). Furthermore, ROP18$_I$ exerts a facilitated effect on the ER stress-induced apoptosis of the host cell by increasing the expression levels of the key molecules involved in the pathway (84). Consistent with this, two human proteins, PPT1 and PSMD10, which were involved in the ER stress-induced apoptosis, were identified as the ROP18$_{II}$-interacting proteins in our HT-BiFC assay. PPT1 is a lysosomal enzyme that is associated with the depalmitoylation and degradation of S-acylated proteins. PSMD10, also named as p28, suppresses ER stress-induced apoptosis by upregulating the expression of GRP78 and promoting the recovery of the cell from ER stress (85). Considering the significant roles of PPT1 and PSMD10 in ER stress-induced apoptosis, disruption of PPT1 and PSMD10 by ROP18$_{II}$ may facilitate the ER stress-induced apoptosis of host cells, leading to restricted immune responses and high parasite burden. Our study suggests a pleiotropic role of *Tg*ROP18 in altering the host cell apoptosis through multiple targets and pathways, providing a new and better understanding of this pathological process.

CONCLUSION

Identification of the host targets of *T. gondii* effectors is important to reveal host-parasite interaction. We used high-throughput PPI screening based on BiFC for the first time to identify the human host proteins targeted by the *T. gondii* key virulence factor *Tg*ROP18. In total, 492 and 141 human proteins were identified as the targets of ROP18$_I$ and ROP18$_{II}$, respectively. These *Tg*ROP18-interacting proteins were involved in crucial pathways related to immune response and apoptosis. Our findings characterized an interactome of *Tg*ROP18 in human cells and described novel regulatory roles of *Tg*ROP18 on host cell functions. The analysis of the ROP18$_I$ and ROP18$_{II}$ PPIs networks would be useful to reveal the strategies of *T. gondii* virulence elicitation and the regulatory mechanisms of human responses to *T. gondii* infection.

AUTHOR CONTRIBUTIONS

JX designed and performed experiments, analyzed data, and drafted manuscript. LK performed FRET and Co-IP assays of IL20RB, and graphed data. L-JZ performed FRET and Co-IP assays of P2RX1. S-ZW performed FRET and Co-IP assays of IL21. L-JY performed FRET assay of UBC. CH performed

FRET and Co-IP assays of vimentin. CYH revised manuscript. H-JP designed experiments, revised manuscript, and submitted manuscript. All the authors read and approved the final version of the manuscript.

SUPPLEMENTARY MATERIAL

FIGURE S1 | Flow cytometry histograms of HTC75 cells co-expressing ROP18$_I$- (upper panel) or ROP18$_{II}$-NYFP (lower panel) and Prey-CYFP, or

expressing control constructs CYFP-EV, showing the ultimate positive sorting rate was more than 90%. EV, empty vector.

TABLE S1 | List of ROP18$_I$-interacting proteins identified by HT-BiFC assay.

TABLE S2 | List of ROP18$_{II}$-interacting proteins identified by HT-BiFC assay.

TABLE S3 | List of significant pathways related to ROP18$_I$ or ROP18$_{II}$-interacting proteins.

REFERENCES

1. Moncada PA, Montoya JG. Toxoplasmosis in the fetus and newborn: an update on prevalence, diagnosis and treatment. *Expert Rev Anti Infect Ther* (2012) 10:815–28. doi:10.1586/eri.12.58
2. Morrison DA. Evolution of the apicomplexa: where are we now? *Trends Parasitol* (2009) 25:375–82. doi:10.1016/j.pt.2009.05.010
3. Nichols BA, Chiappino ML, O'Connor GR. Secretion from the rhoptries of *Toxoplasma gondii* during host-cell invasion. *J Ultrastruct Res* (1983) 83:85–98. doi:10.1016/S0022-5320(83)90067-9
4. Boothroyd JC, Dubremetz JF. Kiss and spit: the dual roles of *Toxoplasma* rhoptries. *Nat Rev Microbiol* (2008) 6:79–88. doi:10.1038/nrmicro1800
5. Howe DK, Sibley LD. *Toxoplasma gondii* comprises three clonal lineages: correlation of parasite genotype with human disease. *J Infect Dis* (1995) 172:1561–6. doi:10.1093/infdis/172.6.1561
6. Barragan A, Sibley LD. Migration of *Toxoplasma gondii* across biological barriers. *Trends Microbiol* (2003) 11:426–30. doi:10.1016/S0966-842X(03)00205-1
7. Howe DK, Summers BC, Sibley LD. Acute virulence in mice is associated with markers on chromosome VIII in *Toxoplasma gondii*. *Infect Immun* (1996) 64:5193–8.
8. Mordue DG, Monroy F, La Regina M, Dinarello CA, Sibley LD. Acute toxoplasmosis leads to lethal overproduction of Th1 cytokines. *J Immunol* (1950) 2001(167):4574–84.
9. Sibley LD, Ajioka JW. Population structure of *Toxoplasma gondii*: clonal expansion driven by infrequent recombination and selective sweeps. *Annu Rev Microbiol* (2008) 62:329–51. doi:10.1146/annurev.micro.62.081307.162925
10. Sibley LD, Boothroyd JC. Virulent strains of *Toxoplasma gondii* comprise a single clonal lineage. *Nature* (1992) 359:82–5. doi:10.1038/359082a0
11. Saeij JP, Boyle JP, Coller S, Taylor S, Sibley LD, Brooke-Powell ET, et al. Polymorphic secreted kinases are key virulence factors in toxoplasmosis. *Science* (2006) 314:1780–3. doi:10.1126/science.1133690
12. Taylor S, Barragan A, Su C, Fux B, Fentress SJ, Tang K, et al. A secreted serine-threonine kinase determines virulence in the eukaryotic pathogen *Toxoplasma gondii*. *Science* (2006) 314:1776–80. doi:10.1126/science.1133643
13. El Hajj H, Lebrun M, Arold ST, Vial H, Labesse G, Dubremetz JF. ROP18 is a rhoptry kinase controlling the intracellular proliferation of *Toxoplasma gondii*. *PLoS Pathog* (2007) 3:e14. doi:10.1371/journal.ppat.0030014
14. Fentress SJ, Behnke MS, Dunay IR, Mashayekhi M, Rommereim LM, Fox BA, et al. Phosphorylation of immunity-related GTPases by a *Toxoplasma gondii*-secreted kinase promotes macrophage survival and virulence. *Cell Host Microbe* (2010) 8:484–95. doi:10.1016/j.chom.2010.11.005
15. Steinfeldt T, Konen-Waisman S, Tong L, Pawlowski N, Lamkemeyer T, Sibley LD, et al. Phosphorylation of mouse immunity-related GTPase (IRG) resistance proteins is an evasion strategy for virulent *Toxoplasma gondii*. *PLoS Biol* (2010) 8:e1000576. doi:10.1371/journal.pbio.1000576
16. Wu L, Wang X, Li Y, Liu Y, Su D, Fu T, et al. *Toxoplasma gondii* ROP18: potential to manipulate host cell mitochondrial apoptosis. *Parasitol Res* (2016) 115:2415–22. doi:10.1007/s00436-016-4993-6
17. Yamamoto M, Ma JS, Mueller C, Kamiyama N, Saiga H, Kubo E, et al. ATF6beta is a host cellular target of the *Toxoplasma gondii* virulence factor ROP18. *J Exp Med* (2011) 208:1533–46. doi:10.1084/jem.20101660
18. Du J, An R, Chen L, Shen Y, Chen Y, Cheng L, et al. *Toxoplasma gondii* virulence factor ROP18 inhibits the host NF-kappaB pathway by promoting p65 degradation. *J Biol Chem* (2014) 289:12578–92. doi:10.1074/jbc.M113.544718

19. Niedelman W, Gold DA, Rosowski EE, Sprokholt JK, Lim D, Farid Arenas A, et al. The rhoptry proteins ROP18 and ROP5 mediate *Toxoplasma gondii* evasion of the murine, but not the human, interferon-gamma response. *PLoS Pathog* (2012) 8:e1002784. doi:10.1371/journal.ppat.1002784
20. Cheng L, Chen Y, Chen L, Shen Y, Shen J, An R, et al. Interactions between the ROP18 kinase and host cell proteins that aid in the parasitism of *Toxoplasma gondii*. *Acta Trop* (2012) 122:255–60. doi:10.1016/j.actatropica.2012.02.065
21. Fields S, Song O. A novel genetic system to detect protein-protein interactions. *Nature* (1989) 340:245–6. doi:10.1038/340245a0
22. Yang Z, Hou Y, Hao T, Rho HS, Wan J, Luan Y, et al. A human proteome array approach to identifying key host proteins targeted by *Toxoplasma* kinase ROP18. *Mol Cell Proteomics* (2017) 16(3):469–84. doi:10.1074/mcp.M116.063602
23. Howell JM, Winstone TL, Coorssen JR, Turner RJ. An evaluation of in vitro protein-protein interaction techniques: assessing contaminating background proteins. *Proteomics* (2006) 6:2050–69. doi:10.1002/pmic.200500517
24. Kerppola TK. Design and implementation of bimolecular fluorescence complementation (BiFC) assays for the visualization of protein interactions in living cells. *Nat Protoc* (2006) 1:1278–86. doi:10.1038/nprot.2006.201
25. Kodama Y, Hu CD. Bimolecular fluorescence complementation (BiFC): a 5-year update and future perspectives. *Biotechniques* (2012) 53:285–98. doi:10.2144/000113943
26. Lee OH, Kim H, He Q, Baek HJ, Yang D, Chen LY, et al. Genome-wide YFP fluorescence complementation screen identifies new regulators for telomere signaling in human cells. *Mol Cell Proteomics* (2011) 10:M110.001628. doi:10.1074/mcp.M110.001628
27. Yang X, Boehm JS, Yang X, Salehi-Ashtiani K, Hao T, Shen Y, et al. A public genome-scale lentiviral expression library of human ORFs. *Nat Methods* (2011) 8:659–61. doi:10.1038/nmeth.1638
28. Na RH, Zhu GH, Luo JX, Meng XJ, Cui L, Peng HJ, et al. Enzymatically active Rho and Rac small-GTPases are involved in the establishment of the vacuolar membrane after *Toxoplasma gondii* invasion of host cells. *BMC Microbiol* (2013) 13:125. doi:10.1186/1471-2180-13-125
29. Balasubramanian S. Solexa sequencing: decoding genomes on a population scale. *Clin Chem* (2015) 61:21–4. doi:10.1373/clinchem.2014.221747
30. Huang da W, Sherman BT, Lempicki RA. Bioinformatics enrichment tools: paths toward the comprehensive functional analysis of large gene lists. *Nucleic Acids Res* (2009) 37:1–13. doi:10.1093/nar/gkn923
31. Huang da W, Sherman BT, Lempicki RA. Systematic and integrative analysis of large gene lists using DAVID bioinformatics resources. *Nat Protoc* (2009) 4:44–57. doi:10.1038/nprot.2008.211
32. Szklarczyk D, Franceschini A, Wyder S, Forslund K, Heller D, Huerta-Cepas J, et al. STRING v10: protein-protein interaction networks, integrated over the tree of life. *Nucleic Acids Res* (2015) 43:D447–52. doi:10.1093/nar/gku1003
33. Shannon P, Markiel A, Ozier O, Baliga NS, Wang JT, Ramage D, et al. Cytoscape: a software environment for integrated models of biomolecular interaction networks. *Genome Res* (2003) 13:2498–504. doi:10.1101/gr.1239303
34. *IBM SPSS Statistics for Windows*. Version 20.0 ed. Armonk, New York: IBM Corporation (2011).
35. He C, Kong L, Zhou L, Xia J, Wei H, Liu M, et al. Host cell vimentin restrains *Toxoplasma gondii* invasion and phosphorylation of vimentin is partially regulated by interaction with TgROP18. *Int J Biol Sci* (2017) 13:1126–37. doi:10.7150/ijbs.21247

36. Vidal M, Cusick ME, Barabasi AL. Interactome networks and human disease. *Cell* (2011) 144:986–98. doi:10.1016/j.cell.2011.02.016

37. Mostafavi S, Ray D, Warde-Farley D, Grouios C, Morris Q. GeneMANIA: a real-time multiple association network integration algorithm for predicting gene function. *Genome Biol* (2008) 9(Suppl 1):S4. doi:10.1186/gb-2008-9-s1-s4

38. Vanunu O, Magger O, Ruppin E, Shlomi T, Sharan R. Associating genes and protein complexes with disease via network propagation. *PLoS Comput Biol* (2010) 6:e1000641. doi:10.1371/journal.pcbi.1000641

39. Barabasi AL, Gulbahce N, Loscalzo J. Network medicine: a network-based approach to human disease. *Nat Rev Genet* (2011) 12:56–68. doi:10.1038/nrg2918

40. Hu CD, Chinenov Y, Kerppola TK. Visualization of interactions among bZIP and Rel family proteins in living cells using bimolecular fluorescence complementation. *Mol Cell* (2002) 9:789–98. doi:10.1016/S1097-2765(02)00496-3

41. Citovsky V, Lee LY, Vyas S, Glick E, Chen MH, Vainstein A, et al. Subcellular localization of interacting proteins by bimolecular fluorescence complementation in planta. *J Mol Biol* (2006) 362:1120–31. doi:10.1016/j.jmb.2006.08.017

42. Morell M, Espargaro A, Aviles FX, Ventura S. Detection of transient protein-protein interactions by bimolecular fluorescence complementation: the Abl-SH3 case. *Proteomics* (2007) 7:1023–36. doi:10.1002/pmic.200600966

43. Silva NM, Vieira JC, Carneiro CM, Tafuri WL. *Toxoplasma gondii*: the role of IFN-gamma, TNFRp55 and iNOS in inflammatory changes during infection. *Exp Parasitol* (2009) 123:65–72. doi:10.1016/j.exppara.2009.05.011

44. Suzuki Y, Conley FK, Remington JS. Importance of endogenous IFN-gamma for prevention of toxoplasmic encephalitis in mice. *J Immunol* (1950) 1989(143):2045–50.

45. Yarovinsky F. Innate immunity to *Toxoplasma gondii* infection. *Nat Rev Immunol* (2014) 14:109–21. doi:10.1038/nri3598

46. Mordue DG, Sibley LD. A novel population of Gr-1+-activated macrophages induced during acute toxoplasmosis. *J Leukoc Biol* (2003) 74:1015–25. doi:10.1189/jlb.0403164

47. Bliss SK, Butcher BA, Denkers EY. Rapid recruitment of neutrophils containing prestored IL-12 during microbial infection. *J Immunol* (1950) 2000(165):4515–21.

48. Del Rio L, Bennouna S, Salinas J, Denkers EY. CXCR2 deficiency confers impaired neutrophil recruitment and increased susceptibility during *Toxoplasma gondii* infection. *J Immunol* (1950) 2001(167):6503–9.

49. Liu CH, Fan YT, Dias A, Esper L, Corn RA, Bafica A, et al. Cutting edge: dendritic cells are essential for in vivo IL-12 production and development of resistance against *Toxoplasma gondii* infection in mice. *J Immunol* (1950) 2006(177):31–5.

50. Wheway J, Herzog H, Mackay F. NPY and receptors in immune and inflammatory diseases. *Curr Top Med Chem* (2007) 7:1743–52. doi:10.2174/156802607782341046

51. Barrionuevo P, Beigier-Bompadre M, Ilarregui JM, Toscano MA, Bianco GA, Isturiz MA, et al. A novel function for galectin-1 at the crossroad of innate and adaptive immunity: galectin-1 regulates monocyte/macrophage physiology through a nonapoptotic ERK-dependent pathway. *J Immunol* (1950) 2007(178):436–45.

52. Levroney EL, Aguilar HC, Fulcher JA, Kohatsu L, Pace KE, Pang M, et al. Novel innate immune functions for galectin-1: galectin-1 inhibits cell fusion by Nipah virus envelope glycoproteins and augments dendritic cell secretion of proinflammatory cytokines. *J Immunol* (1950) 2005(175):413–20.

53. Foell D, Wittkowski H, Kessel C, Luken A, Weinhage T, Varga G, et al. Proinflammatory S100A12 can activate human monocytes via toll-like receptor 4. *Am J Respir Crit Care Med* (2013) 187:1324–34. doi:10.1164/rccm.201209-1602OC

54. Chen M, Zhou H, Cheng N, Qian F, Ye RD. Serum amyloid A1 isoforms display different efficacy at toll-like receptor 2 and formyl peptide receptor 2. *Immunobiology* (2014) 219:916–23. doi:10.1016/j.imbio.2014.08.002

55. Zhong J, Huang W, Deng Q, Wu M, Jiang H, Lin X, et al. Inhibition of TREM-1 and dectin-1 alleviates the severity of fungal keratitis by modulating innate immune responses. *PLoS One* (2016) 11:e0150114. doi:10.1371/journal.pone.0150114

56. Janeway CA Jr, Travers P, Shlomchik MJ, Walport M. *Immunobiology: The Immune System in Health and Disease*. 5th ed. New York: Garland Science (2001).

57. Bacci S, Nakamura T, Streilein JW. Failed antigen presentation after UVB radiation correlates with modifications of Langerhans cell cytoskeleton. *J Invest Dermatol* (1996) 107:838–43. doi:10.1111/1523-1747.ep12330994

58. Kim MT, Harty JT. Impact of inflammatory cytokines on effector and memory CD8+ T cells. *Front Immunol* (2014) 5:295. doi:10.3389/fimmu.2014.00295

59. Haque S, Khan I, Haque A, Kasper L. Impairment of the cellular immune response in acute murine toxoplasmosis: regulation of interleukin 2 production and macrophage-mediated inhibitory effects. *Infect Immun* (1994) 62:2908–16.

60. Villegas EN, Lieberman LA, Carding SR, Hunter CA. Susceptibility of interleukin-2-deficient mice to *Toxoplasma gondii* is associated with a defect in the production of gamma interferon. *Infect Immun* (2002) 70:4757–61. doi:10.1128/IAI.70.9.4757-4761.2002

61. Hwang S, Khan IA. CD8+ T cell immunity in an encephalitis model of *Toxoplasma gondii* infection. *Semin Immunopathol* (2015) 37:271–9. doi:10.1007/s00281-015-0483-7

62. Strack A, Asensio VC, Campbell IL, Schluter D, Deckert M. Chemokines are differentially expressed by astrocytes, microglia and inflammatory leukocytes in *Toxoplasma* encephalitis and critically regulated by interferon-gamma. *Acta Neuropathol* (2002) 103:458–68. doi:10.1007/s00401-001-0491-7

63. Kikumura A, Ishikawa T, Norose K. Kinetic analysis of cytokines, chemokines, chemokine receptors and adhesion molecules in murine ocular toxoplasmosis. *Br J Ophthalmol* (2012) 96:1259–67. doi:10.1136/bjophthalmol-2012-301490

64. Wen X, Kudo T, Payne L, Wang X, Rodgers L, Suzuki Y. Predominant interferon-gamma-mediated expression of CXCL9, CXCL10, and CCL5 proteins in the brain during chronic infection with Toxoplasma gondii in BALB/c mice resistant to development of toxoplasmic encephalitis. *J Interferon Cytokine Res* (2010) 30:653–60. doi:10.1089/jir.2009.0119

65. Davalos-Misslitz AC, Rieckenberg J, Willenzon S, Worbs T, Kremmer E, Bernhardt G, et al. Generalized multi-organ autoimmunity in CCR7-deficient mice. *Eur J Immunol* (2007) 37:613–22. doi:10.1002/eji.200636656

66. Menning A, Hopken UE, Siegmund K, Lipp M, Hamann A, Huehn J. Distinctive role of CCR7 in migration and functional activity of naive- and effector/memory-like Treg subsets. *Eur J Immunol* (2007) 37:1575–83. doi:10.1002/eji.200737201

67. MartIn-Fontecha A, Sebastiani S, Hopken UE, Uguccioni M, Lipp M, Lanzavecchia A, et al. Regulation of dendritic cell migration to the draining lymph node: impact on T lymphocyte traffic and priming. *J Exp Med* (2003) 198:615–21. doi:10.1084/jem.20030448

68. Semple F, Dorin JR. beta-Defensins: multifunctional modulators of infection, inflammation and more? *J Innate Immun* (2012) 4:337–48. doi:10.1159/000336619

69. Denkers EY, Gazzinelli RT. Regulation and function of T-cell-mediated immunity during *Toxoplasma gondii* infection. *Clin Microbiol Rev* (1998) 11:569–88.

70. Sayos J, Wu C, Morra M, Wang N, Zhang X, Allen D, et al. The X-linked lymphoproliferative-disease gene product SAP regulates signals induced through the co-receptor SLAM. *Nature* (1998) 395:462–9. doi:10.1038/26683

71. Sharifi R, Sinclair JC, Gilmour KC, Arkwright PD, Kinnon C, Thrasher AJ, et al. SAP mediates specific cytotoxic T-cell functions in X-linked lymphoproliferative disease. *Blood* (2004) 103:3821–7. doi:10.1182/blood-2003-09-3359

72. Fleisher TA. Apoptosis. *Ann Allergy Asthma Immunol* (1997) 78:245–9; quiz 9–50. doi:10.1016/S1081-1206(10)63176-6

73. Elmore S. Apoptosis: a review of programmed cell death. *Toxicol Pathol* (2007) 35:495–516. doi:10.1080/01926230701320337

74. Schaumburg F, Hippe D, Vutova P, Luder CG. Pro- and anti-apoptotic activities of protozoan parasites. *Parasitology* (2006) 132(Suppl):S69–85. doi:10.1017/S0031182006000874

75. Luder CG, Gross U, Lopes MF. Intracellular protozoan parasites and apoptosis: diverse strategies to modulate parasite-host interactions. *Trends Parasitol* (2001) 17:480–6. doi:10.1016/S1471-4922(01)02016-5

76. Luder CG, Gross U. Apoptosis and its modulation during infection with *Toxoplasma gondii*: molecular mechanisms and role in pathogenesis. *Curr Top Microbiol Immunol* (2005) 289:219–37. doi:10.1007/3-540-27320-4_10

77. An HJ, Shin H, Jo SG, Kim YJ, Lee JO, Paik SG, et al. The survival effect of mitochondrial Higd-1a is associated with suppression of cytochrome C release and prevention of caspase activation. *Biochim Biophys Acta* (2011) 1813:2088–98. doi:10.1016/j.bbamcr.2011.07.017

78. Hou C, Zhu M, Sun M, Lin Y. MicroRNA let-7i induced autophagy to protect T cell from apoptosis by targeting IGF1R. *Biochem Biophys Res Commun* (2014) 453:728–34. doi:10.1016/j.bbrc.2014.10.002

79. Moubarak RS, Planells-Ferrer L, Urresti J, Reix S, Segura MF, Carriba P, et al. FAIM-L is an IAP-binding protein that inhibits XIAP ubiquitinylation and protects from Fas-induced apoptosis. *J Neurosci* (2013) 33:19262–75. doi:10.1523/JNEUROSCI.2479-13.2013

80. Segura MF, Sole C, Pascual M, Moubarak RS, Perez-Garcia MJ, Gozzelino R, et al. The long form of Fas apoptotic inhibitory molecule is expressed specifically in neurons and protects them against death receptor-triggered apoptosis. *J Neurosci* (2007) 27:11228–41. doi:10.1523/JNEUROSCI.3462-07.2007

81. Ron D, Walter P. Signal integration in the endoplasmic reticulum unfolded protein response. *Nat Rev Mol Cell Biol* (2007) 8:519–29. doi:10.1038/nrm2199

82. Wang T, Zhou J, Gan X, Wang H, Ding X, Chen L, et al. *Toxoplasma gondii* induce apoptosis of neural stem cells via endoplasmic reticulum stress pathway. *Parasitology* (2014) 141:988–95. doi:10.1017/S0031182014000183

83. Zhou J, Gan X, Wang Y, Zhang X, Ding X, Chen L, et al. *Toxoplasma gondii* prevalent in China induce weaker apoptosis of neural stem cells C17.2 via endoplasmic reticulum stress (ERS) signaling pathways. *Parasit Vectors* (2015) 8:73. doi:10.1186/s13071-015-0670-3

84. Wan L, Gong L, Wang W, An R, Zheng M, Jiang Z, et al. T. gondii rhoptry protein ROP18 induces apoptosis of neural cells via endoplasmic reticulum stress pathway. *Parasit Vectors* (2015) 8:554. doi:10.1186/s13071-015-1103-z

85. Dai RY, Chen Y, Fu J, Dong LW, Ren YB, Yang GZ, et al. p28GANK inhibits endoplasmic reticulum stress-induced cell death via enhancement of the endoplasmic reticulum adaptive capacity. *Cell Res* (2009) 19:1243–57. doi:10.1038/cr.2009.104

2

Immunoproteomics and Surfaceomics of the Adult Tapeworm *Hymenolepis diminuta*

Daniel Młocicki[1,2], Anna Sulima[1], Justyna Bień[2], Anu Näreaho[3],*
Anna Zawistowska-Deniziak[2], Katarzyna Basałaj[2], Rusłan Sałamatin[1,4],
David Bruce Conn[5,6] and Kirsi Savijoki[7]

[1] Department of General Biology and Parasitology, Medical University of Warsaw, Warsaw, Poland, [2] Witold Stefański Institute of Parasitology, Polish Academy of Sciences, Warsaw, Poland, [3] Department of Veterinary Biosciences, University of Helsinki, Helsinki, Finland, [4] Department of Parasitology and Vector-Borne Diseases, National Institute of Public Health–National Institute of Hygiene, Warsaw, Poland, [5] Department of Invertebrate Zoology, Museum of Comparative Zoology, Harvard University, Cambridge, MA, United States, [6] One Health Center, Berry College, Mount Berry, GA, United States, [7] Division of Pharmaceutical Biosciences, University of Helsinki, Helsinki, Finland

*Correspondence:
Daniel Młocicki
danmlo@twarda.pan.pl

In cestodiasis, mechanical and molecular contact between the parasite and the host activates the immune response of the host and may result in inflammatory processes, leading to ulceration and intestinal dysfunctions. The aim of the present study was to identify antigenic proteins of the adult cestode *Hymenolepis diminuta* by subjecting the total protein extracts from adult tapeworms to 2DE immunoblotting (two-dimensional electrophoresis combined with immunoblotting) using sera collected from experimentally infected rats. A total of 36 protein spots cross-reacting with the rat sera were identified using LC-MS/MS. As a result, 68 proteins, including certain structural muscle proteins (actin, myosin, and paramyosin) and moonlighters (heat shock proteins, kinases, phosphatases, and glycolytic enzymes) were identified; most of these were predicted to possess binding and/or catalytic activity required in various metabolic and cellular processes, and reported here as potential antigens of the adult cestode for the first time. As several of these antigens can also be found at the cell surface, the surface-associated proteins were extracted and subjected to in-solution digestion for LC-MS/MS identification (surfaceomics). As a result, a total of 76 proteins were identified, from which 31 proteins, based on 2DE immunoblotting, were predicted to be immunogenic. These included structural proteins actin, myosin and tubulin as well as certain moonlighting proteins (heat-shock chaperones) while enzymes with diverse catalytic activities were found as the most dominating group of proteins. In conclusion, the present study shed new light into the complexity of the enteric cestodiasis by showing that the *H. diminuta* somatic proteins exposed to the host possess immunomodulatory functions, and that the immune response of the host could be stimulated by diverse mechanisms, involving also those triggering protein export via yet unknown pathways.

Keywords: *Hymenolepis diminuta*, tapeworm, cestoda, host–parasite interactions, proteomics, mass spectrometry, immunoblotting, surface proteins

INTRODUCTION

Cestodes have been recognized for many years as being among the most important human parasites, causing diseases that remain within the top health priorities in many parts of the world (1). Indeed, cestode diseases are explicit targets for control efforts, especially in developing countries (2, 3). Such diseases are emerging threats even in more developed countries, where hymenolepiasis remains among the cestode diseases that have the highest morbidity globally (4, 5).

Similarly to other cestode species the life-cycle of *Hymenolepis diminuta* is complex and involve three morphologically distinct developmental stages: the hexacanth larva, the metacestode juvenile, and the sexual adult stage (6). The hexacanth is enclosed within its oncospheral envelopes, forming the cestode egg (7) that undergoes progressive metamorphosis into the metacestode stage in the intermediate host's body tissues and/or cavities. In most of the cases, the metacestode needs to be ingested to reach the vertebrate definitive host's small intestine and grow into the adult parasite. In the intestinal lumen, developing immature and adult cestodes are exposed to the hostile intestinal environment, including digestive enzymes, immune responses, bacteria, and active peristaltic movements of the small intestine. Adult tapeworms utilize their scolex that is armed with adhesive structures (suckers), for anchoring themselves to the intestinal epithelium. In addition, juvenile, premature and adult cestodes use tegumental surface structures—microtiches—to mediate broad adherence to the intestinal epithelium. In a number of cases, this mechanical contact between the parasite and host intestinal tissue can irritate the intestinal mucosa, which may finally result in inflammatory processes leading to ulceration and intestinal dysfunctions (8). In this way parasite-derived molecules interact with the host immune system as antigens associated with three sources: excretory-secretory, surface, and tegumental proteins (9–11). Many of these molecules are proteins involved in the parasite's metabolism and survival strategies. In our previous study we identified numerous excretory-secretory proteins (ESPs), among which several were found as antigens with potential impact on the parasite–host interaction (10).

However, despite the current progress in understanding the parasite–host cross-talk mechanisms, the immunoparasitology and related proteomes of the adult cestodes have remained largely unknown. The only available data related to immunoproteomics of these organisms is based on the adult tapeworms *Echinococcus granulosus* infecting dogs (9). Comparing the number of reports regarding the immunoparasitology of cestode metacestode stages (predominantly hydatidosis), adult trematodes and nematodes, there is still a gap in our knowledge related to the adult cestode.

Human or other mammalian cestodiases are mostly caused by the metacestode juvenile stages of *Echinococcus* spp. (hydatid cysts) and *Taenia* spp. (cysticerci). Selected *Hymenolepis* species may infect humans in the adult stage, and *H. diminuta* has been extensively studied as it can be maintained in laboratory animal hosts (12). From these species, *H. diminuta* can establish successful invasion in both rodent and human hosts, and has become an important model for studying cestode-host interrelationships. However, from immunological perspectives, the adult stage of this organism has remained largely unexplored (13–23). The presence of adult tapeworms in the host intestine may also influence the function of this organ, thereby affecting the immunity and host condition. In support of this, Kosik-Bogacka et al. (24–31) have reported that *H. diminuta* had impact on ion transport, oxidative stress, the expression and/or activity of toll-like receptors and cyclooxygenases in rat intestines. Due to its low pathogenicity and immunomodulatory activity, *H. diminuta* is also considered a source of potential therapeutic molecules for treating autoimmune and inflammatory diseases activity (32–34).

In the present study, we applied 2DE immunoblotting (two-dimensional gel electrophoresis followed by immunoblotting) of *H. diminuta* proteins using antisera raised against this organism in rats to indicate antigenic proteins with potential role in adaptation and host–parasite interaction. In addition, the surface-associated proteins were identified to complement the 2DE results and to pinpoint the subcellular location of the identified antigens. Our study, besides uncovering plausible antigens in the adult cestodes, demonstrates that gel-based proteomic approach investigating individual proteins still offers an effective way for finding new candidates for immunodiagnostics and therapeutic strategies.

ANIMALS AND METHODS

Experimental Animals

Healthy and pathogen-free male Lewis rats, aged 3 months, were used as definitive hosts for adult *H. diminuta*. They were kept in plastic cages in the laboratory animal facilities of the Institute of Parasitology, PAS. They were provided feed and water *ad libitum*.

Ethics Statement

This study was approved by the 3rd Local Ethical Committee for Scientific Experiments on Animals in Warsaw, Poland (Permit number 51/2012, 30th of May 2012).

Cultivation of *H. diminuta* Adult Cestodes

Six-week-old *H. diminuta* cysticercoids were extracted from dissected *Tenebrio molitor* beetles under a microscope (magnification 100×). Three-month-old rats (10) were infected by voluntary oral uptake of six cysticercoids of *H. diminuta* per rat and the fecal sample direct smears were examined under a microscope (magnification 400×) after 5–6 weeks from the initial infection to verify the presence of adult parasites by finding eggs. Rats were euthanized with 100 mg/kg intraperitoneal tiopenthal anesthesia (Biochemie GmbH, Austria). The rat small intestines were removed immediately, adult parasites were isolated and washed up to five times with 100 mM PBS with antibiotics added (1% penicillin) to remove debris. Before protein extraction and proteomic analysis the parasitic material was stored at −80°C.

Collection of Serum From Infected Rats

Blood samples were collected 4–5 weeks after infection from rats, infected with *H. diminuta* and serum was separated. Sera before the infection at day 0 and from uninfected rats were used as negative controls (**Supplementary Figure 1**). Blood samples were collected to tubes by cardiac puncture at the time of euthanasia from heavily sedated animals. After collection, samples were allow to clot by leaving them undisturbed at room temperature for 20–25 min. The clot was removed by centrifugation (1,500 × g for 15 min, +4°C), serum samples were collected immediately and transferred into a clean polypropylene tube using a pipette. If not used immediately samples were stored at −80°C.

Protein Extraction

Hymenolepis diminuta adult worms in whole (size between 40 and 60 cm in length) were suspended in lysis buffer, containing 8 M Urea, 4% CHAPS and 40 mM Tris-base supplemented with protease inhibitor cocktail (Roche, Germany) and homogenized by sonication on ice until the suspension became clear. The homogenate was centrifuged at 15,000 × g at 4°C for 25 min to collect the supernatant containing soluble proteins, which were either used directly or stored at −80°C until use. The protein concentration was measured using a Spectrometer ND-1000 UV/Vis (NanoDrop Technologies, United States). Three biological replicates (three adult worms at the same age collected from different animals) taken from independent experiments were used in the present study.

Two-Dimensional Gel Electrophoresis (2DE)

The protein samples (150 ±10 μg from each replicate) were rehydrated overnight in 250 μl of the rehydration solution (ReadyPrep™ 2-D Rehydration Buffer, Bio-Rad, USA) with immobilized pH gradient (IPG) gel 7 cm strips having pH ranging from 4 to 7. Isoelectric focusing (IEF) was performed using a Protean IEF Cell (BioRad, United States) at 20°C as follows: 15 min at 250 V, then rapid ramping to 4,000 V for 2 h, and 4,000 V for 16,000 Vh (using a limit of 50 μA/strip). After IEF, the strips were first equilibrated for 25 min in equilibration buffer (ReadyPrep™ 2-D Starter Kit Equilibration Buffer I, Bio-Rad, USA), followed by a 25-min equilibration in the same buffer supplemented with 2.5% iodoacetamide (ReadyPrep™ 2-D Starter Kit Equilibration Buffer II). The second dimension, SDS-PAGE, was run on 12% polyacrylamide gel in the Midi-Protean Tera Cell (Bio-Rad, United States) with 200 V, for approximately 45 min. All the replica gels were run in the same conditions.

After 2DE, the proteomes were visualized using the Silver Staining Kit according to the manufacturer's protocol (Krzysztof Kucharczyk Techniki Elektroforetyczne, Poland), or the 2DE gels were used without staining for immunoblotting. The silver-stained gels were scanned with a GS-800 densitometer (Bio-Rad, United States) and quantitatively analyzed using Quantity One and PDQuest Analysis Software (Bio-Rad, United States). To minimize the risk of protein overstaining, the time used in the developing step was reduced to a minimum.

2DE-Immunoblotting

Proteins from 2DE-gels were transferred by a wet transfer system (Bio-Rad, United States) to a nitrocellulose membrane (Bio-Rad, United States) that was then treated with sera collected from rats experimentally infected with *H. diminuta* diluted 1:500 in Protein-Free T20 (TBS) Blocking Buffer (Thermo Scientific, Rockford, United States) and then with anti-rat IgG-conjugated to horseradish peroxidase (1:8,000, Sigma Aldrich, United States). The blots were developed using the SuperSignal West Pico Chemiluminescent Substrate (ThermoFisher Scientific, United States) according to the provided instructions, and visualized using the GS-800 Densitometer (Bio-Rad, United States) and analyzed by the 1-D Analysis Software Quantity 1 (Bio-Rad, United States). The experiment was performed with three biological replicate samples.

LC-MS/MS Identification

Spots of interest were manually excised from the silver-stained gels and subjected to standard "in-gel digestion" procedure, in which they were first dehydrated with acetonitrile (ACN) and then reduced, alkylated, and digested with trypsin as previously described by Kordan et al. (35). Briefly, the gel pieces were first treated with 10 mM DTT in 100 mM NH_4HCO_3 for 30 min at 57°C, and then with 0.5 M iodoacetamide in 100 mM NH_4HCO_3 (45 min in the dark at room temperature). Proteins were digested overnight with 10 ng/μl trypsin in 25 mM NH_4HCO_3, at pH 8.5 (Promega, Madison, WI, United States) at 37°C. The resulting tryptic peptides were extracted in a solution containing 0.1% formic acid and 2% ACN.

The tryptic peptides were subjected to liquid chromatography and tandem mass spectrometry (LC-MS/MS) in the Laboratory of Mass Spectrometry, Institute of Biochemistry and Biophysics, Polish Academy of Sciences (Warsaw, Poland). Samples were concentrated and desalted on a RP-C18 pre-column (Waters, United States), and further peptide separation was achieved on a nano-Ultra Performance Liquid Chromatography (UPLC) RP-C18 column (Waters, BEH130 C18 column, 75 μm i.d., 250 mm long) of a nanoACQUITY UPLC system, using a 45-min linear acetonitrile gradient. The column outlet was directly coupled to the Electrospray ionization (ESI) ion source of the Orbitrap Velos type mass spectrometer (Thermo, United States), working in the regime of data dependent MS to MS/MS switch with HCD type peptide fragmentation. An electrospray voltage of 1.5 kV was used. Raw data files were pre-processed with Mascot Distiller software (version 2.5, MatrixScience).

The obtained peptide masses and fragmentation spectra were matched to the National Center Biotechnology Information (NCBI) non-redundant database NCBInr 20150115 (57,412,064 sequences; 20,591,031,683 residues), with a Cestoda filter (44,695 sequences) using the Mascot search engine (Mascot Server v. 2.4.1, MatrixScience). The following search parameters were applied: enzyme specificity was set to trypsin, peptide mass tolerance to ± 30 ppm and fragment mass tolerance to ± 0.1 Da. The protein mass was left as unrestricted, and mass values as monoisotopic with one missed cleavage being allowed. Alkylation of cysteine by carbamidomethylation as fixed and oxidation of methionine was set as a variable modification.

Multidimensional protein Identification Technology–type (MudPIT-type) and/or the highest number of peptide sequences, were selected. The expected value threshold of 0.05 was used for analysis, which means that all peptide identifications had a <1 in 20 chance of being a random match. Spectra derived from silver-stained gel pieces usually do not contain enough MS/MS fragmentations to calculate a meaningful FDR, therefore a Mascot score threshold of 30 or above ($p < 0.05$) was used.

Extraction and Identification of Surface-Associated Proteins

Adult *H. diminuta* worms were first washed 3 times in sterile phosphate-buffered saline (PBS), followed by quick wash in sterile PBS with antibiotics (1% penicillin) to remove debris. Then they were washed again in sterile PBS without antibiotics and incubated in 3 ml of 1% Nonidet P-40 (NP-40 [Sigma Aldrich]) in 50 mM Ambic/AMBIC buffer for 30 min on a roller mixer at room temperature. After incubation samples were centrifuged at 15,000 × *g* and the supernatant was collected to a new tube. In order to perform mass spectrometry analysis Nonidet P-40 was removed using detergent Removal Spin Columns (Pierce) according to manufacturer's instructions. Columns were first equilibrated with 50 mM AMBIC without the detergent and then the sample was carefully applied on the column and incubated for 2 min in room temperature and eluted by centrifugation (1,000 × *g*, 2 min) to a new tube. The protein concentration was measured using a Spectrometer ND-1000 UV/Vis (NanoDrop Technologies, United States). Three replicates from the collected surface proteins were subjected to LC-MS/MS identification.

Proteins were identified by LC-MS/MS (Laboratory of Mass Spectrometry, Institute of Biochemistry and Biophysics, Polish Academy of Sciences (Warsaw, Poland) as described above. Protein solutions were subjected to standard procedure of trypsin digestion, during which proteins were reduced with 0.5 M (5 mM f.c.) TCEP for 1 h at 60°C, blocked with 200 mM MMTS (10 mM f.c.) for 10 min at RT and digested overnight with 10 µl of 0.1 ug/ul trypsin. The resulting peptide mixtures were applied in equal volumes of 20 µl to RP-18 pre-column (Waters, Milford, MA) using water containing 0.1% FA as a mobile phase and then transferred to a nano-HPLC RP-18 column (internal diameter 75 µM, Waters, Milford MA) using ACN gradient (0–35% ACN in 160 min) in the presence of 0.1% FA at a flow rate of 250 nl/min. The column outlet was coupled directly to the ion source of the Orbitrap Elite mass spectrometer (Thermo Electron Corp., San Jose, CA, United States) working in the regime of data-dependent MS to MS/MS switch with HCD type peptide fragmentation. A blank run ensuring absence of cross-contamination from previous samples preceded each analysis.

Raw data files were pre-processed with Mascot Distiller software (v. 2.6, MatrixScience, London, UK). The obtained peptide masses and fragmentation spectra were matched to the NCBInr database (167,148,673 sequences; 60,963,227,986 residues), with a *Cestoda* filter (49,619 sequences) using the Mascot Search Engine (MatrixScience, London, UK, Mascot Server 2.5). To reduce mass errors, the peptide and fragment mass tolerance settings were established separately for individual LC-MS/MS runs after a measured mass recalibration, resulting

in values 5 ppm for parent and 0.01 Da for fragment ions. The rest of search parameters were as follows: enzyme, Trypsin; missed cleavages, 1; fixed modifications, Alkylation of cysteine by carbamidomethylation; oxidation of methionine was set as a variable modification. In each Mascot search, the score cutoff was determined automatically to obtain an FDR below 1%? The Decoy Mascot functionality was used for keeping FDR for peptide identifications below 1%.

Proteome Bioinformatics

The presence of potential N-terminal signal peptide cleavage site for the identified proteins was analyzed using the SignalP 4.1 tool (36). The identified proteins were classified according to their predicted molecular function, biological process, and cellular component using the UniProtKB database (http://www.uniprot.org/) and QuickGO (http://www.ebi.ac.uk/QuickGO/). Proteins with enzymatic properties were further classified according to Kyoto Encyclopedia of Genes and Genomes (KEGG) database (http://www.genome.jp/kegg/).

RESULTS

2DE of the *H. diminuta* Adult-Stage Proteins

The stained 2DE-protein patterns in each three biological replica gels were comparable. As our preliminary 2DE analyses indicated that most of the adult-stage proteins migrated with pI values ranging from 4 to 7 (data not shown), the present study focused on proteins covering this proteome region. The PDQuest software analyses of the silver-stained proteomes enabled us to distinguish more than 580 adult-stage protein spots from *H. diminuta*. **Figure 1** showing the representative silver-stained master gel indicates that majority of the protein spots migrated with molecular weights (MWs) between 15 and 130 kDa.

With the use of the 2DE-immunoblotting we detected 36 spots as positively recognized by the *H. diminuta*-infected rat sera, whereas sera collected form uninfected rats were signal free (**Figure 2** and **Supplementary Figure 1**). Potentially immunogenic proteins migrated predominantly with MWs between 35 and 250 kDa and pHs ranging from 4 to 5 and 6 to 7 (**Figure 2**). Several immunoreactive spots were also detected in the area between 10 and 35 kDa. The proteins were organized in eight groups of horizontally adjacent immunoreactive spots as shown in **Figures 1, 2**.

LC-MS/MS Identification of Antigenic and Surface Proteins of *H. diminuta* Adult Stage

Thirty-six protein spots cross-reacting with the rat antisera were excised from the silver-stained replica 2DE-gel and subjected to in-gel tryptic digestion and LC-MS/MS analyses. As a result, 68 potentially antigenic proteins were identified and are listed in **Table 1** and **Supplementary File 1**. As shown in **Table 1** numerous proteins were identified from multiple spots; 38 of the identified proteins were present in more than one spot (**Table 1** and **Supplementary File 1**). Similarly, the number

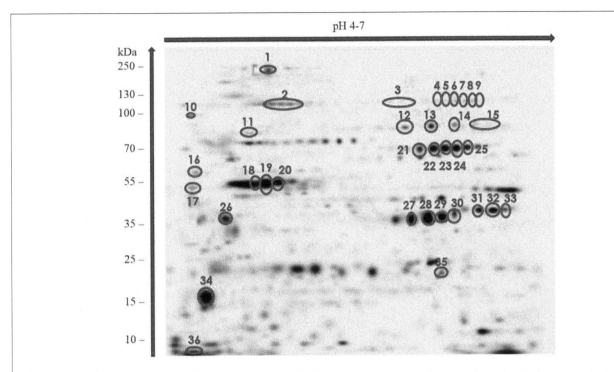

FIGURE 1 | Master gel of silver-stained 2-DE protein maps of *H. diminuta* adult-stage somatic proteome showing spots recognized as immunogenic and excised from the gel for LC-MS/MS analysis (indicated by red color).

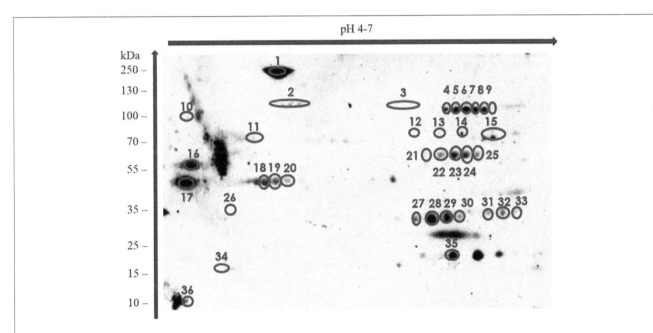

FIGURE 2 | Recognition pattern of *H. diminuta* adult-stage immunoreactive protein spots by antibodies of *H. diminuta*-infected rats visualized using chemiluminescence.

of proteins identified per spot varied from spot to spot; the highest number of proteins were identified from the spot number 12 (with 11 proteins) (**Supplementary File 2**). Only one protein was present in spots 10 (spectrin beta chain) and 36 (myosin essential light chain). Proteins that were most frequently identified from multiple spots included the aldo-keto reductase family 1 (present in 8 spots) proteins, glutamate dehydrogenase (in 9 spots), glyceraldehyde-3-phosphate dehydrogenase—GAPDH (in 8 spots), enolase, phosphoenolpyruvate carboxykinase and pyruvate kinase—PYK (in 7 spots).

TABLE 1 | Alphabetical list of identified adult *Hymenolepis diminuta* antigenic proteins with spot numbers and recognition of potentially signaling/secretory proteins (antigenic proteins identified for the first time in the adult cestode are indicated in bold).

Protein [Organism]	Spot number (Number of spots)	SP*
3-oxoacyl-acyl-carrier-protein reductase# [Hm]	35 (1)	N
Actin, cytoplasmic 2 [Eg]	1, 2, 11, 18, 19, 20 (6)	N
Actin, partial [Dd]	18, 19, 20, 26 (4)	N
Actin-1 [Eg]	19 (1)	N
Actin-5#, partial [Dd]	19 (1)	N
Alanine aminotransferase 2# [Hm]	12, 21, 22 (3)	N
Aldo-keto reductase family 1, member B4# [Hm]	22, 27, 28, 29, 30, 32, 33, 35 (8)	N
Alpha-tubulin [Hd]	11 (1)	N
Annexin A8 [Eg]	18, 25 (2)	N
Aspartyl tRNA synthetase, cytoplasmic [Hm]	12, 13 (2)	N
Calpain A# [Hm]	11 (1)	N
Calumenin-B [Eg]	26 (1)	Y
Capping protein (actin filament) muscle Z line [Hm]	31 (1)	N
Cytosolic malate dehydrogenase# [Hm]	27, 28, 29, 30, 31 (5)	N
Deoxyhypusine hydroxylase:monooxygenase# [Hm]	18, 19 (2)	N
Dnaj subfamily A [Hm]	21 (1)	N
Ef hand family protein [Hm]	27 (1)	Y
Elongation factor 2# [Hm]	15 (1)	N
Enolase# [Hm]	4, 12, 21, 22, 23, 24, 25 (7)	N
Estradiol 17 beta-dehydrogenase [Eg]	27 (1)	N
Eukaryotic initiation factor 4A [Hm]	19, 33 (2)	N
Filamin# [Hm]	1, 2, 11 (3)	N
Fructose-1,6-bisphosphate aldolase# [Hm]	32, 33 (2)	N
Fumarate hydratase class I# [Hm]	14, 15 (2)	N
Glucose-6-phosphate isomerase [Eg]	15, 31 (2)	N
Glutamate dehydrogenase# [Hm]	6, 7, 12, 14, 21, 22, 23, 24, 25 (9)	N
Glutamate dehydrogenase, mitochondrial# [Hm]	12, 23 (2)	N
Glyceraldehyde-3-phosphate dehydrogenase# [Hm]	9, 15, 28, 29, 30, 31, 32, 33 (8)	N
Glycogen phosphorylase# [Hm]	1 (1)	N
GTP-binding nuclear protein Ran [Hm]	35 (1)	N
Heat shock cognate protein [Eg]	2 (1)	N
Heat shock protein [Eg]	2, 11 (2)	N
Heat shock protein 60 [Em]	11 (1)	N
Heat shock protein 70# [Hm]	2, 3 (2)	N
Heterogeneous nuclear ribonucleoprotein 87F [Eg]	31, 32, 33 (3)	N
Hypothetical transcript [Hm]	2, 12, 13 (3)	N
Inosine-5- monophosphate dehydrogenase 2 [Hm]	25 (1)	N
Lactate dehydrogenase# [Hm]	28, 30 (2)	N

(Continued)

TABLE 1 | Continued

Protein [Organism]	Spot number (Number of spots)	SP*
Lamin [Hm]	2, 3 (2)	N
Leucyl aminopeptydase [Eg]	13 (1)	N
Major egg antigen [Hm]	11 (1)	N
Major vault protein# [Hm]	1 (1)	N
Myosin essential light chain [Hm]	36 (1)	N
Myosin heavy chain# [Hm]	1, 2 (2)	N
Myosin regulatory light chain [Eg]	34 (1)	N
NADP-dependent malic enzyme# [Hm]	12, 13, 14, 15 (4)	N
Neuronal calcium sensor [Hm]	12, 13 (2)	N
Paramyosin [Hm]	1, 2, 3, 4, 11 (4)	N
Phosphoenolpyruvate carboxykinase# [Hm]	4, 5, 6, 7, 8, 9, 15 (7)	N
Phosphoglucomutase# [Hm]	12, 14 (2)	N
Pseudouridine metabolizing bifunctional protein [Hm]	9 (1)	N
Pyruvate kinase# [Hm]	6, 9, 12, 13, 14, 15 (7)	N
Spectrin alpha actinin# [Hm]	18, 26 (2)	N
Spectrin beta chain [Hm]	10, 16, 20 (3)	N
Stress-70 protein [Eg]	2 (1)	N
Subfamily T1A non peptidase [Hm]	34 (1)	N
Succinate dehydrogenase flavoprotein# [Eg]	3 (1)	N
Succinyl coenzyme A ligase# [Hm]	19, 20 (2)	N
T-complex protein 1 subunit delta [Hm]	14, 15 (2)	N
T-complex protein 1 subunit zeta [Hm]	12, 13 (2)	N
Transketolase# [Hm]	4, 5 (2)	N
Triosephosphate isomerase# [Hm]	35 (1)	N
Tropomyosin [Hm]	16, 17 (2)	N
Tropomyosin 2 high molecular weight [Mc]	17 (1)	N
Tubulin# [Se]	11 (1)	N
Tubulin beta chain# [Eg]	11, 26 (2)	N
Vacuolar H+ atpase v1 sector subunit A [Hm]	2 (1)	N
V-type proton atpase catalytic subunit A [Eg]	2 (1)	N

*SP - signal peptide; * - the presence of secretory/signal proteins predicted with the use of SignalP 4.1 Server software; Y - potentially secretory protein; N - negative search results; # - protein recognized among surface proteins; Dd - Diphyllobothrium dendriticum; Eg - Echinococcus granulosus; Em - Echinococcus multilocularis; Hd - Hymenolepis diminuta; Hm - Hymenolepis microstoma; Mc - Mesocestoides corti; Se - Spirometra erinaceieuropaei.*

Altogether, 30 proteins were identified from individual spots (**Table 1**).

Figure 1 shows the cross-reactive protein spots numbered with 1, 5–8, 18–20, 22–23, 28–29, and 35. They were found to match with the following proteins: actin, aldo keto reductase family 1 proteins, enolase, filamin, glutamate dehydrogenase, paramyosin, myosin, malate dehydrogenase, phosphoenolpyruvate carboxykinase, succinyl coenzyme-A ligase, spectrin, triosephosphate isomerase (TPI), and 3 oxoacyl

TABLE 2 | Enzymatic proteins identified by LCMS/MS in immunoreactive spots of the adult tapeworm *Hymenolepis diminuta*.

Enzyme classes	Protein names
Fructose-bisphosphate aldolase	Fructose-1,6-bisphosphate aldolase
Hydrolases	Calpain A
	Leucyl aminopeptidase
	Vacuolar H+ ATPase v1 sector subunit A
	V-type proton ATPase catalytic subunit A
Interconverting aldoses and ketoses	Glucose-6-phosphate isomerase
	Triosephosphate isomerase
Isomerases	Phosphoglucomutase
	Triosephosphate isomerase
Ligase	Aspartyl tRNA synthetase cytoplasmic
	Succinyl coenzyme A ligase
Lyases	Enolase
	Fumarate hydratase
	Phosphoenolpyruvate carboxykinase
Oxidoreductases	3-oxoacyl-[acyl-carrier-protein] reductase
	Aldo keto reductase family 1 member B4
	Cytosolic malate dehydrogenase
	Deoxyhypusine hydroxylase
	Estradiol 17 beta-dehydrogenase
	Glutamate dehydrogenase
	Glutamate dehydrogenase, mitochondrial
	Glyceraldehyde-3-phosphate dehydrogenase
	Inosine-5′-monophosphate dehydrogenase
	Lactate dehydrogenase
	NADP-dependent malic enzyme
	Succinate dehydrogenase flavoprotein
Proteasome endopeptidase complex	Proteasome subunit alpha type
Transferases	Alanine aminotransferase 2
	Pyruvate kinase
	Transketolase

acyl carrier protein reductase. The MW and pH values of these potential antigens ranged between 55 and 250 kDa and 4 and 7, respectively.

Several of the potentially antigenic *H. diminuta* adult-stage proteins could be classified as enzymes with 9 different subclasses, structural proteins and heat shock proteins (HSPs) (**Tables 1, 2**). The oxidoreductases were found to be the most dominating enzyme group for the identified proteins (13 proteins) (**Table 2**).

Using non-gel based proteomic approach (in-solution tryptic digestion of proteins coupled with LC-MS/MS identification) we were able to identify 76 proteins from the surface of *H. diminuta* adult stage worms. All these proteins were identified in each replicate with at least three matching peptides (**Supplementary File 3**). Among these surface-associated proteins, enzymes involved in various catalytic activities were suggested to be the most abundant protein group. In addition, heat shock proteins with potential moonlighting functions and classical structural proteins including actins, myosins, and tubulins were also identified. Notably, 31 from these

surface proteins were detected as potential antigens in 2DE immunoblotting (**Table 1**, proteins marked with hashtag), which indicates that several of these antigens are excreted out of the worm.

Gene Ontology (GO) of the Potentially Antigenic Proteins of *H. diminuta* Adult Stage

According to bioinformatics predictions only 2 of the proteins were predicted to be secreted via the classical secretion pathway (calumenin-B, ef-hand family protein) (**Table 1**). Based on the GO annotation the identified proteins were classified into 3 different categories; molecular function (62 proteins), biological process (35 proteins), and as cellular components (30 proteins) (**Figures 3–5**). Twenty subcategories were assigned to molecular functions (**Figure 3**), with predominant groups related to binding, e.g., ion binding (42 proteins), organic cyclic compound binding (29), heterocyclic compound binding (29), and small molecule binding (27). Biological processes could be assigned to 35 proteins, most of them engaged with carboxylic acid metabolism (12), cellular nitrogen compound metabolism (9), aromatic compound metabolism (9), heterocycle (9) and phosphorus (8) metabolic processes (**Figure 4**). **Figure 5** shows the distribution of the identified proteins according to their subcellular location; 30 proteins were associated with cellular structures (**Figure 5**), majority of them predicted to be localized in different cell (25) and organelle parts (9) or macromolecular complexes (9).

According to GO annotation 75 of the identified surface proteins were classified to molecular function, 48 to biological processes and 32 to associated cellular components (**Figures 6–8**). Among molecular functions the recognized proteins could be divided into 21 subcategories related mainly to molecule binding ion binding (43 proteins), organic (35) and heterocyclic compound binding (35), and small molecule binding (33) (**Figure 6**). The identified surface proteins associated with biological processes (**Figure 7**) are involved in cellular processes (40 proteins), organic substance (29) and primary metabolic (26) processes as well as in electron transport chain (25). **Figure 8** illustrates the division of the identified surface proteins into different cellular compartments.

DISCUSSION

The present study shows that somatic proteins of the adult *H. diminuta* tapeworms exhibit immunogenicity in the rat host, and that the revealed immunoproteome could be used to propose new candidate proteins taking part in parasite–host interactions. Our previously published proteomic results of the *H. diminuta* (ESPs) show that the adult cestode immunogenic proteins were involved in stress response, various metabolic processes and structurally related functions (10). Some of these proteins have been considered as potential vaccine candidates and drug targets for treating e.g., schistosomiasis (37–39) and hydatidosis (40–42). Present study indicates slight differences between the protein profiles

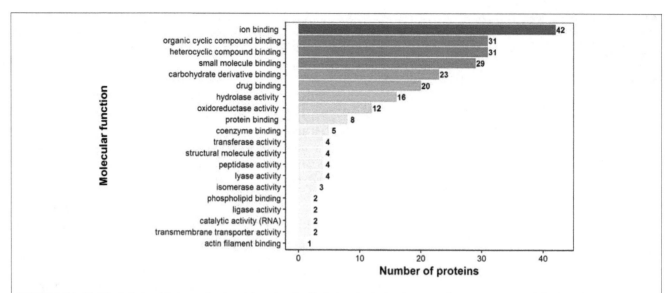

FIGURE 3 | Identified *H. diminuta* adult stage antigenic proteins categorized by their molecular functions according to gene ontology (GO) information obtained from UniProtKB and QuickGO databases.

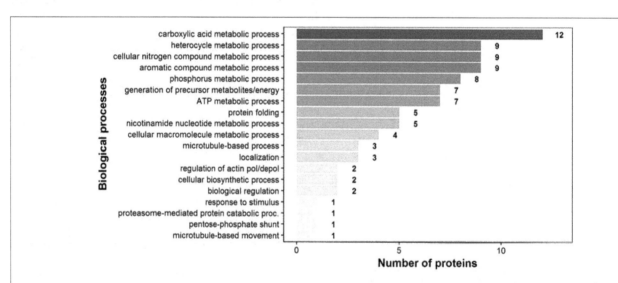

FIGURE 4 | Identified *H. diminuta* adult-stage antigenic proteins categorized by their biological processes according to gene ontology (GO) information obtained from UniProtKB and QuickGO databases.

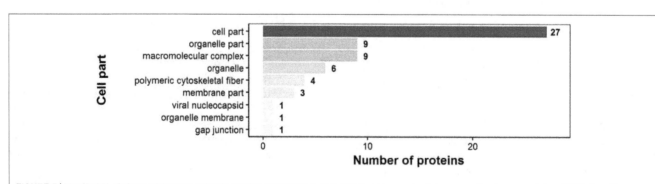

FIGURE 5 | Identified *H. diminuta* adult-stage antigenic proteins categorized by their cellular component category according to gene ontology (GO) information obtained from UniProtKB and QuickGO databases.

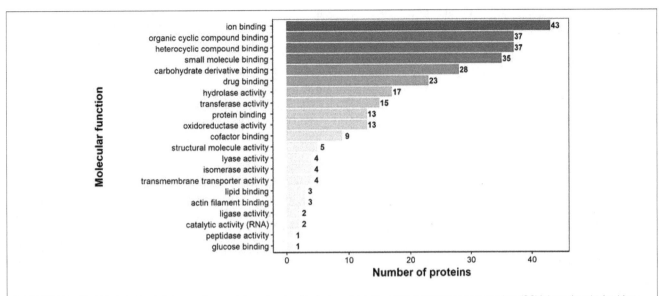

FIGURE 6 | Identified *H. diminuta* adult stage surface proteins categorized by their molecular functions according to gene ontology (GO) information obtained from UniProtKB and QuickGO databases.

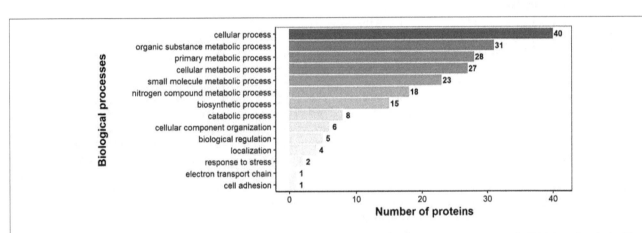

FIGURE 7 | Identified *H. diminuta* adult stage surface proteins categorized by their biological processes according to gene ontology (GO) information obtained from UniProtKB and QuickGO databases.

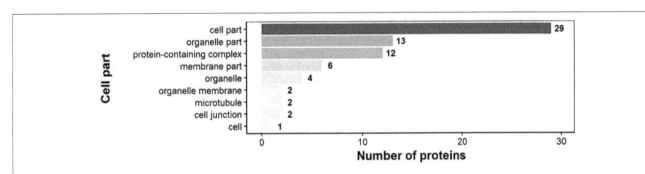

FIGURE 8 | Identified *H. diminuta* adult stage surface proteins categorized by their cellular component category according to gene ontology (GO) information obtained from UniProtKB and QuickGO databases.

obtained from ESPs and somatic proteome. The ESPs, cross-reacting with the specific antibodies and not recognized in the somatic proteome, were predominantly identified as structural proteins (titin, myoferlin, gelsolin, and neurogenic locus notch protein), proteins associated with transport (basement membrane-specific heparan sulfate, phospholipid transporting ATPase, armadillo type fold) and ion-binding and/or ion channels (anoctamin, sarcoplasmic calcium-binding protein).

The identified immunoproteome of the adult *H. diminuta* tapeworm could be divided into two main groups: (i) structural proteins engaged in diverse parasite–host interactions and (ii) enzymes involved in key metabolic processes (NADP dependent malic enzyme, pyruvate kinase–PYK) or conferring moonlighting activity (43, 44) (e.g., triosephosphate isomerase—TPI, glycogen phosphorylase, L- lactate dehydrogenase–L-LDH, glyceraldehyde 3-phosphate dehydrogenase—GAPDH, glucose-6-phosphate isomerase-GPI, fructose 1,6-bisphosphate aldolase-FBA, inosine-5′-monophosphate dehydrogenase-IMP, succinate dehydrogenase, and deoxyhypusine hydroxylase) to the cells. Majority of these proteins are catalytic enzymes with a role in glycolysis, glyconeogenesis, tricarboxylic acid cycle, pyruvate fermentation or purine metabolism, which are cytosolic proteins predicted to be exported via non-classical secretion pathways and having adhesive moonlighting functions after entering the cell surface of an organism (43, 44). Since cestodes take the nutrients through the tegument and directly from the host, the direct contact of the host with the parasite-derived enzymes is highly probable. We may then hypothesize that the constant release of enzymes by the parasite not only influence host immunity but may also change the environment, and could explain the ability of the cestode to modify and alter the microbiome communities of the host intestine (14, 45–47). This is in consistent with the results of Kosik-Bogacka et al. who studied the impact of *H. diminuta* on transepithelial ion transport in intestines, and blood parameters of infected rats at different stages of the infection (24, 26). According to these observations cestodiasis reduced the transepithelial electrical potential and caused a leakage of tight junctions. Another effect of active hymenolepidosis was related to increased lipid peroxidation, changes in anti-oxidant enzyme activity and altered glutathion level in the infected rat gastrointestinal tract (25). This suggests decreased efficiency of intestinal protection against oxidative stress induced by the presence of the parasite. All of the aforementioned processes and the presence of parasite derived molecules may change the intestinal environment and provoke changes in microbiome composition.

On the other hand, as suggested by Kosik-Bogacka (24–26) imbalance between oxidant and anti-oxidant processes can play a major role in pathology associated with hymenolepidosis, including its proinflamatory role associated with the expression and activation of cyclooxygenases in the rat gastrointestinal tract (31). Pathomechanisms observed during infection with *H. diminuta* may be connected with the changes in the expression of toll-like receptors (TLR) important for pathogen recognition. Kosik-Bogacka et al. (28, 29), studying the expression of TLR in *H. diminuta* infected rats, observed increased TLR2 and TLR4 expression compared to the control group, especially in the small intestine. Similarly, the TLR3 snf TLT9 expression was higher in infected rats (30). These analyses confirmed the role of TLR in hymenolepidosis and suggest that *H. diminuta* releases antigens stimulating immune response, which results in adaptation of the host organism to parasite derived molecules (32). Our previous research demonstrated the presence of PYK and GAPDH among the ESP of adult *H. diminuta* (10) and here we confirmed their immunogenic potential. In addition to glycolytic enzymes (PYK and GAPDH), also these taking part in fatty enzyme metabolism are considered important drug targets. Similarly to 3-oxoacyl-ACP reductase, an important candidate in antischistosomal combat (48). As the above mentioned enzymatic proteins have not been identified as immunogenic in the adult *E. granulosus* (9), our study reports their possible antigenicity in an adult tapeworms for the first time. This suggests that similarly to metacestodes, adult tapeworm enzymes (moonlighters) take part in parasite-host interplay. Some of these metabolic enzymes may be derived from the tegument by shedding of glycocalyx (present paper) or are released with secretory vesicles as described by Ancarola et al. (49) for metacestodes.

Our findings suggest that the non-classical protein export, possibly involving protein moonlighters, could contribute to increased viability and interaction with the host. Intriguingly, a recent study reported that this interplay may be mediated by the involvement of extracellular vesicles (EVs) to export cytosolic proteins in a protected and concentrated manner, as proved for metacestodes (49). Similarly, EVs released by hexacanth larvae were proved to be a source of *Taenia ovis* vaccine antigens (50). Since our immunoproteomic approach shows the presence of certain cytosolic and structural proteins as possible antigens, we suppose that the mechanism of their trafficking may have involved EVs. These include for instance antigens considered as vaccine candidates such as calpain (51, 52) and the major egg antigen p40 (mp40) (53–55).

Structural and enzymatic proteins are the most typical immunodominant antigens represented by the somatic proteome of the adult stage of *H. diminuta*. Among cestodes, antigenicity of certain structural proteins was first described in studies focusing on the metacestode stages (40–42, 56–61). Our recent study on antigenic proteins of *H. diminuta* cysticercoid metacestodes (57) supported these findings and confirmed the immunogenic importance of structural proteins, in host's immune response to infection. This indicated that structural proteins, for example beta-tubulin, should be considered as vaccine candidates and/or drug targets against cestode metacestode and adult stages. Another interesting example of structural protein is paramyosin identified at the helminths' surface or among the secreted proteins. This structural protein is believed to function as a multifunctional modulator of the host immune response (62, 63), and together with actin is involved in tegumental repair and considered to represent an important vaccine target molecule. The localization of this protein in the tegument of the parasite is the likely basis for resistance observed in mice immunized with paramyosin (64). Interestingly, it has been speculated that paramyosin protects invading helminths from the immune attack by "decoy" binding proteins of the complement pathway (62). The presence of paramyosin has also been identified as a potential antigen in adult tapeworms (51). Antigenicity of paramyosin was further confirmed by Wang et al. (9), as this protein was one of the major antigens recognized by the antisera from dogs infected with adult *Echinococcus granulosus*.

Immunoproteomic analysis of adult *E. granulosus* has revealed the presence of 12 and 8 potentially antigenic proteins associated, respectively with the somatic proteome and the secretome of this organism (9). Only 7 potentially immunogenic proteins were commonly identified from *E. granulosus* and by us in *H. diminuta* adult worms. These included actin, paramyosin and several moonlighters such as enolase (ENO), malate dehydrogenase (MDH), TPI as well as the stress-related HSP60 and HSP70 proteins. Two other proteins, namely, calreticulin and superoxide dismutase (SOD) were previously identified in *H. diminuta* cysticercoids (11), but they have not been recognized as immunogenic (57). The revealed immunoproteome of the *H. diminuta* indicated potential vaccine candidates against echinococcosis, such as ENO, calpain, and GAPDH and the stress proteins HSP60 and HSP70 (51). Heat shock proteins (HSPs) are known key players in processes associated with development, differentiation, survival, aging, and death. While the antigenic potential of HSPs was shown in previous studies on cestode metacestode stages (56, 57, 65), their immunogenicity in the adult tapeworms has been confirmed only in *E. granulosus* (9), in the present and in our previous studies on *H. diminuta* ESP (10). For as much as HSPs are considered as potential vaccine target proteins (66), their presence throughout the cestode life cycle suggests their importance in cestode biology and survival in the host. The balanced interplay between structural and stress molecules is probably one of the survival factors adopted by parasites during coevolution with their hosts (11). Comparative proteomic analyses of adult and metacestode stages suggest stage-specific mechanisms engaged in the parasite's survival at different life-cycle stages (11, 67). In *H. diminuta*, proteins with antigenic potential, common for these two stages are structural proteins (actins, annexin, lamin, myosin, paramyosin, tubulin), enzymes (calpain, NADP dependent malic enzyme, phosphoenolpyruvate carboxykinase, succinyl co-A), HSPs, and major egg antigen (57). Differences in the expression of immunogenic proteins observed in these two distinct stages are associated predominantly with enzymes and may reflect variability in metabolic activity and stage-specific survival strategies.

There has been interest in targeting metabolic enzymes in the treatment of infectious diseases (68). Fumarate hydratase, involved in canalization of the stereospecific reversible hydration of fumarate to l-malate during the citric acid cycle, was one of the enzymes we have previously identified as one of the immunogens characteristic for the adult *H. diminuta* (11). It has been shown that this enzyme takes part in dismutation of malate in the nematode mitochondria (69), thereby making this enzyme one of the promising targets for designing efficient anthelminthic drugs. The present study also suggests that non-classically exported cytoplasmic proteins, i.e., moonlighters (e.g., enzymes, structural proteins, and HSPs), form another group of proteins playing important roles in host–parasite interactions. One of these moonlighters may be TPI that has also been identified as one of the somatic and surface proteins in *H. diminuta* (9) and in the present study. This enzyme is involved in glycolysis and has been proposed to represent a potential drug target and vaccine candidate to treat schistosomiasis (70).

The potential role of parasite antigens in contributing to increased viability via their immunomodulatory and anti-inflammatory activity has resulted in the concept of helminth-derived molecules as a source of immunomodulatory agents (32, 71, 72). The immunogenic proteins in the crude extract and among the identified surface proteins of *H. diminuta* adult worms may show potential in search of new drug targets and diagnostic methods, since the helminth-derived molecules are considered as potential therapeutics of autoimmune and inflammatory diseases (32–34, 72–74). Recent reports indicated that adult *H. diminuta* tapeworms can effectively modulate the host immune system (15, 16, 20, 47, 75, 76), and that *H. diminuta*-derived molecules can be used to control inflammation (20, 75, 77–79). The results here indicate that *H. diminuta* somatic proteins have been exposed to the host immune system as antigens. However, to uncover full immunomodulatory potential of the identified *H. diminuta* proteins, further studies and finally *in vivo* experiments are needed.

CONCLUSIONS

The somatic proteome and surfaceome of the adult *H. diminuta* with the use of 2DE immunoblotting and LC-MS/MS identification is reported here. The present study proposed a number of new immunogenic proteins involved in key metabolic processes and with likely roles in mediating parasite–host interactions. The identified immunodominant antigens, classified as proteins having structural and enzymatic functions, suggest contributory role of these molecules in mediating host–parasite interaction and during the adult cestode infection. Here we point to enzymes, structural and heat-shock proteins as potential mediators in the interactions between the parasite and the host. Most of these molecules are predicted to trafficate by non-classical ways by motifs or signals that remain to be uncovered. Thus, the present study shed new light on the complexity of the parasite-host interplay during cestodiasis, and highlights the importance of non-classical protein export (e.g., EVs and protein moonlighters) in modulating the parasite–host interaction. This study also provides valuable data not only for understanding the adult cestode biology but also for searching new targets for diagnostic and drug innovations.

AUTHOR CONTRIBUTIONS

DM supervised the work and all its proteomic features and drafted the manuscript. KS and AN participated in the planning of the study. AN, DM, JB, and KS conceived and designed the experiments. AS, JB, and DM conceived and performed the immunological study with rats. KS supported AS and DM in mass spectrometry data analyses. AN, AZ-D, DBC, JB, KB, KS, and RS participated in data analyses and final editing of the manuscript. All authors were actively involved in preparing the manuscript with the responsible author. All authors read and approved the final version of the manuscript.

ACKNOWLEDGMENTS

The equipment used for protein identification by LC-MS/MS analysis was sponsored in part by the Center for Preclinical Research and Technology (CePT), a project co-sponsored by the European Regional Development Fund and Innovative Economy, The National Cohesion Strategy of Poland.

REFERENCES

1. Ito A, Budke CM. Culinary delights and travel? a review of zoonotic cestodiases and metacestodiases. *Travel Med Infect Dis.* (2014) 12:582–91. doi: 10.1016/j.tmaid.2014.06.009
2. Torgerson PR, Devleesschauwer B, Praet N, Speybroeck N, Willingham AL, Kasuga F, et al. World Health Organization estimates of the global and regional disease burden of 11 foodborne parasitic diseases, 2010: a data synthesis. *PLoS Med.* (2015) 12:e1001920. doi: 10.1371/journal.pmed.1001920
3. Thompson RCA. Neglected zoonotic helminths: *Hymenolepis nana, Echinococcus Canadensis,* and *Ancylostoma ceylanicum. Clin Microbiol Infect.* (2015) 21:426–32. doi: 10.1016/j.cmi.2015.01.004
4. Crompton DWT. How much human helminthiasis is there in the world? *J Parasitol.* (1999) 85:397–403. doi: 10.2307/3285768
5. Rabiee MH, Mahmoudi A, Siahsarvie R, Kryštufek B, Mostafavi E. Rodent-borne diseases and their public health importance in Iran. *PLoS Negl Trop Dis.* (2018) 12:e0006256. doi: 10.1371/journal.pntd.0006256
6. Conn DB. *Atlas of Invertebrate Reproduction and Development.* 2nd ed. New York, NY: John Wiley & Sons (2000).
7. Conn DB, Swiderski Z. A standardised terminology of the embryonic envelopes and associated developmental stages of tapeworms (Platyhelminthes: *Cestoda). Folia Parasitol.* (2008) 55:42–52. doi: 10.14411/fp.2008.006
8. Webb C, Cabada MM. Intestinal cestodes. *Curr Opin Infect Dis.* (2017) 30:504–10. doi: 10.1097/QCO.0000000000000400
9. Wang Y, Xiao D, Shen Y, Han X, Zhao F, Li X, et al. Proteomic analysis of the excretory/secretory products and antigenic proteins of *Echinococcus granulosus* adult worms from infected dogs. *BMC Vet Res.* (2015) 11:1–7. doi: 10.1186/s12917-014-0312-6
10. Bien J, Sałamatin R, Sulima A, Savijoki K, Conn DB, Näreaho A, et al. Mass spectrometry analysis of the excretory-secretory (E-S) products of the model cestode *Hymenolepis diminuta* reveals their immunogenic properties and the presence of new E-S proteins in *cestodes. Acta Parasitol.* (2016) 61:429–42. doi: 10.1515/ap-2016-0058
11. Sulima A, Savijoki K, Bien J, Näreaho A, Salamatin R, Conn DB, et al. Comparative proteomic analysis of *Hymenolepis diminuta* cysticercoid and adult stages. *Front Microbiol.* (2018) 8:2672. doi: 10.3389/fmicb.2017.02672
12. Siles-Lucas M, Hemphill A. *Cestode* parasites: application of *in vivo* and *in vitro* models for studies on the host-parasite relationship. *Adv Parasitol.* (2002) 51:133–230. doi: 10.1016/S0065-308X(02)51005-8
13. Graepel R, Leung G, Wang A, Villemaire M, Jirik FR, Sharkey KA, et al. Murine autoimmune arthritis is exaggerated by infection with the rat tapeworm, *Hymenolepis diminuta. Int J Parasitol.* (2013) 43:593–601. doi: 10.1016/j.ijpara.2013.02.006
14. McKenney EA, Williamson L, Yoder AD, Rawls JF, Bilbo SD, Parker W. Alteration of the rat cecal microbiome during colonization with the helminth *Hymenolepis diminuta. Gut Microbes* (2015) 6:182–93. doi: 10.1080/19490976.2015.1047128
15. Hunter MM, Wang A, Parhar KS, Johnston MJG, Van Rooijen N, Beck PL, et al. In vitro-derived alternatively activated macrophages reduce

colonic inflammation in mice. *Gastroenterology* (2010) 138:1395–405. doi: 10.1053/j.gastro.2009.12.041
16. Zawistowska-Deniziak A, Basałaj K, Strojny B, Młocicki D. New data on human macrophages polarization by *Hymenolepis diminuta* tapeworm-An *in vitro* study. *Front Immunol.* (2017) 8:148. doi: 10.3389/fimmu.2017.00148
17. Melon A, Wang A, Phan V, McKay DM. Infection with *Hymenolepis diminuta* is more effective than daily corticosteroids in blocking chemically induced colitis in mice. *J Biomed Biotechnol.* (2010) 2010:384523. doi: 10.1155/2010/384523
18. Jones P, Binns D, Chang H-Y, Fraser M, Li W, McAnulla C, et al. InterProScan 5: genome-scale protein function classification. *Bioinformatics* (2014) 30:1236–40. doi: 10.1093/bioinformatics/btu031
19. Aira N, Andersson AM, Singh SK, McKay DM, Blomgran R. Species dependent impact of helminth-derived antigens on human macrophages infected with *Mycobacterium tuberculosis*: direct effect on the innate anti-mycobacterial response. *PLoS Negl Trop Dis.* (2017) 11: e0005390. doi: 10.1371/journal.pntd.0005390
20. Reyes JL, Fernando MR, Lopes F, Leung G, Mancini NL, Matisz CE, et al. IL-22 restrains tapeworm-mediated protection against experimental colitis via regulation of IL-25 expression. *PLoS Pathog.* (2016) 12:e1005481. doi: 10.1371/journal.ppat.1005481
21. Wang A, McKay DM. Immune modulation by a high molecular weight fraction from the rat tapeworm *Hymenolepis diminuta. Parasitology* (2005) 130:575–85. doi: 10.1017/S0031182004006985
22. Persaud R, Wang A, Reardon C, McKay DM. Characterization of the immuno-regulatory response to the tapeworm *Hymenolepis diminuta* in the non-permissive mouse host. *Int J Parasitol.* (2007) 37:393–403. doi: 10.1016/j.ijpara.2006.09.012
23. Matisz CE, McDougall JJ, Sharkey KA, McKay DM. Helminth parasites and the modulation of joint inflammation. *J Parasitol Res.* (2011) 2011:942616. doi: 10.1155/2011/942616
24. Kosik-Bogacka DI, Baranowska-Bosiacka I, Salamatin R. *Hymenolepis diminuta*: effect of infection on ion transport in colon and blood picture of rats. *Exp Parasitol.* (2010) 124:285–94. doi: 10.1016/j.exppara.2009.10.014
25. Kosik-Bogacka DI, Baranowska-Bosiacka I, Nocen I, Jakubowska K, Chlubek D. *Hymenolepis diminuta*: activity of anti-oxidant enzymes in different parts of rat gastrointestinal tract. *Exp Parasitol.* (2011) 128:265–71. doi: 10.1016/j.exppara.2011.02.026
26. Kosik-Bogacka DI, Kolasa A, Baranowska-Bosiacka I, Marchlewicz M. *Hymenolepis diminuta*: the effects of infection on transepithelial ion transport and tight junctions in rat intestines. *Exp Parasitol.* (2011) 127:398–404. doi: 10.1016/j.exppara.2010.09.001
27. Kosik-Bogacka DI, Kolasa A. Histopathological changes in small and large intestines during hymenolepidosis in rats. *Folia Biol.* (2012) 60:195–8. doi: 10.3409/fb60_3-4.195-198
28. Kosik-Bogacka DI, Wojtkowiak-Giera A, Kolasa A, Czernomysy-Furowicz D, Lanocha N, Wandurska-Nowak E, et al. *Hymenolepis diminuta*: analysis of the expression of Toll-like receptor genes (TLR2 and TLR4) in the small and large intestines of rats. Part II. *Exp Parasitol.* (2013) 130:261–6. doi: 10.1016/j.exppara.2013.08.002

SUPPLEMENTARY MATERIAL

Supplementary Figure 1 | Negative control showing Western blot recognition pattern of *H. diminuta* adult-stage proteins with sera collected from *H. diminuta*-uninfected rats and visualized using chemiluminescence.

Supplementary File 1 | Results of the LC-MS/MS analysis of immunoreactive protein spots of the adult tapeworm somatic proteome recognized by sera from *Hymenolepis diminuta* infected rats.

Supplementary File 2 | *Hymenolepis diminuta* adult stage proteins identified from immunoreactive spots selected for LC-MS/MS analysis.

Supplementary File 3 | Results of the LC-MS/MS analysis of collected surface proteins of the adult tapeworm *Hymenolepis diminuta*

29. Kosik-Bogacka DI, Wojtkowiak-Giera A, Kolasa A, Salamatin R, Jagodzinski PP, Wandurska-Nowak E. *Hymenolepis diminuta*: analysis of the expression of Toll-like receptor genes (TLR2 and TLR4) in the small and large intestines of rats. *Exp Parasitol*. (2012) 130:261–6. doi: 10.1016/j.exppara.2011.12.002

30. Kosik-Bogacka DI, Wojtkowiak-Giera A, Kolasa A, Baranowska-Bosiacka I, Lanocha N, Wandurska-Nowak E, et al. *Hymenolepis diminuta*: analysis of the expression of Toll-like receptor genes and protein (TLR3 and TLR9) in the small and large intestines of rats. *Exp Parasitol*. (2014) 145:61–7. doi: 10.1016/j.exppara.2014.07.009

31. Kosik-Bogacka DI, Baranowska-Bosiacka I, Kolasa-Wołosiuk A, Lanocha-Arendarczyk N, Gutowska I, Korbecki J, et al. The inflammatory effect of infection with *Hymenolepis diminuta* via the increased expression and activity of COX-1 and COX-2 in the rat jejunum and colon. *Exp Parasitol*. (2016) 169:69–76. doi: 10.1016/j.exppara.2016.07.009

32. Maizels RM, McSorley HJ. Regulation of the host immune system by helminth parasites. *J Allergy Clin Immunol*. (2016) 138:666–75. doi: 10.1016/j.jaci.2016.07.007

33. Smallwood TB, Giacomin PR, Loukas A, Mulvenna JP, Clark RJ, Miles JJ. Helminth immunomodulation in autoimmune disease. *Front Immunol*. (2017) 8:453. doi: 10.3389/fimmu.2017.00453

34. Wang M, Wu L, Weng R, Zheng W, Wu Z, Lv Z. Therapeutic potential of helminths in autoimmune diseases: helminth-derived immune-regulators and immune balance. *Parasitol Res*. (2017) 116:2065–74. doi: 10.1007/s00436-017-5544-5

35. Kordan W, Malinowska A, Lecewicz M, Wysocki P, Fraser L, Strzezek J. The structure of platelet-activating factor acetylhydrolase (PAF-AH) isolated from boar seminal plasma and examined using mass spectrometry. *Anim Sci Pap Rep*. (2007) 25:289–95.

36. Nielsen H. Predicting secretory proteins with signalP. *Methods Mol Biol*. (2017) 1611:59–73. doi: 10.1007/978-1-4939-7015-5_6

37. Sotillo J, Pearson M, Becker L, Mulvenna J, Loukas A. A quantitative proteomic analysis of the tegumental proteins from *Schistosoma mansoni* schistosomula reveals novel potential therapeutic targets. *Int J Parasitol*. (2015) 45:505–16. doi: 10.1016/j.ijpara.2015.03.004

38. DeMarco R, Verjovski-Almeida S. Schistosomes-proteomics studies for potential novel vaccines and drug targets. *Drug Discov Today* (2009) 14:472–78. doi: 10.1016/j.drudis.2009.01.011

39. Verjovski-Almeida S, DeMarco R. Current developments on *Schistosoma* proteomics. *Acta Trop*. (2008) 108:183–5. doi: 10.1016/j.actatropica.2008.04.017

40. Chemale G, Van Rossum AJ, Jefferies JR, Barrett J, Brophy PM, Ferreira HB, et al. Proteomic analysis of the larval stage of the parasite *Echinococcus granulosus*: causative agent of cystic hydatid disease. *Proteomics* (2003) 3:1633–6. doi: 10.1002/pmic.200300487

41. Virginio VG, Monteiro KM, Drumond F, De Carvalho MO, Vargas DM, Zaha A, et al. Excretory/secretory products from *in vitro*-cultured *Echinococcus granulosus* protoscoleces. *Mol Biochem Parasitol*. (2012) 183:15–22. doi: 10.1016/j.molbiopara.2012.01.001

42. Monteiro KM, De Carvalho MO, Zaha A, Ferreira HB. Proteomic analysis of the *Echinococcus granulosus* metacestode during infection of its intermediate host. *Proteomics* (2010) 10:1985–99. doi: 10.1002/pmic.200900506

43. Jeffery CJ. Moonlighting proteins – nature's Swiss army knives. *Sci Prog*. (2017) 100:363–73. doi: 10.3184/003685017X15063357842574

44. Chen C, Zabad S, Liu H, Wang W, Jeffery C. MoonProt 2.0: an expansion and update of the moonlighting proteins database. *Nucleic Acids Res*. (2018) 46:D640–4. doi: 10.1093/nar/gkx1043

45. Aivelo T, Norberg A. Parasite-microbiota interactions potentially affect intestinal communities in wild mammals. *J Anim Ecol*. (2018) 87:438–47. doi: 10.1111/1365-2656.12708

46. Wegener Parfrey L, Jirku M, Šíma R, Jalovecká M, Sak B, Grigore K, et al. A benign helminth alters the host immune system and the gut microbiota in a rat model system. *PLoS ONE* (2017) 12:e0182205. doi: 10.1371/journal.pone.0182205

47. Kapczuk P, Kosik-Bogacka D, Łanocha-Arendarczyk N, Gutowska I, Kupnicka P, Chlubek D, et al. Selected molecular mechanisms involved in the parasite–host system *Hymenolepis diminuta–Rattus norvegicus*. *Int J Mol Sci*. (2018) 19:2435. doi: 10.3390/ijms19082435

48. Liu J, Dyer D, Wang J, Wang S, Du X, Xu B, et al. 3-Oxoacyl-ACP reductase from *Schistosoma japonicum*: integrated *in silico-in vitro* strategy

for discovering antischistosomal lead compounds. *PLoS ONE* (2013) 8:e64984. doi: 10.1371/journal.pone.0064984

49. Ancarola ME, Marcilla A, Herz M, Macchiaroli N, Pérez M, Asurmendi S, et al. Cestode parasites release extracellular vesicles with microRNAs and immunodiagnostic protein cargo. *Int J Parasitol*. (2017) 47:675–86. doi: 10.1016/j.ijpara.2017.05.003

50. Jabbar A, Swiderski Z, Mlocicki D, BeveridgeEI, Lightowlers MW. The ultrastructure of taeniid cestode oncospheres and localization of host-protective antigens. *Parasitology* (2010) 137:521–35. doi: 10.1017/S0031182009991260

51. Cui SJ, Xu LL, Zhang T, Xu M, Yao J, Fang CY, et al. Proteomic characterization of larval and adult developmental stages in *Echinococcus granulosus* reveals novel insight into host-parasite interactions. *J Proteomics* (2013) 84:158–75. doi: 10.1016/j.jprot.2013.04.013

52. Zhang Y, Taylor MG, Johansen MV, Bickle QD. Vaccination of mice with a cocktail DNA vaccine induces a Th1-type immune response and partial protection against Schistosoma japonicum infection. *Vaccine* (2001) 20:724–30. doi: 10.1016/S0264-410X(01)00420-0

53. Anthony RM, Rutitzky LI, Urban JF, Stadecker MJ, Gause WC, Urban JF Jr, et al. Protective immune mechanisms in helminth infection. *Nat Rev Immunol*. (2007) 7:975–87. doi: 10.1038/nri2199

54. Cass CL, Johnson JR, Califf LL, Xu T, Hernandez HJ, Stadecker MJ, et al. Proteomic analysis of *Schistosoma mansoni* egg secretions. *Mol Biochem Parasitol*. (2007) 155:84–93. doi: 10.1016/j.molbiopara.2007.06.002

55. Abouel-Nour MF, Lotfy M, Attallah AM, Doughty BL. *Schistosoma mansoni* major egg antigen Smp40: molecular modeling and potential immunoreactivity for anti-pathology vaccine development. *Mem Inst Oswaldo Cruz*. (2006) 101:365–72. doi: 10.1590/S0074-02762006000400004

56. Aziz A, Zhang W, Li J, Loukas A, McManus DP, Mulvenna J. Proteomic characterisation of *Echinococcus granulosus* hydatid cyst fluid from sheep, cattle and humans. *J Proteomics* (2011) 74:1560–72. doi: 10.1016/j.jprot.2011.02.021

57. Sulima A, Bien J, Savijoki K, Näreaho A, Sałamatin R, Conn DB, et al. Identification of immunogenic proteins of the cysticercoid of *Hymenolepis diminuta*. *Parasit. Vectors* (2017) 10:577. doi: 10.1186/s13071-017-2519-4

58. Vendelova E, Camargo de Lima J, Lorenzatto KR, Monteiro KM, Mueller T, Veepaschit J, et al. Proteomic analysis of excretory-secretory products of *mesocestoides corti* metacestodes reveals potential suppressors of dendritic cell functions. *PLoS Negl Trop Dis*. (2016) 10:e0005061. doi: 10.1371/journal.pntd.0005061

59. Cantacessi C, Mulvenna J, Young ND, Kasny M, Horak P, Aziz A, et al. A deep exploration of the transcriptome and "Excretory/Secretory" proteome of adult *Fascioloides magna*. *Mol Cell Proteomics* (2012) 11:1340–53. doi: 10.1074/mcp.M112.019844

60. Liu F, Hu W, Cui SJ, Chi M, Fang CY, Wang ZQ, et al. Insight into the host-parasite interplay by proteomic study of host proteins copurified with the human parasite, *Schistosoma japonicum*. *Proteomics* (2007) 7:450–62. doi: 10.1002/pmic.200600465

61. Wang Y, Cheng Z, Lu X, Tang C. *Echinococcus multilocularis*: proteomic analysis of the protoscoleces by two-dimensional electrophoresis and mass spectrometry. *Exp Parasitol*. (2009) 123:162–7. doi: 10.1016/j.exppara.2009.06.014

62. Santivañez SJ, Hernández-González A, Chile N, Oleaga A, Arana Y, Palma S, et al. Proteomic study of activated *Taenia solium* oncospheres. *Mol Biochem Parasitol*. (2010) 171:32–9. doi: 10.1016/j.molbiopara.2010.01.004

63. Laschuk A, Monteiro KM, Vidal NM, Pinto PM, Duran R, Cerveñanski C, et al. Proteomic survey of the cestode *Mesocestoides corti* during the first 24 hours of strobilar development. *Parasitol Res*. (2011) 108:645–56. doi: 10.1007/s00436-010-2109-2

64. Matsumoto Y, Perry G, Levine RJ, Blanton R, Mahmoud AA, Aikawa M. Paramyosin and actin in schistosomal teguments. *Nature* (1988) 333:76–8. doi: 10.1038/333076a0

65. Kouguchi H, Matsumoto J, Katoh Y, Suzuki T, Oku Y, Yagi K. *Echinococcus multilocularis*: two-dimensional Western blotting method for the identification and expression analysis of immunogenic proteins in infected dogs. *Exp Parasitol*. (2010) 124:238–43. doi: 10.1016/j.exppara.2009.09.016

66. Colaco CA, Bailey CR, Walker KB, Keeble J. Heat shock proteins: stimulators of innate and acquired immunity. *Biomed Res Int*. (2013) 2013:461230. doi: 10.1155/2013/461230

67. Camargo de Lima J, Monteiro KM, Basika Cabrera TN, Paludo GP, Moura H, Barr JR, et al. Comparative proteomics of the larval and adult stages of the model cestode parasite *Mesocestoides corti*. *J Proteomics* (2018) 175:127–35. doi: 10.1016/j.jprot.2017.12.022

68. Srinivasan V, Morowitz HJ. Ancient genes in contemporary persistent microbial pathogens. *Biol Bull.* (2006) 210:1–9. doi: 10.2307/4134531

69. Kulkarni G, Sabnis NA, Harris BG. Cloning, expression, and purification of fumarase from the parasitic nematode *Ascaris suum*. *Protein Expr Purif.* (2004) 33:209–13. doi: 10.1016/j.pep.2003.09.005

70. Zinsser VL, Farnell E, Dunne DW, Timson DJ. Triose phosphate isomerase from the blood fluke *Schistosoma mansoni* : biochemical characterisation of a potential drug and vaccine target. *FEBS Lett.* (2013) 587:3422–7. doi: 10.1016/j.febslet.2013.09.022

71. Harnett W. Secretory products of helminth parasites as immunomodulators. *Mol Biochem Parasitol.* (2014) 195:130–6. doi: 10.1016/j.molbiopara.2014.03.007

72. McSorley HJ, Maizels RM. Helminth infections and host immune regulation. *Clin Microbiol Rev.* (2012) 25:585–608. doi: 10.1128/CMR.05040-11

73. Vendelova E, Lutz MB, Hrčková G. Immunity and immune modulation elicited by the larval cestode *Mesocestoides vogae* and its products. *Parasite Immunol.* (2015) 37:493–504. doi: 10.1111/pim.12216

74. Steinfelder S, O'Regan NL, Hartmann S. Diplomatic assistance: can helminth-modulated macrophages act as treatment for inflammatory disease? *PLOS Pathog.* (2016) 12:e1005480. doi: 10.1371/journal.ppat.10 05480

75. Matisz CE, Leung G, Reyes JL, Wang A, Sharkey KA, McKay DM. Adoptive transfer of helminth antigen-pulsed dendritic cells protects against the development of experimental colitis in mice. *Eur J Immunol.* (2015) 45:3126–39. doi: 10.1002/eji.201545579

76. Hernandez JLR, Leung G, McKay DM. Cestode regulation of inflammation and inflammatory diseases. *Int J Parasitol.* (2013) 43:233–43. doi: 10.1016/j.ijpara.2012.09.005

77. Johnston MJG, MacDonald JA, McKay DM. Parasitic helminths: a pharmacopeia of anti-inflammatory molecules. *Parasitology* (2009) 136:125–47. doi: 10.1017/S0031182008005210

78. Johnston MJG, Wang A, Catarino MED, Ball L, Phan VC, MacDonald JA, et al. Extracts of the rat tapeworm, *Hymenolepis diminuta*, suppress macrophage activation *in vitro* and alleviate chemically induced colitis in mice. *Infect Immun.* (2010) 78:1364–75. doi: 10.1128/IAI. 01349-08

79. Reyes JL, Wang A, Fernando MR, Graepel R, Leung G, van Rooijen N, et al. Splenic B cells from *Hymenolepis diminuta*- infected mice ameliorate colitis independent of T cells and via cooperation with macrophages. *J Immunol.* (2015) 194:364–78. doi: 10.4049/jimmunol.1400738

3

Unravelling the Immunity of Poultry Against the Extracellular Protozoan Parasite *Histomonas meleagridis* is a Cornerstone for Vaccine Development

Taniya Mitra [1], Fana Alem Kidane [1], Michael Hess [1,2] and Dieter Liebhart [1]*

[1] *Clinic for Poultry and Fish Medicine, Department for Farm Animals and Veterinary Public Health, University of Veterinary Medicine Vienna, Vienna, Austria,* [2] *Christian Doppler Laboratory for Innovative Poultry Vaccines (IPOV), University of Veterinary Medicine Vienna, Vienna, Austria*

*Correspondence:
Dieter Liebhart
dieter.liebhart@vetmeduni.ac.at

The protozoan parasite *Histomonas meleagridis* is the causative agent of histomonosis in gallinaceous birds, predominantly in turkeys and chickens. Depending on the host species the outcome of the disease can be very severe with high mortality as observed in turkeys, whereas in chickens the mortality rates are generally lower. The disease is known for more than 100 years when *in vitro* and *in vivo* investigations started to understand histomonosis and the causative pathogen. For decades histomonosis could be well-controlled by effective drugs for prevention and therapy until the withdrawal of such chemicals for reasons of consumer protection in Europe, the USA and additional countries worldwide. Consequently, research efforts also focused to find new strategies against the disease, resulting in the development of an efficacious live-attenuated vaccine. In addition to efficacy and safety several studies were performed to obtain a deeper understanding of the immune response of the host against *H. meleagridis*. It could be demonstrated that antibodies accumulate in different parts of the intestine of chickens following infection with *H. meleagridis* which was much pronounced in the ceca. Furthermore, expression profiles of various cytokines revealed that chickens mounted an effective cecal innate immune response during histomonosis compared to turkeys. Studying the cellular immune response following infection and/or vaccination of host birds showed a limitation of pronounced changes of B cells and T-cell subsets in vaccinated birds in comparison to non-protected birds. Additionally, numbers of lymphocytes including cytotoxic T cells increased in the ceca of diseased turkeys compared to infected chickens suggesting an immunopathological impact on disease pathogenesis. The identification of type 1 and type 2 T-helper (Th) cells in infected and lymphoid organs by *in situ* hybridization did not show a clear separation of Th cells during infection but revealed a coherence of an increase of interferon (IFN)-γ mRNA positive cells in ceca and protection. The present review not only summarizes the research performed on the immune response of host birds in the course of histomonosis but also highlights the specific features of *H. meleagridis* as a model organism to study immunological principles of an extracellular organism in birds.

Keywords: *Histomonas meleagridis*, histomonosis, immunity, vaccination, immune response, extracellular parasite, poultry

INTRODUCTION

Histomonas meleagridis is an important flagellated parasite of poultry causing the disease histomonosis (syn. blackhead disease, histomoniasis, or infectious typhlohepatitis) (1). Historically, the disease was extensively investigated in the first half of the last century and thereby effective chemotherapeutics were identified to prevent and treat birds from infection. This success neglects that for a long time the true etiology of the disease was questioned and under debate. Difficulties to determine the real cause of histomonosis in earlier studies are comprehensively recapitulated elsewhere (2). However, to date the disease is of high relevance in poultry flocks as effective prophylactic and therapeutic options are not available anymore in many countries for reasons of food safety. As a consequence research was intensified in recent years and with it several reviews were published addressing different features of the parasite or the disease. This includes a general overview on the disease (3), updated findings of the recent years (4), a summary of experimental infections (5), a recapitulation on previous and current strategies for prevention and therapy (6), and assumptions how the disease might be controlled in the future (7).

The purpose of this review is to emphasize on studies investigating mechanisms of the immune response of host birds against the disease. This includes early studies describing inflammatory reactions of birds' up to recent investigations on specific immune cells and signaling proteins involved in host defense. Furthermore, the host reaction due to vaccination and its functional aspects are reviewed. Finally, *H. meleagridis* might be a model to unravel peculiar immune mechanisms of extracellular pathogens considering that the avian immune response against these organisms is not as investigated in depth compared to viral or bacterial infections.

Histomonosis, an Important Poultry Disease

Histomonosis was firstly described in turkeys by Cushman (8) more than a century ago. Infection with *H. meleagridis* can occur directly or via embryonated eggs of the nematode *Heterakis gallinarum* which was already described by Graybill and Smith (9). Horizontal transmission was hypothesized to occur by active uptake via the cloaca (10) or orally, based on successful oral application of cultured histomonads (11).The first signs of histomonosis are reflected by clinical changes such as reduced appetite, depression, drowsiness, droopy wings, and ruffled feathers. Infected birds might suffer from yellowish diarrhea and

succumb to death (4). The pathogenesis generally varies between species of gallinaceous birds: in turkeys (*Meleagris gallopavo*) the disease can cause high mortality due to severe necrotic inflammation of the ceca and the liver, while in chickens (*Gallus gallus*) clinical signs are milder and pathological manifestations are often restricted to the ceca of infected birds.

Following infection, *H. meleagridis* migrates into the mucosa and deeper layers of the cecal wall leading to inflammation and ulceration, resulting in a thickening of the cecal tissue and formation of fibrin. Occasionally, ulcers erode throughout the cecal wall leading to peritonitis. Following destruction of cecal tissue, the parasite is able to infiltrate into blood vessels and to reach the liver via the portal vein. As a consequence, areas of inflammation and necrosis can occur in the liver. Liver lesions are highly variable in appearance: they may be up to 4 cm in diameter and can involve parts or the entire organ. Liver and cecal lesions together are a strong hint during post mortem investigations. The disease causes generally less severe lesions in chickens. Especially changes in the liver occur less frequently in chickens as compared to turkeys. In the final stage, the disease may become systemic when DNA of histomonads can be found in the blood and in the tissues of many organs, whether lesions are present or not (12). Lesions can be observed in different organs beside cecum and liver, such as kidneys, bursa of Fabricius, spleen, and pancreas (13–15). Apart from turkeys and chickens, other members of the galliformes, including pheasants, partridges, and farm-reared bobwhite quails can serve as hosts (16–19). In contrary, other avian species like ostriches and ducks show a high resistance to disease even though they may contribute to the transmission of the parasite (20, 21).

Histomonas meleagridis, a Unique Protozoan Parasite

H. meleagridis is a member of the family *Dientamoebidae*, order Tritrichomonadida (22). The parasite mainly possesses cell organelles that are typical for trichomonads (3). It is pleomorphic and generally two forms of the parasite are known: (i) the tissue form and (ii) the cecal lumen dwelling form. The tissue form is almost round with 6–20 μm in size and capable of forming pseudopodia (23, 24). Unlike the tissue form the cecal lumen form (3–16 μm) has a single flagellum although early during cell division, two may be observed (25). It was observed that the flagellum is getting lost during the invasion in the host tissue (26). In culture, *H. meleagridis* exhibits the morphology of the lumen-dwelling form. More recently, the occurrence of a cyst-like stage was reported (27). Later on, this resistant stage of *H. meleagridis* was investigated *in vitro* and it could be observed independent of the passage level and pathogenicity *in vivo* indicating an early adaption to *in vitro* conditions (28).

H. meleagridis is antigenetically (29) closely related to the intestinal parasite *Dientamoeba fragilis*, a trichomonad with a wider host range in mammals which is suspected to be associated with gastrointestinal disorders in humans. *Dientamoeba fragilis* is a protozoan parasite often described as "neglected parasite" (30). Recently, several major advances have been made with respect to this organism's life cycle and molecular biology, although knowledge on immune response against the pathogen is scant. The pathogenic potential of *D. fragilis* is still debatable. However, because of the close relativity to histomonads, the immunological research on *H. meleagridis* can give an indication to the immunological responsiveness of host against *D. fragilis*.

Hyperimmune antisera raised in rabbits against the two flagellates cross-reacted in an indirect fluorescent antibody test (31), although in agar gel immune-diffusion test (32) species-specific precipitin lines were seen. Both, antigenic differences and some cross-reactivity could also be demonstrated by immunoelectrophoresis (33). The nucleotide sequence analysis of a small subunit rRNA of the organism showed a close relationship between *D. fragilis* and *H. meleagridis* (34). First investigations on specific proteins of *H. meleagridis* were performed by Mazet et al. (35). The authors characterized genes encoding three proteins involved in hydrogenosomal carbon metabolism: a nicotinamide adenine dinucleotide phosphate-dependent hydrogenosomal malic enzyme, an α-subunit of a succinyl coenzyme-A synthetase and an iron-only hydrogenase. Afterwards, Bilic et al. (36) identified a broad spectrum of partial protein-coding sequences with homology to both intracellular and surface proteins. The antigenic potential of α-actinins of the parasite in host animals was later on demonstrated (37). Lynn and Beckstead, (38) applied splinkerette PCR to identify new genes. Their sequence analysis identified the 5′ coding portions of the β-tubulin genes, the intergenic regions, and two different open reading frames encoding for a putative serine/threonine phosphatase and a putative ras-related protein, racG. They predicted that these intergenic regions contain polyadenylation and cleavage signals for the two open reading frames and initiator elements for the β-tubulin genes. These regulatory elements are necessary for gene transcription in *H. meleagridis*. Most recently, sequencing of a cDNA library reported sequences of 3425 *H. meleagridis* genes (39). These analyses identified 81 genes coding for putative hydrogenosomal proteins and determined the codon usage frequency. That study also suggested that *H. meleagridis* α-actinins strongly contribute to the immune-reaction of host birds. Recently, *de novo* transcriptome sequencing of a virulent and an attenuated *H. meleagridis* strain provided novel insights into the parasite's biological processes, such as metabolism, locomotion, cell signaling and its ability to adapt to dynamic environmental changes (40). In addition, the study elucidated potential pathogenic mechanisms in respect to cytoadherence and host cell membrane disruption, together with the possible regulation of such processes. Monoyios et al. (41) addressed differences between *in vivo* cultivated virulent and attenuated *H.*

meleagridis parasites on protein expression level. Based on mass spectrometry data it could be shown that eight different proteins, with the majority related to cellular stress management, have been found up-regulated in virulent histomonads compared to the attenuated strain which potentially affect the host-pathogen interaction between the two strains. Additionally, a virulence factor named legumain cysteine peptidase was detected. Applying two-dimensional electrophoresis in combination with mass spectrometric analysis 32 spots were identified as specific for the attenuated strain. These spots were described to correspond to the increased metabolism due to *in vitro* adaptation of the parasite and the amoeboid morphology.

IMMUNOLOGICAL RESPONSES AGAINST HISTOMONOSIS

Modulations of the innate and adaptive immune responses of the host by pathogens are known to be major determinants in the outcome of certain infectious diseases. Histomonosis causes severe disease in turkeys whereas less clinical signs occur in chickens as described above. This outcome can be linked with the host defense, indicating substantial differences between these two phylogenetically closely related species against *H. meleagridis*. Elucidating these differences in host response does not only unravel a certain host reaction it is also useful to understand protection and susceptibility in a broader context. Important studies investigating distinct parameter of the immune response against *H. meleagridis* are listed in **Table 1**.

Innate Immune Response

The first arm of the innate immune system against histomonosis is the anatomical barrier in the gastrointestinal tract. The parasite can infect its host via cloacal or oral route. However, oral inoculation was not always successful probably due to the acidity of the gizzard (10, 11, 54–56). The acid environment in the gizzard is a physiological barrier against pathogens and it was reported earlier that an effective infection depends upon the pH of the gizzard and the upper intestine (55). In the last mentioned work it was observed that the severity of lesions increased in chickens that have starved or were fed with an alkali mixture before the oral infection. Feed restriction after the application of live histomonads was shown to be an additional parameter which should be considered in the context of a successful oral infection (11).

Concerning the innate cellular response, first observations were made by histopathology in birds infected with *H. gallinarum* and *H. meleagridis* (57). Thereby, larvae of the cecal worm and an influx of heterophilic granulocytes were visible already from day 1 post infection (p.i.), even though first histomonads were only visualized after 5 days p.i.. First lesions in the liver, characterized by lymphocytic infiltration with few heterophils at the portal area, were observed at the same time point (13). Specific detection of the parasite in tissue sections was described to be accompanied with infiltrations of mononuclear and polymorphonuclear cells in the infected organs cecum and liver (58, 59). In recent studies, quantitative analyses using specific

TABLE 1 | Year wise experimental studies in turkeys and/or chickens investigating important immunological parameters of histomonosis.

Parameter	Components	Technique	Tissue	Host	Strain or antigenic preparation	Year of publication (reference)
Serum antibodies	Precipitating antibodies	Agar gel immunodiffusion (Ouchterlony test)	Serum	Turkeys (Beltsville White) and chicken (Light Sussex cockerels)	Homogenate of cecum and liver tissues harvested from an infected turkey or ceca contents of an infected chicken	1963 (42)
Serum antibodies	IgG	Indirect immunofluorescence assay	Serum	Turkeys (breed BIG 6)	Virulent $H.$ $meleagridis$ (strain mdc), and a lysed (by sonication) preparation of the same strain	2009 (43)
Serum antibodies	IgG	indirect sandwich ELISA	Serum	Turkeys and chickens	Virulent $H.$ $meleagridis$ Turkey/Austria/2922-C6/04 or the same clones passaged for 95, 215 and 295 times	2009 (44)
Chemokine and cytokine mRNA	IL-1β, IL-6, CXCL2, IL-10, TGF-β4, IFN-γ, IL-4, and IL-13	RT-qPCR	Cecal tonsil, liver and spleen	Turkeys and chickens (broilers and breeder cockerels)	A suspension of severely affected cecum and liver tissue homogenate harvested from chickens orally inoculated with embryonated eggs of $H.$ $gallinarum$	2009 (45)
β-defensin mRNA	AvBD2		Cecal tonsil and liver			
Immune cells	CD4$^+$, CD8α$^+$, CD28$^+$ and CD44$^+$ cells	Immunohistochemistry	Liver and spleen			
Serum & mucosal antibodies	IgA, IgG, IgM	Indirect sandwich ELISA	Serum, duodenum, jejunum & cecum	Chickens	Clonal cultures of virulent (passaged for 21 times) $H.$ $meleagridis$ / Turkey/Austria/2922-C6/04	2010 (46)
Serum antibodies	IgG	Blocking ELISA	Serum	Turkeys (BUT 6) and chickens (Isa Brown layers)	A Dutch field strain (strain /Deventer/NL/AL327-type I/03)	2010 (47)
Serum antibodies	IgG	Indirect sandwich ELISA	Serum	Turkeys (BUT 9)	Clonal cultures of virulent (passaged for 21 times) and/or attenuated (passaged for 295 times) $H.$ $meleagridis$ / Turkey/Austria/2922-C6/04	2010 (48)
Serum antibodies	IgG	Indirect sandwich ELISA	Serum	Chickens (layer type)	Clonal cultures of virulent (passaged for 21 times) and/or attenuated (passaged for 295 times) $H.$ $meleagridis$ / Turkey/Austria/2922-C6/04	2013 (49)
Serum antibodies	IgG	indirect sandwich ELISA	Serum	Turkeys	Clonal cultures of attenuated (passaged for 295) $H.$ $meleagridis$ / Turkey/Austria/2922-C6/04 or the same strain back passaged in vivo	2013 (50)
Serum antibodies	IgG	Indirect sandwich ELISA	Serum	Chickens (layer and meat-type)	$H.$ $meleagridis$ strain Turkey/Germany/GB551/04 from an outbreak in a commercial meat turkey flock in Germany	2014 (51)
Immune cells	CD4$^+$, CD8α$^+$, B cells, heterophils, macrophages; Heterophils, macrophages	Flow cytometry	cecum, liver, spleen, PBMC; Whole blood	Turkeys and chickens; Chickens	Clonal cultures of virulent (passaged for 21 times) and/or attenuated (passaged for 295 times) $H.$ $meleagridis$/Turkey/Austria/2922-C6/04	2017 (52)
Immune cells	T cells, B cells and monocytes/macrophages	Immunofluorescence	Cecum, liver, and spleen	Chickens	Clonal cultures of virulent (passaged for 21 times) and/or attenuated (passaged for 295 times) $H.$ $meleagridis$ / Turkey/Austria/2922-C6/04	2018 (53)
Type1/type2 signature cytokines	IFN-γ or IL-13 mRNA positive cells	In situ hybridization		Turkeys and chickens		

markers against chicken macrophages/monocytes revealed that significantly higher amounts of this cell population were present in the blood (52) and the cecum (53) of infected chickens from the early stage of infection until the time period when most severe lesions were observed. The ability of macrophages to incorporate cells by phagocytosis indicates efforts to contain the parasite during the initial stage of infection in chickens. Furthermore, a lower presence of heterophils in the infected chickens' blood can be explained by the infiltration of these granulocytes to the local site of infection (52). Due to the lack of specific or cross-reactive antibodies for innate immune cells of turkeys it was so far not possible to generate comparative data in this more affected host species.

To investigate the innate cell signaling following infection, mRNA expression of the pro-inflammatory innate cytokines IL-1beta, IL-6, and CXCLi2 were measured in chickens and in turkeys after infection with histomonads (45). It was found that the immune response in the chicken was initiated in the cecal tonsils already after 1 day p.i. Interestingly, mRNA expression levels of these pro-inflammatory cytokines in turkeys were not up-regulated locally during the initial phase of infection even until the protozoa were already detectable in the liver. This depicts that an initial induced innate inflammatory response in the cecal tonsils may be critical to limit the dissemination of the parasite to the liver, with consequences on the clinical outcome within the different poultry species.

Adaptive Immune Response
Pathogen-Specific Antibodies
The first study on specific antibodies against *H. meleagridis* was reported by Clarkson (42), who detected serum precipitins 7 days after infection. The attempt to transfer protective immunity by injections of serum from infected turkeys to naïve birds failed in the last mentioned study. Several years later, Powell et al. (45), observed increased antibody levels in sera of infected chickens compared to infected turkeys, but no further information on the methodology was given. More recently, vaccination against histomonosis using killed vaccines which elicit a dominantly antibody-mediated immune response was shown to be ineffective in providing protection (60). Similarly, Bleyen et al. (43) confirmed the inadequacy of serum antibodies in protecting turkeys from histomonosis, although the same immune component was shown to induce complement-mediated lysis of *H. meleagridis in vitro*. In recent years, an indirect sandwich ELISA (44), as well as a blocking ELISA using monoclonal antibodies (47) for the detection of antibodies against histomonads have been established. In these studies, an increase of antibodies in sera could be demonstrated in experimentally infected chickens and turkeys. Field studies on the prevalence of histomonads-specific antibodies in chicken flocks revealed a wide dissemination of the parasite in European countries (61, 62). In experimental studies, it was demonstrated that pathogen-specific serum antibodies increased already 2 weeks p.i. (44) and 3 weeks post vaccination with attenuated parasites above the cut off value until the following 13 weeks when the experiment was finished (48).

In a single study, the occurrence of different types of systemic and intestinal antibodies of chickens following infection with *H. meleagridis* was investigated by ELISA (46). Thereby, first optical density values for IgG above the cut-off in the serum were detected at 14 days p.i., whereas IgA and IgM levels remained low. Furthermore, it could be revealed that the intestinal tissue showed an intense humoral response in the parasitized ceca with an initial peak of IgM, high levels of IgG as well as a continuous increase of IgA and similar high levels of IgG together with IgA in the small intestine. Unfortunately, comparative results to the last mentioned studies in turkeys are not available which might be due to the lack of suitable reagents. However, along with an elevated level of antibodies the numbers of B cells increased in infected organs and systemically during infection were also reported recently in chickens and turkeys (52), which is outlined in the following chapter.

Another study, involving different lines of chickens, reported that antibody production differ due to the genetic background of the host (51). The study reported that the humoral immune response against actinin 1 started sooner and was significantly more pronounced in layer-type chickens than in meat-type chickens.

Cell-Mediated Immune Response
First investigations on leukocytes were based on histopathology and indicated an influx of different populations of immune cells including lymphocytes in the infected organs cecum and liver (57). However, until recently there was no detailed information on the phenotype of immune cells that are involved in an adapted immune response and the link with the appearance following infection. In the last few years different studies were performed to investigate the mechanisms of the cellular modulation by detailed characterization of the involved leukocytes as well as cytokines triggering specific changes in the cellular response.

In general, the polarization of CD4$^+$ T-helper (Th) and CD8$^+$ T-cytotoxic (Tc) cells plays a major role in host-pathogen interaction. CD3$^+$CD4$^+$CD8α^- T cells are predominantly of helper phenotype, act as coordinators of the immune response by producing a variety of cytokines and secrete soluble molecules to the extracellular space which affects other cells of the immune system. In contrast, CD3$^+$CD4$^-$CD8α^+ T cells are cytotoxic cells, promoting the cytolytic pathway. A protective immune response may rely on the ability of CD4$^+$ T cells to accumulate high numbers of effector cells in order to activate a response against an invading pathogen. They can promote B cell-immunity with antibody production or, on the opposite, directly modulate, respectively control, the activity of different types of T cells. Secreted cytokines can activate macrophages and other cells through cell to cell signal communication. Powell et al. (45) used immunohistochemical stainings to specifically detect CD4$^+$, CD8α^+, CD28$^+$, and CD44$^+$ cells in the spleen as well as liver of chickens and turkeys infected with *H. meleagridis*. With this, they noticed an influx of the mentioned T cell-subpopulations into the liver of turkeys and chickens in coincidence with parasite infiltration. These cellular changes were more pronounced in turkeys and correlated with a decrease in numbers of such cells in

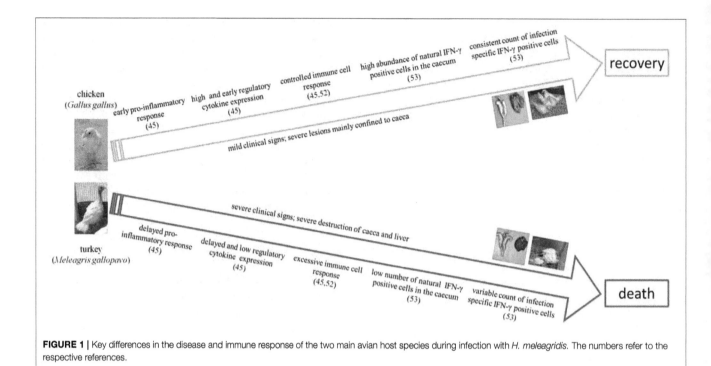

FIGURE 1 | Key differences in the disease and immune response of the two main avian host species during infection with *H. meleagridis*. The numbers refer to the respective references.

spleens whereas no obvious changes were observed in the spleen of chickens.

By investigating T-cell subsets of chickens co-infected with *H. gallinarum* and *H. meleagridis*, a decrease of splenic CD4$^+$ T cells together with a destruction of the cecal mucosa in association with a severe T cell infiltration in the cecal lamina propria was described (63).

In a more recent work, different populations of lymphocytes of host birds were analyzed by flow cytometry after vaccination with attenuated histomonads and/or infection using virulent parasites (52). Thereby, a detailed investigation on the adaptive immune system by investigating quantitative changes of CD4$^+$, CD8α^+ T cells and B cells in different organs and blood of turkeys and chickens was performed. In that study, all infected turkeys died by 14 days p.i. due to severe histomonosis whereas infected chickens or vaccinated birds were not clinically affected. It was hypothesized that the excessive necrosis of caecum and liver in infected tissues of turkeys might be an effect of cytotoxic activity of effector CD8$^+$ T cells which still needs to be verified. The predominance of CD8α^+ T cells might contribute to the destruction of the host tissue and the local suppression of other immune responses including the inhibition of CD4$^+$ T-cell proliferation (52). This is supported by the finding that CD4$^+$ T cells were significantly decreased in the cecum of infected turkeys. On the other hand, the challenge of vaccinated turkeys led to a significant increase of CD4$^+$, CD8α^+, and B cells in the blood already at 4 days post inoculation, indicating an effective and fast recall response of the primed immune system. In infected chickens the analyzed immune cells in cecum and liver were mostly in the range of values of non-infected birds matching with the lower lesion scores. However, a continuing recruitment of

CD4$^+$ and CD8α^+ T cells was observed in the blood of infected chickens. Beside the translocation of these cells to the target organs of infection, this finding might also be explained by the presence of the parasite in the blood of infected host birds (14, 64, 65). In vaccinated as well as vaccinated and challenged chickens, changes of cecal B cells, CD4$^+$ and CD8α^+ T cells were in general even lower compared to infected chickens (52). Overall, such findings demonstrated that vaccination of turkeys and chickens using clonal cultures of *H. meleagridis* limits severe changes of B cells and T cell-subsets as compared to the exacerbated influx observed in non-protected animals. Additionally, a more intense cellular immune response in infected organs of turkeys in comparison to chickens was concluded to contribute to the fatal clinical outcome of the infection in turkeys.

Immunofluorescence and quantification of lymphocyte populations by image analyses, confirmed an influx of B cells and T cells in the infected chicken's cecum from 4 days p.i. until 10 days p.i. (53). In contrast, chickens that were vaccinated showed a similar range of the above mentioned cell population in the cecum compared to control birds even after challenge. Comparative data on turkey ceca obtained by immunofluorescence have so far not been reported due to the lack of cross-reactivity of those antibodies for this host species (52).

Investigations on cytokines in context of an immune response against *H. meleagridis* were performed in different studies by gene expression analyses and *in situ* hybridization for the detection of cells that contain transcripts of specific cytokines. Along with innate pro-inflammatory cytokines mentioned above, Powell et al. (45) investigated adaptive response-signature cytokines IFN-γ, IL-13, and IL-4 and the regulatory cytokines IL-10 and

TGF-β4 by RT-qPCR in different organs of infected chickens and turkeys. Most important, in chickens, IFN-γ and IL-13 mRNA expression was up-regulated while IL-4 mRNA expression remained unaltered during infection. Expression of the regulatory cytokine IL-10 was up-regulated very early during infection in this host species while TGF-β4 mRNA expression levels were unchanged during the experiment. In turkeys, IFN-γ mRNA expression levels were down-regulated in the cecal tonsils soon after infection but up-regulated during later stages. IL-4 mRNA expression levels were variable while IL-13 again showed a sustained up-regulation. As in chickens, IL-10 did not appear to play a significant role during infection in turkeys, but TGF-β4 mRNA expression levels were increased.

Later on, Schwarz et al. (63) found a significant increase in mRNA expression of IFN-γ in chicken cecal tissue infected with *H. gallinarum* harboring histomonads in contrast to an elevated expression of IL-13 when chickens were infected only with *H. gallinarum*. The authors hypothesized that the IFN-γ over-expression in the co-infection was modulated by the presence of *H. meleagridis*. Nevertheless, based on the experimental setting it is difficult to determine if both parasites together cause a variant immune response.

Recently, Kidane et al. (53) investigated the abundance of Th1 and Th2 cytokines, IFN-γ, respectively IL-13 mRNA positive cells by *in situ* hybridization in vaccinated and/or infected chickens and turkeys. It was demonstrated that changes in the abundance of positive cells following infection or vaccination were less pronounced in chickens compared to turkeys. Infected turkeys showed an early decrease of cytokine mRNA positive cells in cecum which later increased together with a severe destruction of the mucosa and infiltration of cytokine expressing cells up to the muscularis layer. A similar destruction and cytokine distribution was observed in the liver of these birds. In comparison, an increased percentage of IFN-γ mRNA positive cells were noticed in vaccinated and challenged turkeys already 4 days post challenge confirming the priming of an immune response by vaccination. An interesting finding was that IFN-γ mRNA positive cells in the cecum of naïve chickens were distinctly higher than in naïve turkeys. These findings led to the conclusion that IFN-γ positive cells may act as a protective trait against histomonosis. However, no distinct Th1/Th2 separation in the immune response was noticed, indicating a more balanced activation of the Th pathways during infection with an extracellular protozoan parasite in birds. Moreover, it could be demonstrated that the fatal clinical outcome of turkeys due to histomonosis is in coherence with a more intense adaptive immune response in infected organs compared to chickens.

CONCLUSION AND OUTLOOK

The reviewed studies are fundamental in devising prospective immunoprophylactic strategies against histomonosis. Results on different types of vaccine either killed or live, revealed a possible direction into how a vaccine could successfully mount

a protective immune response. Furthermore, it is crucial to understand relevant protective traits as well as the failure of the immune system against an infection with *H. meleagridis*.

The most peculiar and differing changes in the immune response in chickens and turkeys against histomonosis are drafted in **Figure 1**. From the experimental studies on the immune response during histomonosis we can clearly elicited that differing profiles of cytokine expression and abundances of specific immune cells resulted in a varying disease progression and outcome in the two main avian host species, chickens and turkeys. At the early infection phase chickens show an expeditious immune response against the parasite which triggers the immune cascade to restrict the parasite progression. In comparison, the turkey's immune responsiveness is delayed, which obviously allows the parasite to disseminate systematically to the liver and other organs. After the initial phase, the effectiveness of the adaptive immune response is based on the accessibility of natural IFN-γ positive cells and a controlled expression of adaptive immune cells which seem to be further key factors to minimize clinical signs and to induce the recovery of chickens. In contrast, a predominance of the cellular response toward the cytolytic pathway may be involved in aggravating tissue destruction in turkeys. Thus, un-controlled immune response and excessive destruction of the tissue can be understood as a further failure of the immune system with consequences on the fatal outcome of the disease in turkeys. Conclusions on the different immune response in chickens and turkeys are supported by the fact that vaccination triggered a similar enhanced allocation of IFN-γ cells and controlled adaptive cell response for both host species. Overall, it can be concluded that an early and locally induced immune response is the crucial factor behind the survival of chickens and immunoprophylaxis induced by vaccination independent of the host.

Further studies on the immune response of poultry against *Histomonas meleagridis* should consider both host and pathogen factors. Given the fact that turkeys and chickens display a different involvement of the immune response to *H. meleagridis*, it could be beneficial to use these contrasting host features in further exploring traits of the immune response. So far, there is hardly any information on the innate immune response against histomonosis. Especially the role of toll-like receptors (TLRs), with possible consequences on modulation of the immune response following vaccination and/or infection, needs to be understood. Furthermore, mechanisms on the function of innate immunity, particularly pro-inflammatory cytokines and antigen-presenting cells, could be useful to link the transition from the innate to the adaptive stage of the immune response. This can unveil essential features such as the quality and persistence of the acquired immune response which is helpful in establishing vaccination schedules. Data collected in experimental studies investigating histomonosis or following vaccination against the disease revealed important changes in the immune response but further identification on pathogen-specific mechanisms would be valuable. Hence, determining specific immunological correlates of protection e.g., the role and function of pathogen-specific T cells would contribute in pin-pointing features that mediate protection. Consequently, unraveling selective mechanisms that induce protection would be useful to promote such effector functions for facilitating new prospects in research on vaccination against histomonosis. Finally, along with studies on screening virulence factors of the protozoa, further explorations on the molecular plethora for potential immunogenic components are necessary to explain pathogen-directed immune reactions of the host.

AUTHOR CONTRIBUTIONS

TM, FK, MH, and DL conceived and designed the review. All authors read and approved the final manuscript.

REFERENCES

1. Smith T. An infectious disease among turkeys caused by protozoa (infectious entero-hepatitis). *USDA Bur Anim Ind Bull.* (1895) 8:3–27.
2. Hess M. Commensal or pathogen—A challenge to fulfil Koch's Postulates. *Br Poult Sci.* (2017) 58:1–12. doi: 10.1080/00071668.2016.1245849
3. McDougald LR. Blackhead disease (histomoniasis) in poultry: a critical review. *Avian Dis.* (2005) 49:462–76. doi: 10.1637/7420-081005R.1
4. Hess M, Liebhart D, Bilic I, Ganas P. Histomonas meleagridis— New insights into an old pathogen. *Vet Parasitol.* (2015) 208:67–76. doi: 10.1016/j.vetpar.2014.12.018
5. Hauck R, Hafez HM. Experimental infections with the protozoan parasite *Histomonas meleagridis*: a review. *Parasitol Res.* (2013) 112:19–34. doi: 10.1007/s00436-012-3190-5
6. Liebhart D, Ganas P, Sulejmanovic T, Hess M. Histomonosis in poultry: previous and current strategies for prevention and therapy. *Avian Pathol.* (2017) 46:1–18. doi: 10.1080/03079457.2016.1229458
7. Clark S, Kimminau E. Critical review: future control of blackhead disease (histomoniasis) in poultry. *Avian Dis.* (2017) 61:281–8. doi: 10.1637/11593-012517-ReviewR
8. Cushman S. *The Production of Turkeys.* Kingston, RI: Bulletin 25, Agricultural Experiment Station, Rhode Island College of Agriculture and Mechanical Arts (1893). 89–123.
9. Graybill HW, Smith T. Production of fatal blackhead in turkeys by feeding embryonated eggs of *Heterakis papillosa*. *J Exp Med.* (1920) 31:647–55. doi: 10.1084/jem.31.5.647
10. Hu J, Fuller L, McDougald LR. Infection of turkeys with *Histomonas meleagridis* by the cloacal drop method. *Avian Dis.* (2004) 48:746–50. doi: 10.1637/7152
11. Liebhart D, Hess M. Oral infection of turkeys with *in vitro*-cultured *Histomonas meleagridis* results in high mortality. *Avian Pathol.* (2009) 38:223–7. doi: 10.1080/03079450902912192
12. Huber K, Reynaud M-C, Callait MP, Zenner L. Histomonas meleagridis in turkeys: dissemination kinetics in host tissues after cloacal infection. *Poult Sci.* (2006) 85:1008–14. doi: 10.1093/ps/85.6.1008
13. Malewitz TD. The pathology of experimentally produced histomoniasis in turkeys. *Am J Vet Res.* (1958) 19:181–5.
14. McGuire WC, Morehouse NF. Blood-induced blackhead. *J Parasitol.* (1958) 44:292–6.
15. Peardon DL, Ware JE. Atypical foci of histomoniasis lesions in a study of direct oral transmission. *Avian Dis.* (1969) 13:340–4. doi: 10.2307/1588502
16. Potts GR. Long-term changes in the prevalences of caecal nematodes and histomonosis in gamebirds in the UK and the interaction with poultry. *Vet Rec.* (2009) 164:715–8. doi: 10.1136/vr.164.23.715
17. Reis Jr JL, Beckstead RB, Brown CC, Gerhold RW. Histomonas meleagridis and capillarid infection in a captive chukar (*Alectoris chukar*). *Avian Dis.* (2009) 53:637–9. doi: 10.1637/8678-030409-Case.1
18. McDougald LR, Abraham M, Beckstead RB. An outbreak of blackhead disease (*Histomonas meleagridis*) in farm-reared bobwhite quail (*Colinus virginianus*). *Avian Dis.* (2012) 56:754–6. doi: 10.1637/10140-032212-Case.1
19. Liebhart D, Neale S, Garcia-Rueda C, Wood AM, Bilic I, Wernsdorf P, et al. A single strain of *Tetratrichomonas gallinarum* causes fatal typhlohepatitis in red-legged partridges (*Alectoris rufa*) to be distinguished from histomonosis. *Avian Pathol.* (2014) 43:473–80. doi: 10.1080/03079457.2014.959435

20. Gordo FP, Herrera S, Castro AT, Durán BG, Diaz RAM. Parasites from farmed ostriches (*Struthio camelus*) and rheas (*Rhea americana*) in Europe. *Vet Parasitol.* (2002) 107:137–60. doi: 10.1016/S0304-4017(02)00104-8
21. Callait-Cardinal MP, Chauve C, Reynaud MC, Alogninouwa T, Zenner L. Infectivity of *Histomonas meleagridis* in ducks. *Avian Pathol.* (2006) 35:109–16. doi: 10.1080/03079450600597626
22. Cepicka I, Hampl V, Kulda J. Critical taxonomic revision of parabasalids with description of one new genus and three new species. *Protist* (2010) 161:400–33. doi: 10.1016/j.protis.2009.11.005
23. Tyzzer EE. Developmental phases of the protozoon of "Blackhead" in turkeys. *J Med Res.* (1919) 40:1–30.
24. Tyzzer EE. The flagellate character and reclassification of the parasite producing "Blackhead" in turkeys: Histomonas (gen. nov.) *meleagridis* (Smith). *J Parasitol.* (1920) 6:124–31. doi: 10.2307/3271065
25. Honigberg BM, Benett CJ. Lightmicroscopic observations on structure and division of *Histomonas meleagridis* (Smith). *J Eukaryot Microbiol.* (1971) 18:687–97.
26. Bishop A. Histomonas meleagridis in domestic fowls (*Gallus gallus*). Cultivation and experimental infection. *Parasitology* (1938) 30:181–94. doi: 10.1017/S0031182000025749
27. Zaragatzki E, Hess M, Grabensteiner E, Abdel-Ghaffar F, Al-Rasheid KAS, Mehlhorn H. Light and transmission electron microscopic studies on the encystation of *Histomonas meleagridis*. *Parasitol Res.* (2010) 106:977–83. doi: 10.1007/s00436-010-1777-2
28. Gruber J, Ganas P, Hess M. Long-term *in vitro* cultivation of *Histomonas meleagridis* coincides with the dominance of a very distinct phenotype of the parasite exhibiting increased tenacity and improved cell yields. *Parasitology* (2017) 144:1253–63. doi: 10.1017/S0031182017000646
29. Dwyer DM. Analysis of the antigenic relationships among *Trichomonas, Histomonas, Dientamoeba*, and *Entamoeba*. I. Quantitative fluorescent antibody methods. *J Eukaryot Microbiol.* (1972) 19:316–25. doi: 10.1111/j.1550-7408.1972.tb03467.x
30. Stark D, Barratt J, Chan D, Ellis JT. *Dientamoeba fragilis*, the neglected trichomonad of the human bowel. *Clin Microbiol.* (2016) 29(3):553–80. doi: 10.1128/CMR.00076-15
31. Dwyer DM, Honigberg BM. Immunologic analysis by quantitative fluorescent antibody methods of effects of prolonged cultivation on *Histomonas meleagridis* (Smith). *Z Parasitenkd* (1972) 39:39–52.
32. Dwyer DM. Analysis of the antigenic relationships among *Trichomonas, Histomonas, Dientamoeba*, and *Entamoeba*. II. Gel diffusion methods. *J Eukaryot Microbiol.* (1972) 19:326–32. doi: 10.1111/j.1550-7408.1972.tb03468.x
33. Dwyer DM. Analysis of the antigenic relationships among *Trichomonas, Histomonas, Dientamoeba*, and *Entamoeba* III. immunoelectrophoresis technics. *J Eukaryot Microbiol.* (1974) 21:139–45. doi: 10.1111/j.1550-7408.1974.tb03628.x
34. Gerbod D, Edgcomb VP, Noël C, Zenner L, Wintjens R, Delgado-Viscogliosi P, et al. Phylogenetic position of the trichomonad parasite of turkeys, Histomonas meleagridis (smith) tyzzer, inferred from small subunit rRNA sequence1. *J Eukaryot Microbiol.* (2005) 48:498–504. doi: 10.1111/j.1550-7408.2001.tb00185.x
35. Mazet M, Diogon M, Alderete JF, Vivares CP, Delbac F. First molecular characterisation of hydrogenosomes in the protozoan parasite *Histomonas meleagridis*. *Int J Parasitol.* (2008) 38:177–90. doi: 10.1016/j.ijpara.2007.06.006

36. Bilic I, Leberl M, Hess M. Identification and molecular characterization of numerous *Histomonas meleagridis* proteins using a cDNA library. *Parasitology* (2009) 136:379–91. doi: 10.1017/S0031182008005477

37. Leberl M, Hess M, Bilic I. *Histomonas meleagridis* possesses three alpha-actinins immunogenic to its hosts. *Mol Biochem Parasitol.* (2010) 169:101–7. doi: 10.1016/j.molbiopara.2009.10.007

38. Lynn EC, Beckstead RB. Identification of gene expression elements in *Histomonas meleagridis* using splinkerette PCR, a variation of ligated adaptor PCR. *J Parasitol.* (2012) 98:135–41. doi: 10.1645/GE-2916.1

39. Klodnicki ME, McDougald LR, Beckstead RB. A genomic analysis of *Histomonas meleagridis* through sequencing of a cDNA library. *J Parasitol.* (2013) 99:264–9. doi: 10.1645/GE-3256.1

40. Mazumdar R, Endler L, Monoyios A, Hess M, Bilic I. Establishment of a *de novo* reference transcriptome of *Histomonas meleagridis* reveals basic insights about biological functions and potential pathogenic mechanisms of the parasite. *Protist* (2017) 168:663–85. doi: 10.1016/j.protis.2017.09.004

41. Monoyios A, Patzl M, Schlosser S, Hess M, Bilic I. Unravelling the differences: comparative proteomic analysis of a clonal virulent and an attenuated *Histomonas meleagridis* strain. *Int J Parasitol.* (2018) 48:145–57. doi: 10.1016/j.ijpara.2017.08.017

42. Clarkson MJ. Immunological responses to *Histomonas meleagridis* in the turkey and fowl. *Immunology* (1963) 6:156–68.

43. Bleyen N, Ons E, De Gussem M, Goddeeris BM. Passive immunization against *Histomonas meleagridis* does not protect turkeys from an experimental infection. *Avian Pathol.* (2009) 38:71–6. doi: 10.1080/03079450802641255

44. Windisch M, Hess M. Establishing an indirect sandwich enzyme-linked-immunosorbent-assay (ELISA) for the detection of antibodies against *Histomonas meleagridis* from experimentally infected specific pathogen-free chickens and turkeys. *Vet Parasitol.* (2009) 161:25–30. doi: 10.1016/j.vetpar.2008.12.014

45. Powell FL, Rothwell L, Clarkson MJ, Kaiser P. The turkey, compared to the chicken, fails to mount an effective early immune response to *Histomonas meleagridis* in the gut. *Parasite Immunol.* (2009) 31:312–27. doi: 10.1111/j.1365-3024.2009.01113.x

46. Windisch M, Hess M. Experimental infection of chickens with *Histomonas meleagridis* confirms the presence of antibodies in different parts of the intestine. *Parasite Immunol.* (2010) 32:29–35. doi: 10.1111/j.1365-3024.2009.01159.x

47. van der Heijden HMJF, Stegeman A, Landman WJM. Development of a blocking-ELISA for the detection of antibodies against *Histomonas meleagridis* in chickens and turkeys. *Vet Parasitol.* (2010) 171:216–22. doi: 10.1016/j.vetpar.2010.03.028

48. Liebhart D, Windisch M, Hess M. Oral vaccination of 1-day-old turkeys with *in vitro* attenuated *Histomonas meleagridis* protects against histomonosis and has no negative effect on performance. *Avian Pathol.* (2010) 39:399–403. doi: 10.1080/03079457.2010.506906

49. Liebhart D, Sulejmanovic T, Grafl B, Tichy A, Hess M. Vaccination against histomonosis prevents a drop in egg production in layers following challenge. *Avian Pathol.* (2013) 42:79–84. doi: 10.1080/03079457.2012.760841

50. Sulejmanovic T, Liebhart D, Hess M. *In vitro* attenuated *Histomonas meleagridis* does not revert to virulence, following serial *in vivo* passages in turkeys or chickens. *Vaccine* (2013) 31:5443–50. doi: 10.1016/j.vaccine.2013.08.098

51. Lotfi A, Hauck R, Olias P, Hafez HM. Pathogenesis of histomonosis in experimentally infected specific-pathogen-free (SPF) layer-type chickens and SPF meat-type chickens. *Avian Dis.* (2014) 58:427–32. doi: 10.1637/10782-012814-Reg.1

52. Mitra T, Gerner W, Kidane FA, Wernsdorf P, Hess M, Saalmüller A, et al. Vaccination against histomonosis limits pronounced changes of B cells and T-cell subsets in turkeys and chickens. *Vaccine* (2017) 35:4184–96. doi: 10.1016/j.vaccine.2017.06.035

53. Kidane FA, Mitra T, Wernsdorf P, Hess M, Liebhart D. Allocation of interferon (IFN)-gamma mRNA positive cells in caecum hallmarks a protective trait against histomonosis. *Front Immunol.* (2018) 9:1164. doi: 10.3389/fimmu.2018.01164

54. Farmer RK, Stephenson J. Infectious enterohepatitis (blackhead) in turkeys; a comparative study of methods of infection. *J Comp Pathol Ther.* (1949) 59:119–26.

55. Horton-Smith C, Long PL. Studies in histomoniasis: I. The infection of chickens (*Gallus gallus*) with histomonad suspensions. *Parasitology* (1956) 46:79–90. doi: 10.1017/S0031182000026354

56. Lund EE. Oral transmission of Histomonas in turkeys. *Poult Sci.* (1956) 35:900–4.

57. Tyzzer EE. A study of immunity produced by infection with attenuated culture-strains of *Histomonas meleagridis*. *J Comp Pathol Ther.* (1936) 49:285–303. doi: 10.1016/S0368-1742(36)80025-3

58. Liebhart D, Grabensteiner E, Hess M. A virulent mono-eukaryotic culture of *Histomonas meleagridis* is capable of inducing fatal histomonosis in different aged turkeys of both sexes, regardless of the infective dose. *Avian Dis.* (2008) 52:168–72. doi: 10.1637/8107-090707-ResNote

59. Singh A, Weissenböck H, Hess M. *Histomonas meleagridis*: immunohistochemical localization of parasitic cells in formalin-fixed, paraffin-embedded tissue sections of experimentally infected turkeys demonstrates the wide spread of the parasite in its host. *Exp Parasitol.* (2008) 118:505–13. doi: 10.1016/j.exppara.2007.11.004

60. Hess M, Liebhart D, Grabensteiner E, Singh A. Cloned *Histomonas meleagridis* passaged *in vitro* resulted in reduced pathogenicity and is capable of protecting turkeys from histomonosis. *Vaccine* (2008) 26:4187–93. doi: 10.1016/j.vaccine.2008.05.071

61. Grafl B, Liebhart D, Windisch M, Ibesich C, Hess M. Seroprevalence of *Histomonas meleagridis* in pullets and laying hens determined by ELISA. *Vet Rec.* (2011) 168:160. doi: 10.1136/vr.c6479

62. van der Heijden HMJF, Landman WJM. High seroprevalence of *Histomonas meleagridis* in Dutch layer chickens. *Avian Dis.* (2011) 55:324–7. doi: 10.1637/9609-120610-ResNote.1

63. Schwarz A, Gauly M, Abel H, Daş G, Humburg J, Weiss ATA, et al. Pathobiology of *Heterakis gallinarum* mono-infection and co-infection with *Histomonas meleagridis* in layer chickens. *Avian Pathol.* (2011) 40:277–87. doi: 10.1080/03079457.2011.561280

64. Clarkson MJ. The progressive pathology of Heterakis-produced histomoniasis in turkeys. *Res Vet Sci.* (1962) 3:443–8.

65. Farmer RK, Hughes DL, Whiting G. Infectious enterohepatitis (blackhead) in turkeys: a study of the pathology of the artificially induced disease. *J Comp Pathol Ther.* (1951) 61:251–62. doi: 10.1016/S0368-1742(51)80025-0

4

Parasitic Nematodes Exert Antimicrobial Activity and Benefit from Microbiota-Driven Support for Host Immune Regulation

4

Sebastian Rausch [1*], Ankur Midha [1], Matthias Kuhring [2,3,4,5], Nicole Affinass [1], Aleksandar Radonic [6,7], Anja A. Kühl [8], André Bleich [9], Bernhard Y. Renard [2] and Susanne Hartmann [1*]

[1] Department of Veterinary Medicine, Institute of Immunology, Freie Universität Berlin, Berlin, Germany, [2] Bioinformatics Unit (MF 1), Robert Koch Institute, Berlin, Germany, [3] Core Unit Bioinformatics, Berlin Institute of Health (BIH), Berlin, Germany, [4] Berlin Institute of Health Metabolomics Platform, Berlin Institute of Health (BIH), Berlin, Germany, [5] Max Delbrück Center for Molecular Medicine, Berlin, Germany, [6] Centre for Biological Threats and Special Pathogens (ZBS 1), Robert Koch Institute, Berlin, Germany, [7] Genome Sequencing Unit (MF 2), Robert Koch Institute, Berlin, Germany, [8] IPATH.Berlin, Core Unit for Immunopathology for Experimental Models, Berlin Institute of Health, Charité - Universitätsmedizin Berlin, Corporate Member of Freie Universität Berlin, Humboldt-Universität zu Berlin, Berlin, Germany, [9] Institute for Laboratory Animal Science, Hannover Medical School, Hannover, Germany

*Correspondence:
Sebastian Rausch
sebastian.rausch@fu-berlin.de
Susanne Hartmann
susanne.hartmann@fu-berlin.de

Intestinal parasitic nematodes live in intimate contact with the host microbiota. Changes in the microbiome composition during nematode infection affect immune control of the parasites and shifts in the abundance of bacterial groups have been linked to the immunoregulatory potential of nematodes. Here we asked if the small intestinal parasite *Heligmosomoides polygyrus* produces factors with antimicrobial activity, senses its microbial environment and if the anti-nematode immune and regulatory responses are altered in mice devoid of gut microbes. We found that *H. polygyrus* excretory/secretory products exhibited antimicrobial activity against gram$^{+/-}$ bacteria. Parasites from germ-free mice displayed alterations in gene expression, comprising factors with putative antimicrobial functions such as chitinase and lysozyme. Infected germ-free mice developed increased small intestinal Th2 responses coinciding with a reduction in local Foxp3$^+$RORγt$^+$ regulatory T cells and decreased parasite fecundity. Our data suggest that nematodes sense their microbial surrounding and have evolved factors that limit the outgrowth of certain microbes. Moreover, the parasites benefit from microbiota-driven immune regulatory circuits, as an increased ratio of intestinal Th2 effector to regulatory T cells coincides with reduced parasite fitness in germ-free mice.

Keywords: parasite, nematode, immune regulation, germ-free, microbiota, antimicrobial, Treg, Th2

INTRODUCTION

Infections with enteric nematodes are associated with changes in the composition of the host intestinal microbiota in mice, pigs, and primates (1–5). Our previous work showed that nematode-infected mice deficient in IL-4Rα-signaling, hence refractory to IL-4/IL-13-dependent immune sequelae, experience similar microbiota alterations as fully immune-competent mice (2), leaving open the question of the mechanistic basis for structural changes in microbial communities associated with nematode infections. Our and other groups have shown that products released by parasitic nematodes possess antimicrobial activity (6–8), prompting the question if enteric nematodes sense and actively shape their microbial environment.

To ensure prolonged survival and reproduction, parasitic nematodes have developed strategies suppressing host immune responses, in part driven by the release of immunomodulators interfering with innate and adaptive immune effector mechanisms (9–11), but also by supporting the *de novo* generation, expansion and activation of regulatory T cells (Treg) (12–16). Recent studies provide evidence for a contribution of microbiota alterations to immune regulation during nematode infection. More specifically, the increased abundances of Lactobacilli and Clostridiales family members during nematode-infection have been linked to the expansion and activation of Treg (1, 17), which in turn control the magnitude of anti-parasite and unrelated inflammatory responses (13–16, 18).

Here we focused on the interaction of an enteric parasite infection, microbiota, and host immunity. We surveyed fitness and gene expression of the small intestinal nematode *Heligmosomoides polygyrus* reared in conventional and germ-free mice and investigated products released by the parasite for antimicrobial activity against gram$^-$ and gram$^+$ bacterial species. Furthermore, we compared anti-parasite Th2 immunity and the expansion, cytokine production and phenotypic heterogeneity of Treg in conventional and germfree mice. Our data demonstrate that (I) *H. polygyrus* may actively shape the composition of the host microbiota by releasing antimicrobials and that (II) nematode fitness is compromised in the absence of host microbes. Furthermore, our data suggest that the nematode senses the microbiota, as indicated by differential gene expression of worms from germ-free and conventional hosts, and finally, that microbes support Treg responses regulating anti-parasite Th2 immunity.

MATERIALS AND METHODS

Mice and Parasites

The experiments performed followed the National Animal Protection Guidelines and were approved by the German Animal Ethics Committee for the protection of animals (G0176/16). Female specific pathogen-free (SPF) and germfree C57BL/6 mice were kept in individually ventilated, filter-topped cages with autoclaved bedding, chow and water. Infections with 200 *H. polygyrus* larvae were performed aseptically in a laminar flow. *H. polygyrus* L3 were freshly isolated from fecal cultures of infected mice and treated for 1 week with an antibiotic cocktail (5 mg/ml streptomycin, 1 mg/ml ampicillin, 0.5 mg/ml gentamicin, 1 mg/ml neomycin, 0.5 mg/ml vancomycin; all from AppliChem, Darmstadt, Germany). L3 were shown to be free of aerobic microbes as determined by lack of bacterial growth in antibiotic-free LB medium. Infected and naïve control GF mice received antibiotics (as specified above) via the drinking water. To further reduce the risk of contamination, SPF and GF C57BL/6 mice were kept without bedding change until the dissection 2 weeks post-infection. The axenic status of GF mice was confirmed by qPCR of eubacterial 16s rRNA with colon content collected on the day

of infection and dissection. Adult worms were removed from the small intestine, counted and eight females per mouse were kept at 37°C in RPMI-1640 medium containing 200 U/mL penicillin, 200 µg/mL streptomycin (all from PAN Biotech, Aidenbach, Germany) and 1% glucose for 24 h for the determination of individual egg counts. Female worm length was determined after culture.

Parasite Excretory/Secretory Products

Excretory/secretory products of *H. polygyrus* (HES) were collected from adult worms extensively washed before being cultured in phenol-red free RPMI-1640 medium containing 200 U/mL penicillin, 200 µg/mL streptomycin. After 24 h in culture, worms were washed extensively with antibiotic-free worm growth media (RPMI-1640 medium with 1% glucose) and maintained in this medium with daily media changes. Spent media from the first 48 h were discarded. Thereafter, supernatants were harvested every 48 h and sterile filtered through a 0.22 µm syringe-driven filter system, and stored at −20°C until further use.

Bacterial Strains

The strains used to evaluate antibacterial activities of HES in the radial diffusion assay included *Escherichia coli* IMT19224, *Salmonella enterica* serovar Typhimurium ATCC14028, and *Staphylococcus aureus* IMT29828 obtained from the strain collection of the Institute of Microbiology and Epizoonotics, Freie Universität Berlin and *Enterococcus faecium* DSM20477 provided by Dr. Markus Heimesaat (Institute of Microbiology, Charité—Universitätsmedizin Berlin). *E. coli* IMT19224 was used to assess agglutinating activity of HES.

Radial Diffusion Assay

Antibacterial activities of HES were assessed using the radial diffusion assay (19). Overnight bacterial cultures were diluted 1:100 in Mueller-Hinton broth (Carl Roth, Karlsruhe, Germany) and incubated at 37°C with shaking at 250 rpm until reaching an optical density of 0.3–0.4 at 600 nm. Bacteria were washed and resuspended in cold sodium phosphate buffer (100 mM, pH 7.4) by centrifugation (880 × g, 10 min, 4°C). Bacteria were then resuspended in warm (50°C), sterile underlay agar [10 mM sodium phosphate buffer, 1% (v/v) Mueller-Hinton broth, 1.5 (w/v) agar] at 4×10^5 colony forming units per mL. Fifteen milliliter of bacteria-infused underlay agar was poured into 120 mm square petri dishes and allowed to solidify. Evenly spaced wells (5 mm) were formed in the agar using the blunt ends of P10 pipet tips, and treatments and controls added (5 µL/well). Five microliter native HES corresponded to 5 µg protein. The antimicrobial peptide Pexiganan (kindly provided by Jens Rolff, Institute of Biology, Freie Universität Berlin, 0.0125 µg/well) was applied as positive control. PBS and RPMI-1640 medium were included as negative controls. Plates were incubated at 37°C for 3 h and then overlaid with double-strength Mueller-Hinton agar [4.2% (w/v) Mueller-Hinton broth, 1.5% agar]. Petri dishes were incubated for 18 h at 37°C and the growth inhibition zones around each well were measured. Antibacterial activity is represented as the diameter of the inhibition zone (mm) beyond the 5 mm well.

Agglutination Assay

Agglutinating activity of HES was assessed as described previously (20) using *E. coli* IMT19224. Bacteria were collected at mid-logarithmic phase by centrifugation at 880 × g for 5 min, then washed and resuspended in Tris-buffered saline (50 mM Tris-HCl, 150 mM NaCl, pH 7.5) at approximately 10^9 cells/mL. Thirty microliter of bacteria were mixed with 30 μL of treatments in the presence and absence of 10 mM $CaCl_2$ and incubated for 1 h at room temperature on a glass slide. Concanavalin A from *Canavalia ensiformis* (Con A) and Lectin from *Triticum vulgaris* (Wheat germ agglutinin; WGA, both from Sigma-Aldrich) were included as positive controls. Samples were then visualized and photographed using the 40X objective on a Leica DM750 microscope equipped with an ICC50HD digital camera (Leica Microsystems, Wetzlar, Germany).

Parasite RNA-Isolation and Quality Check

Small intestines and the bulk of removed parasites were kept in ice-cold physiological NaCl solution. Thirty worms (15 males/15 females) were quickly isolated from three individual SPF and GF mice, washed repeatedly in cold physiological NaCl solution, inspected for physical integrity, and absence of host tissue and then snap frozen in liquid nitrogen before storage at −80°C. Samples were homogenized using shredder columns filled with 200 mg sterile sea sand and the FastPrep®-24 instrument (MP Biomedicals, Eschwege, Germany) at 5 m/s for 35 s. Supernatants of homogenized worms were further processed for RNA isolation (InnuPREP RNA isolation, Analytik Jena AG, Germany), DNase treatment (Analytik Jena AG, Germany), and RNA quality control (Agilent 2100 Bioanalyzer, RNA 6000 Nano Kit, Agilent Technologies, Waldbronn, Germany). All RNA samples displayed RIN values of 10.

Sequencing and Data Processing

For transcriptome sequencing on an Illumina platform a TruSeq RNA library generation was utilized. The library was generated by using the TruSeq RNA Sample Prep Kit v2 (Illumina, San Diego, CA, USA) following the manufacturer's instructions. The library was quantified by using the KAPA Library Quantification Kit for Illumina (Kapa Biosystems, Wilmington, MA, USA). The library size was determined by using the High Sensitivity DNA Analysis Kit for the 2100 Bioanalyzer Instrument (Agilent Technologies, Waldbronn, Germany). Libraries were adjusted to a concentration of 12 pM and sequenced on a HiSeq 1500 instrument (Illumina, San Diego, CA, USA) in rapid mode. For cluster generation, the TruSeq Rapid PE Cluster Kit v2 was used. Cluster generation was performed on board. For sequencing the HiSeq Rapid SBS kit v2 was used to sequence 100 + 100 bases.

We sequenced three isolates from SPF and GF mice with a mean library size of 40.15 million paired-end reads and a standard deviation of 10.74. Raw reads were subjected to quality control and trimming via the QCumber pipeline (version 1.0.14, https://gitlab.com/RKIBioinformaticsPipelines/QCumber) utilizing FastQC

(v0.11.5, https://www.bioinformatics.babraham.ac.uk/projects/fastqc/), Trimmomatic (0.36) (21) and Kraken (0.10.5-beta) (22). On average, 91.77% of reads remained after trimming.

Preprocessed reads were mapped to a reference genome (as specified below) and corresponding sequence features using the TopHat split-read mapper (v2.1.1) (23) and reference as well as novel features were extracted and merged with the aid of Cufflinks and Cuffmerg (24) (v2.2.1) to obtain one integrated and unified transcriptome for *H. polygyrus* samples. The *H. polygyrus* draft genome nHp_v2.0 was applied as reference genome (database version WBPS10, annotation version 2016-09-WormBase), as available at WormBase ParaSite (25). For each sample, raw expression values were created by counting uniquely mapped reads on gene level using featureCounts (v1.5.0-p3) (26). To identify differentially expressed genes (DEGs) between SPF and GF mice isolates, respectively, DESeq2 (1.12.4) (27) was applied with a classic pairwise design model and a p-value threshold of 0.05. In addition, normalized and transformed expression values were extracted from DESeq2 (regularized log transformation) and corrected for batch effects via Limma (3.28.21, removeBatchEffect) (28) to allow for sample comparison with clustered heatmaps and principal component analysis (PCA).

Reference as well as novel transcripts were functionally (re-)annotated using an iterative annotation strategy. First, transcripts were either first-frame translated (reference) or examined for ORFs (novels, Cuffcompare class code "u") using EMBOSS transeq (6.6.0.0) (29) and TransDecoder (v2.1), respectively. Next, resulting protein sequences were passed through a series of database searches until successfully annotated with Gene Ontology (GO) terms (30), either via blastp (2.6.0+) (31), and Blast2GO (4.0.7) (32) or by a final InterProScan (33). Databases used for annotation included (in this order) the UniProt (34) *Heligmosomoides polygyrus bakeri* proteome (UP000050761, downloaded at 07.04.2017), UniProt Swiss-Prot Nematoda proteins, UniProt TrEMBL Nematoda proteins as well as the complete Swiss-Prot database and the complete TrEMBL database (all downloaded at 16.02.2017).

Cell Isolation, Stimulation, and Flow Cytometry

Lymph node single cell suspensions and small intestinal tissue digestion for the isolation of siLP cells were performed as described previously (35). Cultures were kept for 6 h with brefeldin A added after 1 h before surface and intracellular staining. Surface and intracellular markers were stained according to the manufacturer's instructions with the following antibodies obtained from ThermoFisher/eBioscience, if not stated otherwise: CD4-PerCP/-BV510/-A700 (RM4-5), Foxp3-FITC/-PerCP-Cy5.5 (FJK-16s), GATA-3-A660/-PE/-PE-eF610 (TWAJ), T-bet-PE/-PE-Cy7 (eBio4B10), RORγt-BV421 (Q31-378, BD biosciences), IL-10-APC (JES5-16E3), IL-4-PE/-PE-Cy7 (11B11), and IL-17A-PerCP-Cy5.5 (eBio17B7). Live/dead discrimination was performed using fixable viability dye eF780 (ThermoFisher/eBioscience). Unspecific binding was prevented by addition of 20 μg/ml FcgRII/III blocking antibody (2.4G2).

Histology

Formalin-fixed, paraffin-embedded sections (1–2 μm) of duodenum were de-waxed and stained with hematoxylin and eosin for overview, with periodic acid Schiff for goblet cell quantification and by Direct red 80 (Sigma) for the detection of eosinophils. Enteritis was scored using hematoxylin and eosin-stained section as described before (16). PAS$^+$ goblet cells were counted along five villi per section. Images were acquired using the AxioImager Z1 microscope (Carl Zeiss MicroImaging, Inc., Göttingen, Germany). All evaluations were performed blinded.

Statistical Analyses

Data were assessed for normality using GraphPad Prism software (La Jolla, CA, USA). For comparison between two groups, an unpaired T-test was used. Testing of multiple groups was performed using a one-way analysis of variances followed by Tukey's multiple comparison or the Kruskall-Wallis test combined with Dunn's multiple comparison test.

RESULTS

Antimicrobial Activity of Nematode Excretory/Secretory Products

Infection with *H. polygyrus* alters the composition of the intestinal microbiota alongside the intestine, including an increase in gram⁻ Enterobacteriaceae (2, 17, 36). Similar changes occurred in IL-4Rα$^{-/-}$ mice, hence independently of Th2-mediated changes in gut physiology (2). As both free-living and parasitic nematodes defend themselves against potentially harmful microbes by the production of antimicrobial factors (7), we asked if *H. polygyrus* releases active antimicrobials, possibly interfering with its microbial environment. We used the radial diffusion assay to test the antibacterial activity of *H. polygyrus* excretory/secretory products (HES) in comparison to the antimicrobial peptide Pexiganan. Five micrograms of native HES collected from *H. polygyrus* cultures inhibited the growth of gram⁻ and gram⁺ bacteria, including *E. coli*, *S. enterica* var. Typhimurium, *E. faecium*, and *S. aureus* (**Table 1**).

TABLE 1 | Antimicrobial activity* of excretory/secretory products from adult *Heligmosomoides polygyrus* nematodes in the radial diffusion assay.

	E. coli IMT19224	S. typhimurium ATCC14028	E. faecium DSM20477	S. aureus IMT29828
H. polygyrus E/S (5 μg)	5.3 ± 3.1	4.3 ± 0.6	3.7 ± 1.5	5.7 ± 1.5
Pexiganan (0.0125 μg)	9.0 ± 0.0	8.0 ± 0.0	12.0 ± 0.0	13.0 ± 0.0
PBS	–	–	–	–
RPMI-1640	–	–	–	–

*Activity reported as inhibition zone (mm; mean ± standard deviation) produced by 5 μL treatments (n = 3 biological replicates with independent batches of HES). "–"indicates no detectable activity. Data are representative for two independent experiments.

C-type lectin domain-containing proteins are known to agglutinate bacteria and are important in nematode immune defense against microbial infection (37). As *H. polygyrus* produces a C-type lectin protein (38) we tested the agglutinating activity of nematode products by treating *E. coli* with increasing amounts of native HES in the presence and absence of CaCl$_2$. We observed dose- and calcium-dependent agglutinating activity (**Figure 1**), suggestive of C-type lectin-mediated bacterial agglutination. These data indicate that *H. polygyrus* employs defense mechanisms via released products during its interactions with microbes which may contribute to shaping its microbial environment in the murine gut.

Altered Parasite Gene Expression in Germ-Free Mice

Having demonstrated the ability of nematode products to influence bacterial growth, we sought to investigate if intestinal nematodes sense their microbial environment and hence asked if the complete absence of microbes in the host gut resulted in altered parasite gene expression. To that end, we infected germfree (GF) and conventional (specific pathogen-free; SPF) mice and performed RNA-sequencing with parasites isolated 2 weeks post-infection. Samples clearly clustered according to SPF vs. GF parasite origin (**Figures 2A,B**). We found that a surprisingly small set of 52 genes was differentially expressed in adult worms isolated from GF compared to SPF mice (**Supplementary Table 1**). The majority of genes were upregulated, comprising a venom-like allergen (VAL-1), chitinase-1, lysozyme-3, and orthologs of putative *Caenorhabditis elegans* glutathione S-transferase and *C. elegans*/*C. briggsae* UDP-glucuronosyl- transferases, amongst others (**Supplementary Table 1**). Only four of ten genes downregulated in parasites isolated from GF mice were annotated, including a putative *C. elegans* UDP-glucuronosyl-transferase. Hence, parasitic nematodes reared in a germ-free environment display a distinct gene expression pattern.

Reduced Parasite Fitness in Germ-Free Mice

Previous studies reported on impeded survival and fecundity of intestinal nematodes in the absence of gut microbes (39–41); therefore, we assessed if parasite burden and fitness were altered depending on the host microbial status. While adult worm burdens were similar in SPF and GF mice at 2 weeks post-infection (**Figure 3A**), female worms developing in GF mice were significantly smaller and produced fewer eggs (**Figures 3B,C**). Importantly, *H. polygyrus* resides in the proximal small intestine harboring few microbes and the parasite mainly relies on host tissue as food source (42). Thus, we investigated next if the reduced parasite fitness in GF mice coincided with immune changes.

Altered Treg Responses in Nematode-Infected Germ-Free Mice

The microbiota supports the induction and maintenance of regulatory T cells (Treg) (43–46) and infections with *H. polygyrus*

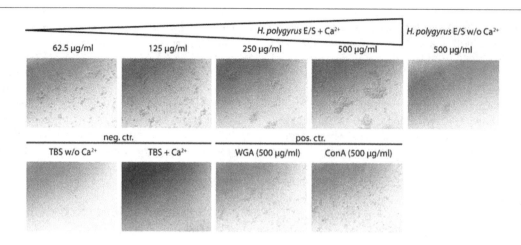

FIGURE 1 | *H. polygyrus* excretory/secretory products cause bacterial agglutination. **(Top)** Bacterial agglutination in the presence and absence of native adult *H. polygyrus* E/S products (HES) and 10 mM CaCl$_2$. Representative images of agglutination of *E. coli* IMT19224 with serial dilutions of *H. polygyrus* E/S products are shown. **(Bottom)** controls of agglutination include tris-buffered saline (TBS) with and without CaCl$_2$ as well as the C-type lectins wheat germ agglutinin (WGA) and concanavalin A (Con A). Magnification ×400. Data are representative for two individual experiments performed with two independent HES batches.

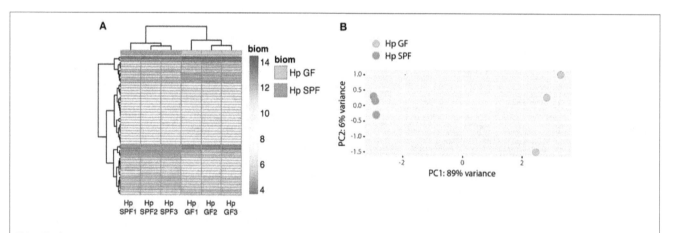

FIGURE 2 | Principle component analysis (PCA) and clustering of differentially expressed genes (DEGs). **(A)** Unsupervised clustering heatmap of differentially expressed genes (DEG, *n* = 52) in *H. polygyrus* samples isolated from SPF and GF mice. Red intensity indicates high gene expression, whereas blue intensity indicates low gene expression. **(B)** Principle component (PC) analysis revealed that 89% of the data variation is explained by the difference between SPF and GF isolates. Data are from one experiment with three biological replicates.

lead to the activation and expansion of regulatory T cells suppressing local immunopathology, but also host protective Th2 immunity (1, 15–17). Therefore, we surveyed if Treg expansion, phenotype and cytokine production in *H. polygyrus* infected mice differed depending on the microbial status.

The overall frequencies of Foxp3$^+$ Treg were similar in mLN of naive SPF and GF mice and did not change significantly upon infection (**Figure 4A**). While Treg frequencies in the small intestinal lamina propria (siLP) were stably maintained in infected SPF mice, Treg frequencies dropped significantly in the small intestines of infected GF mice compared to the respective naive controls (**Figure 4B**).

Intestinal Foxp3$^+$ Treg form a functional heterogeneous population comprising subsets marked by the elevated expression of GATA-3 or RORγt, respectively (47). While GATA-3 expression is necessary for Treg stability under inflammatory

conditions (48, 49), RORγt$^+$ Treg exhibit a highly activated phenotype and limit the Th2-driven control of helminth infection and immune pathology in intestinal inflammation (43, 50). Hence, we investigated if the reduced fitness of worms isolated from GF mice was associated with phenotypic alterations in the Treg population. Fewer Treg in mLN and siLP of naïve and infected GF mice expressed RORγt compared to the respective SPF controls (**Figures 4C,D**). Steady state GATA-3 expression by Treg and the expansion of GATA-3$^+$ Treg upon infection was similar in mLN of SPF and GF mice (**Figure 4C**). Upon infection, the increase in GATA-3$^+$Treg reached significance in the small intestine of SPF mice (**Figure 4D**). Thus, naïve and infected GF mice harbored significantly less RORγt$^+$ Treg compared to SPF mice, while GATA-3$^+$Treg expanded similarly.

Next, we asked if Treg activation differed depending on the microbial status and hence assessed their cytokine production.

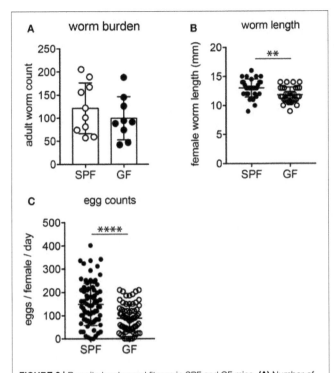

FIGURE 3 | Parasite burden and fitness in SPF and GF mice. **(A)** Number of luminal adults isolated 2 weeks post-*H. polygyrus* infection from SPF and GF mice. **(B)** Length of female parasites. **(C)** Fecundity of female worms determined as egg production within 24 h after isolation. Data are pooled from two independent experiments each performed with four to five infected mice per group. Mean, SD, and individual data points are shown. **p < 0.01, ****p < 0.0001.

IL-10 production by Treg in mLN increased similarly and strongly in SPF and GF mice upon infection (**Figure 4E**). IL-10 production by siLP Treg of SPF mice did not change in response to infection (**Figure 4F**). Small intestinal Treg of GF mice were rather poor IL-10 producers at steady state and upon infection (**Figure 4F**). As intestinal RORγt⁺ Treg have been reported as superior in IL-10 production compared to other gut Treg (43), we next surveyed IL-10⁺ Treg of SPF and GF mice for co-expression of RORγt and GATA-3. Expectedly, the reduced frequencies of RORγt⁺ cells in the Foxp3⁺Treg pool (**Figures 4C,D**) was reflected by their underrepresentation in the IL-10 producing Treg population of naïve and infected GF mice (**Figures 4G,H**). GATA-3⁺Treg expanding in mLN of infected SPF and GF mice (**Figure 4C**) clearly dominated the IL-10-expressing Treg pool in both groups upon infection (**Figure 4G**). Reflecting their high frequencies in the total siLP Treg population (**Figure 4D**), GATA-3⁺Treg dominated in the small intestinal IL-10⁺ population irrespective of microbial and nematode-infection status (**Figure 4H**). Finally, we investigated if the reduction in RORγt⁺ Treg in the intestine and the poor IL-10 expression by gut Treg in GF mice was associated with differences in local immunopathology. Duodenal enteritis scores were, however, similar in SPF and GF nematode-infected mice (**Figure 4I**).

Taken together our data show that Treg activation in gut-associated lymphoid tissue seen as increased IL-10 production

occurs independently of the presence of gut microbes. Naïve and nematode-infected GF mice display a reduction in RORγt⁺ Treg in the gut and gut-draining lymph nodes, while GATA-3⁺ Treg expanded similarly in SPF and GF mice and formed the major IL-10 producing Treg subset upon infection irrespective of the microbial status.

Increased Th2/Treg Ratios in Nematode-Infected Germ-Free Mice

To see if the reduction in RORγt⁺ Treg and the lower IL-10 expression by small intestinal Treg in GF mice coincided with deregulated Th2 responses we quantified Th2 cells based on GATA-3 expression and IL-4 expression. Significantly more GATA-3⁺ Th2 cells were present in the small intestines of infected GF mice compared to SPF mice, while IL-4 production was significantly increased in mLN (**Figures 5A,B**). Calculating the ratios of Th2 cells to Treg based on their frequencies in CD4⁺ T cells, we found significantly elevated Th2 effector to Treg ratios in the small intestine of infected GF compared to SPF mice (**Figure 5C**). We have previously shown that intestinal nematode infections lead to the differentiation of GATA-3⁺ Th2 and GATA-3⁺T-bet⁺ Th2/1 hybrid cells (51, 52). Th2/1 cells developed in infected SPF as well as GF mic, hence microbial signals were dispensable for their induction (**Figures 5D,E**). The increase in intestinal GATA-3⁺Th2 cells coincided with trends of increased goblet cell and eosinophil counts in the duodenum (**Figures 5F,G**). As the microbiota supports Th17 differentiation (53, 54) we assessed RORγt and IL-17A expression by Foxp3⁻CD4⁺ T effector cells. Expectedly, GF mice harbored very few Th17 cells in mLN and small intestine (**Figure S1**). In conclusion, nematode-induced local Th2 responses were significantly increased in the absence of gut microbes and decreased parasite fitness in GF mice was associated with elevated Th2 to Treg ratios at the site of infection.

DISCUSSION

Over the last decade, several studies have shown that intestinal parasite infections lead to changes in the gut microbiota of the host [reviewed in (55, 56)]. Enteric nematodes such as *H. polygyrus*, *Nippostrongylus brasiliensis*, and *Trichuris* species alter the abundance of numerous bacterial genera in the host gut (2–4, 36, 57). Changes in the microbiota composition also result from infections with the protozoan parasites *Toxoplasma gondii* and *Giardia lamblia* (58, 59). Though the mechanistic basis for the microbiome changes provoked by the infections is not well understood, it is speculated that parasites may directly influence the composition of the microbiota. Parasite-driven immune responses resulting from tissue damage (3, 59) and leading to changes in gut physiology and epithelial barrier function (60–63) are likely to be involved. Nutrient competition and changes in host antimicrobial peptide production upon parasite infection may also contribute to structural changes in gut microbial communities (3, 64).

Here, we show that the excretory/secretory (E/S) products of the small intestinal nematode *H. polygyrus* exert antimicrobial

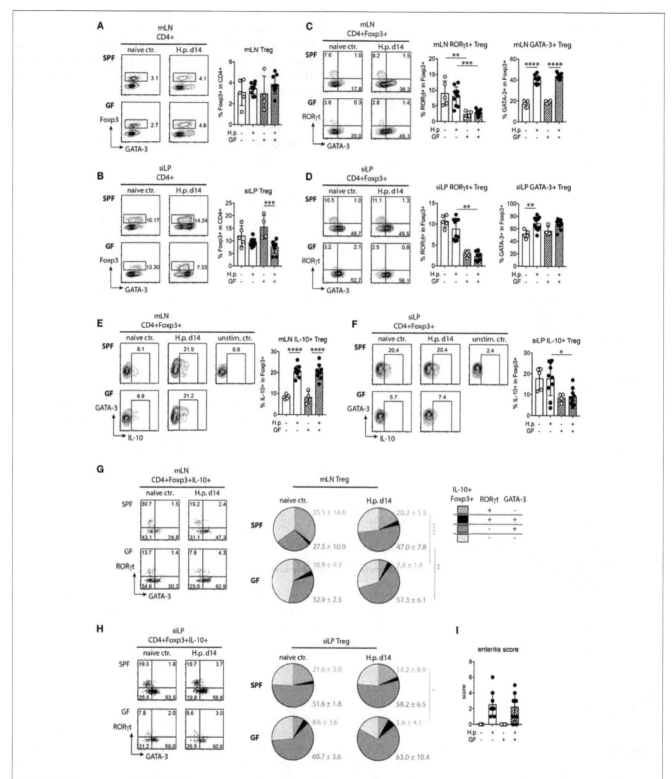

FIGURE 4 | Treg responses in SPF and GF mice infected with *H. polygyrus*. **(A,B)** Representative plots of Foxp3$^+$ Treg detection in CD4$^+$ T cells and Treg frequencies in mesenteric lymph nodes (mLN, **A**) and small intestinal lamina propria (siLP, **B**) of uninfected controls and mice infected with *H. polygyrus* for 2 weeks. **(C,D)** Representative plots of RORγt and GATA-3 expression by Treg and frequencies of RORγt$^+$ and GATA-3$^+$ Treg in mLN **(C)** and siLP **(D)**. **(E,F)** Representative plots of IL-10 expression and frequencies of IL-10$^+$ Treg in mLN **(E)** and siLP **(F)**. **(G,H)** Representation of RORγt$^+$, RORγt$^+$GATA-3$^+$, GATA-3$^+$, and RORγt$^-$GATA-3$^-$ Treg in the IL-10$^+$ Treg population in mLN and siLP of naïve and infected mice. Numbers express group means and SD. **(I)** Duodenal enteritis scores. Data are pooled from two independent experiments each performed with two to three uninfected and four to five infected mice per group. Mean, SD, and individual data points are shown in **(A–H)**. *$p < 0.05$; **$p < 0.01$, ***$p < 0.001$, ****$p < 0.0001$.

Parasitic Nematodes Exert Antimicrobial Activity and Benefit from Microbiota-Driven...

45

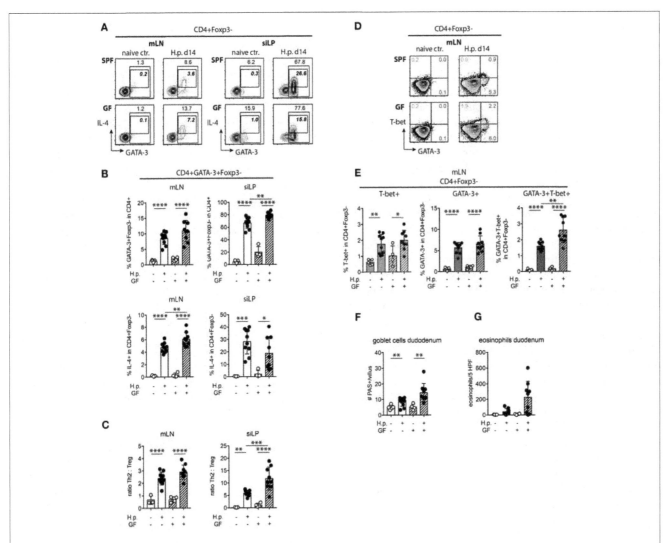

FIGURE 5 | Th2 response and Th2/Treg ratios in SPF and GF mice. **(A,B)** Representative plots of GATA-3 and IL-4 expression by CD4+Foxp3− T cells **(A)** and frequencies **(B)** of GATA-3+ and IL-4+ Th2 cells in mLN and siLP. Bold italic numbers in FACS plots refer to IL-4+ cells. **(C)** Ratios of GATA-3+ Th2 cells to Foxp3+ Treg in mLN and siLP determined based on frequencies in CD4+ T cells. **(D,E)** Representative plots of GATA-3 and T-bet expression by CD4+Foxp3− T cells **(D)** and frequencies of T-bet+ Th1, GATA-3+ Th2, and GATA-3+T-bet+ Th2/1 cells in mLN **(E)**. **(F,G)** Histological goblet cell **(F)** and eosinophil **(G)** quantification in the small intestine of naïve and infected mice. Data are pooled from two independent experiments each performed with two to three uninfected and four to five infected mice per group. Mean, SD, and individual data points are shown. *$p < 0.05$; **$p < 0.01$, ***$p < 0.001$, ****$p < 0.0001$.

activities seen as inhibited growth of several bacterial species including commensal intestinal species such as *E. faecium*, and agglutination of *E. coli*. Previous studies have reported on antimicrobial activity of nematode products, such as *Ascaris suum* antibacterial factors (ASABF) and cecropins (65, 66). We have recently shown that E/S products of the porcine roundworm *A. suum* possess antibacterial and agglutinating activity and impair biofilm formation (8). *Ascaris* E/S products comprise proteins and peptides with known and predicted antimicrobial activity, such as cecropins, ASABF, lysozymes, and C-type lectins (8). As our previous studies showed that changes in the gut microbiota of *H. polygyrus*-infected mice occurred independently of the parasite-driven Th2 response and subsequent changes in gut physiology (2), the detection of antimicrobial activities of

nematode E/S products offers an attractive explanation of how these parasites may directly shape their microbial environment. On the other hand, strong Th2 responses, and the subsequent changes in host antimicrobial peptide and mucin production have been shown to be related to the decrease of segmented filamentous bacteria during infections with *N. brasiliensis* (3).

Of note, our previous studies showed an increase in Enterobacteriaceae along the small and large intestine upon infection with *H. polygyrus* (2). Whether the antimicrobial activity of *H. polygyrus* E/S products against Enterobacteriaceae family members such as *E. coli* and *S. enterica* prevents a more vigorous increase of such potentially pathogenic bacteria benefitting from intestinal inflammation can only be speculated on. It is conceivable that during coevolution, parasitic worms have not only developed intricate mechanisms interfering with host immunity, but also adapted to directly support or restrict the growth of commensal families which might be beneficial or detrimental to parasite survival and host health via the release of antimicrobial factors. Furthermore, the parasites may benefit from the support of immune regulatory circuits fostered by microbiome changes upon infection. Indeed, others have shown that *H. polygyrus* infection leads to the outgrowth of *Lactobacillus* species and members of the Clostridiales family, which in turn support the expansion and activation of regulatory T cells (1, 17). Our unpublished data show strong and selective antimicrobial activity of E/S products of *A. suum* on several members of the porcine microbiota, whereas *Clostridia* species displayed a growth advantage in presence of *A. suum* E/S. It hence seems that nematode infections provoke fine-tuned changes in the structure of the gut microbiome in favor of commensals supporting anti-inflammatory circuits, assisting host health and facilitating parasite survival. Future work will address if nematode antimicrobial factors such as cecropins, ASABF, lysozymes, and c-type lectins present in nematode E/S products differentially affect the growth of commensal and potentially pathogenic gut bacteria.

The release of antimicrobial factors by enteric nematodes and potential interference with the growth of certain bacterial species suggest that the parasites sense their microbial environment similar to free living worms such as *C. elegans* or *Pristionchus pacificus* (67, 68). However, whether intestinal parasites react by the differential expression of antimicrobial factors to environmental changes has not been assessed before. Here, we show that nematode gene expression is altered in the absence of host microbes. Our data provide evidence for microbial sensing by *H. polygyrus*, as factors with putative antimicrobial defense functions, such as chitinase (69) and lysozyme (70), were differentially expressed in nematodes isolated from germ-free in comparison to conventional mice, in addition to xenobiotic detoxification genes which are upregulated during bacterial infection of *C. elegans* (71). Interestingly, while lysozymes are thought to play an important role in nematode antimicrobial defenses (72), lysozyme-3 was upregulated in nematodes isolated from germ-free mice. Compared to worms reared in conventional mice, nematodes from germ-free mice develop in the face of a stronger Th2 response and are likely negatively impacted by the lack of a host microbiota, as evidenced by their reduced size and fecundity. Hence, upregulation of defense factors such as lysozyme-3 may be due to a stress response rather than a lack of microbial stimulation. This view is supported by the fact that also putative detoxification genes were upregulated in parasites isolated from germ-free mice. The altered gene expression of nematodes from germ-free mice might further result from the lack of microbial metabolic factors in the germ-free host gut. A direct dependence of *H. polygyrus* on small intestinal microbes as food source appears, however, unlikely, as host tissue, but not ingesta provide the main food source of the adult worms (42).

Several reports linked the host microbial status to differences in susceptibility for infections with intestinal helminths [reviewed in (56)]. We show here that *H. polygrus* adult worms display signs of reduced fitness when developing in GF mice, confirming early studies reporting impeded nematode infectivity and fitness in the absence of gut microbes (39–41). *H. polygyrus* fitness is determined by the magnitude of the anti-parasite Th2 response, evident as disparate worm fecundity and duration of infection in inbred mouse lines differing in Th2 reactivity (73). Anti-nematode immune responses are regulated by Treg, seen as increased Th2 and associated innate responses after Treg depletion, leading to lower worm burdens or shortened retention of adult worms in some experimental systems (12, 15, 74). Microbial signals are important for the activation and instruction of thymus-derived and peripherally induced Foxp3$^+$ Treg in the gut (75). Here we show that the frequencies of Foxp3$^+$ Treg were similar in conventional and GF mice infected with *H. polygyrus*, but the phenotypic composition of Foxp3$^+$ Treg was altered in the small intestine and gut-associated lymphoid tissue of germ-free mice. Confirming a previous report (43), RORγt$^+$Foxp3$^+$ Treg were reduced in GF mice at steady state and after *H. polygyrus* infection, while the expansion of GATA-3$^+$Foxp3$^+$ Treg did not differ between infected SPF and GF mice. Whereas the complete absence of microbiota-induced RORgt$^+$Foxp3$^+$ Treg during *H. polygyrus* infection has been shown to result in the overt production of Th2 cytokines and reduced parasite fitness (43), our study provides evidence that more subtle changes in the intestinal Th2/Treg ratio are resulting from the germ-free status and, presumably, a reduction of microbiota-induced RORγt$^+$Treg is sufficient to significantly stunt parasite fitness.

The production of IL-10 by regulatory T cells has been shown to be of central importance for the prevention of gut inflammation at steady state and in experimental settings of lung and skin inflammation (76). We show here that while IL-10 production by mLN-derived Treg increased significantly upon nematode infection irrespective of the host microbial status, IL-10 production by small intestinal Treg was not altered in response to infection. Furthermore, small intestinal Treg of GF mice displayed reduced IL-10 production at steady state and after nematode infection. The reduced IL-10 expression by small intestinal Treg of GF mice may in part be explained by the reduction in RORγt$^+$ Treg, which have been previously reported as superior in IL-10 production compared to other intestinal Treg (43). Upon infection, however, we detected GATA-3$^+$Treg as the dominant IL-10$^+$ Treg source in the small intestine and mLN of SPF as well as GF mice. While our earlier studies have shown that Treg depletion during *H. polygyrus* infection results in increased small intestinal immunopathology (16), neither the decreased IL-10 production nor the reduction in RORγt$^+$ Treg detected in nematode-infected GF mice reported here were associated with signs of increased gut inflammation.

In conclusion, the antimicrobial activity of nematode products reported here suggests that enteric helminths actively shape their microbial environment, possibly facilitating the outgrowth of microbes supporting immune regulatory circuits, and restricting the expansion of potentially harmful species. Our finding of stunted parasite fitness in germ-free mice associated with locally increased Th2 and blunted Treg responses is in line with previous reports on gut microbes affecting host susceptibility and Th2 reactivity during nematode infection. Future studies should assess if altering the gut microbiota could be used to shift the Th2/Treg balance in favor of parasite-specific effector cells and if parasite products may be employed to counteract states of pathological dysbiosis resulting from and perpetuating inflammation in intestinal inflammatory disorders.

DATA DEPOSITION

All sequencing data generated in this project are available from the NCBI Sequence Read Archive (SRA) and collectively available via the BioProject: PRJNA486010 and the SRA accession SRP157940, available at https://www.ncbi.nlm.nih.gov/bioproject/486010 and https://www.ncbi.nlm.nih.gov/sra/SRP157940.

AUTHOR CONTRIBUTIONS

SH and SR conceptualized and designed the research. SR, AM, NA, and AR performed all the experiments. SR, AM, MK, NA, AR, AK and BR analyzed the data. SR, AM, MK, and SH wrote the manuscript. AR, AK, AB, and BR provided additional resources and edited the manuscript. All authors approved the final manuscript version.

ACKNOWLEDGMENTS

The excellent support by the technicians Y. Weber, B. Sonnenburg, M. Müller, C. Palissa, and S. Spieckermann and by the Robert Koch sequencing lab (ZBS1/MF 2) is acknowledged gratefully. Bacterial strains were generously provided by Prof. Marcus Fulde, Institute of Microbiology and Epizoonotics, Freie Universität Berlin and Dr. Markus Heimesaat, Institute of Microbiology, Charité – Universitätsmedizin Berlin. Pexiganan was generously provided by Prof. Jens Rolff, Institute of Biology, Freie Universität Berlin.

REFERENCES

1. Zaiss MM, Rapin A, Lebon L, Dubey LK, Mosconi I, Sarter K, et al. The intestinal microbiota contributes to the ability of helminths to modulate allergic inflammation. *Immunity* (2015) 43:998–1010. doi: 10.1016/j.immuni.2015.09.012
2. Rausch S, Held J, Fischer A, Heimesaat MM, Kühl AA, Bereswill S, et al. Small intestinal nematode infection of mice is associated with increased enterobacterial loads alongside the intestinal tract. *PLoS ONE* (2013) 8:e74026. doi: 10.1371/journal.pone.0074026
3. Fricke WF, Song Y, Wang A-J, Smith A, Grinchuk V, Pei C, et al. Type 2 immunity-dependent reduction of segmented filamentous bacteria in mice infected with the helminthic parasite *Nippostrongylus brasiliensis*. *Microbiome* (2015) 3:40. doi: 10.1186/s40168-015-0103-8
4. Li RW, Wu S, Li W, Navarro K, Couch RD, Hill D, et al. Alterations in the porcine colon microbiota induced by the gastrointestinal nematode *Trichuris suis*. *Infect Immun.* (2012) 80:2150–7. doi: 10.1128/IAI.00141-12
5. Broadhurst MJ, Ardeshir A, Kanwar B, Mirpuri J, Gundra UM, Leung JM, et al. Therapeutic helminth infection of macaques with idiopathic chronic diarrhea alters the inflammatory signature and mucosal microbiota of the colon. *PLoS Pathog.* (2012) 8:e1003000. doi: 10.1371/journal.ppat.1003000
6. Abner SR, Parthasarathy G, Hill DE, Mansfield LS. *Trichuris suis*: detection of antibacterial activity in excretory-secretory products from adults. *Exp Parasitol.* (2001) 99:26–36. doi: 10.1006/expr.2001.4643
7. Midha A, Schlosser J, Hartmann S. Reciprocal interactions between nematodes and their microbial environments. *Front. Cell. Infect. Microbiol.* (2017) 7:144. doi: 10.3389/fcimb.2017.00144
8. Midha A, Janek K, Niewienda A, Henklein P, Guenther S, Serra DO, et al. The intestinal roundworm ascaris suum releases antimicrobial factors which interfere with bacterial growth and biofilm formation. *Front. Cell. Infect. Microbiol.* (2018) 8:271. doi: 10.3389/fcimb.2018.00271.
9. Maizels RM, Hewitson JP, Murray J, Harcus YM, Dayer B, Filbey KJ, et al. Immune modulation and modulators in *Heligmosomoides polygyrus* infection. *Exp Parasitol.* (2012) 132:76–89. doi: 10.1016/j.exppara.2011.08.011
10. Maizels RM, McSorley HJ. Regulation of the host immune system by helminth parasites. *J Allergy Clin Immunol.* (2016) 138:666–75. doi: 10.1016/j.jaci.2016.07.007
11. Ziegler T, Rausch S, Steinfelder S, Klotz C, Hepworth MR, Kühl AA, et al. A novel regulatory macrophage induced by a helminth molecule instructs IL-10 in CD4+ T cells and protects against mucosal inflammation. *J Immunol.* (2015) 194:1555–64. doi: 10.4049/jimmunol.1401217
12. Blankenhaus B, Reitz M, Brenz Y, Eschbach M-L, Hartmann W, Haben I, et al. Foxp3+ regulatory T cells delay expulsion of intestinal nematodes by suppression of IL-9-driven mast cell activation in BALB/c but not in C57BL/6 mice. *PLoS Pathog.* (2014) 10:e1003913. doi: 10.1371/journal.ppat.1003913
13. Finney CAM, Taylor MD, Wilson MS, Maizels RM. Expansion and activation of CD4+CD25+ regulatory T cells in *Heligmosomoides polygyrus* infection. *Eur J Immunol.* (2007) 37:1874–86. doi: 10.1002/eji.200636751
14. Grainger JR, Smith KA, Hewitson JP, McSorley HJ, Harcus Y, Filbey KJ, et al. Helminth secretions induce de novo T cell Foxp3 expression and regulatory function through the TGF-β pathway. *J Exp Med.* (2010) 207:2331–41. doi: 10.1084/jem.20101074
15. Rausch S, Huehn J, Kirchhoff D, Rzepecka J, Schnoeller C, Pillai S, et al. Functional analysis of effector and regulatory T cells in a parasitic nematode infection. *Infect Immun.* (2008) 76:1908–19. doi: 10.1128/IAI.01233-07
16. Rausch S, Huehn J, Loddenkemper C, Hepworth MR, Klotz C, Sparwasser T, et al. Establishment of nematode infection despite increased Th2 responses and immunopathology after selective depletion of Foxp3+ cells. *Eur. J. Immunol.* (2009) 39:3066–77. doi: 10.1002/eji.200939644
17. Reynolds LA, Smith KA, Filbey KJ, Harcus Y, Hewitson JP, Redpath SA, et al. Commensal-pathogen interactions in the intestinal tract. *Gut Microb.* (2014) 5:522–32. doi: 10.4161/gmic.32155
18. Wilson MS, Taylor MD, Balic A, Finney CAM, Lamb JR, Maizels RM. Suppression of allergic airway inflammation by helminth-induced regulatory T cells. *J Exp Med.* (2005) 202:1199–212. doi: 10.1084/jem.20042572
19. Takemura H, Kaku M, Kohno S, Hirakata Y, Tanaka H, Yoshida R, et al. Evaluation of susceptibility of gram-positive and -negative bacteria to human defensins by using radial diffusion assay. *Antimicrob Agents Chemother.* (1996) 40:2280–4.
20. Gasmi L, Ferré J, Herrero S. High bacterial agglutination activity in a single-CRD C-type lectin from *Spodoptera exigua* (Lepidoptera: Noctuidae). *Biosensors* (2017) 7:12. doi: 10.3390/bios7010012
21. Bolger AM, Lohse M, Usadel B. Trimmomatic: a flexible trimmer for Illumina sequence data. *Bioinformatics* (2014) 30:2114–20. doi: 10.1093/bioinformatics/btu170

22. Wood DE, Salzberg SL. Kraken: ultrafast metagenomic sequence classification using exact alignments. *Genome Biol.* (2014) 15:R46. doi: 10.1186/gb-2014-15-3-r46

23. Kim D, Pertea G, Trapnell C, Pimentel H, Kelley R, Salzberg SL. TopHat2: accurate alignment of transcriptomes in the presence of insertions, deletions and gene fusions. *Genome Biol.* (2013) 14:R36. doi: 10.1186/gb-2013-14-4-r36

24. Trapnell C, Hendrickson DG, Sauvageau M, Goff L, Rinn JL, Pachter L. Differential analysis of gene regulation at transcript resolution with RNA-seq. *Nat Biotechnol.* (2013) 31:46–53. doi: 10.1038/nbt.2450

25. Howe KL, Bolt BJ, Shafie M, Kersey P, Berriman M. WormBase ParaSite – a comprehensive resource for helminth genomics. *Mol Biochem Parasitol.* (2017) 215:2–10. doi: 10.1016/j.molbiopara.2016.11.005

26. Liao Y, Smyth GK, Shi W. featureCounts: an efficient general purpose program for assigning sequence reads to genomic features. *Bioinformatics* (2014) 30:923–30. doi: 10.1093/bioinformatics/btt656

27. Love MI, Huber W, Anders S. Moderated estimation of fold change and dispersion for RNA-seq data with DESeq2. *Genome Biol.* (2014) 15:550. doi: 10.1186/s13059-014-0550-8

28. Ritchie ME, Phipson B, Wu D, Hu Y, Law CW, Shi W, et al. limma powers differential expression analyses for RNA-sequencing and microarray studies. *Nucleic Acids Res.* (2015) 43:e47. doi: 10.1093/nar/gkv007

29. Rice P, Longden I, Bleasby A. EMBOSS: the European molecular biology open software suite. *Trends Genet.* (2000) 16:276–7. doi: 10.1016/S0168-9525(00)02024-2

30. Ashburner M, Ball CA, Blake JA, Botstein D, Butler H, Cherry JM, et al. Gene ontology: tool for the unification of biology. *Nat. Genet.* (2000) 25:25–9. doi: 10.1038/75556

31. Camacho C, Coulouris G, Avagyan V, Ma N, Papadopoulos J, Bealer K, et al. BLAST+: architecture and applications. *BMC Bioinformatics* (2009) 10:421. doi: 10.1186/1471-2105-10-421

32. Conesa A, Götz S, García-Gómez JM, Terol J, Talón M, Robles M. Blast2GO: a universal tool for annotation, visualization and analysis in functional genomics research. *Bioinformatics* (2005) 21:3674–6. doi: 10.1093/bioinformatics/bti610

33. Jones P, Binns D, Chang H-Y, Fraser M, Li W, McAnulla C, et al. InterProScan 5: genome-scale protein function classification. *Bioinformatics* (2014) 30:1236–40. doi: 10.1093/bioinformatics/btu031

34. The UniProt Consortium (2017). UniProt: the universal protein knowledgebase. *Nucleic Acids Res.* 45: D158–69.

35. Strandmark J, Steinfelder S, Berek C, Kühl AA, Rausch S, Hartmann S. Eosinophils are required to suppress Th2 responses in Peyer's patches during intestinal infection by nematodes. *Mucosal Immunol.* (2017) 10:661–72. doi: 10.1093/nar/gkh131

36. Walk ST, Blum AM, Ewing SA-S, Weinstock JV, Young VB. Alteration of the murine gut microbiota during infection with the parasitic helminth *Heligmosomoides polygyrus*. *Inflamm Bowel Dis.* (2010) 16:1841–9. doi: 10.1002/ibd.21299

37. Miltsch SM, Seeberger PH, Lepenies B. The C-type lectin-like domain containing proteins Clec-39 and Clec-49 are crucial for *Caenorhabditis elegans* immunity against *Serratia marcescens* infection. *Dev Comp Immunol.* (2014) 45:67–73. doi: 10.1016/j.dci.2014.02.002

38. Harcus Y, Nicoll G, Murray J, Filbey K, Gomez-Escobar N, Maizels RM. C-type lectins from the nematode parasites *Heligmosomoides polygyrus* and *Nippostrongylus brasiliensis*. *Parasitol Int.* (2009) 58:461–70. doi: 10.1016/j.parint.2009.08.011

39. Chang J, Wescott RB. Infectivity, fecundity, and survival of Nematospiroides dubius in gnotobiotic mice. *Exp Parasitol.* (1972) 32:327–34. doi: 10.1016/0014-4894(72)90060-4

40. Wescott RB. Experimental Nematospiroides dubius infection in germfree and conventional mice. *Exp Parasitol.* (1968) 22:245–9. doi: 10.1016/0014-4894(68)90099-4

41. Wescott RB, Todd AC. A Comparison of the development of *Nippostrongylus brasiliensis* in germ-free and conventional mice. *J Parasitol.* (1964) 50:138–43. doi: 10.2307/3276048

42. Bansemir AD, Sukhdeo MV. The food resource of adult *Heligmosomoides polygyrus* in the small intestine. *J Parasitol.* (1994) 80:24–8. doi: 10.2307/3283340

43. Ohnmacht C, Park J-H, Cording S, Wing JB, Atarashi K, Obata Y, et al. The microbiota regulates type 2 immunity through RORγt+ T cells. *Science* (2015) 349:989–93. doi: 10.1126/science.aac4263

44. Smith PM, Howitt MR, Panikov N, Michaud M, Gallini CA, Bohlooly YM, et al. The microbial metabolites, short-chain fatty acids, regulate colonic treg cell homeostasis. *Science* (2013) 341:569–73. doi: 10.1126/science.1241165

45. Round JL, Mazmanian SK. Inducible Foxp3+ regulatory T-cell development by a commensal bacterium of the intestinal microbiota. *Proc Natl Acad Sci USA.* (2010) 107:12204–9. doi: 10.1073/pnas.0909122107

46. Korn LL, Hubbeling D, Porrett PM, Yang Q, Barnett LG, Laufer TM. Regulatory T cells occupy an isolated niche in the intestine that is antigen independent. *Cell Rep.* (2014) 9:1567–73. doi: 10.1016/j.celrep.2014.11.006

47. Luu M, Steinhoff U, Visekruna A. Functional heterogeneity of gut-resident regulatory T cells. *Clin Transl Immunol.* (2017) 6:e156. doi: 10.1038/cti.2017.39

48. Wang Y, Su MA, Wan YY. An essential role of the transcription factor GATA-3 for the function of regulatory t cells. *Immunity* (2011) 35:337–48. doi: 10.1016/j.immuni.2011.08.012

49. Wohlfert EA, Grainger JR, Bouladoux N, Konkel JE, Oldenhove G, Ribeiro CH, et al. GATA3 controls Foxp3+ regulatory T cell fate during inflammation in mice. *J Clin Invest.* (2011) 121:4503–15. doi: 10.1172/JCI57456

50. Yang B-H, Hagemann S, Mamareli P, Lauer U, Hoffmann U, Beckstette M, et al. Foxp3+ T cells expressing RORγt represent a stable regulatory T-cell effector lineage with enhanced suppressive capacity during intestinal inflammation. *Mucosal Immunol.* (2016) 9:444–57. doi: 10.1038/mi.2015.74

51. Bock CN, Babu S, Breloer M, Rajamanickam A, Boothra Y, Brunn M-L, et al. Th2/1 hybrid cells occurring in murine and human strongyloidiasis share effector functions of Th1 cells. *Front. Cell. Infect. Microbiol.* (2017) 7:261. doi: 10.3389/fcimb.2017.00261

52. Peine M, Rausch S, Helmstetter C, Fröhlich A, Hegazy AN, Kühl AA, et al. Stable T-bet(+)GATA-3(+) Th1/Th2 hybrid cells arise *in vivo*, can develop directly from naive precursors, and limit immunopathologic inflammation. *PLoS Biol.* (2013) 11:e1001633. doi: 10.1371/journal.pbio.1001633

53. Atarashi K, Tanoue T, Ando M, Kamada N, Nagano Y, Narushima S, et al. Th17 cell induction by adhesion of microbes to intestinal epithelial cells. *Cell* (2015) 163:367–80. doi: 10.1016/j.cell.2015.08.058

54. Ivanov II, Atarashi K, Manel N, Brodie EL, Shima T, Karaoz U, et al. Induction of intestinal Th17 cells by segmented filamentous bacteria. *Cell* (2009) 139:485–98. doi: 10.1016/j.cell.2009.09.033

55. Burgess SL, Gilchrist CA, Lynn TC, Petri WA. Parasitic protozoa and interactions with the host intestinal microbiota. *Infect Immun.* (2017) 85:e00101–17. doi: 10.1128/IAI.00101-17

56. Zaiss MM, Harris NL. Interactions between the intestinal microbiome and helminth parasites. *Parasite Immunol.* (2016) 38:5–11. doi: 10.1111/pim.12274

57. Holm JB, Sorobetea D, Kiilerich P, Ramayo-Caldas Y, Estellé J, Ma T, et al. Chronic trichuris muris infection decreases diversity of the intestinal microbiota and concomitantly increases the abundance of Lactobacilli. *PLOS ONE* (2015) 10:e0125495. doi: 10.1371/journal.pone.0125495

58. Barash NR, Maloney JG, Singer SM, Dawson SC. Giardia alters commensal microbial diversity throughout the murine gut. *Infect Immun.* (2017) 85:e00948–16. doi: 10.1128/IAI.00948-16

59. Heimesaat MM, Bereswill S, Fischer A, Fuchs D, Struck D, Niebergall J, et al. Gram-negative bacteria aggravate murine small intestinal Th1-type immunopathology following oral infection with *Toxoplasma gondii*. *J Immunol.* (2006) 177:8785–95. doi: 10.4049/jimmunol.177.12.8785

60. Zhao A, McDermott J, Urban JF, Gause W, Madden KB, Yeung KA, et al. Dependence of IL-4, IL-13, and nematode-induced alterations in murine small intestinal smooth muscle contractility on Stat6 and enteric nerves. *J Immunol.* (2003) 171:948–54. doi: 10.4049/jimmunol.171.2.948

61. Marillier RG, Michels C, Smith EM, Fick LC, Leeto M, Dewals B, et al. IL-4/IL-13 independent goblet cell hyperplasia in experimental helminth infections. *BMC Immunol.* (2008) 9:11. doi: 10.1186/1471-2172-9-11

62. McKay DM, Shute A, Lopes F. Helminths and intestinal barrier function. *Tissue Barr.* (2017) 5:e1283385. doi: 10.1080/21688370.2017.1283385

63. Finkelman FD, Shea-Donohue T, Morris SC, Gildea L, Strait R, Madden KB, et al. Interleukin-4- and interleukin-13-mediated host protection against intestinal nematode parasites. *Immunol. Rev.* (2004) 201:139–55. doi: 10.1111/j.0105-2896.2004.00192.x

64. Manko A, Motta J-P, Cotton JA, Feener T, Oyeyemi A, Vallance BA, et al. Giardia co-infection promotes the secretion of antimicrobial peptides beta-defensin 2 and trefoil factor 3 and attenuates attaching and

Parasitic Nematodes Exert Antimicrobial Activity and Benefit from Microbiota-Driven...

49

effacing bacteria-induced intestinal disease. *PLOS ONE* (2017) 12:e0178647. doi: 10.1371/journal.pone.0178647

65. Pillai A, Ueno S, Zhang H, Kato Y. Induction of ASABF (*Ascaris suum* antibacterial factor)-type antimicrobial peptides by bacterial injection: novel members of ASABF in the nematode *Ascaris suum*. *Biochem J.* (2003) 371:663–8. doi: 10.1042/bj20021948

66. Pillai A, Ueno S, Zhang H, Lee JM, Kato Y. Cecropin P1 and novel nematode cecropins: a bacteria-inducible antimicrobial peptide family in the nematode *Ascaris suum*. *Biochem J.* (2005) 390:207–14. doi: 10.1042/BJ200 50218

67. Samuel BS, Rowedder H, Braendle C, Félix M-A, Ruvkun G. *Caenorhabditis elegans* responses to bacteria from its natural habitats. *Proc Natl Acad Sci USA.* (2016) 113:E3941–9. doi: 10.1073/pnas.1607183113

68. Sinha A, Rae R, Iatsenko I, Sommer RJ. System wide analysis of the evolution of innate immunity in the nematode model species *Caenorhabditis elegans* and *Pristionchus pacificus*. *PLoS ONE* (2012) 7:e44255. doi: 10.1371/journal.pone.0044255

69. Chung MC, Dean S, Marakasova ES, Nwabueze AO, van Hoek ML. Chitinases are negative regulators of *Francisella novicida* biofilms. *PLoS ONE* (2014) 9:e93119. doi: 10.1371/journal.pone.0093119

70. Dierking K, Yang W, Schulenburg H. Antimicrobial effectors in the nematode *Caenorhabditis elegans*: an outgroup to the Arthropoda. *Philos Trans R Soc B Biol Sci.* (2016) 371:20150299. doi: 10.1098/rstb.2015.0299

71. Pukkila-Worley R. Surveillance immunity: an emerging paradigm of innate defense activation in *Caenorhabditis elegans*. *PLOS Pathog.* (2016) 12:e1005795. doi: 10.1371/journal.ppat.1005795

72. Schulenburg H, Boehnisch C. Diversification and adaptive sequence evolution of Caenorhabditislysozymes (Nematoda: Rhabditidae). *BMC Evol Biol.* (2008) 8:114. doi: 10.1186/1471-2148-8-114

73. Filbey KJ, Grainger JR, Smith KA, Boon L, van Rooijen N, Harcus Y, et al. Innate and adaptive type 2 immune cell responses in genetically controlled resistance to intestinal helminth infection. *Immunol Cell Biol.* (2014) 92:436–48. doi: 10.1038/icb.2013.109

74. Smith KA, Filbey KJ, Reynolds LA, Hewitson JP, Harcus Y, Boon L, et al. Low-level regulatory T-cell activity is essential for functional type-2 effector immunity to expel gastrointestinal helminths. *Mucosal Immunol.* (2016) 9:428–43. doi: 10.1038/mi.2015.73

75. Geuking MB, Cahenzli J, Lawson MAE, Ng DCK, Slack E, Hapfelmeier S, et al. Intestinal bacterial colonization induces mutualistic regulatory T cell responses. *Immunity* (2011) 34:794–806. doi: 10.1016/j.immuni.2011.03.021

76. Rubtsov YP, Rasmussen JP, Chi EY, Fontenot J, Castelli L, Ye X, et al. Regulatory T cell-derived interleukin-10 limits inflammation at environmental interfaces. *Immunity* (2008) 28:546–58. doi: 10.1016/j.immuni.2008.02.017

5

To B or Not to B: Understanding B Cell Responses in the Development of Malaria Infection

Eduardo L. V. Silveira*, Mariana R. Dominguez and Irene S. Soares

Department of Clinical and Toxicological Analyses, School of Pharmaceutical Sciences, University of São Paulo, São Paulo, Brazil

*Correspondence:
Eduardo L. V. Silveira
eduardosilveira@usp.br

Malaria is a widespread disease caused mainly by the *Plasmodium falciparum* (Pf) and *Plasmodium vivax* (Pv) protozoan parasites. Depending on the parasite responsible for the infection, high morbidity and mortality can be triggered. To escape the host immune responses, *Plasmodium* parasites disturb the functionality of B cell subsets among other cell types. However, some antibodies elicited during a malaria infection have the potential to block pathogen invasion and dissemination into the host. Thus, the question remains, why is protection not developed and maintained after the primary parasite exposure? In this review, we discuss different aspects of B cell responses against *Plasmodium* antigens during malaria infection. Since most studies have focused on the quantification of serum antibody titers, those B cell responses have not been fully characterized. However, to secrete antibodies, a complex cellular response is set up, including not only the activation and differentiation of B cells into antibody-secreting cells, but also the participation of other cell subsets in the germinal center reactions. Therefore, a better understanding of how B cell subsets are stimulated during malaria infection will provide essential insights toward the design of potent interventions.

Keywords: B cell biology, malaria, antibodies, effective mechanism, protective immunity

MALARIA INFECTION AND IMMUNITY

Malaria is a widespread disease mainly caused by the *Plasmodium falciparum* (Pf) and *Plasmodium vivax* (Pv) parasites in tropical countries. Currently, half of the world population lives in areas at risk of a malaria infection. In 2016, a global estimative enumerated 216 million clinical cases and 445,000 deaths associated with this disease (1), portraying the real magnitude of this public health problem. Most cases of malaria morbidity and mortality have been attributed to Pf infections, prevalent in sub-Saharan Africa and characterized by high parasitemias and severe complications, especially in children (2). Contrarily, Pv infections are more disseminated in American and Asian countries and induce lower parasitemia levels and milder symptoms. Rarely, Pv infections can elicit severe symptoms and kill like Pf infections (2–4).

Plasmodium parasites have a complex life cycle, with sporozoites transmitted from the *Anopheles* mosquito salivary glands to the human skin dermis during mosquito blood meals. These motile parasites cross layers of the skin and enter the bloodstream, reaching the liver within hours upon infection. Then, they invade the hepatocytes, replicating and differentiating into schizonts. In the case of a Pv infection, part of the sporozoites are transformed into dormant forms called hypnozoites, which can be activated even after a long term of parasite infection. As a result of the hepatocyte burst, the merozoites are released in the bloodstream and invade the erythrocytes (Pf parasites) or the reticulocytes (Pv parasites), initiating the asexual blood stage of the cycle. These parasitic forms undergo several rounds of multiplication and differentiation, increasing the parasitemia levels in the host. Those forms found in infected red blood cells (iRBCs) have been identified as rings, trophozoites, schizonts, and gametocytes. Whereas the newly-released merozoites can keep re-invading the erythrocytes, a small fraction of them differentiate directly into gametocytes, giving rise to the sexual blood stage. Gametocytes are ingested during the mosquito blood meal and fuse to each other within the digestive tract, forming a zygote. The zygote differentiates into an ookinete, followed by oocyst forms, previously to the generation of infectious sporozoites that can be found in a mosquito's salivary glands (5, 6). Interestingly, the bone marrow has been described as the major parasite reservoir for early blood stage (asexual and sexual) and gametocytes in Pv infections (7, 8).

Regarding the mechanisms of immunity naturally induced by malaria, the humoral response has been described as the most important for the establishment of protection. This concept has been solidified after the finding that a passive transfer of serum samples from malaria-immune adults controlled the Pf parasitemia levels and ameliorated symptoms in acutely infected children (9). Although the elicitation of the humoral response is critical to reduce malaria morbidity and mortality, antibody-dependent protective immunity usually takes multiple parasitic exposures and may take even years to be established. The extensive genetic diversity of clinical Pf and Pv malaria episodes (10, 11) and the low frequency of malaria-specific memory B cells (MBCs) detected in residents of high endemic areas (12, 13) corroborate this statement. Considering that antibodies represent a snapshot of B cell responses at a single cell level (14), it is fundamental to understand how this cellular component is stimulated upon *Plasmodium* infection to improve vaccine formulations and consequently generate more effective antibodies against human malaria. In this review, we present the distinct aspects of B cell immunity derived from a malaria infection, ranging from the activation of naive B cells to the generation of antibody-secreting cells and the mechanisms of action by protective antibodies.

MALARIA-SPECIFIC B CELL RESPONSES

During malaria infection, thousands of parasitic antigens are expressed in each stage of the parasite life cycle (15). However, the anti-malarial humoral responses are preferentially headed to blood stage antigens rather than the liver counterparts. Besides the differences on the antigen density, a malaria murine model has shown that the blood stage of infection weakens the humoral immunity against the liver stage antigens through the modification of lymphoid structures and the expression of cytokines and chemokines (16). Overall, these responses are mainly characterized by the generation of the antibody-secreting cells (ASCs), memory B cells (MBCs), and antibody titers. Whereas, the MBCs and antibody titers have been

found with steady levels for years in individuals living in low Pf and Pv malaria-endemic areas without the evidence of reinfection (17), these parameters are not sustained for longer periods, especially in younger individuals from high Pf-endemic areas (12, 13).

The question arises, disregarding the timing that antibodies can be detected in serum samples, how is their secretion triggered upon malaria infection? Usually, the antigen-specific antibodies are expected to be detected in the serum in <2 weeks upon any pathogen exposure. During this period, the naive B cells are activated upon B cell receptor (BCR) interaction with a parasitic antigen in the periphery, eliciting cell proliferation and differentiation into multiple subsets such as the MBCs, follicular B cells (FoBs), major players of the germinal center (GC) reactions, or marginal zone B cells (MZBs). Although all these B cell subsets express immunoglobulin (Ig) genes, only the ASCs secrete antibodies. Regarding FoBs, they form and maintain structures called the germinal centers (GCs) together with the follicular T helper cells (TFh), dendritic cells (FDCs), cytokines [IL-21, IL-6, and B cell activating factor (BAFF)], and the critical participation of co-stimulatory molecules (CD40L and ICOS). During the germinal center reactions, the GC B cells are activated and undergo several rounds of antigen selection, acquiring a mature status through the somatic hypermutations and class-switch in Ig genes. Thus, it prompts the production of high-affinity, class-switched antibodies. Models of human and murine malaria infections point to higher numbers of GC B cells and lower for MZB-like cells (18, 19). Terminal signaling triggered by activation guides the FoB cells to exit the follicles and differentiate into high-affinity, atypical, or classical MBCs (20) or short-lived, class-switched ASCs. However, there is evidence from a malaria murine model that high affinity, somatic hypermutated IgM+ MBCs dominate a recall response, being differentiated either into IgM+ or IgG+ ASCs and MBCs (21). The higher the frequency of the antigen-specific MBCs during that second encounter with the antigen, the higher will be the frequency of the antigen-specific ASCs generated. It is still controversial whether the unswitched or switched MBCs enter the GCs or form the ASCs: [reviewed by (22)]. Once generated, the ASCs migrate through circulation to the bone marrow or secondary lymphoid organs. More specifically, their physical contact with bone marrow stroma cells and the recognition of cytokines described above lead to modifications in their transcriptome profile, upregulating preferentially the expression of anti-apoptotic genes. This process culminates in their transformation from short-lived to long-lived ASCs, whose function results in the increased titers of serum antibodies (23).

On the other hand, malaria infection affects the generation of some critical cell subsets for humoral responses. Repeated parasitic exposures drive the expansion and accumulation of atypical MBCs in individuals from Pf malaria-endemic areas (24, 25). Although these cells have been mostly associated with the impaired B cell responses in this infection context, some groups have stated that atypical MBCs present a similar function as classical MBCs (26). Furthermore, this was demonstrated in an impaired GC response in a murine model of severe malaria due to the inhibition of TFh cell differentiation (27).

In addition, the murine conventional DCs presented lower BAFF expression, culminating in a reduced ASC number in the spleen (28). Noteworthily, the bone marrow ASCs have serious restrictions for sampling due to their location, being avoided in malaria clinical trials. This issue has impaired our complete understanding around the immune response triggered by malaria infection in humans.

ACTIVATION OF B CELLS

Similar to pathogenic infections such as *Trypanosoma cruzi* (the etiologic agent of Chagas disease) or HIV, malaria infection elicits the polyclonal activation of B cells. Among the major factors contributing to this condition are the parasite-specific antigens and cytokines. Consequently, malaria patients present hypergammaglobulinemia, i.e., the increased serologic IgG titers. Furthermore, asymptomatic individuals with high parasitemia usually display broader antibody responses than the asymptomatic individuals with low parasitemia or symptomatic individuals (29). Thus, the malarial parasite load derived from the acute phase of infection seems to drive the ASC response as described for HIV and SIV (30) and Silveira et al., manuscript in preparation. A primary parasite exposure elicits the activation and differentiation of naive B cells into *Plasmodium*-specific MBCs and ASCs. These antigen-specific MBCs, activated through engagement of BCR or Toll-like receptors (31), can also be differentiated into ASCs, enhancing the antibody secretion upon Pf infection (32–35). Alternatively, MBCs induced by *S. mansion* worms may cross-react with Pf antigens and become activated in an malarial-specific manner (36, 37). However, this humoral response does not reach enough concentration in the serum to provide protection. As already mentioned, the individuals from malaria-endemic areas develop an antibody-derived natural immunity only after multiple parasite exposures.

Among the several potential parasite antigens that could induce hypergammaglobulinemia under infection, the domain C1DR1a of EMP1 from a cloned strain (FCR3S1.2), a blood-stage antigen, has been identified in Pf (38). It remains elusive whether the same antigen derived from Pf isolates can also trigger hypergammaglobulinaemia. Interestingly, the domain C1DR1a of PfEMP1 preferentially promotes the MBC activation and proliferation (39). Another *Plasmodium* variant antigen (MSP-1) has been described to activate antigen-specific IgM+ MBCs as the earlier responders upon a malaria re-challenge in mice. Both IgM- and IgG-secreting cells can be generated from the differentiation of those IgM+ MBCs (21). It is still obscure whether the domain C1DR1a is capable of eliciting a similar response during malaria infection in humans. Considering that autoimmunity has been commonly detected during malaria infection as a result of hypergammaglobulinemia, molecular mimicking cannot be ruled out for parasite antigens. In fact, the serum samples of systemic lupus erythematosus (SLE) patients displayed the ability to recognize the Pf malarial antigens (40). Cardiolipin, histones, and DNA are among the auto-antigens usually targeted by the anti-*Plasmodium* antibodies (41).

Another important piece of the polyclonal B cell activation puzzle is related to the modifications in the cytokine profile during malaria infection. BAFF is known to support B cell differentiation into ASCs and potentially elicit hypergammaglobulinemia. Increased levels of this cytokine have been found in the plasma of volunteers upon the Pf challenge (42), in acute Pf-infected children (43), in pregnant women (44), and in Pv infection (45). Moreover, the IL-10 has shown increased levels detected upon the Pf or Pv infections (46) and can influence the serological BAFF levels (47).

B Cell Subsets

Strikingly, human and murine malaria infections strongly alter the composition of B cell subsets. A murine malaria model showed severe reductions in the bone marrow-derived B cell progenitor numbers (48). Alternately, the infection enhances the numbers of atypical hematopoietic stem and progenitor cells (HSPCs) in the murine spleen. Considering their potential to differentiate into B cells and generate the GC B cells, MBCs, and antigen-specific ASCs *in vivo* (49), the HSPCs could repopulate the immune cell repertoire by counteracting the deficiency in B cell progenitors. Besides progenitor B cells, the Pf and Pv infections also affect the frequency of the peripheral B cells. Whereas the kinetics of classical MBCs and ASCs seem paradoxical in infected individuals living in endemic or non-endemic areas, the transitional B cells (TBCs) and atypical MBCs consistently have shown increased numbers in the blood of all individuals (42, 50).

In terms of TBCs, their frequency has been directly correlated to high parasitemias and an impaired immunity to Pf infection (50). Interestingly, the BAFF receptor signaling has been connected to the control of the immature B cell differentiation to TBCs (51). Considering that BAFF levels are significantly higher during the acute phase of Pf and Pv malaria (43, 45), this cytokine could indeed stimulate a stronger TBC proliferation. Regarding the atypical MBCs in malaria, these cells have been mainly characterized as exhausted cells with a decreased capability to differentiate into ASCs and secrete antibodies (24, 25), as for HIV infection (52). However, the monoclonal antibodies cloned out from those cells majorly recognized the Pf-infected RBCs and neutralized Pf parasites. Furthermore, it has been speculated that their contribution for the neutralizing IgG titers would be similar to the classical MBCs (26). Although total atypical MBCs significantly expand upon Pf or Pv malaria infections, parasitic-specific atypical MBCs still present similar frequencies to classical counterparts (26). In terms of longevity, it remains undetermined whether atypical MBCs represent the majority of the malarial-specific MBCs detected years after parasite exposure in primed individuals without reinfection (17). In infected mice, malarial-specific atypical MBCs were recently associated to short-lived responses that were dependent on the presence of the parasite (53). It would be plausible that the atypical MBCs are high-affinity, somatic hypermutated MBCs in human malaria. Indeed, these cells have been described as the first cells to expand during a recall malaria challenge in mice (21) and both cell subsets can differentiate into IgG+ ASCs, strongly related to malaria immunity.

Follicular T Helper Cells

To clear microbial infections, the immune system simultaneously triggers cellular and humoral responses that converge to the onset of a long-lasting, protective response. Although it correlates with the titers of high-affinity, class-switched antibodies, B cells are not the unique players in this scenario. In fact, the generation of these antibodies relies on assistance from a particular CD4+ T cell subset called the follicular T helper (TFh) cells. More specifically, the germinal center (GC) B cells physically interact with the activated CD4+ T cells in structures of lymphoid organs called follicles. Within the GCs, B-T cell talk leads to B cell activation, which mature through somatic hypermutations in V(D)J Ig genes as well as the Ig isotype switch, and differentiation into ASCs. Importantly, some TFh cytokines have shown to be critical in this process, such as the IL-6 and IL-21 that regulate B cell survival and cell differentiation.

It has been demonstrated that Pv malaria stimulates the expansion of the TFh cells and secretion of the TFh cytokines (54). Interestingly, Pf infection stimulates a less-functional Th1-like Tfh cell subset, whose function does not correlate to ASC differentiation and antibody secretion. Due to the increased secretion of IFNγ and TNFα during the Pf acute malaria, TFh cell precursors increase the T-bet expression and hinder their differentiation into mature TFh cells (55). Moreover, B cells are also affected by that IFNγ secretion, expressing high levels of T-bet and mainly expanding IgG3 class-switched cells that have the phenotype of atypical MBCs (20). Similarly, this issue is also seen in murine malaria models, implicating lower frequencies of the GC B cells and ASCs as well as the decreased antibody titers. Noteworthily, the murine bone marrow reconstituted with T-bet KO CD4+ T cells had the TFh cell functionality restored, followed by the elicitation of GC formation and higher antibody titers (27). Alternately, IL-10 signaling restricts the T-bet expression and rescues the GC formation and antibody responses upon malaria infection in mice (56). Hence, the IL-21 has also demonstrated an important role during this process since the IL-21 KO mice showed decreased numbers of splenic GC B cells and ASCs in the bone marrow, lower antibody titers, and, consequently, a failure to control the parasitemia levels upon challenge (57).

Moreover, other factors can disturb the TFh cell differentiation and influence the effectiveness of humoral responses, such as the expression of particular MHC class II molecules by B cells or co-infections. Regarding the MHC class II expression, humanized mice expressing only HLA-DR0401 as the only MHC class II molecules had impaired antibody responses and could not clear parasitemia after a challenge with a strain causing murine malaria. An expanded subset of the regulatory T cells (Tregs) was found to interact with B cells in those mice, rather than the TFh cells. However, the Treg depletion or HLA-DR0401 co-expression with murine MHC class II molecules boosted the antibody titers and, consequently, the parasitemia dropped to undetectable levels in these mice (58). The expression of T-bet and the influence of Th1 cytokines,

such as IFNγ, have been associated with that Treg expansion which impairs the Tfh cell differentiation and survival as well as wanes the secretion of malaria-specific antibodies (59, 60). In terms of co-infections, an acute gammaherpesvirus (MHV68) infection decreased the resistance against a non-lethal malaria in mice. This co-infection diminished the frequencies of the Tfh cells, GC B cells, and ASCs, suppressing the humoral response to malaria (61).

Antibody-dependent Protective Immunity

The malarial-specific antibody responses derived from Pf exposure are usually transient since their titers decrease by the next parasitic transmission season. After their contraction, the antibody levels are still maintained in a higher magnitude than the respective titers detected in the previous parasite exposure (62). For the Pv infection, it follows an opposite pattern (17, 54). However, once secreted at a certain level in the serum, the antibodies can provide protection against human malaria. Serology data against blood stage antigens have determined an inverse correlation between the antibody titers specific for Pf MSP-2-, MSP-3-, and AMA-1 and Pf morbidity in the infected individuals. Thus, an increased breadth of antibody specificity would be associated with a lower chance to experience a clinical episode or be admitted to hospital with severe Pf malaria (63).

To provide antibody-dependent protection, the immune system launches different mechanisms of action upon malaria infection. Considering that the blood stage of infection breaks humoral immunity against the liver stage antigens in murine malaria models (16), malaria-specific antibodies would preferentially opsonize the merozoites. Subsequently, they could trigger effector functions, such as inhibition of cell invasion, phagocytosis, activation of respiratory burst, or complement-derived parasite death [reviewed by (64)]. In the context of the inhibition of cell invasion, it has been challenging to study the breadth of antibody responses which could block sporozoite or merozoite invasion into the hepatocytes or erythrocytes (Pf) / reticulocytes (Pv), respectively. To assess the antigens linked to protective humoral responses against Pf malaria, the high-throughput technologies have been utilized. Among the identified antigens were liver and blood-stage antigens (65). Regarding the reactivity against the *Plasmodium* liver stage antigens, most of such response is driven to the circumsporozoite protein (CSP). The most immunogenic region of Pf CSP for antibodies consists of the central repeat-region. Recently, a Pf CSP-specific mAb (CIS43) displayed a high capacity of parasite neutralization, with its binding region identified in the junction between the N-terminal and central repeat regions of CSP (66). Another anti-Pf CSP repeat-region mAb (2A10) has been shown to elicit protection in mice challenged with chimeric Pb-Pf sporozoites. After being cloned into a adeno-associated virus vector, 2A10 was expressed for long-term and reduced parasite burden, providing protection in mice either by sporozoite injection or mosquito bites (67). The N-terminal region flanking those Pf CSP repeat-regions also possess a linear protective B cell epitope recognized by the mAb 5D5. The antibody-binding inhibits the CSP proteolytic cleavage, neutralizing the hepatocyte invasion. Whenever administered in combination with mAb 2A10, these mAbs enhanced the sporozoite neutralization *in vivo* (68). Contrarily, the antibody reactivity had multiple targets against the blood stage antigens. Anti-EBA-175 mAbs (R217 and R218) have been described as inhibitory for Pf invasion in RBCs. Whereas R217, the more inhibitory mAb, engages fundamental antigen residues for RBC binding, R218 interacts with F1 region residues, irrelevant for RBC binding (69). The subdomains I and II of Duffy binding protein (DBP) have also been targeted by the neutralizing antibodies detected in high concentration in the serum of individuals from Pv malaria-endemic areas. Mutations in those antibody sequences accumulate over parasitic exposures, enhancing their breadth and potency (70). Furthermore, although barely recognized during infection even in residents of Pf malaria-endemic areas (71), the anti-RH5 antibodies have demonstrated a great capacity of inhibiting invasion of the Pf merozoites in erythrocytes (72–76). Due to a subcellular location, the RH5 antigen has been detected around the moving junction that is assembled just before the erythrocyte invasion. Thus, RH5 would be accessible to antibodies only during the short contact between Pf merozoites and erythrocytes. Crystallography data showed that anti-RH5 bNAbs bind at or close to the basigin-binding site, blocking the interaction

between RH5 and basigin (77) that is critical for Pf merozoite invasion. However, this protein interaction does not seem to be the unique spot for the anti-RH5 mAb neutralizing activity. Considering that distinct RH5-derived B cell epitopes have been described with those bNAbs, it suggests that the RH5 sequences may suffer some immunological pressure (78). Other Pf antigens have been described as stimulators of malaria bNAbs, such as EXP1, MSP-3, GLURP, RAMA, SEA, and EBA-181. Those antigens were discovered after an investigation of serum samples from the cured Pf malaria patients and individuals with subsequent recrudescent infection. The cured patient samples had higher antibody titers against all those antigens and consequently, a higher capacity to inhibit the erythrocytes invasion by Pf merozoites (79). Recently, a mechanism based on interchromosomal DNA transposition was described as the contributor to the antibody diversity in the context of Pf malaria infection. A DNA insertion from a sequence of a collagen-binding inhibitory receptor (LAIR1) into V(D)J Ig genes was described to generate broad reactive antibodies against the Pf-infected erythrocytes (80). Although these LAIR1-containing antibodies were found in 5-10% of residents of Pf malaria-endemic areas and recognized distinct members of the RIFIN family, they did not confer protection against the disease (80, 81).

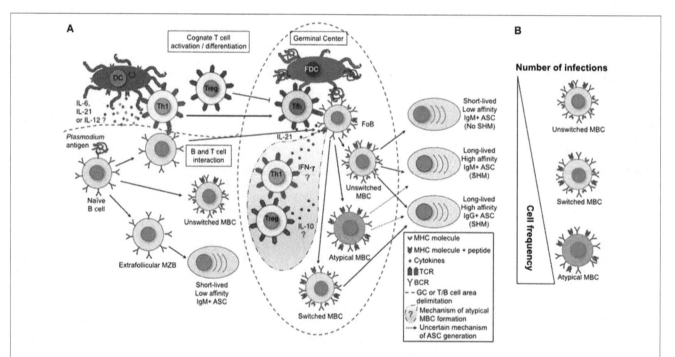

FIGURE 1 | B cell response triggered by malaria infection. (A) During a malaria infection, the naive B cells are activated by a *Plasmodium* antigen through the interaction with B cell receptors (BCR), leading to their differentiation into marginal zone B cells (MZB), follicular B cells (FoB), or unswitched memory B cell (MBCs). The switched and atypical MBCs are derived from the activation of FoBs within the germinal centers (GCs). Either the MZBs, or the unswitched, switched, or atypical MBCs can differentiate into antibody-secreting cells (ASCs). These ASCs range from short-lived, low-affinity, IgM+ to long-lived, high-affinity, IgM+ or IgG+. This variation depends on the type of interaction between a particular B cell with a T cell subset. The activated Th1 T cells migrate to the GCs, becoming follicular T helper cells (TFh) that help the GC reactions (acquisition of somatic hypermutations in V(D)J Ig genes and class switch by activated FoBs). Contrarily, the regulatory T cells (Tregs) have the potential to inhibit TFh cell differentiation and GC reactions. (B) A single parasite infection can induce the differentiation of multiple *Plasmodium*-specific B cell clones. However, the repeated parasite exposures shift the MBC frequencies with an increase for an atypical MBC over the unswitched or switched MBCs. This shift in cell frequency may interfere on the function of the secreted antibodies and, consequently, on the development of protective immunity.

Similar to the importance of immunoglobulin variable regions for effective humoral responses, Fc regions also have a fundamental role in mediating protection against infectious diseases. Receptors for immunoglobulin Fc regions have been described to be involved in cellular processes such as phagocytosis, antibody-dependent cellular cytotoxicity, and inflammation, among others (82). In the context of Pf malaria infection, the inoculations of human anti-MSP1$_{19}$ IgG protected transgenic mice for human Fc gamma receptor after challenge with chimeric Pb-Pf sporozoites. Contrarily, protection was not obtained when the same mAb was tested in non-transgenic mice, suggesting that the antibody interaction with MSP1$_{19}$ is not sufficient, while the presence of the Fc region is critical for parasite clearance (83). Few studies about human single nucleotide polymorphisms (SNPs) of the Fc gamma receptor have already validated the relevance of this opsonizing antibody-dependent phagocytosis for Pf malaria immunity [reviewed by (64)]. Noteworthily, the merozoite opsonisation has been associated with several conserved antigens and induces immunity against multiple Pf parasite strains (84).

Among the cells that can phagocyte and eliminate an opsonised Pf merozoite are neutrophils through the activation of respiratory burst [reviewed by (64)]. A SNP study has associated the increased levels of nitric oxide (NO) to Pf malaria protection (85). Furthermore, ROS levels have been correlated to natural acquired Pf malaria immunity (86). Once secreted to the extracellular medium, NO and ROS can both dampen the growth of Pf parasites *in vitro* (64, 87).

In terms of antibody-dependent complement activation, complement C1q proteins have shown to be deposited on the merozoite surface after the antibody-antigen interaction, allowing the further formation of the membrane attack complex (MAC) for parasite destruction. MSP-1 and MSP-2 have been identified as the main Pf merozoite targets involved in this protective mechanism. The higher is the C1q deposition, the higher is the protection. Interestingly, older children from Pf endemic areas presented higher C1q deposition than the younger children (88).

CONCLUDING REMARKS

After decades of suffering with malaria morbidity and mortality in several tropical areas, the at risk-populations are long overdue for effective strategies to contain this epidemic. The development of *Plasmodium*-specific vaccines already tested in clinical trials has not presented a considerable degree of protection yet. Hence, it has been strongly demonstrated that *Plasmodium* parasites have an enhanced resistance against the anti-malarial drugs on a daily basis. Thus, other alternatives of preventative or therapeutic treatments for malaria should be considered. Following all the characteristics presented in this manuscript about malaria-derived B cell immunity (**Figure 1**), those formulations must prioritize the best conditions for optimal B cell activation and development of the GC, TFh, and ASC responses. In terms of antibodies which are the final and effector products of the potential formulations, there are several reports of neutralizing antibodies identified for human malaria. However, their mechanisms of action have not been elucidated yet. Overall, it has been widely seen that antibody-based prophylaxis or therapeutical approaches possess a great efficacy against multiple pathogens. Therefore, strategies that properly stimulate malarial B cell responses may be beneficial not only in inhibiting infection, but also in reducing the morbidity and mortality numbers and disease transmission.

AUTHOR CONTRIBUTIONS

ELVS and MRD wrote the draft of this manuscript. ISS reviewed the manuscript and contributed significantly to the final draft. All authors read and approved the final manuscript.

ACKNOWLEDGMENTS

The authors thank Feda Masseoud (Centers for Disease Control and Prevention) for the critical reading of this manuscript and Fapesp grants 2012/13032-5 and 2017/11931-6 for the financial support. ELVS and ISS received fellowships from CNPq. MRD is currently receiving CAPES (Coordenação de Aperfeiçoamento de Pessoal de Nível Superior) fellowship.

REFERENCES

1. World Health Organization. *World Malaria Report 2016*. (2016). Available from: http://www.who.int/malaria/publications/world-malaria-report-2016/report/en/ (Accessed February 14, 2017).
2. World Health Organization. *Management of Severe Malaria: A Practical Handbook*. Geneva (2012). p. 1–83.
3. Lacerda MV, Mourão MP, Alexandre MA, Siqueira AM, Magalhães BM, Martinez-Espinosa FE, et al. Understanding the clinical spectrum of complicated *Plasmodium vivax* malaria: a systematic review on the contributions of the Brazilian literature. *Malar J*. (2012) 11:12. doi: 10.1186/1475-2875-11-12
4. Murray CJ, Rosenfeld LC, Lim SS, Andrews KG, Foreman KJ, Haring D, et al. Global malaria mortality between 1980 and 2010: a systematic analysis. *Lancet* (2012) 379:413–31. doi: 10.1016/S0140-6736(12)60034-8
5. Ménard R, Tavares J, Cockburn I, Markus M, Zavala F, Amino R. Looking under the skin: the first steps in malarial infection and immunity. *Nat Rev Microbiol*. (2013) 11:701–12. doi: 10.1038/nrmicro3111
6. Absalon S, Robbins JA, Dvorin JD. An essential malaria protein defines the architecture of blood-stage and transmission-stage parasites. *Nat Commun*. (2016) 7:11449. doi: 10.1038/ncomms11449
7. Obaldia N, Meibalan E, Sa JM, Ma S, Clark MA, Mejia P, et al. Bone marrow is a major parasite reservoir in *Plasmodium vivax* infection. *MBio* (2018) 9:e00625-18. doi: 10.1128/mBio.00625-18
8. Joice R, Nilsson SK, Montgomery J, Dankwa S, Egan E, Morahan B, et al. Plasmodium falciparum transmission stages accumulate in the human bone marrow. *Sci Transl Med*. (2014) 6:244re5. doi: 10.1126/scitranslmed.3008882
9. Cohen S, McGregor IA, Carrington S. Gamma-globulin and acquired immunity to human malaria. *Nature* (1961) 192:733–7. doi: 10.1038/192733a0
10. Ferreira MU, da Silva Nunes M, Wunderlich G. Antigenic diversity and immune evasion by malaria parasites. *Clin Diagn Lab Immunol*. (2004) 11:987–95. doi: 10.1128/CDLI.11.6.987-995.2004

11. Neafsey DE, Galinsky K, Jiang RH, Young L, Sykes SM, Saif S, et al. The malaria parasite *Plasmodium vivax* exhibits greater genetic diversity than *Plasmodium falciparum*. *Nat Genet*. (2012) 44:1046–50. doi: 10.1038/ng.2373

12. Weiss GE, Traore B, Kayentao K, Ongoiba A, Doumbo S, Doumtabe D, et al. The Plasmodium falciparum-specific human memory B cell compartment expands gradually with repeated malaria infections. *PLoS Pathog*. (2010) 6:e1000912. doi: 10.1371/journal.ppat.1000912

13. Nogaro SI, Hafalla JC, Walther B, Remarque EJ, Tetteh KK, Conway DJ, et al. The breadth, but not the magnitude, of circulating memory B cell responses to *P. falciparum* increases with age/exposure in an area of low transmission. *PLoS ONE* (2011) 6:e25582. doi: 10.1371/journal.pone.0025582

14. Wrammert J, Smith K, Miller J, Langley WA, Kokko K, Larsen C, et al. Rapid cloning of high-affinity human monoclonal antibodies against influenza virus. *Nature* (2008) 453:667–71. doi: 10.1038/nature06890

15. Le Roch KG, Johnson JR, Florens L, Zhou Y, Santrosyan A, Grainger M, et al. Global analysis of transcript and protein levels across the *Plasmodium falciparum* life cycle. *Genome Res*. (2004) 14:2308–18. doi: 10.1101/gr.2523904

16. Keitany GJ, Kim KS, Krishnamurty AT, Hondowicz BD, Hahn WO, Dambrauskas N, et al. Blood stage malaria disrupts humoral immunity to the pre-erythrocytic stage circumsporozoite protein. *Cell Rep*. (2016) 17:3193–205. doi: 10.1016/j.celrep.2016.11.060

17. Wipasa J, Suphavilai C, Okell LC, Cook J, Corran PH, Thaikla K, et al. Long-lived antibody and B Cell memory responses to the human malaria parasites, *Plasmodium falciparum* and *Plasmodium vivax*. *PLoS Pathog*. (2010) 6:e1000770. doi: 10.1371/journal.ppat.1000770

18. Ubillos I, Campo JJ, Requena P, Ome-Kaius M, Hanieh S, Rose H, et al. Chronic exposure to malaria is associated with inhibitory and activation markers on atypical memory B cells and marginal zone-like B cells. *Front Immunol*. (2017) 8:966. doi: 10.3389/fimmu.2017.00966

19. Stephens R, Ndungu FM, Langhorne J. Germinal centre and marginal zone B cells expand quickly in a second *Plasmodium chabaudi* malaria infection producing mature plasma cells. *Parasite Immunol*. (2009) 31:20–31. doi: 10.1111/j.1365-3024.2008.01066.x

20. Obeng-Adjei N, Portugal S, Holla P, Li S, Sohn H, Ambegaonkar A, et al. Malaria-induced interferon-γ drives the expansion of Tbethi atypical memory B cells. *PLoS Pathog*. (2017) 13:e1006576. doi: 10.1371/journal.ppat.1006576

21. Krishnamurty AT, Thouvenel CD, Portugal S, Keitany GJ, Kim KS, Holder A, et al. Somatically hypermutated plasmodium-specific IgM(+) memory B cells are rapid, plastic, early responders upon malaria rechallenge. *Immunity* (2016) 45:402–14. doi: 10.1016/j.immuni.2016.06.014

22. Harms Pritchard G, Pepper M. Memory B cell heterogeneity: remembrance of things past. *J Leukoc Biol*. (2018) 103:269–74. doi: 10.1002/JLB.4MR0517-215R

23. Radbruch A, Muehlinghaus G, Luger EO, Inamine A, Smith KG, Dörner T, et al. Competence and competition: the challenge of becoming a long-lived plasma cell. *Nat Rev Immunol*. (2006) 6:741–50. doi: 10.1038/nri1886

24. Weiss GE, Crompton PD, Li S, Walsh LA, Moir S, Traore B, et al. Atypical memory B cells are greatly expanded in individuals living in a malaria-endemic area. *J Immunol*. (2009) 183:2176–82. doi: 10.4049/jimmunol.0901297

25. Portugal S, Tipton CM, Sohn H, Kone Y, Wang J, Li S, et al. Malaria-associated atypical memory B cells exhibit markedly reduced B cell receptor signaling and effector function. *Elife* (2015) 4:e07218. doi: 10.7554/eLife.07218

26. Muellenbeck MF, Ueberheide B, Amulic B, Epp A, Fenyo D, Busse CE, et al. Atypical and classical memory B cells produce *Plasmodium falciparum* neutralizing antibodies. *J Exp Med*. (2013) 210:389–99. doi: 10.1084/jem.20121970

27. Ryg-Cornejo V, Ioannidis LJ, Ly A, Chiu CY, Tellier J, Hill DL, et al. Severe malaria infections impair germinal center responses by inhibiting T follicular helper cell differentiation. *Cell Rep*. (2016) 14:68–81. doi: 10.1016/j.celrep.2015.12.006

28. Xue J, Zhan B, Guo J, He N, Qiang HQ, Hotez P, et al. Acquired hookworm immunity in the golden hamster (*Mesocricetus auratus*) elicited by living *Necator americanus* third-stage infective larvae. *Exp Parasitol*. (2012) 130:6–12. doi: 10.1016/j.exppara.2011.10.007

29. Finney OC, Danziger SA, Molina DM, Vignali M, Takagi A, Ji M, et al. Predicting antidisease immunity using proteome arrays and sera from children naturally exposed to malaria. *Mol Cell Proteomics* (2014) 13:2646–60. doi: 10.1074/mcp.M113.036632

30. Cepok S, von Geldern G, Nolting T, Grummel V, Srivastava R, Zhou D, et al. Viral load determines the B-cell response in the cerebrospinal fluid during human immunodeficiency virus infection. *Ann Neurol*. (2007) 62:458–67. doi: 10.1002/ana.21195

31. Crompton PD, Mircetic M, Weiss G, Baughman A, Huang CY, Topham DJ, et al. The TLR9 ligand CpG promotes the acquisition of *Plasmodium falciparum*-specific memory B cells in malaria-naive individuals. *J Immunol*. (2009) 182:3318–26. doi: 10.4049/jimmunol.0803596

32. Elias SC, Choudhary P, de Cassan SC, Biswas S, Collins KA, Halstead FD, et al. Analysis of human B-cell responses following ChAd63-MVA MSP1 and AMA1 immunization and controlled malaria infection. *Immunology* (2014) 141:628–44. doi: 10.1111/imm.12226

33. Turner L, Wang CW, Lavstsen T, Mwakalinga SB, Sauerwein RW, Hermsen CC, et al. Antibodies against PfEMP1, RIFIN, MSP3 and GLURP are acquired during controlled Plasmodium falciparum malaria infections in naïve volunteers. *PLoS ONE*. (2011) 6:e29025. doi: 10.1371/journal.pone.0029025

34. Walker DM, Oghumu S, Gupta G, McGwire BS, Drew ME, Satoskar AR. Mechanisms of cellular invasion by intracellular parasites. *Cell Mol Life Sci*. (2014) 71:1245–63. doi: 10.1007/s00018-013-1491-1

35. Walker KM, Okitsu S, Porter DW, Duncan C, Amacker M, Pluschke G, et al. Antibody and T-cell responses associated with experimental human malaria infection or vaccination show limited relationships. *Immunology* (2015) 145:71–81. doi: 10.1111/imm.12428

36. Naus CW, Jones FM, Satti MZ, Joseph S, Riley EM, Kimani G, et al. Serological responses among individuals in areas where both schistosomiasis and malaria are endemic: cross-reactivity between *Schistosoma mansoni* and *Plasmodium falciparum*. *J Infect Dis*. (2003) 187:1272–82. doi: 10.1086/368361

37. Pierrot C, Wilson S, Lallet H, Lafitte S, Jones FM, Daher W, et al. Identification of a novel antigen of *Schistosoma mansoni* shared with *Plasmodium falciparum* and evaluation of different cross-reactive antibody subclasses induced by human schistosomiasis and malaria. *Infect Immun*. (2006) 74:3347–54. doi: 10.1128/IAI.01724-05

38. Donati D, Zhang LP, Chêne A, Chen Q, Flick K, Nyström M, et al. Identification of a polyclonal B-cell activator in *Plasmodium falciparum*. *Infect Immun*. (2004) 72:5412–8. doi: 10.1128/IAI.72.9.5412-5418.2004

39. Donati D, Mok B, Chêne A, Xu H, Thangarajh M, Glas R, et al. Increased B cell survival and preferential activation of the memory compartment by a malaria polyclonal B cell activator. *J Immunol*. (2006) 177:3035–44. doi: 10.4049/jimmunol.177.5.3035

40. Zanini GM, De Moura Carvalho LJ, Brahimi K, De Souza-Passos LF, Guimarães SJ, Da Silva Machado E, et al. Sera of patients with systemic lupus erythematosus react with plasmodial antigens and can inhibit the *in vitro* growth of *Plasmodium falciparum*. *Autoimmunity* (2009) 42:545–52. doi: 10.1080/08916930903039810

41. Brahimi K, Martins YC, Zanini GM, Ferreira-da-Cruz MeF, Daniel-Ribeiro CT. Monoclonal auto-antibodies and sera of autoimmune patients react with *Plasmodium falciparum* and inhibit its *in vitro* growth. *Mem Inst Oswaldo Cruz*. (2011) 106(Suppl. 1):44–51. doi: 10.1590/S0074-02762011000900006

42. Scholzen A, Teirlinck AC, Bijker EM, Roestenberg M, Hermsen CC, Hoffman SL, et al. BAFF and BAFF receptor levels correlate with B cell subset activation and redistribution in controlled human malaria infection. *J Immunol*. (2014) 192:3719–29. doi: 10.4049/jimmunol.1302960

43. Nduati E, Gwela A, Karanja H, Mugyenyi C, Langhorne J, Marsh K, et al. The plasma concentration of the B cell activating factor is increased in children with acute malaria. *J Infect Dis*. (2011) 204:962–70. doi: 10.1093/infdis/jir438

44. Muehlenbachs A, Fried M, Lachowitzer J, Mutabingwa TK, Duffy PE. Genome-wide expression analysis of placental malaria reveals features of lymphoid neogenesis during chronic infection. *J Immunol*. (2007) 179:557–65. doi: 10.4049/jimmunol.179.1.557

45. Patgaonkar M, Herbert F, Powale K, Gandhe P, Gogtay N, Thatte U, et al. Vivax infection alters peripheral B-cell profile and induces persistent serum IgM. *Parasite Immunol*. (2018) 40:e12580. doi: 10.1111/pim.12580

46. Rodrigues-da-Silva RN, Lima-Junior JaC, Fonseca BeP, Antas PR, Baldez A, Storer FL, et al. Alterations in cytokines and haematological parameters during the acute and convalescent phases of *Plasmodium falciparum* and

Plasmodium vivax infections. *Mem Inst Oswaldo Cruz.* (2014) 109:154–62. doi: 10.1590/0074-0276140275

47. Craxton A, Magaletti D, Ryan EJ, Clark EA. Macrophage- and dendritic cell–dependent regulation of human B-cell proliferation requires the TNF family ligand BAFF. *Blood* (2003) 101:4464–71. doi: 10.1182/blood-2002-10-3123

48. Bockstal V, Geurts N, Magez S. Acute Disruption of Bone Marrow B Lymphopoiesis and apoptosis of transitional and marginal zone B cells in the spleen following a blood-stage *Plasmodium chabaudi* infection in mice. *J Parasitol Res.* (2011) 2011:534697. doi: 10.1155/2011/534697

49. Ghosh D, Wikenheiser DJ, Kennedy B, McGovern KE, Stuart JD, Wilson EH, et al. An atypical splenic B cell progenitor population supports antibody production during plasmodium infection in mice. *J Immunol.* (2016) 197:1788–800. doi: 10.4049/jimmunol.1502199

50. Sullivan RT, Ssewanyana I, Wamala S, Nankya F, Jagannathan P, Tappero JW, et al. B cell sub-types following acute malaria and associations with clinical immunity. *Malar J.* (2016) 15:139. doi: 10.1186/s12936-016-1190-0

51. Rowland SL, Leahy KF, Halverson R, Torres RM, Pelanda R. BAFF receptor signaling aids the differentiation of immature B cells into transitional B cells following tonic BCR signaling. *J Immunol.* (2010) 185:4570–81. doi: 10.4049/jimmunol.1001708

52. Moir S, Ho J, Malaspina A, Wang W, DiPoto AC, O'Shea MA, et al. Evidence for HIV-associated B cell exhaustion in a dysfunctional memory B cell compartment in HIV-infected viremic individuals. *J Exp Med.* (2008) 205:1797–805. doi: 10.1084/jem.20072683

53. Pérez-Mazliah D, Gardner PJ, Schweighoffer E, McLaughlin S, Hosking C, Tumwine I, et al. Plasmodium-specific atypical memory B cells are short-lived activated B cells. *Elife* (2018) 7:e39800. doi: 10.7554/eLife.39800

54. Figueiredo MM, Costa PAC, Diniz SQ, Henriques PM, Kano FS, Tada MS, et al. T follicular helper cells regulate the activation of B lymphocytes and antibody production during *Plasmodium vivax* infection. *PLoS Pathog.* (2017) 13:e1006484. doi: 10.1371/journal.ppat.1006484

55. Obeng-Adjei N, Portugal S, Tran TM, Yazew TB, Skinner J, Li S, et al. Circulating Th1-cell-type Tfh cells that exhibit impaired B cell help are preferentially activated during acute malaria in children. *Cell Rep.* (2015) 13:425–39. doi: 10.1016/j.celrep.2015.09.004

56. Guthmiller JJ, Graham AC, Zander RA, Pope RL, Butler NS. Cutting Edge: IL-10 is essential for the generation of germinal center B cell responses and anti-plasmodium humoral immunity. *J Immunol.* (2017) 198:617–22. doi: 10.4049/jimmunol.1601762

57. Pérez-Mazliah D, Ng DH, Freitas do Rosário AP, McLaughlin S, Mastelic-Gavillet B, Sodenkamp J, et al. Disruption of IL-21 signaling affects T cell-B cell interactions and abrogates protective humoral immunity to malaria. *PLoS Pathog.* (2015) 11:e1004715. doi: 10.1371/journal.ppat.1004715

58. Wijayalath W, Danner R, Kleschenko Y, Majji S, Villasante EF, Richie TL, et al. HLA class II (DR0401) molecules induce Foxp3+ regulatory T cell suppression of B cells in *Plasmodium yoelii* strain 17XNL malaria. *Infect Immun.* (2014) 82:286–97. doi: 10.1128/IAI.00272-13

59. Zander RA, Obeng-Adjei N, Guthmiller JJ, Kulu DI, Li J, Ongoiba A, et al. PD-1 co-inhibitory and OX40 co-stimulatory crosstalk regulates helper T cell differentiation and anti-plasmodium humoral immunity. *Cell Host Microbe* (2015) 17:628–41. doi: 10.1016/j.chom.2015.03.007

60. Zander RA, Guthmiller JJ, Graham AC, Pope RL, Burke BE, Carr DJ, et al. Type I interferons induce T regulatory 1 responses and restrict humoral immunity during experimental malaria. *PLoS Pathog.* (2016) 12:e1005945. doi: 10.1371/journal.ppat.1005945

61. Matar CG, Anthony NR, O'Flaherty BM, Jacobs NT, Priyamvada L, Engwerda CR, et al. Gammaherpesvirus co-infection with malaria suppresses anti-parasitic humoral immunity. *PLoS Pathog.* (2015) 11:e1004858. doi: 10.1371/journal.ppat.1004858

62. Hviid L, Barfod L, Fowkes FJ. Trying to remember: immunological B cell memory to malaria. *Trends Parasitol.* (2015) 31:89–94. doi: 10.1016/j.pt.2014.12.009

63. Osier FH, Fegan G, Polley SD, Murungi L, Verra F, Tetteh KK, et al. Breadth and magnitude of antibody responses to multiple *Plasmodium falciparum* merozoite antigens are associated with protection from clinical malaria. *Infect Immun.* (2008) 76:2240–8. doi: 10.1128/IAI.01585-07

64. Hill DL, Schofield L, Wilson DW. IgG opsonization of merozoites: multiple immune mechanisms for malaria vaccine development. *Int J Parasitol.* (2017) 47:585–95. doi: 10.1016/j.ijpara.2017.05.004

65. Dent AE, Nakajima R, Liang L, Baum E, Moormann AM, Sumba PO, et al. *Plasmodium falciparum* protein microarray antibody profiles correlate with protection from symptomatic malaria in Kenya. *J Infect Dis.* (2015) 212:1429–38. doi: 10.1093/infdis/jiv224

66. Kisalu NK, Idris AH, Weidle C, Flores-Garcia Y, Flynn BJ, Sack BK, et al. A human monoclonal antibody prevents malaria infection by targeting a new site of vulnerability on the parasite. *Nat Med.* (2018) 24:408–16. doi: 10.1038/nm.4512

67. Deal C, Balazs AB, Espinosa DA, Zavala F, Baltimore D, Ketner G. Vectored antibody gene delivery protects against *Plasmodium falciparum* sporozoite challenge in mice. *Proc Natl Acad Sci USA.* (2014) 111:12528–32. doi: 10.1073/pnas.1407362111

68. Espinosa DA, Gutierrez GM, Rojas-López M, Noe AR, Shi L, Tse SW, et al. Proteolytic cleavage of the *Plasmodium falciparum* circumsporozoite protein is a target of protective antibodies. *J Infect Dis.* (2015) 212:1111–9. doi: 10.1093/infdis/jiv154

69. Chen E, Paing MM, Salinas N, Sim BK, Tolia NH. Structural and functional basis for inhibition of erythrocyte invasion by antibodies that target *Plasmodium falciparum* EBA-175. *PLoS Pathog.* (2013) 9:e1003390. doi: 10.1371/journal.ppat.1003390

70. Chootong P, Ntumngia FB, VanBuskirk KM, Xainli J, Cole-Tobian JL, Campbell CO, et al. Mapping epitopes of the *Plasmodium vivax* Duffy binding protein with naturally acquired inhibitory antibodies. *Infect Immun.* (2010) 78:1089–95. doi: 10.1128/IAI.01036-09

71. Partey FD, Castberg FC, Sarbah EW, Silk SE, Awandare GA, Draper SJ, et al. Kinetics of antibody responses to PfRH5-complex antigens in Ghanaian children with *Plasmodium falciparum* malaria. *PLoS ONE* (2018) 13:e0198371. doi: 10.1371/journal.pone.0198371

72. Douglas AD, Williams AR, Illingworth JJ, Kamuyu G, Biswas S, Goodman AL, et al. The blood-stage malaria antigen PfRH5 is susceptible to vaccine-inducible cross-strain neutralizing antibody. *Nat Commun.* (2011) 2:601. doi: 10.1038/ncomms1615

73. Douglas AD, Baldeviano GC, Lucas CM, Lugo-Roman LA, Crosnier C, Bartholdson SJ, et al. A PfRH5-based vaccine is efficacious against heterologous strain blood-stage Plasmodium falciparum infection in aotus monkeys. *Cell Host Microbe* (2015) 17:130–9. doi: 10.1016/j.chom.2014.11.017

74. Weaver R, Reiling L, Feng G, Drew DR, Mueller I, Siba PM, et al. The association between naturally acquired IgG subclass specific antibodies to the PfRH5 invasion complex and protection from *Plasmodium falciparum* malaria. *Sci Rep.* (2016) 6:33094. doi: 10.1038/srep33094

75. Kapulu MC, Da DF, Miura K, Li Y, Blagborough AM, Churcher TS, et al. Comparative assessment of transmission-blocking vaccine candidates against *Plasmodium falciparum. Sci Rep.* (2015) 5:11193. doi: 10.1038/srep11193

76. Payne RO, Silk SE, Elias SC, Miura K, Diouf A, Galaway F, et al. Human vaccination against RH5 induces neutralizing antimalarial antibodies that inhibit RH5 invasion complex interactions. *JCI Insight.* (2017) 2:96381. doi: 10.1172/jci.insight.96381

77. Wright KE, Hjerrild KA, Bartlett J, Douglas AD, Jin J, Brown RE, et al. Structure of malaria invasion protein RH5 with erythrocyte basigin and blocking antibodies. *Nature* (2014) 515:427–30. doi: 10.1038/nature13715

78. Douglas AD, Williams AR, Knuepfer E, Illingworth JJ, Furze JM, Crosnier C, et al. Neutralization of *Plasmodium falciparum* merozoites by antibodies against PfRH5. *J Immunol.* (2014) 192:245–58. doi: 10.4049/jimmunol.1302045

79. Goh YS, Peng K, Chia WN, Siau A, Chotivanich K, Gruner AC, et al. Neutralizing antibodies against *Plasmodium falciparum* associated with successful cure after drug therapy. *PLoS ONE* (2016) 11:e0159347. doi: 10.1371/journal.pone.0159347

80. Tan J, Pieper K, Piccoli L, Abdi A, Perez MF, Geiger R, et al. A LAIR1 insertion generates broadly reactive antibodies against malaria variant antigens. *Nature* (2016) 529:105–9. doi: 10.1038/nature16450

81. Pieper K, Tan J, Piccoli L, Foglierini M, Barbieri S, Chen Y, et al. Public antibodies to malaria antigens generated by two LAIR1 insertion modalities. *Nature* (2017) 548:597–601. doi: 10.1038/nature23670

82. Pleass RJ, Holder AA. Opinion: antibody-based therapies for malaria. *Nat Rev Microbiol.* (2005) 3:893–9. doi: 10.1038/nrmicro1267

83. McIntosh RS, Shi J, Jennings RM, Chappel JC, de Koning-Ward TF, Smith T, et al. The importance of human FcgammaRI in mediating protection to malaria. *PLoS Pathog.* (2007) 3:e72. doi: 10.1371/journal.ppat.0030072

84. Hill DL, Wilson DW, Sampaio NG, Eriksson EM, Ryg-Cornejo V, Harrison GLA, et al. Merozoite antigens of *Plasmodium falciparum* elicit strain-transcending opsonizing immunity. *Infect Immun.* (2016) 84:2175–84. doi: 10.1128/IAI.00145-16

85. Kun JF, Mordmüller B, Perkins DJ, May J, Mercereau-Puijalon O, Alpers M, et al. Nitric oxide synthase 2(Lambaréné) (G-954C), increased nitric oxide production, and protection against malaria. *J Infect Dis.* (2001) 184:330–6. doi: 10.1086/322037

86. Joos C, Marrama L, Polson HE, Corre S, Diatta AM, Diouf B, et al. Clinical protection from falciparum malaria correlates with neutrophil respiratory bursts induced by merozoites opsonized with human serum antibodies. *PLoS ONE* (2010) 5:e9871. doi: 10.1371/journal.pone.0009871

87. Hodgson SH, Llewellyn D, Silk SE, Milne KH, Elias SC, Miura K, et al. Changes in serological immunology measures in UK and Kenyan adults post-controlled human malaria infection. *Front Microbiol.* (2016) 7:1604. doi: 10.3389/fmicb.2016.01604

88. Boyle MJ, Reiling L, Feng G, Langer C, Osier FH, Aspeling-Jones H, et al. Human antibodies fix complement to inhibit *Plasmodium falciparum* invasion of erythrocytes and are associated with protection against malaria. *Immunity* (2015) 42:580–90. doi: 10.1016/j.immuni.2015.02.012

6

Age-Related Differential Stimulation of Immune Response by *Babesia microti* and *Borrelia burgdorferi* During Acute Phase of Infection Affects Disease Severity

Vitomir Djokic[†], Shekerah Primus[†], Lavoisier Akoolo[†], Monideep Chakraborti and Nikhat Parveen*

Department of Microbiology, Biochemistry and Molecular Genetics, Rutgers New Jersey Medical School, Newark, NJ, United States

Correspondence:
Nikhat Parveen
Parveeni@njms.rutgers.edu

[†] *These authors have contributed equally to this work*

Lyme disease is the most prominent tick-borne disease with 300,000 cases estimated by CDC every year while ~2,000 cases of babesiosis occur per year in the United States. Simultaneous infection with *Babesia microti* and *Borrelia burgdorferi* are now the most common tick-transmitted coinfections in the U.S.A., and they are a serious health problem because coinfected patients show more intense and persisting disease symptoms. *B. burgdorferi* is an extracellular spirochete responsible for systemic Lyme disease while *B. microti* is a protozoan that infects erythrocytes and causes babesiosis. Immune status and spleen health are important for resolution of babesiosis, which is more severe and even fatal in the elderly and splenectomized patients. Therefore, we investigated the effect of each pathogen on host immune response and consequently on severity of disease manifestations in both young, and 30 weeks old C3H mice. At the acute stage of infection, Th1 polarization in young mice spleen was associated with increased IFN-γ and TNF-α producing T cells and a high Tregs/Th17 ratio. Together, these changes could help in the resolution of both infections in young mice and also prevent fatality by *B. microti* infection as observed with WA-1 strain of *Babesia*. In older mature mice, Th2 polarization at acute phase of *B. burgdorferi* infection could play a more effective role in preventing Lyme disease symptoms. As a result, enhanced *B. burgdorferi* survival and increased tissue colonization results in severe Lyme arthritis only in young coinfected mice. At 3 weeks post-infection, diminished pathogen-specific antibody production in coinfected young, but not older mice, as compared to mice infected with each pathogen individually may also contribute to increased inflammation observed due to *B. burgdorferi* infection, thus causing persistent Lyme disease observed in coinfected mice and reported in patients. Thus, higher combined proinflammatory response to *B. burgdorferi* due to Th1 and Th17 cells likely reduced *B. microti* parasitemia significantly only in young mice later in infection, while the presence of *B. microti* reduced humoral immunity later in infection and enhanced tissue colonization by Lyme spirochetes in these mice even at the acute stage, thereby increasing inflammatory arthritis.

Keywords: *Babesia microti*, age-related immunity, babesiosis, *Borrelia burgdorferi*, Lyme disease, immunity to tick-borne coinfections

INTRODUCTION

Concomitant coinfections with parasites and bacteria in humans are common in the developing world (1); however, reports of such coinfections in the developed world are rare. In contrast, coinfections with tick-borne protozoan parasite of *Babesia* species and *Borrelia burgdorferi* sensu lato group of spirochetes have been emerging more recently (2–5). The CDC estimates that ~300,000 cases of Lyme disease and ~2,000 cases of babesiosis occur in the U.S.A. every year. Lyme disease is caused by *B. burgdorferi* spirochetes while the Apicomplexan protozoan parasite *Babesia microti* is the major causative agent of babesiosis in the United States and *B. divergence* is prevalent in Europe. Coinfections of *Ixodes* species ticks with *B. burgdorferi* and *B. microti* have been increasing steadily over the years (6–10). Reservoir hosts and tick-feeding habits determine the spread of these pathogens to humans. The most commonly recognized tick-borne coinfection in most of the Eastern United States is Lyme spirochetes and *B. microti* with detection levels of concurrent infections by these pathogens in New York as high as 67% (11).

B. burgdorferi is responsible for systemic Lyme disease that affects the skin, musculoskeletal system, heart, joints, and nervous system. Babesiosis remains asymptomatic in healthy individuals such that donation of blood by these infected persons can often lead to transfusion-transmitted babesiosis, raising serious health care problems for already sick recipients of this tainted blood or blood products (12–14). Severe babesiosis in splenectomized patients result in high morbidity and even mortality indicating that the spleen plays a critical role in resolution of *Babesia* infection (15–19). Several immunological deficiencies emerge with age, resulting in an increased susceptibility of the elderly to various infections. Innate immune response in both humans and mice affect clearance of infections that changes with age (20–23). For example, declines in function of neutrophils and defect in macrophage (mφ) response with in aged humans in responses to infection have been described previously (24, 25). Therefore, it is not surprising that severe babesiosis is most common in people >40 years of age, especially in the elderly individuals (2, 26). Severe disease requires patient hospitalization, and can even cause death due to multi-organ failure (27). In contrast, Lyme disease severity has not been reported to be age dependent in humans but older mice are somewhat resistant to inflammatory Lyme disease. These observations underscore the need for a comprehensive evaluation of the effect of coinfections on overall disease severity using the susceptible mouse model of infection.

The lack of symptoms in patients and unavailability of cost-effective and sensitive diagnostic tests often results in underestimation of babesiosis prevalence. Epidemiological studies demonstrated that *B. microti-B. burgdorferi* coinfected patients suffer from significantly more diverse and intense symptoms, which persist longer than those in patients infected with each pathogen individually (28–30). Symptoms, such as chronic fatigue and headache have been reported to persist in coinfected patients for months and were significantly higher than patients with Lyme disease alone (28). In the United States, 10% of patients with initial erythema migrans show persistent flu-like symptoms, joint and muscular pain, and fatigue even after completion of antibiotic treatment regimen (31). Physicians in the endemic regions are encouraged to recommend additional blood tests for concurrent infection with *B. microti* because the treatment approach for this parasitic disease is different from bacterial infections and testing for babesiosis is not often conducted to determine coinfection (11).

Susceptible C3H mouse strain infection system has provided significant information about immune responses against *B. burgdorferi* and *B. microti* and the impact of these infections on respective disease manifestations. Splenic cells of *B. burgdorferi* infected C3H mice showed an increase in B and CD4+ lymphocytes, increase in IFN-γ levels and diminished levels of IL-4 production (32–36). IFN-γ production together with increase in IL-17 producing Th17 cells, which produce TNF-α simultaneously, were shown to contribute to Lyme arthritis severity, while primarily antibodies against *B. burgdorferi* facilitated clearance of the spirochetes, reducing their burden in tissues (32, 36–38). Both Th1 and Th2 responses are indicative of the development of the adaptive immune response including their contribution to humoral immunity. Innate immune response, involving macrophage and NK cells, has been found to be critical for control of protozoan infections, including intracellular pathogen *B. microti* during acute phase (39–44). Cytokines IFN-γ and TNF-α contribute to infection-associated inflammatory complications; however, they also help in elimination of protozoan pathogens with the help of Nitric oxide (NO) produced during infection (39–44). Increase in IL-10 levels was found to exacerbate *Plasmodium* parasitemia but this cytokine suppressed hepatic pathology (45). Thus, balance between these 3 cytokines; IFN-γ, TNF-α, and IL-10 levels are critical for moderating parasitic disease severity, and establishment of long-term, non-fatal diseases (43, 46). Macrophage and NK cells were also shown to play critical roles in conferring resistance in C57BL/6 mice to highly infectious WA-1 strain of *Babesia* species (21), while both CD4+ cells and IFN-γ contributed to resolution of parasitemia of *B. microti*, which causes milder disease in mice (47).

Only limited murine studies have been conducted to study tick-borne coinfections until now. Two previous investigations reported contradictory outcomes of coinfections particularly as demonstrated by Lyme disease severity (48, 49). We decided to conduct a comprehensive study to understand the effect of simultaneous *B. burgdorferi* and *B. microti* infections on acute immune responses of inbred mice during parasitemia upward incline phase, and consequentially, on survival and persistence of each pathogen later as affected by the age of mice. We selected C3H mice for our coinfection studies because young mice of this strain exhibit Lyme arthritis and carditis (50, 51), as well as *B. microti* parasitemia and anemia (48, 49) similar to humans. We hypothesized that using a mouse model of Borrelia-Babesia coinfection, we will be able to understand why patients with these coinfections show more persistent subjective symptoms. We describe here the impact of coinfection on the splenic immune response in C3H young and mature, older mice at acute phase of infection and its effect on parasitemia and Lyme disease due to modulation of immune response by *B. microti* particularly in coinfected mice.

MATERIALS AND METHODS

Ethical Statement

This study was carried out in accordance with the guidelines of the Animal Welfare Act and the Institute of Laboratory Animal Resources Guide for the Care and Use of Laboratory Animals, and Public Health Service Policy with the recommendations of Newark Institutional Animal Care and Use Committee (IACUC) designated members. The protocol number D-14011-A1 of the corresponding author was approved by the Newark IACUC and study was conducted at Rutgers-New Jersey Medical School following this approved protocol.

Culture and Maintenance of *B. burgdorferi* and *B. microti* and Injection of Mice

C3H/SCID female mice were first injected with *B. microti* infected RBCs stock to obtain inoculum for subsequent experiments. Parasitemia was determined daily using the approved guidelines as described previously (52, 53). *B. burgdorferi* N40 strain carrying a firefly luciferase gene (Bbluc) (54), which is a derivative of the N40D10/E9 clone (55), was used in this study and is labeled as N40 throughout. N40 was cultured at 33°C in Barbour-Stoenner-Kelly-II (BSK-II) medium supplemented with 6% rabbit serum (BSK-RS). The spirochetes were harvested and count adjusted to 10^4 N40 per ml of medium. Only female mice were used in all experiments to avoid the effect of testosterone on parasitemia and innate immune response reported for parasitic diseases (56).

To assess the mechanistic details of coinfections, we conducted experiments in susceptible C3H mice. Young mice were used because they display both Lyme disease and babesiosis disease manifestations while middle age, mature 30 weeks old mice (referred as old mice throughout) were included to determine if they show different immune response in acute phase and display higher parasitemia as observed in humans. Three weeks or Twenty-Nine weeks old female C3H mice were purchased from Rutgers approved reputable vendor(s) and were used in the experiments after acclimatization for one week. The mice were randomly divided into 4 experimental groups in each set with each group containing 5 mice, thus a total of 40 mice were used, 20 young mice at 4 weeks of age and 20 mice that were 30 weeks old. The first group of mice in each age category remained uninfected, second group were injected with *B. burgdorferi* (N40) alone, third group received both N40 strain and *B. microti* and fourth group was inoculated with *B. microti* alone. Mice were injected with 1×10^4 gray strain of *B. microti* (ATCC30221 strain) infected RBCs/mouse diluted in Phosphate Buffered Saline (PBS) intraperitoneally (ip), or injected with 10^3 *B. burgdorferi* diluted in 100 μl BSK-RS subcutaneously (sc) in each mouse on the lateral aspect of the right thigh, or injected with both pathogens at the respective sites. Naïve mice received BSK-RS and PBS, sc and ip, respectively. BSK-RS does not interfere in live imaging of mice and allows light emission to occur *in vivo* for 10 min. Based upon our experience, we do

not expect any impact of the vehicles, if any, beyond a few days post-infection. Due to different vehicles suitable for each microbe survival and dissemination in host after injection, both pathogens were injected at different sites using the established protocols for each pathogen.

We determined the effect of coinfections during the acute phase of infection before the development of peak parasitemia and adaptive immune response. Our goal was to analyze the effect of *B. burgdorferi* impact on *B. microti* parasitemia and consequently on splenic immunity during pre-convalescence period. Mice were euthanized when *B. microti* parasitemia was ~20%, i.e., before reaching the peak parasitemia. Thus, for determination of immune response at early stage of infection, young mice were euthanized at 11 days post-infection and old mice at 17th day of infection because parasitemia and Lyme spirochetes colonization was slower in the older as compared to the young mice. Dose and mode of injection for each pathogen is described above.

Monitoring of Infected Mice

Infected mice were monitored closely for both N40 and *B. microti* infection progression for up to 21 days post infection in the initial experiment to determine the acute phase of infection before peak parasitemia develops. Based upon the parasitemia profile, a thorough investigation of acute phase of infection on immune response and evaluation of disease severity is presented here. Plasma was also recovered for antibody response determination at 3 weeks of infection. Samples collected from mice at acute phase were then evaluated further for splenic immune response, tissue colonization, and disease pathology. Mice infected with *B. microti* were monitored for parasitemia every day by examination of Giemsa stained blood smears.

Assessment of Tissue Colonization Levels by *B. burgdorferi* and Disease Pathology

To eliminate microbiome on skin surface after euthanasia, mice were soaked in Betadine for 30–40 min followed by soaking in 70% ethyl alcohol for 30 min and then dissected in biosafety hood to aseptically remove organs to recover live spirochetes. The skin at the injection site, ear, blood and urinary bladder were transferred to tubes containing BSK-II+RS medium and antibiotic mixture for Borreliae with 100x stock containing 2 mg Phosphomycin, 5 mg Rifampicin and 250 μg of Amphotericin B in 20% DMSO (HI-MEDIA Laboratories, PA) and grown at 33°C to recover live *B. burgdorferi* from each tissue. In each experiment, right joint and heart were fixed in neutral buffered formalin, processed by routine histological methods, sectioned and scored in a blinded manner for carditis and arthritis severity caused by *B. burgdorferi*. DNA was isolated from the left joint and brain of mice in each experiment to use for qPCR. The qPCR was carried out using *B. burgdorferi recA* amplicon and the specific molecular beacon probes tagged with FAM fluorophore in the duplex assay developed in our laboratory (57). To determine spirochete burden in each organ, nidogen amplicon copy number using the specific molecular beacon tagged with TET fluorophore was used for normalization of *B. burgdorferi* copy number. After euthanasia, aseptically removed liver and spleens were weighed, and splenocytes collected for flow cytometry as described below.

HISTOPATHOLOGY

Two graduates of veterinary medicine (LA and VD) evaluated sections of joints and hearts independently in a blinded manner and scored for inflammation. Briefly, severity of arthritic manifestation was measured by assessing (i) synovial hyperplasia and (ii) erosion of cartilage, (iii) increase in lymphocytic infiltration and (iv) change in synovial space as observed in N40-infected and coinfected mice compared to the naïve or mice infected with *B. microti* alone. Scoring of joint inflammation ranged from "–" (for naïve mice) to "+ + +" in *B. burgdorferi* infected/coinfected mice based upon display of all four criteria. Carditis is considered severe (+) in mice if mixed leukocyte infiltration (primarily macrophage) and fibroblastic proliferation of the connective tissue around the aortic valve and origin of the coronary artery are observed. Infiltration of macrophages and lymphoid cells may also appear around the aorta or in focal areas of the auricular or ventricular epicardium to the apex of the heart (50). These manifestations are usually observed between 2 and 3 weeks of infection with our N40 strain. Manifestations (+/-) are considered milder if consistently reduced distribution of these features is observed. The lack of these characteristics is indicative of no (-) carditis.

Analyses of Splenic Cells by Flow Cytometry

Single cell suspensions of the splenocytes was obtained by slicing the organ into small pieces and straining it into 50 ml conical tube using a 70 μm nylon sterile cell strainer. The cells were then washed with PBS by centrifugation at 350 xg and RBCs lysed by Ammonium-Chloride–Potassium (ACK) lysis buffer (Thermo Fisher # A10492201). The cells were then resuspended in fluorescence-activated cell sorting (FACS) buffer (PBS +5%FBS), and stained with specific antibodies diluted 1:50. Using hemocytometer cell number was adjusted to 10^8 for each individual sample in 2 separate tubes. In the first tube, B cells were detected with Brilliant violet 421 conjugated anti-mouse CD19 antibodies (BioLegend, #115537) and macrophages with PE conjugated anti-mouse F4/80 antibodies (BioLegend, # 123110) followed by FACS. In the second tube, splenocytes were incubated with APC-Cy7 conjugated anti-NK1.1 mouse monoclonal (PK136) antibodies (Bilegend # 108724), T cells with PE/Cy7 conjugated anti-mouse CD3 antibodies (BioLegend #100220), T helper cells with FITC conjugated anti-mouse CD4 antibodies (BioLegend #100406) and cytotoxic T cells with Alexafluor-700 conjugated anti-mouse CD8a antibodies (BioLegend #1000730) by incubation for 30 min in the dark on ice. The cells were washed three time with PBS containing 5% FBS (FACS Buffer) by centrifugation and resuspended in Fixation buffer (BioLegend # 420801) for 20 min at room temperature, and then permeabilized twice in 1x Intracellular Staining Permeabilization Wash Buffer (BioLegend # 421002). After centrifugation, for intracellular cytokines staining, cells

were incubated with anti-mouse IFN-γ antibodies conjugated with Pacific Blue (BioLegend #505818), anti-mouse TNF-α antibodies conjugated with PE (BioLegend #506306), anti-mouse IL-4 antibodies conjugated with BV605 (BioLegend #504126), anti-mouse IL-10 antibodies conjugated with PerCP-Cy5.5 (BioLegend #505028), anti-mouse IL-21 antibodies conjugated with eFluor 660 (ThermoFisher #50-7211-82) all used at 1:50 dilution, for 20 min on RT in dark. The samples were then washed twice with Intracellular Staining Permeabilization Wash Buffer and centrifuged at 350 xg for 5 min. Fixed and labeled cells were then resuspended in 0.5 ml of FACS Buffer and analyzed using BD LSRFortessa™ X-20 (BD Biosciences) driven by software FACS DiVa (BD Biosciences). For each fluorophore, appropriate compensation was made using one of the naïve mice splenocytes. Acquired data was analyzed using FlowJo, Version 10.3 software. After analysis of samples, ratio between CD19+ and F4/80+ was determined from the first tube while FcR+ cells were distinguished from CD3+ cells in the second tube. Furthermore, subpopulation of CD4+ and CD8+ were quantified among these CD3+ cells. Intracellular cytokine profile was used to quantify Th1 cells by identifying IFN-γ+ label only, Th2 cells marked with IL-4+, IL-10+, Th17 with IL-21+ only and Tregs labeled for only IL-10+.

In vitro Stimulation of Splenic T Cells

Splenic cells separated as described above were suspended in 5 ml cell staining buffer (BioLegend #420201). All further treatments were done in this buffer. After counting live cells, splenocytes from each mouse were labeled with 1:50 dilutions of APC.Cy7 anti-NK1.1 mouse antibodies (BioLegend #108724), and anti-mouse CD45 coupled with PE (BioLegend #103106). Anti-NK1.1 mouse monoclonal IgGa2 antibodies (PK136 clone), binds to mouse FcR+ cells such as high affinity FcγRI possessing macrophages and neutrophils, and cells that are primarily involved in inflammatory response and display low affinity FcγRII and FcγRIII on myeloid cells and platelets (58). Since NK1.1 marker is lacking in C3H mice, anti-NK1.1 mouse monoclonal antibodies helped us quantify splenic FcR+ cells because Fc rather than Fab region of antibodies bound to the cells. DAPI (1 mg/ml) was also included in the buffer at 1:50 dilution to separate dead cells. Cell suspensions were incubated on ice in dark for 30 min for staining. After washing three times with the buffer by centrifugation at 350 xg for 5 min each, cell pellets were suspended in 1 ml buffer and 5 samples from each mouse group pooled. Cell sorting was done using BD AREA II (BD Biosciences) by first gating for appropriate cell size, then for DAPI negative, live cells followed for APC.Cy7 positive in first tube, and PE positive cells for the second tube.

For *in vitro* stimulation, six aliquots of 50,000 cells suspended in 200 μl of RPMI with 10% FBS and 5% penicillin-streptomycin (cell suspension medium) were prepared for pooled cells from spleens from each mouse group in 96-well plate. Three wells served as untreated control and the other three replicates treated with 100 ng/ml phorbol 12 myristate 13-acetate (PMA) for stimulation, 1 μg/ml ionomycin to increase intracellular levels of calcium, 5 μg/ml monestin as protein transport blocker that helps retention of intracellular cytokines in stimulated lymphoid

Age-Related Differential Stimulation of Immune Response by Babesia microti and Borrelia...

63

cells in the Golgi complex and 5 μg/ml brefeldin A, a lactone antiviral that inhibits protein transport from the endoplasmic reticulum to the Golgi apparatus, i.e., in the presence of the mixture of ionomycin-monestin-brefeldin A or IMB. The plates were incubated at 37°C with 5% CO_2 for 10 h. Cells from each well were transferred to 4 ml tube and wells washed twice to recover all untreated/treated cells. After centrifugation at 350 xg for 5 min, supernatant was removed and cells washed twice with cell staining buffer. Cell pellets were then resuspended in 1 ml buffer and then stained for surface markers using 1:50 dilution of anti-mouse CD4 antibodies labeled with FITC (BioLegend #100406) and anti-mouse CD8a antibodies labeled with AlexaFluor 647 (BioLegend #100724) by incubation on ice in dark for 30 min. After three washings, cells were fixed using BioLegend Intracellular Flow Cytometry Staining protocol. Briefly, after two incubations of cells in 0.5 ml of fixation buffer at room temperature for 20 min in dark, cells were recovered by centrifugation, washed twice in 1 × Intracellular Staining and Permeabilization Wash Buffer (BioLegend #421002). Cocktail of 1:50 dilution of anti-mouse IFN-γ antibodies labeled with Pacific Blue (BioLegend #505818), anti-TNF-α antibodies labeled with APC.Cy7 (BioLegend #506344), anti-IL-21 antibodies labeled with e-Fluor 711 (ThermoFisher #50-7211-82), anti-IL-10 antibodies labeled with PerCP/Cy5.5 (BioLegend #505028) and IL-4 coupled with Brilliant Violet 605 (BioLegend #504125) was prepared and after adding to cells in each tube, incubated at room temperature in dark for 20 min to mark intracellular cytokines present in each cell type. Cells were then washed twice using 2 ml buffer to remove unbound antibodies and then resuspended in 0.5 ml of cell staining buffer for Flow cytometry. Cell identifications were carried out on BD LSRFortessa™ X-20 (BD Biosciences) driven by software FACS DiVa (BD Biosciences). Acquired data was analyzed using FloxJo, software Version 10.3.

B. microti Protein Extract Preparation

When parasitemia in infected C3H/SCID mice reached to approximately 30%, blood was collected and centrifuged at 2,000 ×g at 4°C for 5 min. Free parasites that were released were recovered from the supernatant by centrifugation at 10,000 ×g for 5 min. The remaining RBC pellet was treated with 0.15% saponin on ice for 30 min and centrifuged at 2,900 ×g for 25 min to recover the parasite pellet. The pellet was washed three times with ice cold PBS by centrifugation at 10,000 ×g for 5 min and resuspended in 1.5 ml of 5 mM MgCl2 solution in PBS in an Eppendorf tube. Parasites were treated with detergent to lyse and incubated with 10 μl DNAse at 37 C for 30 min. The antigen preparation was kept frozen at −20°C and was thawed to use in ELISA.

Humoral Response

ELISA was used to determine antibody response against each pathogen. Plates were coated with either 50 μL B. burgdorferi N40 lysate or with B. microti total protein extract (concentration adjusted to 0.3 mg/ml) and incubated at 37°C overnight. Wells without protein coating (buffer only) were included as controls. Plates were then blocked with 1% BSA containing PBS for

1 h and then incubated for 1 h with plasma recovered from all mice diluted at 1:5,000 for B. burgdorferi or 1:200 for B. microti. After washing three times with PBS containing 5% Tween-20 (PBST), bound mouse antibodies were reacted with 1:2,500 anti-mouse-IgG HRP-conjugated secondary antibody. After washing with PBST, 50 μL of TMB substrate (KPL SureBlue, #520001) was added to each well to detect antibody reactivity. Absorbance was measured at OD_{620} using a SpectraMax M2 plate reader.

Statistical Analysis

All data collected was analyzed by Prism version 8.0 for Mac, GraphPad Software (La Jolla, CA). Data is presented as mean ± standard deviation (s.d.). Comparisons were made between groups using one-way ANOVA with binomial 95% confidence interval. In post-hoc analysis, when ANOVA P-value was below 0.05, unpaired, two-tailed student t-tests with Welch's correction for unequal s.d. was conducted to determine significant differences between respective groups. Thus, values below 0.05 were considered statistically significant for a paired group comparison at 95% confidence interval. Two tailed unpaired parametric student t-test was used to compare two variables between groups, and P-values bellow 0.05 were found to be statistically significant.

RESULTS

Effect of Coinfections on B. microti Parasitemia in C3H Mice

In our initial experiment, young mice infected with B. microti alone, or coinfected with B. microti and N40 exhibited similar temporal patterns of parasitemia such that peak parasitemia was reached on 13th day post infection. In that experiment, peak parasitemia levels were significantly higher by ~10% in mice infected with B. microti as compared to coinfected mice while difference was not significant in old mice (data not shown). Based upon this data, we selected time points here for euthanasia at acute phase before peak parasitemia was obtained. We show here that on 11th day post infection, there was no statistically significant difference in parasitemia levels between single and coinfected young mice (Figure 1A). Older mice previously showed delay in development of parasitemia after B. microti infection (59). We conducted experiments here to determine age-related differences in the host immune response at acute phase of both infections to find reason for differences between young and old mice later in infection. In our experiment with 30-week old mice, parasitemia developed slightly slower as compared to young infected mice because 20%parasitemia was obtained on 17th day compared to on 11th day in young mice (Figure 1B). These results agree with previous finding of delayed peak parasitemia in old B. microti infected mice (60). Therefore, we euthanized mice when the parasitemia reached ~20% in young and old mice, i.e., on 11th and 17th day post-infection, respectively (Figures 1A,B).

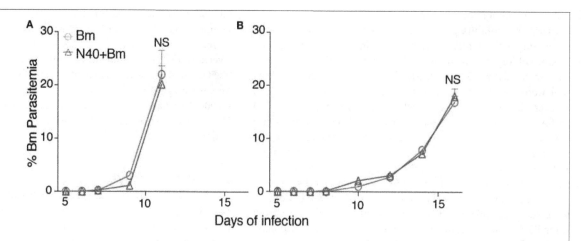

FIGURE 1 | *B. microti* (Bm) and *B. burgdorferi* (N40) coinfection and their impact on the host. **(A)** Bm parasitemia in young female C3H mice at different time points until euthanasia at 11th day post-infection. Each point represents average parasitemia in each group of mice (mean ± s.d.) **(B)** Determination of parasitemia in *B. microti* infected and coinfected old female mice until euthanasia on 17th day post-infection. In each case **(A,B)**, mice were euthanized when parasitemia was ~20%.

B. microti-Mediated Splenomegaly and Hepatomegaly During Acute Phase of Infection

We examined the effect of *B. microti* infection on liver and spleen of mice during acute phase because these organs of the reticuloendothelial system are also involved in clearance of blood-borne pathogens and help in disease resolution (61, 62). Damaged or parasitized erythrocytes are also removed from circulation by macrophages located primarily within these organs. Although spleen size was slightly larger in N40 infected vs. naïve young mice at 11 days post-infection (**Figure 2A**), size of spleen was not significantly different in old N40 infected mice (**Figure 2B**). In young mice, moderate but significant splenomegaly was observed in *B. microti* infected and coinfected mice (**Figure 2A**) while pronounced splenomegaly was apparent in the old mice (**Figure 2B**). Surprisingly, we did not see a change in the size of liver in any infected mouse group at this stage of infection (data not shown).

We previously showed that marginal zone disappears 3 weeks after infection with *B. microti* (53). Our results here show that disruption of marginal zone starts during the acute phase of *B. microti* infection (**Figures 2C,E**) and erosion of marginal zone is more pronounced during coinfection of both in young and old C3H mice (**Figures 2D,F**). Both young and old mice infected with *B. burgdorferi* alone show normal splenic architecture (data not shown). These results suggest that changes in splenic immunity modulation also begin at the acute stage of infection, particularly in response to protozoan infection. Therefore, we further examined the splenic innate and adaptive immune response more in detail at this stage.

Effect of *B. burgdorferi* and *B. microti* on Splenic Leukocytes at Acute Phase of Infection

To determine the effect of each infection on splenic cells that affects parasitemia development and Lyme spirochetes

colonization before adaptive immune response establishment, total splenocytes were analyzed by flow cytometry during pre-peak parasitemia (upward incline phase of parasitemia) and acute phase of Lyme disease (**Table 1**). To understand the impact of innate immune response during infections, we first analyzed numbers of macrophages. A significant increase in myeloid cell numbers in infected as compared to naïve mice was noticed in young mice with total macrophage numbers increased at higher levels in *B. microti* infected or coinfected young mice (27.6 and 28.9%) relative to N40 infected and naïve mice (18.1 and 7.79%) while increase in macrophage numbers in old infected mice (7–9%) was not as pronounced (**Figure 3B**). Moreover, in both single and coinfection macrophage numbers were significantly higher in young compared to old mice (N40 infection p-value = 0.0286; *B. microti* infection p-value = 0.0008; coinfection p-value < 0.0001). A significant proliferation in FcR+, representing primarily phagocytic cell total numbers and their percent in young and old infected mice suggests that these cells are potentially involved in clearance of both *B. burgdorferi* and *B. microti* at acute phase of infection in young and old mice (**Table 1**). Only N40 infection of young mice resulted in production of significantly higher FcR+ cells compared to old mice (p value = 0.0407). Statistically significant increase in CD3+ T cells was observed in all infected young but not old mice with highest change in total T cells observed in *B. microti* infected and coinfected young mice relative to naïve mice (**Table 1**). In contrast, there was almost no change in CD19+ B cells in young mice compared to controls, and greatest change in B cells were observed in N40 and *B. microti* infected old mice individually (approximately 3-fold and 2-fold increase, respectfully) relative to naïve mice that reduced significantly (from 14.3 and 11.2% to 8.32%) during coinfection with these pathogens (**Table 1**). Although the CD19+ proliferation varied greatly among old single and coinfected mice, still these numbers are statistically higher than in young infected mice with the same pathogens (N40 infection p-value < 0.0001; *B. microti* infection p-value < 0.0001; coinfection p-value = 0.0063). Not surprising, the numbers of CD4+ and CD8+ cells remained similar to naïve

Age-Related Differential Stimulation of Immune Response by Babesia microti and Borrelia...

65

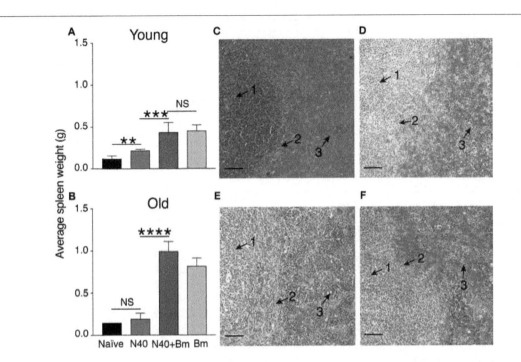

FIGURE 2 | B. microti (Bm) infection causes enlargement of the spleen in both young and old C3H mice at acute phase of infection. **(A)** Spleen weights of Bm infected and coinfected mice showed a significant increase over spleens of N40 infected mice on 11th day of infection in young mice, and **(B)** on 17th (pre-peak parasitemia) day of infection in 30 weeks old mice. Each bar represents the mean ± s.d. (*p <0.01, ***p < 0.001, ****p < 0.001). **(C–F)** H & E stained spleen sections showed erosion of marginal zone (arrow 2) between white (arrow 1) and red pulp (arrow 3) regions in B. microti infected **(C)** young, and **(E)** old mice. Disruption of marginal zone was found to have progressed more significantly in coinfected **(D)** young, and **(F)** old mice at this stage of infection, resulting in the absence of clear demarcation between red and white pulp in these **(D,F)** mice. Bar in microscopic images represents 100 μm.

mice, without any statistically significant difference between young and old mice at this stage of infections. These results suggest differential splenic T and B cell response to infection with B. microti and B. burgdorferi in young vs. old mice at acute phase of infection.

The pattern observed with total splenic cells was also reflected in the percentage of each cell type. One representative infected mouse from each group with data normalized to 5,000 cells is shown in **Figure 3A**. In sets of old mice, infection with N40 caused a significant and most pronounced increase in CD19+ B cells likely because it was a little later in infection (17th day post-infection) as compared to young mice (11th day of infection). B cells percentage also increased in B. microti infected old mice (11.2%) but not as high as that after N40 infection (14.3%). Increase in total CD3+ T cell percentage was moderately but significantly higher in N40 infected as compared to the naïve young mice with p-values of 0.021 (**Figure 3B**). A significantly higher stimulation of CD3+ cells in B. microti infected and coinfected young mice (with p < 0.0001 for both) indicates that T cells could play a prominent role in elimination of the intracellular protozoan pathogens. Although the previous reports showed that CD4+ cells are critical for clearance of B. microti infected erythrocytes (47, 63), the change in total CD4+ T cell percentage was neither significantly different in infected young nor old mice as compared to the uninfected controls (**Figures 3A,B**) suggesting that during pre-adaptive immune response development period at which point this

experiment was concluded, CD4+ T cells were not yet fully stimulated.

Response of Splenic T-Helper (TH), CD4+ Cells During Acute Phase of Infection

The experimental scheme for determining different cytokines production after *in vitro* stimulation by PMA+IMB, and identification of different types of CD4+ cells is shown in **Figure 4**. Briefly, to understand the priming and T-cell mediated immune mechanism involved during acute phase of infection, we stained splenocytes with anti-CD45 antibodies to label all leukocytes and NK1.1 for FcR+ cells, and cells sorted by FACS. The remaining leukocytes mixtures containing macrophages, CD4+ and CD8+ cells were used for *in vitro* stimulation with PMA+IMB. After stimulation, cells were marked with individual cell-type markers, then fixed, permeabilized and stained for different intracellular cytokines. **Figure 4** shows the example of CD4+ cells producing each cytokine, data for which is shown in **Figure 5A**, and outline for identification of each category of CD4+ cell type based upon specific or combination of cytokines production with results shown in **Figure 5B**. Furthermore, various cytokines production by the sorted and stimulated CD8+ cells from infected and naïve, young and old, mice were also determined (top right of **Figure 4**) and results are shown in **Figure 6**.

CD4+ cell numbers that produced IL-10 were not significantly different between uninfected naïve and various

TABLE 1 | Analyses of splenocytes and determination of lymphocytes and myeloid cells by flow cytometry at parasitemia between 15 and 20%.

	Young (Average values)				Old (Average values)			
	Cells	Total No	Percentage		Cells	Total No	Percentage	t-test Young vs. Old, p-values
N40	Splenocytes	89446.8	89.4		Splenocytes	89891.0	89.9	
	F4/80	16187.0	18.1		F4/80	7832.3	8.71	0.0286(*)
	Nk1.1/FcR+	38793.6	43.4		Nk1.1/FcR+	36438.8	40.5	0.0407(*)
	CD19	2548.6	2.83		CD19	12855.7	14.3	<0.0001(****)
	CD3	6299.6	7.04		CD3	4073.3	4.53	0.0117(*)
	CD8a	1311.2	1.46		CD8a	1661.3	1.85	0.7278(NS)
	CD4	2333.4	2.59		CD4	3780.0	4.20	0.2127(NS)
N40+Bm	Splenocytes	90755.6	90.8		Splenocytes	92252.6	92.3	
	F4/80	26300.0	28.9		F4/80	6901.3	7.48	<0.0001(****)
	Nk1.1/FcR+	37486.8	41.3		Nk1.1/FcR+	38820.0	42.1	0.2876(NS)
	CD19	2742.0	3.02		CD19	7679.0	8.32	0.0063(**)
	CD3	10599.0	11.7		CD3	3091.3	3.35	<0.0001(****)
	CD8a	2225.8	2.45		CD8a	1750.3	1.89	0.4594(NS)
	CD4	4459.4	4.91		CD4	3062.5	3.32	0.5896(NS)
Bm	Splenocytes	90480.2	90.5		Splenocytes	98637.2	98.6	
	F4/80	25000.6	27.6		F4/80	9461.5	9.59	0.0008(***)
	Nk1.1/FcR+	37720.8	41.7		Nk1.1/FcR+	41822.2	42.4	0.1853(NS)
	CD19	3107.8	3.44		CD19	11047.4	11.2	0.0130(*)
	CD3	9758.7	10.8		CD3	3915.9	3.97	0.0001(***)
	CD8a	2104.0	2.32		CD8a	1361.2	1.38	0.0716(NS)
	CD4	4192.4	4.64		CD4	3166.3	3.21	0.1251(NS)
Naïve	Splenocytes	82605.6	82.6		Splenocytes	85431	85.4	
	F4/80	6436.7	7.79		F4/80	5007	5.86	
	Nk1.1/FcR+	30209.4	36.5		Nk1.1/FcR+	15922	28.7	
	CD19	1876.0	2.26		CD19	4268	4.99	
	CD3	3507.7	4.24		CD3	4678	5.47	
	CD8a	837.3	1.01		CD8a	1364	1.59	
	CD4	3319.2	4.02		CD4	2857	3.34	

Statistical analyses: (*p < 0.05, **p <0.01, ***p <0.001, ****p <0.0001, NS-Not significant).

infected old mice. Whereas, young coinfected mice have significantly higher number of CD4+ cells produced IL-10 as compared to naïve mice. At the same time the level of cells producing IL-10 was significantly lower in mice infected with N40 and *B. microti* individually (**Figure 5A**). Even untreated CD4+ cells from uninfected and infected mice produced IL-10 but increase in numbers of these IL-10 producing cells was higher in young N40 infected and coinfected mice as compared to *B. microti* infected mice. IL-10 producing cell numbers were indistinguishable in uninfected and infected old mice. After *in vitro* stimulation, a significantly higher number of CD4+ T cells obtained from all infected mice irrespective of age showed production of TNF-α, IFN-γ, IL-4, and IL-21 as compared to the cells from naïve uninfected mice demonstrating high proliferation of T cells as a response on infection with N40 and *B. microti* individually or together. Surprisingly, increase in stimulated CD4+ cells producing IL-4 and IL-21 cytokines was higher in young as compared to all respective old infected mice. IFN-γ producing CD4+ cells representing Th1 cells were

particularly higher in response to infection of young mice with *B. microti* after *in vitro* stimulation. This response is likely due to the high levels of *B. burgdorferi* lipoproteins presence, thus offering a potent proinflammatory ligand to induce Th1 polarization and also potentially by yet to be identified Pathogen Associated Membrane Patterns (PAMPs) of *B. microti* (**Figure 5A**).

Th1 cellular proliferation and response (**Figure 5B**) demonstrated by intracellular IFN-γ production was most pronounced in both young and old mice infected with *B. microti* early in infection indicating that these cells likely play important role in resolution of parasitemia. Increase in Th1 cells was also significant in N40 infected and coinfected mice suggesting contribution of these cells in potential clearance of both pathogens during acute phase of infection. Interestingly, Th2 cells increase in response to both infections was higher in old mice compared to naïve mice, suggesting a faster activation by more mature and fully developed immune system in these mice. Th2 response was highest in response to N40 infection followed by that in *B. microti* infected old mice; however, IL-4

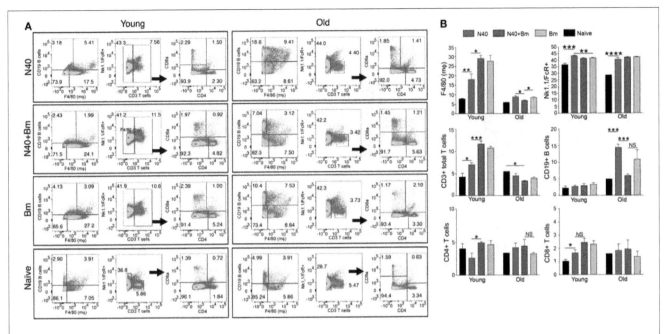

FIGURE 3 | N40 and *B. microti* infection affects splenic leukocytes of young and old mice differently. **(A)** Analyses of one young and one old representative mouse spleen cells from each infection group is shown at 11th and 17th day post-infection, respectively. **(B)** Although percentage of all splenic leukocytes increased in infected mice, growth was highest in B cells in N40 infected old mice, CD3+ T cells in young *B. microti* and coinfected mice, and CD8+ T cells in all young infected mice. Macrophage increased most prominently in *B. microti* infected and coinfected young mice while total FcR+ cells increased in all young and old infected mice. Each bar represents the mean ± s.d. (*$p < 0.05$, **$p < 0.01$, ***$p < 0.001$, ****$p < 0.0001$).

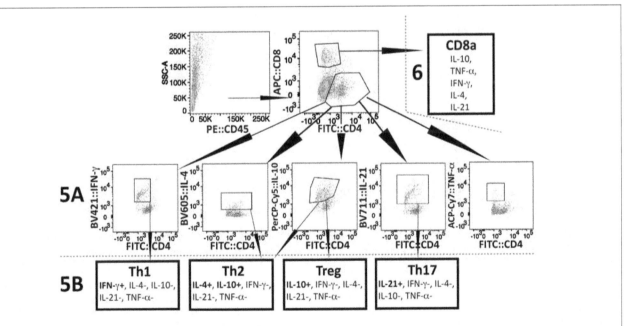

FIGURE 4 | Scheme of Flow-based quantification of various intracellular cytokines production, and of different types of CD4+ cell, and different cytokine producing CD8+ cells in infected mice after *in vitro* stimulation with PMA+IMB. After cell sorting for CD45+ cells (top left), cells were stimulated and then marked with antibodies against mouse CD4 (FITC), and CD8 (AF 647) cells (top center). Cells were then fixed, permeabilized, and stained for intracellular cytokines: IFN-γ-PB, TNF-α-APC.Cy7, IL-21-e-Fluor 711, IL-10-PerCP/Cy5.5, and IL-4-BV605 (2nd row). Then CD4+ cells producing different cytokines were quantified (results presented in **Figure 5A**). In CD4+ subpopulation, cells that were positive for IFN-γ, but negative for other four cytokines were identified as Th1 cells (bottom left). CD4+ cells that had IL-10 but no other cytokines were defined as Tregs, whereas cells producing both IL-4 and IL-10 cytokines, but not IL-21, IFN-γ, and TNF-α were identified as Th2 (bottom center two boxes). CD4+ cells that produced only IL-21 were identified as Th17 (bottom right) and results are presented in **Figure 5B**. CD8 cells producing different cytokines are presented in **Figure 6**.

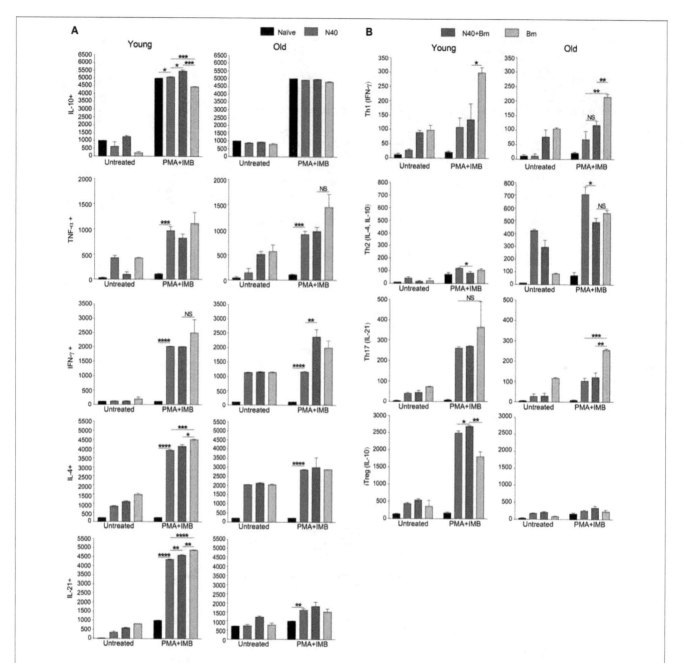

FIGURE 5 | Delineation and quantification of different types of CD4+ T cells based upon their cytokines production by FACS after *ex-vivo* stimulation of splenic leukocytes by PMA. Intracellular cytokines transport blockers IMB were included during stimulation. **(A)** Various cytokines, IL-10, TNF-α, IFN-γ, IL-4, and IL-21 producing CD4+ T cells increased significantly in young mice after PMA stimulation while high levels of IFN-γ and IL-4 cytokine producing CD4+ T cells are observed in old mice even without PMA stimulation. High numbers of IL-10 cytokine producing CD4+ cells were observed in all young and old mice irrespective of infection. **(B)** Th1 response was stimulated in all infected mice with most pronounced change in T cells of *B. microti* infected mice after PMA stimulation. Th2 response was most pronounced in all infected old C3H mice. High Th17 cells stimulation in young infected mice could indicate inflammatory response; however, a much higher Tregs response in these mice appears to maintain splenic immune cells homeostasis preventing fatal disease. Lowest ratio of Tregs/Th17 cells was observed in old *B. microti* infected mice but mice did not appear sick or lethargic at this stage of infection. Each bar represents the mean ± s.d. (*p < 0.05, **p <0.01, ***p <0.001, ****p <0.0001).

production only occurred after *in vitro* stimulation. Analysis of CD4+ cells after PMA stimulation showed highest Th1 response by *B. microti* infected mice cells as seen in other intracellular protozoa in both young and old mice (**Figure 5B**) that could not be detected in the unstimulated fresh splenocytes (**Table 2**).

More pronounced Th2 response was observed in spleens of old mice with and without PMA stimulation (**Figure 5B**, **Table 2**).

We analyzed splenic leukocytes based upon surface markers and respective cytokines production to further determine the specific T helper cell types that increase in numbers during

Age-Related Differential Stimulation of Immune Response by Babesia microti and Borrelia...

69

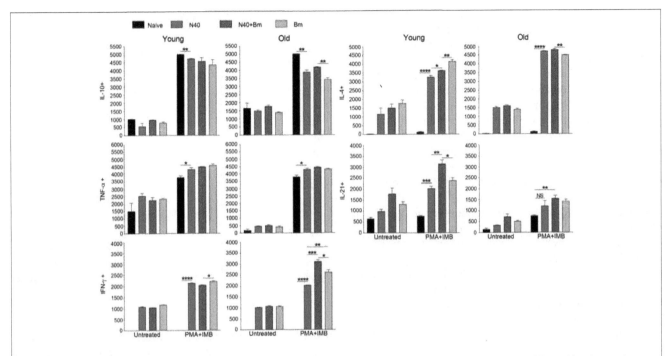

FIGURE 6 | Analysis of splenic CD8+ cells from young and old mice collected at acute phase and stimulated *ex-vivo* by PMA. Intracellular cytokines transport blockers IMB were included during stimulation. Response of CD8+ T cells observed in young mice infected with *B. microti*, N40 or both was comparable to respective infected old mice except IL-21 producing cells numbers were higher in young infected mice. Each bar represents the mean ± s.d. (*p <0.05, **p <0.01, ***p <0.001, ****p <0.0001).

infection with N40 and *B. microti*. Increase in Th17 and T-regulatory (Treg) cells were observed in all young infected mice as compared to the naïve mice. Interestingly, Th17 cells proliferation was most pronounced in *B. microti* infected old mice and was more than double in numbers of those observed in old mice infected with either N40 or *B. microti* alone. Increase in Th17 cells in N40 infected and coinfected mice were significantly higher as compared to naïve mice after stimulation with PMA (**Figure 5B**). High ratio of Tregs/Th17 fresh splenocytes in N40 infected and coinfected young mice, 9.5 ± 0.53 and 9.84 ± 0.04, respectively at acute phase of infection suggests maintenance of immune homeostasis in spleen of these mice that prevents excessive inflammation by these infections (**Table 2**). Even though ratio of Tregs/Th17 was not as high (6.19 ± 0.63) in *B. microti* infected young mice, it was sufficient to prevent excessive inflammation by Th17 cells. Increase in Tregs was substantially lower in all infected old mice with Tregs/Th17 ratio of 2.44 ± 0.25, 2.88 ± 0.73, and 0.89 ± 0.29 in N40 infected, coinfected and *B. microti* infected mice, respectively. Th17 stimulation was highest in old *B. microti* infected mice suggesting possible occurrence of a more severe splenic pathology at later day of infection.

Cytokines Production by CD8+ Cells During Acute Phase of N40 and *B. microti* Infection

PMA stimulated CD8+ cells producing IL-10 and TNF-α between uninfected naïve and various infected young or old mice were similar in numbers (**Figure 6**); however, higher cell

numbers producing IL-10 and TNF-α were detected after PMA stimulation. More of CD8+ T cells obtained from all infected mice irrespective of age showed production of IFN-γ, and IL-4 after PMA stimulation as compared to the cells from naïve uninfected mice demonstrating that infection with N40 and *B. microti* individually or together caused priming and proliferation of these T cells in mice that increased further on *in vitro* stimulation. Interestingly, IL-21 producing CD8+ cells were significantly higher in numbers in young as compared to old infected mice even without PMA treatment.

Lyme Disease at Acute Phase of Infection

We were able to recover live spirochetes by culture into BSK-RS from all tissues examined from mice infected with N40 alone, or with *B. microti* from the skin at the injection site, ear, blood, and urinary bladder. We observed light emission due to the presence of bioluminescent spirochetes in joints and head region of N40 infected and coinfected mice on the day of euthanasia (**Figure 7A**). Brain colonization by *B. burgdorferi* N40 strain has been reported in mice in studies conducted in early nineties (64–66); however thorough investigation of brain colonization has not been conducted until now. Therefore, to further assess the burden of *B. burgdorferi* in joints and potentially brain, we isolated DNA from these organs and conducted duplex qPCR (**Figure 7B**). Spirochete copy number normalized to 10^5 mouse nidogen copies indicated high *B. burgdorferi* burden in joints and brain of all mice infected with N40 alone or coinfected with *B. microti*, likely because mice have not yet fully developed adaptive immune response that is critical for clearance of extracellular spirochetes. N40 quantities were slightly higher in young as compared to old mice. Interestingly, young coinfected mice showed significantly higher *B. burgdorferi* burden in joints relative to those in the N40 infected mice.

Although we found high burden of spirochetes in joints, inflammation in tibiotarsus was not yet fully developed in N40 infected young or old mice (**Table 3**, **Figure 7C**). Coinfected young mice showed more pronounced inflammation with 2/5 mice showing maximum (+++) arthritic severity and 3/5 with moderate (++) inflammatory arthritis (**Table 3**). Neither N40 infected, nor coinfected old mice showed joints swelling visually and exhibited only moderate arthritis in some mice such that all criteria demonstrating fully developed arthritis were not detected. Lymphocytes infiltration was observed in the tibiotarsus of old N40 infected mice, but they did not show as pronounced synovial hyperplasia, erosion of cartilage, and change in synovial space as observed in 2/5 young coinfected mice despite euthanasia of old mice at 17th day post-infection as compared to the 11th day of infection of young mice (**Figure 7C** top vs. bottom, and **Table 3**). Carditis was not observed in either young or old mice either infected with N40 alone, or coinfected with *B. microti*.

Immunomodulation of Humoral Response by *B. microti*

At 3 weeks of infection, antibody response against both pathogens could be detected. Antibody production by B cells is facilitated by CD4+ T helper cells. To determine the effect of significant and consistent reduction in splenic B and T cells caused by *B. microti* infection on *B. burgdorferi* and to determine association of the pathogen specific antibodies production with the change in percentage of B cells, we used ELISA to determine reactivity of mouse antibodies to total protein extract of N40 strain or *B. microti* coated on plates as antigenic cocktail. There was a significant reduction in absorbance when plasma from coinfected young mice were used as compared to plasma from young mice infected with *B. burgdorferi* alone, indicating apparent subversion of the humoral immune response against *B. burgdorferi* by *B. microti* only in young mice (**Figure 8**). A moderate but significant decrease in antibody production against *B. microti* was also observed in coinfected as compared to *B. microti* infected young mice. The specific antibody reactivity against each pathogen was comparable among old mice infected by each pathogen individually and coinfected. However, Overall antibody production against each pathogen was lower in the older mice. Although slightly higher burden of spirochetes was observed in young N40 infected and coinfected mice as compared to old mice, this data is not sufficient to explain the reason for the lack of inflammatory Lyme disease manifestations observed here or was previously reported in old C3H mice (51).

DISCUSSION

Our studies here demonstrate the age-related immune response against two tick-borne pathogens in the susceptible C3H mice. Reduction in erythrocytes population observed in

TABLE 2 | Specific splenic CD4+ cells response in Naïve and infected young and old mice.

	Average ± SD			
Young	**Naïve**	**N40**	**N40 + Bm**	**Bm**
Treg	164.7 ± 48.4	2492.0 ± 103.2	2681.0 ± 37.5	1809.0 ± 243.7
Th17	8.33 ± 2.08	262.7 ± 12.4	271.7 ± 5.03	366.3 ± 41.5
Treg/Th17	31.7 ± 9.77	9.50 ± 0.53	9.84 ± 0.04	6.19 ± 0.63
Th1	21.0 ± 6.08	108.0 ± 9.54	168.3 ± 19.7	298.3 ± 31.0
Th2	71.3 ± 25.7	121.7 ± 7.51	83.7 ± 12.1	106.7 ± 18.8
Th1/Th2	0.30 ± 0.03	0.87 ± 0.43	2.03 ± 0.47	2.82 ± 0.23
Old				
Treg	164.7 ± 48.4	248.7 ± 46.4	336.3 ± 97.6	229.7 ± 82.6
Th17	15.0 ± 3.61	103.3 ± 15.9	121.3 ± 14.5	255.3 ± 10.5
Treg/Th17	10.9 ± 0.56	2.44 ± 0.25	2.88 ± 0.73	0.89 ± 0.29
Th1	21.0 ± 6.08	68.0 ± 20.2	117.3 ± 25.7	215.3 ± 17.01
Th2	71.33 ± 19.0	706.7 ± 107.8	490.0 ± 55.05	560.7 ± 41.8
Th1/Th2	0.39 ± 0.22	0.09 ± 0.06	0.24 ± 0.03	0.38 ± 0.006

blood of *B. microti* infected mice agree with that previously reported in gerbils infected with *B. divergens* (67). Hematologic abnormalities, such as anemia and thrombocytopenia are also associated with babesiosis in humans, often requiring blood transfusion and even hospitalization (19, 68, 69). To evaluate differences between old and young mice, we determined host response to each infection at acute phase. Immune response at this stage affects peak parasitemia and inflammatory Lyme disease later in infection. For example, a lower peak *B. microti* parasitemia was observed later in infection in coinfected as compared to *B. microti* young infected mice and not in old mice suggesting that innate immune response at early phase of infection against *B. burgdorferi* in young susceptible mice, likely induced by abundance of spirochetal lipoproteins and TLR2 signaling, contributes to decrease in erythrocytic infection cycles by this protozoan only in these mice (data not shown).

Splenic immunity plays an important role in resolution of parasitic diseases. For example, splenomegaly shown here irrespective of age of mice and reported previously during infection with *B. microti* has also been observed on infection with other vector-borne, blood protozoan pathogens, such as *Trypanosoma congolense*, *Plasmodium falciparum*, and *Plasmodium yoeli* and can even lead to rupture of spleen in humans (49, 70–76) demonstrating consistent splenic involvement in response to various parasitic diseases (67, 77–79). In humans, babesiosis can be a life-threatening disease particularly in the elderly, immunodeficient or immunosuppressed and in asplenic patients, further emphasizing the importance of the spleen in babesiosis resolution (13, 80). In acute phase, we observed moderate but significant splenomegaly in *B. microti* infected and coinfected young mice (**Figure 2A**) while pronounced splenomegaly was apparent in the old mice (**Figure 2B**). This is likely because it took longer to reach the same level of parasitemia in these mice (euthanasia at 17th day post-infection rather than 11th day), allowing spleen to clear parasitized and damaged blood cells for slightly longer

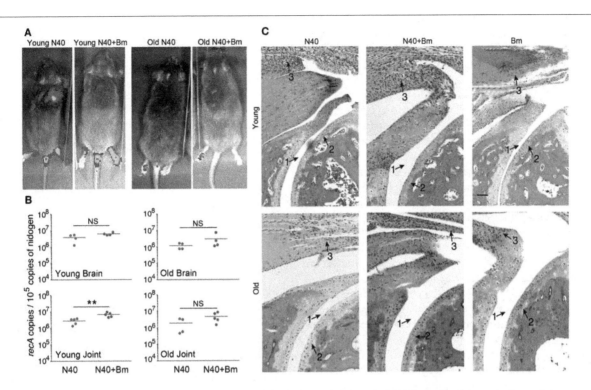

FIGURE 7 | *B. microti* (Bm) and N40 coinfection increases colonization of joints by *B. burgdorferi* causing joint inflammation during acute phase only in young mice. **(A)** Although significant spirochetes-associated bioluminescence was observed in joints and brains of both young and old infected mice, **(B)** burden of N40 was significantly (**p < 0.01) higher in joint of coinfected compared to N40 infected young mice. **(C)** *B. burgdorferi* infection causes only mild inflammation of the joints at acute phase of disease as indicated by synovial hyperplasia and erosion of cartilage (arrow 2), lymphocytic infiltration (arrow 3) and change in synovial space (arrow 1) while respective markers show higher inflammation in coinfected young mice. Although lymphocytes infiltration is observed in old mice, cartilage erosion and change in synovial space was not noticeable in joints of different mice. Bar represents 100 μm in all panels.

period and thus, causing a significant enlargement of spleen. The inflammation of liver in response to *B. divergens* infection has been reported to occur due to hemorrhage, hyperplasia of Kupffer cells and infiltration of lymphocytes (67, 81). Our observation of the absence of hepatomegaly in C3H mice infected with *B. microti* alone or with N40 (data not shown) agrees with that reported in rats (82). We did not visually observe any difference in vitality of these two sets of young or old mice suggesting that either the effect of age on babesiosis is minimum in mice or the difference becomes more obvious only in very old mice (≥18 months).

Innate immune response is critical to curb various infectious diseases. Aguilar-Delfin showed that innate immunity is crucial for determining the fate of *Babesia* infection and development of resistance to babesiosis in mice (83). Since the spleen is a major reservoir of undifferentiated, immature monocytes in mice that can mature into macrophages and dendritic cells *in vitro* (84), it is conceivable that infection of mice with *B. microti* could result in development of these cells *in vivo* into macrophages, which then facilitate clearance of the infected erythrocytes. Indeed, IFN-γ stimulated macrophages have been considered critical for inhibiting growth of *B. microti* and for offering cross-protection against *B. rodhaini* in mice (85, 86). Depletion of macrophages at different stages of infection using drugs resulted in a significant increase in *B. microti* parasitemia and even led to mortality

TABLE 3 | Histopathological scoring of joints of mice at acute phase of infection.

Experimental groups	Knee			Tibiotarsus				
Score	–	±	+	–	±	+	++	+++
Young–N40	1	2	2	0	0	1	4	0
Old–N40	0	3	1	0	1	1	2	0
Young–N40+Bm	1	0	4	0	0	0	3	2
Old–N40+Bm	2	1	2	0	0	3	2	0
Young–Bm	5	0	0	5	0	0	0	0

in mice (87). Furthermore, *in vivo* depletion of NK cells did not significantly impair protection against *Babesia* species in mice, indicting their minor role in conferring resistance to this protozoan (86) further emphasizing the importance of splenic macrophages in clearance of *Babesia* infected erythrocytes.

To better understand the immunological responses during acute phase of infection, we conducted both FACS analyses and *in vitro* stimulation of splenic leukocytes (CD45 labeled) mixture excluding FcR+ cells (**Figures 3, 5, 6**). An increase in levels of innate and Th1-associated cytokines and chemokines, IFN-γ, IL-8, IL-6, and TNF-α has recently been reported in Lyme disease patients (88, 89). A positive association of type I, and III IFN with Lyme arthritis in humans and production of IFN-γ and IL-23 in response to *B. burgdorferi* infection in animal model systems has also been reported previously (90, 91). IFN-γ is also produced in response to *B. microti* infection by activated T cells that help in killing ingested pathogens by activated macrophage (92). Our results support the reported critical role of cell-mediated immunity and Type 1 cytokine response, although it may not always be sufficient in generating protective immunity for controlling intracellular protozoan pathogens (93–98). A comparison of persisting symptoms reported in humans with coinfections, such as fatigue, in which Th1 response may contribute, cannot be determined in mice to fully appreciate the consequence of concurrent infection on overall disease manifestations. We observed more prominent Th2 response in older mice. Th2 response has been known to exacerbate diseases by some protozoan pathogens and could contribute to sustenance of *B. microti* in old hosts reported previously (59, 99). Higher levels of IL-4 production in the young mice at acute phase could lead to significant stimulation of B cells and antibody production later in infection that is critical for *B. burgdorferi* clearance.

Th17 cells play an important role in inflammation as well as clearance of extracellular pathogens, including Borreliae, while they counteract the action of Tregs that prevent excessive inflammatory response caused by Th17 cells (100). Although a high level of regulatory cytokine IL-10 producing CD4+ cells were detected in both young and old mice, the cytokine was associated with Th2 cells in old and Tregs in young mice. A significant Tregs/Th17 ratio was observed during the acute phase of infection by both *B. burgdorferi* and *B. microti* individually or together in young mice. No death associated with babesiosis was observed unlike that by highly infectious WA-1 strain of *Babesia* during acute phase of infection in mice and hamsters (101–103). Mice fatality by WA-1 infection was reported to be associated with prolific pro-inflammatory response including intravascular aggregation of large mononuclear inflammatory cells and multifocal coagulative necrosis in various organs (101–103). Although we cannot determine the molecular mechanism involved, a higher Tregs/Th17 ratio in coinfected mice as compared to *B. microti* infected young mice at acute phase of infection (**Table 2**) could play a role in significantly lower peak parasitemia observed in coinfected young mice (data not shown). High levels of Tregs were also found to be associated with milder, nonlethal malaria with *Plasmodium yoelii* infection in mice, as compared to low levels of Treg cells observed during disease by the lethal strain of *P. berghei* ANKA strain (104). Higher numbers of IL-10 producing CD4+ cells (**Figure 4**) together with increased Treg cell numbers supports participation of these immune responses in suppression of excessive inflammation during simultaneous infection by *B. burgdorferi* and *B. microti* in C3H mice. Thus, despite development of high parasitemia levels by *B. microti*, combined anti-inflammatory response promoted by IL-10 and Tregs could partially explain why this infection does not result in death of mice unlike infection with *Babesia* strain WA-1, which displays fatal outcomes that showed association with the high levels of IFN-γ and TNF-α production in spleen and lungs, heavy intravascular hemolysis, and multiorgan failure (101–103).

Our results here agree with the previous report that mainly young C3H mice, but not old, show more pronounced

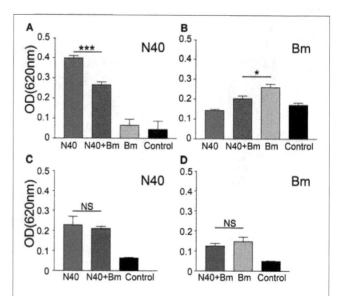

FIGURE 8 | Determination of the specific antibody response in young and old mice at 3 weeks of infection. **(A–C)** N40 protein extract probed with pooled plasma of either young **(A)**, or old **(C)** from each group of infected mice by ELISA indicated a significant reduction in the specific antibodies in plasma of only young coinfected mice with no reactivity observed with plasma from *B. microti* (Bm) infected mice. **(B–D)** Bm protein extract probed with pooled mice plasma from young **(B)**, or old **(D)** mice by ELISA showed that Bm-specific antibodies reduced significantly but moderately in coinfected mice only in young mice. Each bar represents the mean ± s.d. (*$p < 0.05$, ***$p < 0.001$).

inflammatory Lyme arthritis manifestations (51) indicating inherent development of resistance to Lyme disease in older mice. Unlike previously reported independent courses of infection by *B. burgdorferi* and *B. microti* in young C3H mice (49), we observed a major influence of *B. microti* infection on increased survival and tissue colonization by *B. burgdorferi*. Significant increase in joint colonization by *B. burgdorferi* in coinfected mice resulting in inflammatory Lyme arthritis even at acute phase indicates consequence of *B. microti* infection on increased *B. burgdorferi* survival and adverse effect on severity of inflammatory Lyme disease. B cells play a role as professional antigen presenting cells, display regulatory function through cytokine production and play a critical role in humoral immunity by producing protective antibodies. Based upon the infecting pathogen, subversion of different B-cell subsets during parasitic and viral infections has been summarized recently (105). In many protozoan diseases, specific B-cell responses against parasites were delayed or abrogated due to B cell apoptosis and their depletion in spleen (72, 106). Antibodies play an important role in clearance of *B. burgdorferi* by encompassing different effector mechanisms, such as complement activation, neutralization and opsonization that results in phagocytosis facilitated by interaction of the Fc-region of antibodies and Fc-receptors on the professional phagocytes (107). Immunoglobulin levels are elevated in response to *B. burgdorferi* infection and after antibodies maturation, they persist for long periods of time (108). We found reduction in antibody response against both *B. burgdorferi* and *B. microti* only in young coinfected

Age-Related Differential Stimulation of Immune Response by Babesia microti and Borrelia...

73

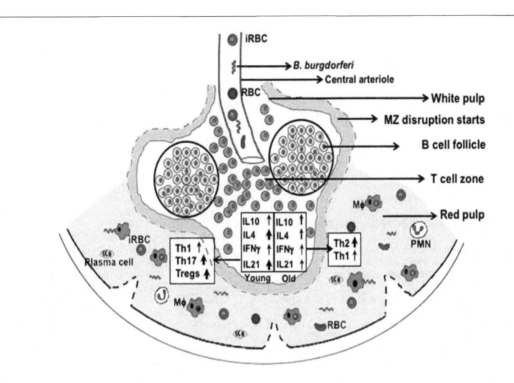

FIGURE 9 | C3H mice splenic immune response at acute phase of coinfection with *B. microti* and *B. burgdorferi*. RBCs and *B. microti* infected RBCs (iRBC) together with *B. burgdorferi* from blood are released in spleen. These pathogens then trigger a differential immune response with more pronounced induction of Th17 cells and Tregs in young mice and significantly higher Th2 cells in the older mice. Disruption of marginal zone (MZ) and atrophy of B cells are also stimulated by *B. microti* such that fewer B cells develop into plasma cells resulting in lower antibody production against both pathogens. Splenic macrophages (Mφ) are the major player in clearance of both pathogens but because of hematopoiesis and phagocytosis of iRBCs, fewer of them are available for clearance of *B. burgdorferi*, causing better survival of these spirochetes.

mice relative to those infected with each pathogen separately. Antibody reduction was most pronounced in coinfected young mice relative to N40 infected mice (**Figure 8**). This reduction could result in better survival of *B. burgdorferi* even at later stages of infection causing increase in inflammatory Lyme disease.

CONCLUSIONS

In our studies, the adverse effect of infection with N40 on *B. microti* was subtle, but we consistently observed diminished parasitemia in coinfected young C3H mice. Th2 polarization at acute phase of infection could play a more effective role in preventing Lyme disease symptoms in coinfected older mice, even at the acute phase of infection. Conversely, despite high Tregs/Th17 ratio and moderate Th1 response in spleens of coinfected young mice, inflammatory arthritis is observed, suggesting that tissue specific colonization by *B. burgdorferi* triggers different immune responses. Based upon these results and our observation of complete disruption of marginal zone of spleen after parasitemia resolution (53), we propose that both marginal zone disruption and B cell atrophy starts at the acute phase of coinfection (**Figure 9**) while *B. microti* infection

ultimately results in reduction in splenic B cells and pathogens specific antibody production. Furthermore, phagocytosis of infected RBCs and hematopoiesis in the red pulp region may overwhelm macrophages, making them less available for Lyme spirochetes phagocytosis. Thus, each pathogen affects disease severity by the other microbe directly, or indirectly by influencing the host immune response with a more pronounced effect seen in the young mice. Despite some differences observed in severity of diseases in mice and humans during coinfection with *B. burgdorferi* and *B. microti*, our results indicate that a thorough understanding of these coinfections can be obtained by study of pathogenesis and immunity at different stages of infection using the susceptible animal model system(s).

AUTHOR CONTRIBUTIONS

The first 3 authors contributed equally to this work. NP conceived the study while VD and SP designed and carried out all animal experiments. VD analyzed and interpreted FACS data, LA carried out all parasitemia determinations and ELISA and SP and MC prepared and analyzed samples as relevant to Lyme spirochetes. All authors read and approved the manuscript before submission.

ACKNOWLEDGMENTS

We acknowledge valuable assistance provided by the technical Director, Sukhwinder Singh of Flow cytometry core laboratory of Rutgers New Jersey Medical School. We also greatly appreciate assistance by Luke Fritzky and Joel Pierre in organ samples preparation, sectioning, and H & E staining for the histopathological examination.

REFERENCES

1. Cox FE. Concomitant infections, parasites and immune responses. *Parasitology* (2001) 122:S23–38. doi: 10.1017/S003118200001698X
2. Diuk-Wasser MA,Vannier E, Krause PJ. Coinfection by *Ixodes* tick-borne pathogens: ecological, epidemiological, and clinical consequences. *Trends Parasitol.* (2016) 32l:30–42. doi: 10.1016/j.pt.2015.09.008
3. Knapp KL, Rice NA. Human coinfection with *Borrelia burgdorferi* and *Babesia microti* in the United States. *J Parasitol Res.* (2015) 2015:587131. doi: 10.1155/2015/587131
4. Rizzoli A, Silaghi C, Obiegala A, Rudolf I, Hubalek Z, Foldvari G, et al. *Ixodes ricinus* and Its transmitted pathogens in urban and peri-urban areas in Europe: new hazards and relevance for public health. *Front Public Health* (2014) 2:251. doi: 10.3389/fpubh.2014.00251
5. Dunn JM, Krause PJ, Davis S, Vannier EG, Fitzpatrick MC, Rollend L, et al. *Borrelia burgdorferi* promotes the establishment of *Babesia microti* in the northeastern United States. *PLoS ONE* (2014) 9:e115494. doi: 10.1371/journal.pone.0115494
6. Moutailler S, Valiente Moro C, Vaumourin E, Michelet L, Tran FH,Devillers E, et al. Co-infection of ticks: the rule rather than the exception. *PLoS Negl Trop Dis.* (2016) 10:e0004539. doi: 10.1371/journal.pntd.0004539
7. Lommano E, Bertaiola L, Dupasquier C, Gern L. Infections and coinfections of questing *Ixodes ricinus* ticks by emerging zoonotic pathogens in Western Switzerland. *Appl Environ Microbiol.* (2012) 78:4606–12. doi: 10.1128/AEM.07961-11
8. Piesman J, Mather TN,Donahue JG,Levine J, Campbell JD,Karakashian SJ, et al. Comparative prevalence of *Babesia microti* and *Borrelia burgdorferi* in four populations of *Ixodes dammini* in eastern Massachusetts. *Acta Trop.* (1986) 43:263–70.
9. Hersh MH,Ostfeld RS,McHenry DJ,Tibbetts M, Brunner JL,Killilea ME,et al. Co-infection of blacklegged ticks with *Babesia microti* and *Borrelia burgdorferi* is higher than expected and acquired from small mammal hosts. *PLoS ONE* (2014) 9:e99348. doi: 10.1371/journal.pone.0099348
10. Schulze TL,Jordan RA,Healy SP, Roegner VE. Detection of *Babesia microti* and *Borrelia burgdorferi* in host-seeking *Ixodes scapularis* (Acari: Ixodidae) in Monmouth County, New Jersey. *J Med Entomol.* (2013) 50:379–83. doi: 10.1603/ME12088
11. Swanson SJ,Neitzel D, Reed KD, Belongia EA. Coinfections acquired from Ixodes ticks. *Clin Microbiol Rev.* (2006) 19:708–27. doi: 10.1128/CMR.00011-06
12. Krause PJ, Spielman A, Telford SR 3rd, Sikand VK, McKay K, Christianson D, et al. Persistent parasitemia after acute babesiosis. *N Engl J Med.* (1998) 339:160–5. doi: 10.1056/NEJM199807163390304
13. Krause PJ, Gewurz BE, Hill D, Marty FM, Vannier E, Foppa IM, et al. Persistent and relapsing babesiosis in immunocompromised patients. *Clin Infect Dis.* (2008) 46:370–6. doi: 10.1086/525852
14. Herwaldt BL, Linden JV, Bosserman E, Young C, Olkowska D, Wilson M. Transfusion-associated babesiosis in the United States: a description of cases. *Ann Int Med.* (2011) 155:509–19. doi: 10.7326/0003-4819-155-8-201110180-00362
15. Ruebush TK 2nd, Collins WE, Warren M. Experimental *Babesia microti* infections in *Macaca mulatta*: recurrent parasitemia before and after splenectomy. *Am J Trop Med Hyg.* (1981) 30:304–7. doi: 10.4269/ajtmh.1981.30.304
16. Wormser GP, Lombardo G, Silverblatt F, El Khoury MY, Prasad A, Yelon JA, et al. Babesiosis as a cause of fever in patients undergoing a splenectomy. *Am Surg.* (2011) 77:345–7.
17. Wudhikarn K, Perry EH, Kemperman M, Jensen KA, Kline SE. Transfusion-transmitted babesiosis in an immunocompromised patient: a case report and review. *Am J Med.* (2011) 124:800–5. doi: 10.1016/j.amjmed.2011.03.009

18. Homer MJ,Aguilar-Delfin I, Telford SR 3rd, Krause PJ, Persing DH. Babesiosis. *Clin Microbiol Rev.* (2000) 13:451–69. doi: 10.1128/CMR.13.3.451
19. White DJ, Talarico J, Chang HG, Birkhead GS, Heimberger T, Morse DL. Human babesiosis in New York State: review of 139 hospitalized cases and analysis of prognostic factors. *Arch Intern Med.* (1998) 158:2149–54. doi: 10.1001/archinte.158.19.2149
20. Shaw AC, Joshi S, Greenwood H, Panda A, Lord JM. Aging of the innate immune system. *Curr Opin Immunol.* (2010) 22:507–13. doi: 10.1016/j.coi.2010.05.003
21. Aguilar-Delfin I, Wettstein PJ, Persing DH. Resistance to acute babesiosis is associated with interleukin-12- and gamma interferon-mediated responses and requires macrophages and natural killer cells. *Infect Immun.* (2003) 71:2002–8. doi: 10.1128/IAI.71.4.2002-2008.2003
22. Beerman I, Bhattacharya D, Zandi S, Sigvardsson M, Weissman IL,Bryder D, et al. Functionally distinct hematopoietic stem cells modulate hematopoietic lineage potential during aging by a mechanism of clonal expansion. *Proc Natl Acad Sci USA.* (2010) 107:5465–70. doi: 10.1073/pnas.1000834107
23. Beerman I, Maloney WJ,Weissmann IL, Rossi DJ. Stem cells and the aging hematopoietic system. *Curr Opin Immunol.* (2010) 22:500–6. doi: 10.1016/j.coi.2010.06.007
24. Wenisch C, Patruta S, Daxbock F, Krause R, Horl W. Effect of age on human neutrophil function. *J Leukoc Biol.* (2000) 67:40–5. doi: 10.1002/jlb.67.1.40
25. Agius E, Lacy KE,Vukmanovic-Stejic M, Jagger AL, Papageorgiou AP, Hall S, et al. Decreased TNF-alpha synthesis by macrophages restricts cutaneous immunosurveillance by memory CD4+ T cells during aging. *J Exp Med.* (2009) 206:1929–40. doi: 10.1084/jem.20090896
26. Akoolo L, Schlachter S, Khan R, Alter L, Rojtman AD, Gedroic K, et al. A novel quantitative PCR detects *Babesia* infection in patients not identified by currently available non-nucleic acid amplification tests. *BMC Microbiol.* (2017) 17:16. doi: 10.1186/s12866-017-0929-2
27. Martinez-Balzano C, Hess M, Malhotra A, Lenox R. Severe babesiosis and *Borrelia burgdorferi* co-infection. *QJM* (2015) 108:141–3. doi: 10.1093/qjmed/hcs100
28. Krause PJ, Telford SR 3rd, Spielman A, Sikand V, Ryan R, Christianson D, et al. Concurrent Lyme disease and babesiosis. Evidence for increased severity and duration of illness. *JAMA* (1996) 275:1657–60. doi: 10.1001/jama.1996.03530450047031
29. Krause PJ, McKay K, Gadbaw J, Christianson D, Closter L, Lepore T, et al. Increasing health burden of human babesiosis in endemic sites. *Am J Trop Med Hygiene* (2003) 68:431–6. doi: 10.4269/ajtmh.2003.68.431
30. Krause PJ, McKay K, Thompson CA, Sikand VK, Lentz R, Lepore T, et al. Disease-specific diagnosis of coinfecting tickborne zoonoses: babesiosis, human granulocytic ehrlichiosis, and Lyme disease. *Clin Infect Dis.* (2002) 34:1184–91. doi: 10.1086/339813
31. Shapiro ED, Baker PJ, Wormser GP. False and misleading information about Lyme disease. *Am J Med.* (2017) 130:771–2. doi: 10.1016/j.amjmed.2017.01.030
32. Keane-Myers A, Nickell SP. Role of IL-4 and IFN-gamma in modulation of immunity to *Borrelia burgdorferi* in mice. *J Immunol.* (1995) 155:2020–8.
33. Anguita J, Persing DH, Rincon M, Barthold SW, Fikrig E. Effect of anti-interleukin 12 treatment on murine lyme borreliosis. *J Clin Invest.* (1996) 97:1028–34. doi: 10.1172/JCI118494
34. Zeidner N, Mbow ML, Dolan M, Massung R, Baca E, Piesman J. Effects of *Ixodes scapularis* and *Borrelia burgdorferi* on modulation of the host immune response: induction of a TH2 cytokine response in Lyme disease-susceptible (C3H/HeJ) mice but not in disease-resistant (BALB/c) mice. *Infect Immun.* (1997) 65:3100–6.
35. Kang I, Barthold SW, Persing DH, Bockenstedt LK. T-helper-cell cytokines in the early evolution of murine Lyme arthritis. *Infect Immun.* (1997) 65:3107–11.

36. Glickstein L, Edelstein M, Dong JZ. Gamma interferon is not required for arthritis resistance in the murine Lyme disease model. *Infect Immun.* (2001) 69:3737–43. doi: 10.1128/IAI.69.6.3737-3743.2001

37. Infante-Duarte C, Horton HF, Byrne MC, Kamradt T. Microbial lipopeptides induce the production of IL-17 in Th cells. *J Immunol.* (2000) 165:6107–15. doi: 10.4049/jimmunol.165.11.6107

38. Hu LT, Klempner MS. Host-pathogen interactions in the immunopathogenesis of Lyme disease. *J Clin Immunol.* (1997) 17:354–65. doi: 10.1023/A:1027308122565

39. Basso B. Modulation of immune response in experimental Chagas disease. *World J Exp Med.* (2013) 3:1–10. doi: 10.5493/wjem.v3.i1.1

40. Dunay IR, Damatta RA, Fux B, Presti R, Greco S, Colonna M, et al. Gr1(+) inflammatory monocytes are required for mucosal resistance to the pathogen *Toxoplasma gondii*. *Immunity* (2008) 29:306–17. doi: 10.1016/j.immuni.2008.05.019

41. Hunter CA, Sibley LD. Modulation of innate immunity by *Toxoplasma gondii* virulence effectors. *Nat Rev Microbiol.* (2012) 10:766–78. doi: 10.1038/nrmicro2858

42. Pifer R, Yarovinsky F. Innate responses to *Toxoplasma gondii* in mice and humans. *Trends Parasitol.* (2011) 27:388–93. doi: 10.1016/j.pt.2011.03.009

43. Magez S, Caljon G. Mouse models for pathogenic African trypanosomes: unravelling the immunology of host-parasite-vector interactions. *Parasite Immunol.* (2011) 33:423–9. doi: 10.1111/j.1365-3024.2011.01293.x

44. Liese J, Schleicher U, Bogdan C. The innate immune response against *Leishmania* parasites. *Immunobiology* (2008) 213:377–87. doi: 10.1016/j.imbio.2007.12.005

45. Niikura M, Inoue S, Kobayashi F. Role of interleukin-10 in malaria: focusing on coinfection with lethal and nonlethal murine malaria parasites. *J Biomed Biotechnol.* (2011) 2011:383962. doi: 10.1155/2011/383962

46. Stevenson MM, Tam MF, Wolf SF, Sher A. IL-12-induced protection against blood-stage *Plasmodium chabaudi* AS requires IFN-gamma and TNF-alpha and occurs via a nitric oxide-dependent mechanism. *J Immunol.* (1995) 155:2545–56.

47. Skariah S, Arnaboldi P, Dattwyler RJ, Sultan AA, Gaylets C, Walwyn O, et al. Elimination of *Babesia microti* is dependent on intraerythrocytic killing and CD4+ T cells. *J Immunol.* (2017) 199:633–42. doi: 10.4049/jimmunol.1601193

48. Moro MH, Zegarra-Moro OL, Bjornsson J, Hofmeister EK, Bruinsma E, Germer JJ, et al. Increased arthritis severity in mice coinfected with *Borrelia burgdorferi* and *Babesia microti*. *J Infect Dis.* (2002) 186:428–31. doi: 10.1086/341452

49. Coleman JL, LeVine D, Thill C, Kuhlow C, Benach JL. *Babesia microti* and *Borrelia burgdorferi* follow independent courses of infection in mice. *J Infect Dis.* (2005) 192:1634–41. doi: 10.1086/496891

50. Armstrong AL, Barthold SW, Persing DH, Beck DS. Carditis in Lyme disease susceptible and resistant strains of laboratory mice infected with *Borrelia burgdorferi*. *Am J Trop Med Hyg.* (1992) 47:249–58. doi: 10.4269/ajtmh.1992.47.249

51. Barthold SW, Beck DS, Hansen GM, Terwilliger GA, Moody KD. Lyme borreliosis in selected strains and ages of laboratory mice. *J Infect Dis.* (1990) 162:133–8. doi: 10.1093/infdis/162.1.133

52. Garcia LS, Bullock-Iacullo SL, Fritsche TR, Grady KK, Healy GR, Palmer J, et al. *Laboratory Diagnosis of Blood-borne Parasitic Diseases; Approved Guideline*. Clinical and Laboratory Standards Institute (2000) p. 1–36.

53. Djokic V, Akoolo L, Parveen N. *Babesia microti* infection changes host spleen architecture and is cleared by a Th1 immune response. *Front Microbiol.* (2018) 9:85. doi: 10.3389/fmicb.2018.00085

54. Chan K, Alter L, Barthold SW, Parveen N. Disruption of bbe02 by insertion of a luciferase gene increases transformation efficiency of *Borrelia burgdorferi* and allows live imaging in Lyme disease susceptible C3H mice *PLoS ONE* (2015) 10:e0129532. doi: 10.1371/journal.pone.0129532

55. Chan K, Casjens S, Parveen N. Detection of established virulence genes and plasmids to differentiate *Borrelia burgdorferi* strains. *Infection Immunity* (2012) 80:1519–29. doi: 10.1128/IAI.06326-11

56. Sasaki M, Fujii Y, Iwamoto M, Ikadai H. Effect of sex steroids on *Babesia microti* infection in mice. *Am J Trop Med Hyg.* (2013) 88:367–75. doi: 10.4269/ajtmh.2012.12-0338

57. Chan K, Marras SA, Parveen N. Sensitive multiplex PCR assay to differentiate Lyme spirochetes and emerging pathogens *Anaplasma phagocytophilum* and *Babesia microti*. *BMC Microbiol.* (2013) 13:295. doi: 10.1186/1471-2180-13-295

58. Takai T, Li M, Sylvestre D, Clynes R, Ravetch JV. FcR gamma chain deletion results in pleiotrophic effector cell defects. *Cell* (1994) 76:519–29. doi: 10.1016/0092-8674(94)90115-5

59. Vannier E, Borggraefe I, Telford SR 3rd, Menon S, Brauns T, Spielman A, et al. Age-associated decline in resistance to *Babesia microti* is genetically determined. *J Infect Dis.* (2004) 189:1721–8. doi: 10.1086/382965

60. Habicht GS, Benach JL, Leichtling KD, Gocinski BL, Coleman JL. The effect of age on the infection and immunoresponsiveness of mice to *Babesia microti*. *Mech Ageing Dev.* (1983) 23:357–69. doi: 10.1016/0047-6374(83)90036-2

61. Wong CH, Jenne CN, Petri B, Chrobok NL, Kubes P. Nucleation of platelets with blood-borne pathogens on Kupffer cells precedes other innate immunity and contributes to bacterial clearance. *Nat Immunol.* (2013) 14:785–92. doi: 10.1038/ni.2631

62. Cousens LP, Wing EJ. Innate defenses in the liver during Listeria infection. *Immunol Rev.* (2000) 174:150–9. doi: 10.1034/j.1600-0528.2002.017407.x

63. Igarashi I, Suzuki R, Waki S, Tagawa Y, Seng S, Tum S, et al. Roles of CD4(+) T cells and gamma interferon in protective immunity against *Babesia microti* infection in mice. *Infect Immun.* (1999) 67:4143–8.

64. Pachner AR, Itano A. *Borrelia burgdorferi* infection of the brain: characterization of the organism and response to antibiotics and immune sera in the mouse model. *Neurology* (1990) 40:1535–40. doi: 10.1212/WNL.40.10.1535

65. Pachner AR, Ricalton N, Delaney E. Comparison of polymerase chain reaction with culture and serology for diagnosis of murine experimental Lyme borreliosis. *J Clin Microbiol.* (1993) 31:208–14.

66. Barthold SW, Sidman CL, Smith AL. Lyme borreliosis in genetically resistant and susceptible mice with severe combined immunodeficiency. *Am J Trop Med Hygiene* (1992) 47:605–13. doi: 10.4269/ajtmh.1992.47.605

67. Dkhil MA, Al-Quraishy S, Abdel-Baki AS. Hepatic tissue damage induced in *Meriones ungliculatus* due to infection with *Babesia divergens*-infected erythrocytes. *Saudi J Biol Sci.* (2010) 17:129–32. doi: 10.1016/j.sjbs.2010.02.005

68. Hatcher JC, Greenberg PD, Antique J, Jimenez-Lucho VE. Severe babesiosis in Long Island: review of 34 cases and their complications. *Clin Infect Dis.* (2001) 32:1117–25. doi: 10.1086/319742

69. Joseph JT, Roy SS, Shams N, Visintainer P, Nadelman RB, Hosur S, et al. Babesiosis in lower hudson valley, New york, USA. *Emerg Infect Dis.* (2011) 17:843–7. doi: 10.3201/eid1705.101334

70. Oz HS, Hughes WT. Acute fulminating babesiosis in hamsters infected with Babesia microti. *Int J Parasitol.* (1996) 26:667–70. doi: 10.1016/0020-7519(96)00022-7

71. Semel ME, Tavakkolizadeh A, Gates JD. Babesiosis in the immediate postoperative period after splenectomy for trauma. *Surg Infect.* (2009) 10:553–6. doi: 10.1089/sur.2008.001

72. Obishakin E, de Trez C, Magez S. Chronic *Trypanosoma congolense* infections in mice cause a sustained disruption of the B-cell homeostasis in the bone marrow and spleen. *Parasite Immunol.* (2014) 36:187–98. doi: 10.1111/pim.12099

73. Buffet PA, Safeukui I, Deplaine G, Brousse V, Prendki V, Thellier M, Turner GD,and Mercereau-Puijalon O. The pathogenesis of *Plasmodium falciparum* malaria in humans: insights from splenic physiology. *Blood* (2011) 117:381–92. doi: 10.1182/blood-2010-04-202911

74. Weiss L, Geduldig U, Weidanz W. Mechanisms of splenic control of murine malaria: reticular cell activation and the development of a blood-spleen barrier. *Am J Anat.* (1986) 176:251–85. doi: 10.1002/aja.1001760303

75. Dumic I, Patel J, Hart M, Niendorf ER, Martin S, Ramanan P. Splenic rupture as the first manifestation of *Babesia Microti* infection: report of a case and review of literature. *Am J Case Rep.* (2018) 19:335–41. doi: 10.12659/AJCR.908453

76. Imbert P, Rapp C, Buffet PA. Pathological rupture of the spleen in malaria: analysis of 55 cases (1958-2008). (2009) *Travel Med Infect Dis.* 7:147–59. doi: 10.1016/j.tmaid.2009.01.002

77. Wilson S, Vennervald BJ, Dunne DW. Chronic hepatosplenomegaly in African school children: a common but neglected morbidity associated with schistosomiasis and malaria. *PLoS Negl Trop Dis.* (2011) 5:e1149. doi: 10.1371/journal.pntd.0001149

78. Kuna A, Gajewski M, Szostakowska B, Nahorski WL,Myjak P, Stanczak J. Imported malaria in the material of the institute of maritime and tropical medicine: a review of 82 patients in the years 2002-2014. *Biomed Res Int.* (2015) 2015:941647. doi: 10.1155/2015/941647

79. Kafetzis DA. An overview of paediatric leishmaniasis. *J Postgrad Med.* (2003) 49:31-8. doi: 10.4103/0022-3859.930

80. Raffalli J, Wormser GP. Persistence of babesiosis for >2 years in a patient on rituximab for rheumatoid arthritis. *Diagn Microbiol Infect Dis.* (2016) 85:231-2. doi: 10.1016/j.diagmicrobio.2016.02.016

81. Dkhil MA, Abdel-Baki AS, Al-Quraishy S, Abdel-Moneim AE. Hepatic oxidative stress in Mongolian gerbils experimentally infected with *Babesia divergens*. *Ticks Tick Borne Dis.* (2013) 4:346-51. doi: 10.1016/j.ttbdis.2013.01.002

82. Okla H, Jasik KP, Slodki J, Rozwadowska B, Slodki A, Jurzak M, et al. Hepatic tissue changes in rats due to chronic invasion of *Babesia microti*. *Folia Biol.* (2014) 62:353-9. doi: 10.3409/fb62_4.353

83. Aguilar-Delfin I, Homer MJ, Wettstein PJ, Persing DH. Innate resistance to *Babesia* infection is influenced by genetic background and gender. *Infect Immun.* (2001) 69:7955-8. doi: 10.1128/IAI.69.12.7955-7958.2001

84. Swirski FK, Nahrendorf M, Etzrodt M, Wildgruber M, Cortez-Retamozo V, Panizzi P, et al. Identification of splenic reservoir monocytes and their deployment to inflammatory sites. *Science* (2009) 325:612-6. doi: 10.1126/science.1175202

85. Chen D, Copeman DB, Hutchinson GW, Burnell J. Inhibition of growth of cultured *Babesia microti* by serum and macrophages in the presence or absence of T cells. *Parasitol Int.* (2000) 48:223-31. doi: 10.1016/S1383-5769(99)00022-7

86. Li Y, Terkawi MA, Nishikawa Y, Aboge GO, Luo Y, Ooka H, et al. Macrophages are critical for cross-protective immunity conferred by *Babesia microti* against *Babesia rodhaini* infection in mice. *Infect Immun.* (2012) 80:311-20. doi: 10.1128/IAI.05900-11

87. Terkawi MA, Cao S, Herbas MS, Nishimura M, Li Y, Moumouni PF, et al. Macrophages are the determinant of resistance to and outcome of nonlethal *Babesia microti* infection in mice. *Infect Immun.* (2015) 83:8-16. doi: 10.1128/IAI.02128-14

88. Strle K, Sulka KB, Pianta A, Crowley JT, Arvikar SL, Anselmo A, et al. T-Helper 17 cell cytokine responses in Lyme disease correlate with *Borrelia burgdorferi* antibodies during early infection and with autoantibodies late in the illness in patients with antibiotic-refractory Lyme arthritis. *Clin Infect Dis.* (2017) 64:930-8. doi: 10.1093/cid/cix002

89. Fallahi P, Elia G, Bonatti A. Interferon-gamma-induced protein 10 in Lyme disease. *Clin Ter.* (2017) 168:e146-50. doi: 10.7417/CT.2017.1997

90. Bachmann M, Horn K, Rudloff I, Goren I, Holdener M, Christen U, et al. Early production of IL-22 but not IL-17 by peripheral blood mononuclear cells exposed to live *Borrelia burgdorferi*: the role of monocytes and interleukin-1. *PLoS Pathog.* (2010) 6:e1001144. doi: 10.1371/journal.ppat.1001144

91. Love AC, Schwartz I, Petzke MM. *Borrelia burgdorferi* RNA induces type I and III interferons via Toll-like receptor 7 and contributes to production of NF-kappaB-dependent cytokines. *Infect Immun.* (2014) 82:2405-16. doi: 10.1128/IAI.01617-14

92. Vannier E, Krause PJ. Human babesiosis. *N Engl J Med.* (2012) 366:2397-407. doi: 10.1056/NEJMra1202018

93. Sher A, Reis e Sousa C. Ignition of the type 1 response to intracellular infection by dendritic cell-derived interleukin-12. *Eur Cytokine Netw.* (1998) 9(3 Suppl):65-8.

94. Park AY, Scott P. Il-12: keeping cell-mediated immunity alive. *Scand J Immunol.* (2001) 53:529-32. doi: 10.1046/j.1365-3083.2001.00917.x

95. Moll H, Berberich C. Dendritic cell-based vaccination strategies: induction of protective immunity against leishmaniasis. *Immunobiology* (2001) 204:659-66. doi: 10.1078/0171-2985-00105

96. Rogers KA, DeKrey GK, Mbow ML, Gillespie RD, Brodskyn CI, Titus RG. Type 1 and type 2 responses to *Leishmania major*. *FEMS Microbiol Lett.* (2002) 209:1-7. doi: 10.1111/j.1574-6968.2002.tb11101.x

97. Rogers WO, Weiss WR, Kumar A, Aguiar JC, Tine JA, Gwadz R, et al. Protection of rhesus macaques against lethal *Plasmodium knowlesi* malaria by a heterologous DNA priming and poxvirus boosting immunization regimen. *Infect Immun.* (2002) 70:4329-35. doi: 10.1128/IAI.70.8.4329-4335.2002

98. Scott P. Development and regulation of cell-mediated immunity in experimental leishmaniasis. *Immunol Res.* (2003) 27:489-98. doi: 10.1385/IR:27:2-3:489

99. Ruebush TK 2nd, Juranek DD, Spielman A, Piesman J, Healy GR. Epidemiology of human babesiosis on Nantucket Island. *Am J Trop Med Hyg.* (1981) 30:937-41. doi: 10.4269/ajtmh.1981.30.937

100. Bettelli E, Korn T, Oukka M, Kuchroo VK. Induction and effector functions of T(H)17 cells. *Nature* (2008) 453:1051-7. doi: 10.1038/nature 07036

101. Dao AH, Eberhard ML. Pathology of acute fatal babesiosis in hamsters experimentally infected with the WA-1 strain of Babesia. *Lab Invest.* (1996) 74:853-9.

102. Hemmer RM, Ferrick DA, Conrad PA. Up-regulation of tumor necrosis factor-alpha and interferon-gamma expression in the spleen and lungs of mice infected with the human Babesia isolate WA1. *Parasitol Res.* (2000) 86:121-8. doi: 10.1007/s004360050021

103. Wozniak EJ, Lowenstine LJ, Hemmer R, Robinson T, Conrad PA. Comparative pathogenesis of human WA1 and *Babesia microti* isolates in a Syrian hamster model. *Lab Anim Sci.* (1996) 46:507-15.

104. Keswani T, Bhattacharyya A. Differential role of T regulatory and Th17 in Swiss mice infected with *Plasmodium berghei* ANKA and *Plasmodium yoelii*. *Exp Parasitol.* (2014) 141:82-92. doi: 10.1016/j.exppara.2014.03.003

105. Borhis G, Richard Y. Subversion of the B-cell compartment during parasitic, bacterial, and viral infections. *BMC Immunol.* (2015) 16:15. doi: 10.1186/s12865-015-0079-y

106. Radwanska M, Guirnalda P, De Trez C, Ryffel B, Black S, Magez S. Trypanosomiasis-induced B cell apoptosis results in loss of protective anti-parasite antibody responses and abolishment of vaccine-induced memory responses. *PLoS Pathog.* (2008) 4:e1000078. doi: 10.1371/journal.ppat.1000078

107. Connolly SE, Benach JL. The versatile roles of antibodies in Borrelia infections. *Nat Rev Microbiol.* (2005) 3:411-20. doi: 10.1038/nrmicro1149

108. Kalish RA, Kaplan RF, Taylor E, Jones-Woodward L, Workman K, Steere AC. Evaluation of study patients with Lyme disease 10-20-year follow-up. *J Infect Dis.* (2001) 183:453-60. doi: 10.1086/318082

7

Innate Lymphoid Cells in Protection, Pathology and Adaptive Immunity During Apicomplexan Infection

Daria L. Ivanova[1], Stephen L. Denton[1], Kevin D. Fettel[1], Kerry S. Sondgeroth[2], Juan Munoz Gutierrez[3], Berit Bangoura[2], Ildiko R. Dunay[4] and Jason P. Gigley[1]*

[1] Molecular Biology, University of Wyoming, Laramie, WY, United States, [2] Veterinary Sciences, University of Wyoming, Laramie, WY, United States, [3] Microbiology, Immunology and Pathology, College of Veterinary Medicine and Biomedical Sciences, Colorado State University, Fort Collins, CO, United States, [4] Institute of Inflammation and Neurodegeneration, Otto-von-Guericke Universität Magdeburg, Magdeburg, Germany

*Correspondence:
Jason P. Gigley
jgigley@uwyo.edu

Apicomplexans are a diverse and complex group of protozoan pathogens including *Toxoplasma gondii*, *Plasmodium* spp., *Cryptosporidium* spp., *Eimeria* spp., and *Babesia* spp. They infect a wide variety of hosts and are a major health threat to humans and other animals. Innate immunity provides early control and also regulates the development of adaptive immune responses important for controlling these pathogens. Innate immune responses also contribute to immunopathology associated with these infections. Natural killer (NK) cells have been for a long time known to be potent first line effector cells in helping control protozoan infection. They provide control by producing IL-12 dependent IFNγ and killing infected cells and parasites via their cytotoxic response. Results from more recent studies indicate that NK cells could provide additional effector functions such as IL-10 and IL-17 and might have diverse roles in immunity to these pathogens. These early studies based their conclusions on the identification of NK cells to be CD3−, CD49b+, NK1.1+, and/or NKp46+ and the common accepted paradigm at that time that NK cells were one of the only lymphoid derived innate immune cells present. New discoveries have lead to major advances in understanding that NK cells are only one of several populations of innate immune cells of lymphoid origin. Common lymphoid progenitor derived innate immune cells are now known as innate lymphoid cells (ILC) and comprise three different groups, group 1, group 2, and group 3 ILC. They are a functionally heterogeneous and plastic cell population and are important effector cells in disease and tissue homeostasis. Very little is known about each of these different types of ILCs in parasitic infection. Therefore, we will review what is known about NK cells in innate immune responses during different protozoan infections. We will discuss what immune responses attributed to NK cells might be reconsidered as ILC1, 2, or 3 population responses. We will then discuss how different ILCs may impact immunopathology and adaptive immune responses to these parasites.

Keywords: innate lymphoid cells (ILC), IL-12 family, IFN-gamma, IL-17, apicomplexan parasites

INTRODUCTION

Apicomplexa are a large family of protozoan parasites, which are obligate intracellular parasites of warm-blooded animals. Almost all of them are considered to be major health threats to humans and livestock throughout the world. These include but are not limited to *Toxoplasma gondii* (*T. gondii*), *Plasmodium* spp., *Cryptosporidium* spp., *Eimeria* spp., and *Babesia* spp. Others do exist, but this review will focus on the genera listed above. They can be generally divided into either vector borne or orally transmitted pathogens. Apicomplexans have reduced genome sizes compared to higher eukaryotes, but they encode several different types effector proteins that allow them to develop a very complex relationship with their hosts and contribute to virulence. The vector borne apicomplexans include the mosquito borne *Plasmodium* spp. and the tick borne *Babesia* spp. Orally infectious apicomplexans include *T. gondii*, *Cryptosporidium* spp. and *Eimeria* spp. *Plasmodium* spp. infects ~200 million people and kills around 400,000 a year (1). *Babesia* spp. is a newly emerging parasitic infection of humans (2, 3). *Toxoplasma gondii* infects ~30% of people worldwide and is the third leading cause of food borne illness in the U.S (4). There are on average 750,000 new cases of *Cryptosporidium* spp. per year in the U.S. alone and the parasite is distributed worldwide (5). *Eimeria* spp. infections can be devastating to chicken and beef farms, but it does not appear to be infectious to humans (6). Many of these protozoan parasites can be problematic for people with compromised immune systems especially those with HIV/AIDS. Moreover, in immune competent individuals the majority of these infections can cause considerable tissue morbidity and pathology resulting in long term damage to the host. In the case of *T. gondii* infection there is increasing evidence that persistent infection could contribute to psychiatric disorders and neurodegenerative disorders (7). Thus, gaining a better understanding of the immune factors involved in control of these pathogens as well as the factors that contribute to immunopathology is important to reduce negative health outcome caused by these common infections.

Immune control of apicomplexans largely depends upon induction of adaptive immunity via a T helper type 1 (Th1) response and production of IFNγ (8). In addition to Th1 response, IL-17 production and associated inflammation also are induced (9–12). In many cases this Th17 response appears to contribute to immune pathology associated with these infections. In order to develop either a Th1 or Th17 response, innate immune cells have to be triggered to produce the cytokines important in directing which types of T helper responses develop. In comparison to viral infections where much is known about innate immune cell composition and how these cells function in protection and immunopathology, less is known in the context of apicomplexan infection. Active areas of research to expand this knowledge in protozoan infection exist including an understanding of how innate immune responses contribute to control, cause pathology and influence the development of adaptive responses. However, a major gap in knowledge still exists in understanding all of the innate immune cell populations that are recruited and activated during protozoan infections and what role they each have in protection, causing pathology and/or regulating adaptive immune responses.

Innate immune responses are critical in setting the stage for how the adaptive immune system responds to infection. Many types of cells of either myeloid or lymphoid origin within the innate immune cell compartment contribute to this process. Common myeloid progenitor derived cells include, granulocytes, monocytes/macrophages, dendritic cells, and mast cells (13). These myeloid populations initiate a response to infection and activate the lymphoid cell populations by producing chemokines and cytokines, presenting antigen, and providing costimulation. Innate immune cells are derived from the common lymphoid progenitor and were originally only thought to include Natural Killer cells and some innate B cell like populations. However, in 2013 after a continuous flow of new discoveries about innate immune responses by lymphoid derived cells, the newly appreciated complexity of lymphoid progenitor derived innate immune cells was acknowledged and the Innate Lymphoid Cell classification was proposed (14). As a result, NK cells were formally recognized to not be the only cell comprising this population and there exist 3 groups of innate lymphoid cells (ILC) (**Figure 1**). Group 1 ILC include what are now considered to be conventional NK (NK) cells and ILC1 (15). Currently, group 2 ILCs include ILC2s, and group 3 ILC include ILC3 and Lymphoid Tissue inducer like cells (LTi-like ILC3) (16, 17). Conventional NK cells appear to be the only cytotoxic cell while all the other ILCs follow the pattern of helper CD4 T cells and produce cytokines and other soluble factors that help adaptive immune responses develop. Conventional NK cells have been studied for years in apicomplexan infection and their importance in producing IFNγ during acute infection is very well-established (1, 4). However, several studies demonstrate that what were considered to be NK cell responses during parasitic infection might be responses of other ILCs to infection. Given the updated view of the diversity of ILC populations, a major gap in knowledge in the apicomplexan field is how do different ILC populations contribute to innate and adaptive immunity and/or immunopathology associated with these infections. Another important question to address is whether and how ILC populations positively and negatively regulate adaptive immunity to apicomplexans. Where published data is available, we will detail what is known about the development, activation, and effector functions of NK cells and other ILCs in the context of different apicomplexan infections. We will also discuss the possible roles of non-NK cell ILC populations in protection or pathology associated with the different apicomplexan infections and how they may impact adaptive immunity during infection with these parasitic protozoans.

GROUP 1 ILC

Group 1 ILCs include the conventional NK cell and ILC1 (**Figure 1**). NK cells have been extensively studied in the context of Apicomplexan infection (1, 4, 18, 19). ILC1 have only recently been investigated (20). Group 1 ILCs can be identified by

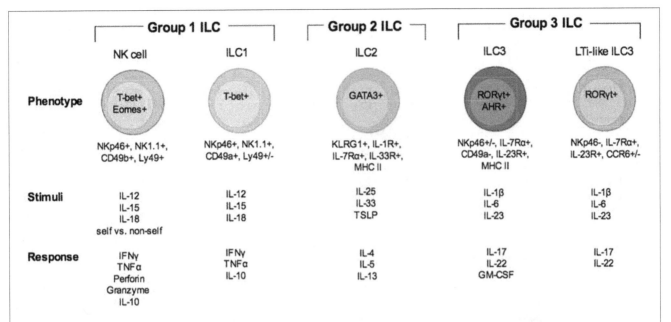

	Group 1 ILC		Group 2 ILC	Group 3 ILC	
	NK cell	ILC1	ILC2	ILC3	LTi-like ILC3
Phenotype	T-bet+ Eomes+	T-bet+	GATA3+	RORγt+ AHR+	RORγt+
	NKp46+, NK1.1+, CD49b+, Ly49+	NKp46+, NK1.1+, CD49a+, Ly49+/-	KLRG1+, IL-1R+, IL-7Rα+, IL-33R+, MHC II	NKp46+/-, IL-7Rα+, CD49a-, IL-23R+, MHC II	NKp46-, IL-7Rα+, IL-23R+, CCR6+/-
Stimuli	IL-12 IL-15 IL-18 self vs. non-self	IL-12 IL-15 IL-18	IL-25 IL-33 TSLP	IL-1β IL-6 IL-23	IL-1β IL-6 IL-23
Response	IFNγ TNFα Perforin Granzyme IL-10	IFNγ TNFα IL-10	IL-4 IL-5 IL-13	IL-17 IL-22 GM-CSF	IL-17 IL-22

FIGURE 1 | Description of ILC subsets. There are three groups of ILC, group 1 ILC, group 2 ILC, and group 3 ILC. Within each of these groups, subsets of cells are indicated (group 1: NK cells and ILC1; group 2: ILC2; group 3 ILC3 and LTi-like ILC3). Each ILC is illustrated with the transcription factors important for their development and function, their surface phenotype, the stimuli that is known to activate them and the immune factors produced when they are activated and responding to infection.

surface expression of the natural cytotoxicity receptor NKp46 and NK1.1 (only in mice that express *NKrp1*). ILC1 can be distinguished from NK cells by their surface expression of very late antigen 1 (VLA-1) or CD49a and TNF—related apoptosis inducing ligand (TRAIL) (15). In the resting state, NK cells are negative for CD49a and positive for very late antigen 2 (VLA-2) or CD49b. Although TRAIL is considered a marker specific for ILC1s, evidence supports that it is also expressed by immature NK cells (iNK) prior to their maturation in the mature NK cells (mNK) which are TRAIL negative (21). NK cells can be found in many tissues and are continuously circulating through the blood. ILC1s are considered to have tissue residence and have been found in both mucosal and non-mucosal tissues (15). These include the spleen, liver, salivary glands, peritoneal cavity, gut, and uterus. NK cells are dependent on expression of T-bet and Eomes for their development and function (21, 22). ILC1 are only dependent upon T-bet (15). Due to the apparent plasticity in ILC populations, ILC1-like cells can arise from both ILC2 and ILC3 (23). Transdifferentiation of ILC2 and ILC3 into ex-ILC2 and ex-ILC3 ILC1 are marked by their increase in NKp46, NK1.1, CD49a, and T-bet expression. These types of ILC1 are also positive for the high affinity IL-7 receptor subunit alpha (IL-7Rα) or CD127 (23). NK cells are the only group 1 ILC that can be cytotoxic. NK cell cytotoxicity is important for killing virally infected cells and tumor cells. The importance of NK cell cytotoxicity in apicomplexan infection is still unclear. NK cells and ILC1 and ex ILC2 and 3 ILC1s produce high levels of IFNγ and TNFα in response to Th1 inducing cytokines IL-12, IL-15, and IL-18 (15). Via their IFNγ production they help control apicomplexan infection.

GROUP 2 ILC

Group 2 ILC includes ILC2 (**Figure 1**) (16). ILC2 could be involved in apicomplexan infection, however, their importance is still not well defined (24, 25). An important distinction between ILC2 and other ILCs is that to date a distinct surface marker has not been identified. ILC2 are lineage (CD3, CD19), NKp46, and NK1.1 negative and CD127, c-Kit(CD117), KLRG1, and the IL-33 receptor (ST2) positive (16, 26). The ILC2 is tissue resident similar to ILC1 and is found at mucosal tissues including the intestine and lungs. ILC2 development and activation depend on the transcription factor GATA3 and they contribute to Th2 responses by producing IL-4, IL-5, IL-9, and IL-13. ILC2 can also express MHC Class II and may be able to prime CD4 T cells (16). ILC2 are known for their importance in immunity against helminth infections to promote tissue repair. Since they express the IL-33 receptor ST2 they can sense tissue damage and respond to promote tissue repair. They are also damaging as they can contribute to allergic inflammation and asthma. As mentioned above, ILC2 demonstrate a high level of plasticity (27–30). IL-1β and IL-12 can drive them to differentiate into an ILC1-like cells. Thus, in addition to their importance in Th2 responses, when given the proper signals they can produce IFNγ and contribute to Th1 dependent immunity. Therefore, ILC2 could contribute to immune protection and immune system regulation during apicomplexan infections.

GROUP 3 ILC

Group 3 ILCs include ILC3 and LTi and LTi-like ILC3 (**Figure 1**) (17). Recent studies suggest that ILC3 can contribute to immunity during apicomplexan infections, however, much is not known about how these cells impact immunity against these parasites (31). Based on surface phenotype ILC3 can be either positive or negative for NKp46 (17). They are also positive for CD127, CD117, and receptors for IL-1(IL-1R) and IL-23 (IL-23R). LTi and LTi-like-ILC3 are NKp46 and CD49a negative, but positive or negative for CCR6 depending on the tissue in which they reside (32). Some LTi cells can also be CD4 positive and ILC3 can express MHC Class II. Group 3 ILC have a wide tissue distribution and reside in mucosal tissues and their associated lymphoid organs. ILC3 and LTi-like-ILC3 differentiation and function depend on the transcription factors RORγt and the aryl hydrocarbon receptor (AHR). Given their tissue residency they are poised to respond to different environmental cues to either maintain barrier homeostasis or provide an inflammatory response against infection. In response to IL-1β and IL-23, ILC3 produce IL-17A, IL-22 and GM-CSF and LTi-like-ILC3s produce IL-17F and IL-22. LTi-like ILC3 also can produce lymphotoxin α/β (LTα/β) to promote lymphoid tissue development. Since group 3 ILC can produce IL-17 and IL-22, they could contribute significantly to Th17 responses observed in many apicomplexan infections, yet their importance is unclear.

ILC PLASTICITY

The border between ILC subtypes has become more defined, however as noted above, ILC are highly plastic and can convert into each other depending on the environment they experience (23). For example, under certain inflammatory conditions, ILC2 and ILC3 can express T-bet and produces Th1 cytokines (27, 29, 33). When the conditions permit, these newly generated ILC1 can convert back into ILC2 and ILC3. This cellular plasticity is likely essential for the generation of optimal responses against pathogens and maintenance of tissue integrity. Due to this new appreciation of ILC diversity, how different ILC populations participate in immunity to apicomplexan infection has not been well defined. We will next discuss what is currently known about ILCs during these parasitic infections and highlight situations where different ILCs may be involved. We will also discuss how different ILCs could be implicated in adaptive immunity to these pathogens.

ILC AND *TOXOPLASMA GONDII*

Even though the ILC classification was recently established to define the innate immune cells of lymphoid lineage, the importance of ILC function for control of *T. gondii* infection has been investigated for many years (4, 34) (**Figure 2**). Infection with *T. gondii* begins after ingestion of oocysts from cat feces or bradyzoite containing tissue cysts from undercooked meat (4, 8). Acute infection is followed by chronic infection in the CNS and muscle for the life of the host. Innate immune responses at mucosal sites and in secondary lymphoid organs are critical for early control of the parasite. In early studies NK cells were shown to be activated by *T. gondii* infection to be cytotoxic (35). Later on NK cells were shown to be a non-T cell source

of IFNγ and were essential for innate immunity to *T. gondii* infection (36, 37). Whether NK cell cytotoxicity is important for early control of *T. gondii* infection is not known and had not been thoroughly tested (4). Importantly, these early studies were some of the first to demonstrate the importance of the IL-12/IFNγ axis in development of Th1 biased immunity (36–38). Indeed IL-12 is required for activation of NK cells to produce IFNγ during *T. gondii* infection (37). Additional cytokines can help stimulate NK cell activation including IL-1β and IL-18 (39, 40). Whether recognition of self-vs. non-self is an important stimulant for NK cells during *T. gondii* infection is not clear (41). To date there have been no observed dominant NK cell populations based on NK cell receptor expression in mice that arise during acute infection suggesting their response is mostly to inflammatory cytokines. Verification of the importance of NK cells in protection against *T. gondii* infection was tested using lymphocyte deficient animals including RAG knockout and SCID mice. In addition NK cell antibody depletion regimes *in vivo* targeting asialo ganglio-N-tetraosylceramide (anti-ASGM1) or anti-NK1.1 were used. These studies laid the foundation for the importance of NK cells in control of *T. gondii* infection.

More recently, studies have addressed how NK cells are involved in immunity against *T. gondii* infection through their impact on other immune cells. NK cell IFNγ can help prime CD8 T cells in the absence of CD4 T cell help (42). NK cell IFNγ can also help activate CD4 T cells during acute *T. gondii* infection (43). Infection of TAP1$^{-/-}$ mice results in reduced CD4 T cell IFNγ production. Adoptive transfer of IFNγ+ but not IFNγ- NK cells restore this deficient CD4+ T cell response. NK cell activity during early during infection could also impact the myeloid cell compartment (44–46). NK cells may enhance DC maturation via NKG2D on the NK cell resulting in more robust CD8 T cell priming during acute infection (44). NK cell IFNγ may be required for the loss of resident mononuclear phagocytes followed by recruitment of circulating monocytes that locally differentiate into macrophages and monocyte derived DC (MoDC) (45). These MoDC then serve as the main source of IL12p40 at the site of infection, which in this study was the peritoneum. Early NK cell (CD49b+CD49a-CD45+TCRb-NK1.1+) IFNγ production during *T. gondii* infection has also been shown to educate the myeloid compartment in the bone marrow. The IFNγ generated by NK cells in the bone marrow skewed monocyte development at that site into a more regulatory phenotype (46). In summary, NK cells via their IFNγ production are able to both positively and negatively regulate other immune cells during *T. gondii* infection. The impact of NK cells on other immune cells could therefore positively or negatively impact the generation of adaptive immune responses to the parasite.

A small number of studies have investigated whether parasite infection of NK cells affects their behavior (47–49). NK cells can be parasitized, however, this occurs at a very low frequency *in vitro* and *in vivo*. These infected NK cells display a hypermotility phenotype and defective function. A recent study indicates that infected NK cells do not contribute to parasite dissemination in the mouse (47). Thus, how direct parasite infection of NK cells impacts the disease course is not known and needs to be further explored.

Innate Lymphoid Cells in Protection, Pathology and Adaptive Immunity During Apicomplexan...

81

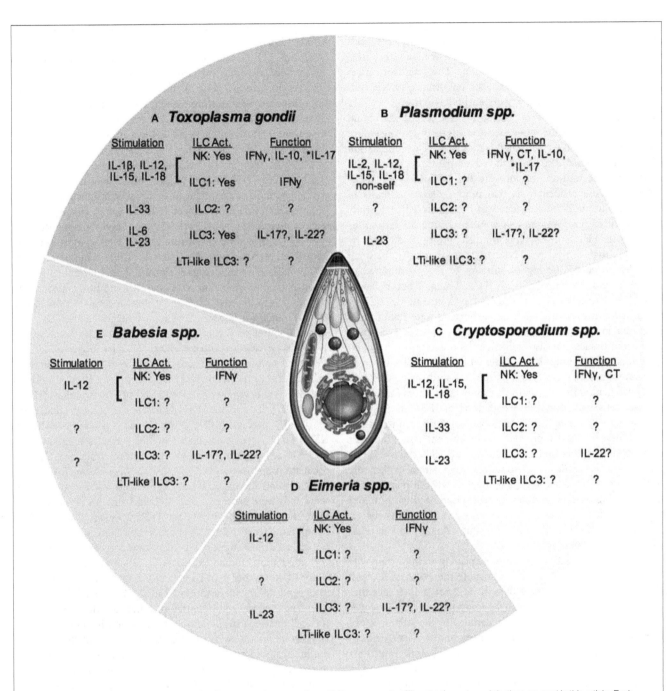

FIGURE 2 | ILC and apicomplexan infection. This figure presents an overview of ILC responses to different apicomplexan infections covered in this article. Each section represents one parasitic protozoan. Under each genus heading there are listed 3 subheadings indicating; (1) Stimuli for each ILC subset (stimulation), (2) The ILC subpopulation activated (ILC Act.), and (3) The function of the activated ILC subset. Question marks indicate where there is no or limited data available. An *denotes where function attributed to NK cells may be from a different ILC population. **(A)** *Toxoplasma gondii* stimulates the production of IL-1β, IL-12, IL-15, and IL-18 that activate NK cells and possibly ILC1 to produce IFNγ and IL-10. IL-17 produced by NK cells may also be produced by other ILC. IL-33 is produced and may activate ILC2. IL-6 and IL-23 are produced and could activate ILC3 for IL-17 and IL-22 production. The importance of LTi-like ILC3 are not known. **(B)** *Plasmodium spp.* stimulates IL-2, IL-12, IL-15, and IL-18, which activate NK cells to produce IFNγ. Recognition of non-self may stimulate NK cell cytotoxicity (CT). These cytokines also stimulate NK cells to produce IL-10. NK cell IL-17 may also be produced by other ILC. The role of ILC2, ILC3, and LTi-like ILC3 are not clear. **(C)** *Cryptosporidium* spp. infection stimulates the production of IL-12, IL-15, and IL-18. These cytokines can activate NK cells to produce IFNγ. NK cell cytotoxicity is also increased after infection, but the stimulus is not known. The importance of ILC1, ILC2, ILC3, and LTi-like ILC3 has not been tested. **(D)** *Eimeria* spp. infection induces IL-12 production that activates NK cells to produce IFNγ. The importance of ILC1, ILC2, ILC3, and LTi-like ILC3 are not known, however evidence suggests IL-17 and IL-22 are produced during infection highlighting the potential activity of non-NK cell ILCs. **(E)** *Babesia* spp. infection stimulates the production of IL-12, which activates NK cells to produce IL-12. The importance of other ILCs has not been investigated at this time.

A major question that now needs to be considered based on the increase in knowledge about additional ILC subsets is can the observations discussed above involve other ILC populations during *T. gondii* infection? This question arises because for many of these studies, the importance of NK cells was further demonstrated by using anti-NK1.1 or anti-ASGM1 to deplete the cells *in vivo* (12, 36). These treatments could easily target other ILC types because of their expression of NK1.1 and or asialo GM1 on their surfaces. One population of ILC that could also be involved in parasite control and in shaping the immune response to the parasite is the ILC1. ILC1 are tissue resident cells that produce large amounts of IFNγ (15). Support for this idea was demonstrated by a study that identified the common helper innate lymphoid progenitor cell or CHILP (20). In these studies, ILC1 as defined by their phenotype Lin-NKp46+NK1.1+Tbet+Eomes- in the small intestine produced the highest amount of IFNγ compared to NK cells and NKp46+NK1.1+ ILC3. Using T-bet deficient (Tbx21$^{-/-}$) mice to eliminate ILC1 development, ILC1 IFNγ was significantly reduced and parasite burdens were significantly increased in the gut. These results suggest that ILC1 resident in specific tissues can also influence the outcome of *T. gondii* infection. A good example that different ILC subsets are involved in different tissues was shown by a separate study using the same T-bet deficient animals (50). In this study the authors found that the NK cells still produced a high level of IFNγ in response to *T. gondii* in the spleen in the absence of this transcription factor. These results demonstrate that in different tissues different transcription factors are important for ILC (NK cell vs. ILC1) responses to *T. gondii*. They also suggest the potential critical role of Eomes and not T-bet in development of NK cell responses in the spleen. Thus, where group 1 ILC IFNγ is impacting immunity to *T. gondii* further investigation is needed to distinguish between NK cells and ILC1 as the source of this cytokine and in what tissues they are working.

Other ILC populations may also be playing an important role in immunity to *T. gondii*. These include the ILC2, ILC3, and LTi-like ILC3 populations. Although ILC2 are helper cells that drive Th2 responses, they could be important during *T. gondii* infection. ILC2 could have a role in dampening the inflammatory response to *T. gondii* infection. ILC2 respond to tissue damage at mucosal sites associated with parasitic helminth infections (16). Their response is controlled by alarmins including IL-33 and IL-1β. Interestingly, a previous report using ST2 (IL-33R) deficient mice demonstrated that these mice were more susceptible to developing inflammatory lesions and Toxoplasmic encephalitis associated with increases in iNOS, IFNγ, and TNFα (25). However, a separate study demonstrated that IL-33 and ST2 correlated with greater immunopathology, inflammation and ocular toxoplasmosis (51). Therefore, whether ILC2 are important or not is unclear. It is still possible that as a result of mucosal tissue damage caused by acute *T. gondii* infection, the release of IL-33 and signaling induced via ST2 could dampen the Th1 biased inflammatory response to the parasite by activating ILC2 to produce Th2 biased cytokines. Whether ILC2s are an important cell type involved as a negative regulator of inflammation and T cell responses during *T. gondii* infection

has not been tested and would be important to address in future studies.

Group 3 ILCs could also be an important immune cell involved in *T. gondii* infections, however, very little is known about them. Group 3 ILCs include LTi-like ILC3 and ILC3, both important cell types that are tissue resident and present in several tissues including the gut. They are important for maintaining tissue homeostasis at these sites, but can also promote tissue damage when they are highly activated (17). ILC3 production of IL-22 is thought to help maintain tissue integrity while ILC3 derived IL-17 can be inflammatory and associated with pathology. ILC3 are thought to be resident at mucosal barriers, but are also found in the spleen (32). During *T. gondii* infection a study revealed that IL-17 was produced and signaling through the IL-17 receptor was important for protection by stimulating neutrophil recruitment (52). A separate study demonstrated that IL-17 via IL-17 receptor signaling caused gut immunopathology associated with infection and was important in promoting chronic *T. gondii* infection (53). At this time, the cellular source of IL-17 was not known. One report suggested that NK cells were the source of *T. gondii* induced IL-17 (12). In this study IL-17 levels increased in infected Rag1$^{-/-}$ mice and anti-ASGM1 treatment significantly reduced the levels of this cytokine in these animals. IL-17 production was induced by IL-6, followed by IL-23 and TGFβ, and suppressed by addition of Th1 cytokines (IL-12, 15, and 27). The splenic NK1.1+CD3- cells that produced IL-17 were not secreting IFNγ as no double positive IFNg+IL17+ NK1.1+CD3- cells were detected. These results suggested that this NK cell population might be distinct from the NK cell population involved in early control of the parasite. Taking into consideration the experimental approaches used to define that these cells were NK cells (Rag1$^{-/-}$ and anti-ASGM1) and that these same approaches can target ILC3 may suggest that the ILC3 populations were the IL-17 producers in these studies and not NK cells. Further support for this idea was revealed because the ILC population studied expressed IL-6Ra and the transcription factor RORγt rather than T-bet (12). Group 3 ILC are now known to depend upon expression of RORγt (17). Since ILC3 are also found in the gut, additional studies indicate that an NKp46+ ILC cell develops in the lamina propria and in response to IL-18 recruits inflammatory monocytes into the gut that increase immunopathology associated with *T. gondii* infection (54). A recent study has investigated more specifically the role of ILC3 in the gut during *T. gondii* infection using aryl hydrocarbon receptor deficient mice and demonstrates that these cells appear to negatively regulate T cell activity (31). Thus, again depending on the tissue investigated, ILC3 may have multiple roles including causing disease pathology and potentially as a negative regulator of adaptive immune responses during *T. gondii* infection. Many questions remain unanswered about these cells during this infection including formal dissection of whether ILC3 could positively or negatively impact development and maintenance of T cell responses against *T. gondii*. In addition, ILC3 and LTi-like ILC3 plasticity would be important to investigate during *T. gondii* infection.

As discussed above, ILCs may also play a role as negative regulators of immunity against *T. gondii*. Using systemic *T.*

gondii as a model infection, NK cells were shown to be capable of producing IL-10 (55). These IL-10 producing cells were defined as conventional NK cells because they were lineage negative (CD3-CD19-TCRβ-) and NK1.1 positive. These cells were also CD127 negative suggesting that they were not ILC2 or ILC3. This regulatory NK cell population was induced by systemic inflammation, and IL-12 and NK cell IL-10 limited IL-12 production by DC. These cells were found to produce IL-10 in lung, liver, brain, blood, but not in spleen and MLN during acute *T. gondii* infection. In another study, NK cells (CD3-CD19-DX5+NK1.1+) were shown to be the major source of IL-10 in spleen, PEC, liver during acute infection (56). Both IL-12 and aryl hydrocarbon receptor (AHR) were required for maximal IL-10 production by these cells. These regulatory NK cells also expressed T-bet, KLRG1 and co-produced IFNγ. The presence of the IL-10 producing NK cells reduced the ability of the mice to control *T. gondii* infection. These data suggest that IL-10 producing cells are present during acute *T. gondii* infection, could be members of group 1 ILC and are important for regulating adaptive immune responses to *T. gondii*. A major open question still is where do these cells originate, what are the long term affects of these cells on T cell responses to the parasite and could they have a negative impact on chronic toxoplasmosis.

There are still many open questions about the roles of different populations of ILCs and *T. gondii* infection. The importance of each ILC subtype has not been fully addressed and there are questions about NK cells that will have to be reinvestigated because of the increase in knowledge of the different ILC subsets in the context of infection. Many studies investigating ILCs during *T. gondii* infection have focused on the acute stage of infection. Their importance in long-term control of the parasite is still not clear especially in chronic *T. gondii* infection and the CNS, which is the current focus of our laboratory.

ILC AND PLASMODIUM

As with *T. gondii* infection, investigations of ILCs in *Plasmodium* spp. infection have been ongoing for many years. Of the ILCs researched the majority of data has been generated from NK cell specific studies [reviewed in (1)]. Infection with *Plasmodium* spp. in humans begins with the injection of sporozoites of the parasite from the salivary gland of the mosquito into the blood stream of the host (57). Once the parasite is inside the host, it migrates to the liver where hepatocytes are infected. The parasite transforms as it replicates into the merozoite stage, which is released from the infected hepatocyte after lysis of the cell. The merozoites then infect erythrocytes (RBC) and develop into male and female gametes and the cycle is repeated. The innate immune response is important in early control of the parasite in liver, periphery, and secondary lymphoid structures where many innate immune cells including ILCs reside. Inflammation generated by the innate immune response including ILC may contribute to *Plasmodium* spp. pathogenesis and pathology such as cerebral malaria (58). NK cells are critical immune cell type in early and continuous control of *Plasmodium* spp. infections in both mouse models of infection and humans (1) (**Figure 2**). NK cells and/or other ILC

types may also be pathogenic by contributing to the development of cerebral malaria. Additionally, the diverse life stages and tissue locations of the parasite likely require the involvement of distinct ILC subsets. Much is still not known about how each ILC type contributes to these processes during *Plasmodium* spp. infection.

In mice splenic, hepatic and peripheral NK (NK1.1+) cells protect against early stages of malaria infection by producing IFNγ and TNFα (59–62). After anti-ASGM1 treatment and NK cell depletion there was a decrease in IFNγ production and an increase in parasitemia in mice (59, 60). In humans, NK cells are thought to be some of the first cells to produce IFNγ during infection (1, 58). Human NK cells (CD56+) produce IFNγ and TNFα after *Plasmodium falciparum* infection (63–65). Human NK cells (can produce IFNγ after stimulation with *Plasmodium* infected erythrocytes *in vitro* (66). In addition to IFNγ production, peripheral blood NK cells are thought to be stimulated to be cytotoxic in response to parasite infection (67, 68). Human NK cells release cytotoxic molecules when cultured with infected hepatocytes and erythrocytes *in vitro*. NK cells have been observed to directly interact with infected erythrocytes forming conjugates (66, 69, 70). Human NK cells have been shown to kill infected erythrocytes (71). Whether NK cell specific cytotoxicity is important in controlling the parasite *in vivo* is still unclear and still needs to be formally tested in mouse models of infection or in humans.

NK cell activation during *Plasmodium* spp. infection is mediated by several signals including cytokines produced by other immune cells and potentially via self-vs. non-self-recognition. Generally, the classic IL-12/IFNγ axis applies to this infection as well as it does to other Apicomplexan infections. Studies are consistent in showing that IL-12 is essential for IFNγ production by NK cells during *Plasmodium* spp. infection (72). Not only is IL-12 important for activation, but also there is interplay between several cytokines and the activation of NK cells to produce IFNγ in response to IL-12. IL-18 in combination with IL-12 can enhance NK cell IFNγ production in mice in response to *Plasmodium* spp. infection (73). This is via IL-18 dependent up regulation of CD25 (IL-2Rα) expression on NK cells allowing them to be more sensitive to IL-2 and produce IFNγ. This IL-18-IL-12-IL-2-NK cell IFNγ is thought to also be occurring in humans exposed to *Plasmodium* spp. infection (65, 74, 75). IL-2 produced by antigen-specific CD4 T cells augmented NK cell activation in immunized individuals. These human studies also demonstrated that different individuals had variable NK cell activation after exposure to infected erythrocytes (75). One hypothesis is that the variability in human NK cell responses is caused by polymorphisms in KIR and/or HLA genes. IL-15 is another cytokine important in NK cell development and function. The role of IL-15 in NK cell activation during *Plasmodium* spp. infection is less clear. One study showed that IL-15 enhanced NK cell IFNγ production (76). In another study IL15$^{-/-}$ DC were as good as WT DC in activating NK cell IFNγ production *in vitro* (72). This is similar to a study with *T. gondii* infection that demonstrated IL-15 is dispensable for NK cell activation (77). In response to *Plasmodium* spp. infection, NK cells are also activated by interactions with monocytes and monocyte derived DCs (70, 78). One of the interactions is dependent upon IL-18. Another interaction is dependent upon direct macrophage to NK cell contact. This cell-to-cell interaction is thought to promote NK cell IFNγ production via interaction between LFA-1 on the macrophage and intercellular adhesion molecule-1 (ICAM-1) on the NK cell (79). In regard to cytotoxicity targeted against hepatocytes and erythrocytes, the exact mechanism of NK cell recognition of these cells remains unknown. Several studies addressed whether NK cell expression of ICAM-1, PECAM, VCAM, CD36, CSA, NKp30, NKp44, NKp46, NKG2D, and the expression of PfEMP1 or heat shock protein 70 on infected erythrocytes facilitated this interaction, however, an exact mechanism is still not known and needs further exploration (71, 79–81).

As with *T. gondii* infection, NK cells may also impact the function of other immune cells and development of adaptive immune responses to *Plasmodium* spp. infection. However, very little has been investigated about how NK cells or other ILCs are involved. NK cells may increase DC maturation and cytokine production facilitating T cell priming (72). In one study, after infection with *P. chabaudi* NK cells promoted DC maturation *in vitro*, IL-12 production and ability to prime CD4 T cells to proliferate and produce IFNγ. Another study demonstrated that NK cell activation *in vivo* was not required for DC maturation or DC-mediated priming of CD4$^+$ T cells specific for OVA antigens expressed by *P. berghei* ANKA (82). This study demonstrated that NK cells (NK1.1+) contributed to the DC-mediated priming of CD8$^+$ T cells *via* a mechanism that required IL-12. Although these studies may differ in mechanism, it appears that similar to *T. gondii* infection, activated NK cells are important for DC priming of adaptive immunity against *Plasmodium* spp. This NK cell dependent enhancement of T cell priming appears to depend upon IFNγ. Whether activated NK cells can take the place of helper T cells in helping the priming of CD8 T cells has not been addressed during *Plasmodium* spp. infection. How NK cell IFNγ could impact development of long-term immunity to *Plasmodium* spp. is also not understood. There are still many questions about the importance of NK cells in their role during *Plasmodium* spp. infection.

To date very little is known about other ILCs and *Plasmodium* spp. infection. Many of the observations about NK cells in malaria could also be attributed to other ILC subsets. Again, this is because NK cell targeting experimental strategies (phenotype: NK1.1+, *in vivo* depletion: anti-NK1.1, anti-ASGM1) also can target the other ILC populations. Evidence supporting the involvement of other ILC in immunity to *Plasmodium* spp. is found in studies elucidating the mechanisms involved in development of cerebral malaria (CM) (83). The first ILC to consider is the ILC1 because of its tissue residency in the liver and ability to produce high levels of IFNγ (84). Although NK cell IFNγ production is important for reducing parasite numbers early during infection, the IFNγ producing liver ILCs could be ILC1. T-bet$^{-/-}$ animals have elevated parasitemia after *Plasmodium berghei* ANKA infection (83). T-bet deficiency would implicate ILC1 as a controller of acute infection because development of ILC1 is T-bet dependent (15). Interestingly, although parasite burden was increased, T-bet deficiency reduced the severity of CM suggesting that

T-bet dependent ILC1 development and activation could also cause immunopathology. A recent study indicates that NK cells and ILC1 are lost in peripheral blood of humans infected with *Plasmodium falciparum* and spleens and livers of mice infected with *Plasmodium chaubaudi chabaudi* AS (85). Using NKp46-iCre mice crossed onto myeloid cell leukemia sequence-1 floxed mice (Mcl1) to genetically ablate mature NK cells, there was no difference in parasitemia compared to WT controls. Using NKp46 iCre mice crossed onto TGFβR2 floxed mice to genetically ablate ILC1, again there was no difference in parasitemia. The results of these studies may suggest that early liver control by NK cells and ILC1s is important, but once the parasite reaches the blood, group 1 ILC may be less able to control the infection.

ILCs are not only important for protecting against infection, but they can also cause immunopathology associated with infections (17). As noted above, the data from studies of CM support this hypothesis (58). In CM susceptible C57BL6 mice, experimental CM is characterized by overproduction of Th1 cytokines (IFNγ, IL-12, and TNFα) (83, 86). Therefore, NK cells and ILC1 could promote CM through the production of inflammatory cytokines including IFNγ. NK cell IFNγ production has been shown to help recruit CXCR3+ T cells into the brain (86). T-bet deficient mice survived experimental CM longer but had higher parasite burdens, indirectly suggesting the potential involvement of group I ILC in contributing to CM pathogenesis (83). While group 1 ILC may be both protective and a cause of immune pathology during *Plasmodium* spp. infection, group 2 ILC may help negatively regulate inflammation and thus prevent development of CM. A recent study suggests that ILC2 may contribute to protection against development of CM (24). ILC2 are sensitive to IL-33 via the expression of the IL-33 receptor ST2 (17). Administration of IL-33 prevented development of CM (24). The therapeutic effect of IL-33 was associated with the expansion of ILC2 and their production of IL-4, IL-5, and IL-13. Adoptive transfer of ILC2 into *Plasmodium berghei* ANKA infection mice increased the frequency of alternatively activated macrophages and T regulatory cells and reduced the severity of CM.

To date there have been no published studies on group 3 ILC including ILC3 and LTi-like ILC3 and *Plasmodium* spp. infection. ILC3 can produce IL-17, IL-22 and GM-CSF in response to IL-1β and IL-23 (17, 32). Based on the function of ILC3 there could be support that they are responding during *Plasmodium* spp. infection. Whether they are protective or causing pathology has not been established. However, during malaria infection in mouse experimental models and humans IL-17 levels increase (87–89). In several cases the increased IL-17 was independent of CD4+ Th17 cells. Macrophages may be one source, but another source not measured in this study could be ILC3s (87). Whether IL-17 is protective or pathogenic is not clear because the data from multiple studies is contradictory (9, 87–91). In mice, IL-17 may help in protection because IL-17 KO mice have higher parasitemia (87). However, in a human study looking at the association of inflammation including IL-17 in Plasmodium induced multiple organ dysfunction (MOD) and CM, high levels of IL-17 in patients was associated with the highest level of MOD

(89). *Plasmodium* spp. infection of AhR KO mice, which are deficient in ILC3, were more susceptible to CM and generated higher IL-17 and IL-6 in brain (91). Lastly, IL-17 deficient and IL-23 deficient mice developed CM similarly to WT mice and similar levels of parasitemia (87, 90). Another important function of ILC3 is the maintenance of tissue immune homeostasis through IL-22 production. Two independent studies have demonstrated that in the absence of IL-22 (IL-22 KO mice) pathology cause by *Plasmodium* spp. infection is more severe (88, 92). Again, whether this IL-22 is coming from ILC3 is not known. Current information about IL-17 and IL-22 produced during *Plasmodium* spp. infection does not definitively suggest ILC3 are an important cell type for immunity. However, given the lack of ILC3 specific studies performed, their production of these cytokines may make these studies important to explore. LTi-like ILC3 have not been explored in *Plasmodium* spp. infection. Overall, even though a recent study suggests that ILCs are irrelevant (85), there are still substantial gaps in knowledge about ILCs and *Plasmodium* spp. that would be important to investigate.

Another open question that has not been investigated in *Plasmodium* spp. infection is whether and how ILC populations can regulate adaptive immune responses. ILCs can both positively and negatively regulate adaptive immunity. NK cell IFNγ may help prime T cell responses during *Plasmodium* spp. infection (72). During *T. gondii* infection, NK cells and/or other ILC produce IL-10 (55, 56). This NK cell IL-10 may negatively regulate the adaptive immune response against the parasite likely to prevent immunopathology. A recent study has now demonstrated that treatment of mice with an IL-15 complex (IL-15C) stimulates NK cells to produce IL-10 during *Plasmodium berghei* ANKA infection (93). This NK cell IL-10 was required to protect against CM. Whether NK cell or other ILC IL-10 production in response to *Plasmodium* spp. infection has an impact on development of adaptive immunity to *Plasmodium* spp. infection will be important to further explore.

ILC AND *CRYPTOSPORIDIUM*

There is very limited information of the importance of ILCs during *Cryptosporidium* spp. infection (**Figure 2**). Infection with *Cryptosporidium* spp. occurs via ingestion of oocysts in contaminated water (5). The parasite remains in the small intestine living inside of gut epithelial cells and is a major cause of diarrhea in people. Innate immunity against the parasite is important for control of the parasite, however there is still limited knowledge about the factors that are critical for this response. This is especially important to investigate because of the mucosal barrier location of the infection where NK cell, ILC1, ILC2, ILC3, and LTi-like ILC3 can all be present (15–17). The level of inflammation generated by these cells could have a positive and or negative impact on infection pathology with this parasite. Results from an early study suggested that a non T cell source of IFNγ was important for control of *Cryptosporidium* spp. infection in mice (94). Subsequent studies suggested that NK cells were not involved into the control of infection (95, 96). Anti-ASGM1 treatment of SCID mice to deplete NK

cells did not result in increased infection pathology. However, more recent studies indicate that innate lymphoid cells are protective against *Cryptosporidium* spp. infection (97). Both adult Rag2$^{-/-}$ and Rag2$^{-/-}$γc$^{-/-}$ mice developed chronic infection but parasite burdens were higher and intestinal pathology was worse in Rag2$^{-/-}$γc$^{-/-}$ mice, which eventually succumbed to the infection. Interestingly, in contrast to adult mice, neonatal mice of both genotypes were able to survive the infection, however, Rag2$^{-/-}$γc$^{-/-}$ had higher parasite burdens for a more extended period of time as compared to Rag2$^{-/-}$ (18). Neonatal C57BL6 mice treated with anti-NK1.1 were slower in controlling the infection and had higher parasite burdens (97). In Rag2$^{-/-}$γc$^{-/-}$ protection was attributed to IFNγ produced by peritoneal macrophages that were IL-18 and IL-12-dependent (98). Whether NK cell IFNγ is also important for control of *Cryptosporidium* spp. infection is still not clear and needs further investigation. In addition the mechanisms by which NK cells could be activated in *Cryptosporidium* spp. infection have not been thoroughly tested. IL-12, one of the potent activators of NK cell IFNγ production, is produced and is needed for immunity against *Cryptosporidium* spp. in mice (99, 100). In humans, peripheral blood NK cells (CD3-CD16+CD56+) were shown to be cytotoxic against cryptosporidium infected intestinal epithelial cells in the presence of IL15 *in vitro* (101). IL-15 induced increased expression of NKG2D receptor on NK cells and that correlated with increased expression of the NKG2D ligands MHC class I-related molecules MICA and MICB on infected intestinal epithelial cells. This data suggests that there may be direct recognition of the infected epithelium by NK cells during this infection (101). Therefore, it is possible that IL-12 and IL-15 are important NK cell activation signals during *Cryptosporidium* spp. infection. However, this has not been thoroughly tested and whether these signals are critical for parasite control is still unclear.

Beyond this very basic knowledge about NK cells and their involvement in protection against *Cryptosporidium* spp. infection, nothing is known about other ILCs and their role in immunity against infection. In addition it has not been tested whether and how ILCs can (1) impact the function of other immune cells (monocytes, macrophages, DCs and T cells); (2) affect the pathology associated with disease; (3) positively or negatively regulate adaptive immunity to this parasite. A small hint that other ILCs may be involved was discovered in a neonatal lamb infection model of *Cryptosporidium parvum* (102). After infection of neonatal lambs, total NKp46+ cells increased in numbers. The frequency of perforin+ cells increased in NKp46+CD16+ and NKp46+CD16- subsets. In addition, IL-22 mRNA expression was upregulated in small intestines of infected lambs. Whether these NKp46+ cells were ILC3s or other ILC is not known (102). ILC3 could be responding to infection because IL-17 is produced in response to *Cryptosporidium* spp. Infection (10, 103, 104). However, no clear links have been established and more research is needed to dissect the roles of different ILCs in *Cryptosporidium* spp. infection. Elucidating the role of different ILCs in control of *Cryptosporidium* spp. could lead to better therapy and vaccine design to help treat this infection.

ILC AND *EIMERIA*

Similar to *Cryptosporidium* spp., very little is known about NK cells and other ILC and their role in protection vs. pathology during *Eimeria* spp. infection. This is a difficult infection to study ILCs because the host animals are chickens and other livestock and thus have limited reagents available. However, this is another important apicomplexan infection that could provide more insight into how the immune system functions in response to other gut tropic apicomplexans. Infection with *Eimeria* spp. occurs via ingestion of fecal matter containing oocysts of the parasite, which then cause severe inflammation in the mucosa of the gut (105). *Eimeria* spp. is a major cause of disease that can impair productivity in livestock including chickens. Similar to other apicomplexan infections, *Eimeria* spp. stimulates a very strong Th1 response that is initiated by innate immune cells that could include ILC (105). Studies investigating innate immunity to this parasite have focused mainly on NK cells and not other ILCs (**Figure 2**). Early investigations of the importance of NK cells in *Eimeria* spp. infection in mice suggested that NK cells were not involved in providing protection (106). Even though infection of BALBC mice with *E. vermiformis* induced an increase in splenic and mesenteric lymph node (MLN) NK cell cytolytic activity, treatment with anti-ASGM1 to deplete the NK cells did not increase parasite burdens in BALBC mice. A later study demonstrated that in chickens, splenic and intestinal NK cell activity via cytotoxicity as measured by ^{51}Cr-release assay decreased after primary infection followed by recovery of this activity (19). However, during secondary *Eimeria* spp. infection, NK cell activity was increased. Secondary intraepithelial lymphocyte derived NK cell activity was accompanied by increase in number of ASGM1-expressing cells. In beige/beige (bg) mice that are NK cell deficient, replication of *E. vermiformis* was reduced (107). A protective role of NK cells in the immune response against *Eimeria* spp. was demonstrated using SCID, SCID/bg and C57BL6 mice treated with anti-NK1.1 (108). After primary infection with *E. papillata*, WT mice depleted of their NK cells with anti-NK1.1 had higher parasite shedding compared to isotype control treated animals. This NK cell dependent protection may have been due to IFNγ production however this was not test directly. The mechanisms underlying the activation of NK cells during *Eimeria* spp. infection most likely involve IL-12 as it is upregulated after infection, however there are no studies that have tested this directly (109). Whether and how other cytokines and signals impact the development of NK cells responses to *Eimeria* spp. infection have not been addressed.

The role of non-NK cell ILCs has not been addressed in *Eimeria* spp. Given the gut pathology that develops in infected animals ILC1, ILC2, and ILC3 (both ILC3 and LTi-like ILC3) may be involved. Based on research into IL-17 and IL-22 production and its importance in this disease implicates ILC3 may be responding to infection (11, 110). In the absence of IFNγ signaling, mice infected with *Eimeria falciformis* had greater body weight loss and gut pathology, but had a lower parasite burden (110). In these animals IL-17A and IL-22 expression was significantly increased. Importantly antibody blockade of IL-17

and IL-22 reduced the pathology associated with infection. This infection pathology was thought to be CD4 T cell dependent because Th17 CD4 T cells expanded in the absence of IFNγ. Whether ILC3 were also producing IL-17 and IL-22 was not tested in this study. A second also demonstrated that IL-17 was a cause of gut pathology in chickens (11). Since ILC3 can help maintain tissue integrity and also cause pathology at mucosal sites, it is possible they contribute to *Eimeria* spp. associated pathology. Outstanding questions are the importance of ILC in protection and immunopathology, impact of ILC on other immune cells function and impact of ILC on positive and negative regulation of adaptive immune responses to *Eimeria* spp. Understanding their role in infection may help to develop therapies to treat this infection.

ILC AND *BABESIA*

Knowledge about ILCs and *Babesia* spp. infection is very limited. How ILC function in response to this infection is still not thoroughly explored, however, based on other apicomplexan infections, they could be very important for at least early control of *Babesia* spp. infection (**Figure 2**). *Babesia* spp. infection of humans begins after the tick *Ixodes scapularis* harboring sporozoites of the parasite has a blood meal from the host (3). Sporozoites infect RBCs where they replicate as trophozoites eventually transforming into merozoites. Blood stage infection causes hemolysis, fever and fatigue in individuals infected. Increasing rates of infection in people have been observed in endemic regions and *Babesia* spp. has severe health consequences for immunocompromised people. Interestingly, this parasite remains in the blood stream during infection and immunity seems to depend upon the spleen as splenectomyzed people are more susceptible to infection (3). NK cell activity was increased in spleen and peritoneal excudate cells (PEC) of infected with *Babesia microti* mice. However, the course of infection in NK cell deficient bg mice was unaltered (111). NK cell frequencies increased in blood, spleen, and liver of BALBC mice infected with *Babesia* spp. (112). Experiments performed in SCID mice on the C57BL6 background indicated that control of *Babesia* spp. was independent of adaptive immune cells (113). Control of *Babesia* spp. in mice was shown to be dependent upon IL-12 and IFNγ signaling because STAT4 and IFNγR2 deficient animals were more susceptible to infection (114). Loss of NK cells from anti-ASGM1 treatment also resulted in elevated susceptibility to *Babesia* spp. Infection (114). *Babesia* spp. is a dangerous pathogen for cattle (3). NK-like cells proliferated in the spleens of young calves during early response to *B. bovis* (115). Bovine splenic NK cells (NKp46+CD3-CD2+/-CD8+/-) produced IFNγ in the presence of supernatants from *Babesia bovis*-exposed monocytes in an IL-12 dependent manner (116). Bovine NK cell IFNγ production required direct cell-to-cell contact with DCs in co-culture after cytokine stimulation (117). Interestingly, bovine NK cells were more cytotoxic when co-cultured with non-cytokine stimulated DCs. Taken together as with other apicomplexans, group 1 ILCs and specifically NK cells play an important role in early control of *Babesia* spp. infection.

Whether other ILCs are responding and playing a role in *Babesia* spp. infection is not known. However, due to the location of this infection (blood and spleen) other ILC may be less important for this infection. Interestingly, *Babesia* spp. appears to predominantly induce a Th1 response as IL-17 and IL-22 levels did not significantly change in a mouse model of infection (2). More in depth investigation of ILC subsets will be needed to fully assess the role of these cells in immunity against *Babesia* spp. infection. This would include studies exploring how ILC can positively and negatively impact adaptive immune responses.

ILCS AND APICOMPLEXA CONCLUSIONS AND FUTURE DIRECTIONS

ILCs are important cells for the early control of Apicomplexan infections via their production of IFNγ (**Figure 2**). NK cells and possibly ILC1 in many of these infections are the source of this cytokine, which is made in response to IL-12, IL-15, IL-18, and IL-2. Although very few studies have dissected the importance of ILC2 and ILC3 in apicomplexan infection, there are hints that these cells are responding to these infections and could either be protective, helping to dampen inflammation (NK-ILC1-IL-10, ILC2-IL-33, ILC3-IL22) or potentiating inflammatory pathology (NK-ILC1-IFNγ ILC3-IL-17). However, there are still major gaps in knowledge for apicomplexan infections about all of the ways ILC contribute to protection and impact overall immunity to these protozoan pathogens. ILC not only provide early protection, but could also participate in the generation and maintenance of adaptive immune responses against these important parasitic infections. ILCs are important in priming T cell responses either indirectly by maturing APCs or directly via their cytokine production. Immune factors such as cytokines or signaling molecules produced by ILC could have a positive or negative impact on primed T cell long-term fate and memory differentiation. ILC could also contribute to long-term protection by developing memory-like responses to

these protozoan pathogens as they do to viral infections (118). Interestingly, during *Plasmodium* spp. vaccination, memory CD4 T cells directed memory-like NK cell responses during secondary infection in vaccinated people (65). How important the ILC contribution to adaptive recall responses during all apicomplexan infections is not well-understood. Lastly, ILC could be cells that are important in honing the adaptive response against these pathogens either making the memory T cell pools better or decreasing their ability to protect against these infections and promoting parasite persistence or susceptibility to reinfection. There are several situations now known during viral infections, in the tumor microenvironment and in autoimmunity where ILC appear to have a negative impact on adaptive immune responses in these different disease situations (4, 119–129). All of these questions will be an important area of research to investigate. Results from future studies of ILC and apicomplexan infections could help improve knowledge of the biology of these complex cells and promote better therapeutic development against these important parasitic pathogens.

AUTHOR CONTRIBUTIONS

JG conceived the review. JG, DI, SD, and KF wrote the review. JG, DI, SD, KF, KS, JM, BB, and ID helped edit the review.

FUNDING

This work is supported by grants from the American Heart Association (AHA 17GRNT33700199) and NIH Wyoming INBRE DRPP P20 GM103432 awarded to JG and NIH Wyoming INBRE graduate student GA awarded to DI. This project is supported in part by a grant from the National Institute of General Medical Sciences (2P20GM103432) from the National Institutes of Health. The content is solely the responsibility of the authors and does not necessarily represent the official views of the National Institutes of Health.

REFERENCES

1. Wolf AS, Sherratt S, Riley EM. NK cells: uncertain allies against malaria. *Front Immunol.* (2017) 8:212. doi: 10.3389/fimmu.2017.00212
2. Djokic V, Akoolo L, Parveen N. *Babesia microti* infection changes host spleen architecture and is cleared by a Th1 immune response. *Front Microbiol.* (2018) 9:85. doi: 10.3389/fmicb.2018.00085
3. Westblade LF, Simon MS, Mathison BA, Kirkman LA. *Babesia microti*: from mice to ticks to an increasing number of highly susceptible humans. *J Clin Microbiol.* (2017) 55:2903–12. doi: 10.1128/JCM.00504-17
4. Gigley JP. The diverse role of nk cells in immunity to *Toxoplasma Gondii* infection. *PLoS Pathog.* (2016) 12:E1005396. doi: 10.1371/journal.ppat.1005396
5. Certad G, Viscogliosi E, Chabe M, Caccio SM. Pathogenic mechanisms of cryptosporidium and giardia. *Trends Parasitol.* (2017) 33:561–76. doi: 10.1016/j.pt.2017.02.006
6. Goff WL, Bastos RG, Brown WC, Johnson WC, Schneider DA. The bovine spleen: interactions among splenic cell populations in the innate immunologic control of hemoparasitic infections. *Vet Immunol Immunopathol.* (2010) 138:1–14. doi: 10.1016/j.vetimm.2010.07.006
7. Donley DW, Olson AR, Raisbeck MF, Fox JH, Gigley JP. Huntingtons disease mice infected with toxoplasma gondii demonstrate early kynurenine pathway activation, altered Cd8+ T-cell responses, and premature mortality. *PLoS ONE.* (2016) 11:E0162404. doi: 10.1371/journal.pone.0162404
8. Hunter CA, Sibley LD. Modulation of innate immunity by *Toxoplasma Gondii* virulence effectors. *Nat Rev Microbiol.* (2012) 10:766–78. doi: 10.1038/nrmicro2858
9. Raballah E, Kempaiah P, Karim Z, Orinda GO, Otieno MF, Perkins DJ, et al. Cd4 T-cell expression of ifn-gamma and Il-17 in pediatric malarial anemia. *PLoS ONE.* (2017) 12:E0175864. doi: 10.1371/journal.pone.0175864
10. Drinkall E, Wass MJ, Coffey TJ, Flynn RJ. A rapid Il-17 response to *Cryptosporidium parvum* in the bovine intestine. *Vet Immunol Immunopathol.* (2017) 191:1–4. doi: 10.1016/j.vetimm.2017.07.009
11. Zhang L, Liu R, Song M, Hu Y, Pan B, Cai J, et al. *Eimeria tenella*: interleukin 17 contributes to host immunopathology in the gut during experimental infection. *Exp Parasitol.* (2013) 133:121–30. doi: 10.1016/j.exppara.2012.11.009
12. Passos ST, Silver J S, O'hara AC, Sehy D, Stumhofer JS, Hunter CA. Il-6 promotes Nk cell production of Il-17 during toxoplasmosis. *J Immunol.* (2010) 184:1776–83. doi: 10.4049/jimmunol.0901843

13. Iwasaki H, Akashi K. Myeloid lineage commitment from the hematopoietic stem cell. *Immunity.* (2007) 26:726–40. doi: 10.1016/j.immuni.2007.06.004

14. Spits H, Artis D, Colonna M, Diefenbach A, Di Santo JP, Eberl G, et al. Innate lymphoid cells–a proposal for uniform nomenclature. *Nat Rev Immunol.* (2013) 13:145–9. doi: 10.1038/nri3365

15. Cortez VS, Colonna M. Diversity and function of group 1 innate lymphoid cells. *Immunol Lett.* (2016) 179:19–24. doi: 10.1016/j.imlet.2016.07.005

16. Schuijs MJ, Halim TYF. Group 2 innate lymphocytes at the interface between innate and adaptive immunity. *Ann N Y Acad Sci.* (2018) 1417:87–103. doi: 10.1111/nyas.13604

17. Withers DR, Hepworth MR. Group 3 innate lymphoid cells: communications hubs of the intestinal immune system. *Front Immunol.* (2017) 8:1298. doi: 10.3389/fimmu.2017.01298

18. Barakat FM, Mcdonald V, Di Santo JP, Korbel DS. Roles for NK cells and an NK cell-independent source of intestinal gamma interferon for innate immunity to *Cryptosporidium parvum* infection. *Infect Immun.* (2009) 77:5044–9. doi: 10.1128/IAI.00377-09

19. Lillehoj HS. Intestinal intraepithelial and splenic natural killer cell responses to eimerian infections in inbred chickens. *Infect Immun.* (1989) 57:1879–84.

20. Klose CSN, Flach M, Mohle L, Rogell L, Hoyler T, Ebert K, et al. Differentiation of type 1 Ilcs from a common progenitor to all helper-like innate lymphoid cell lineages. *Cell.* (2014) 157:340–56. doi: 10.1016/j.cell.2014.03.030

21. Gordon SM, Chaix J, Rupp LJ, Wu J, Madera S, Sun JC, et al. The transcription factors T-bet and eomes control key checkpoints of natural killer cell maturation. *Immunity.* (2012) 36:55–67. doi: 10.1016/j.immuni.2011.11.016

22. Daussy C, Faure F, Mayol K, Viel S, Gasteiger G, Charrier E, et al. T-bet and Eomes instruct the development of two distinct natural killer cell lineages in the liver and in the bone marrow. *J Exp Med.* (2014) 211:563–77. doi: 10.1084/jem.20131560

23. Lim AI, Verrier T, Vosshenrich CA, Di Santo JP. Developmental options and functional plasticity of innate lymphoid cells. *Curr Opin Immunol.* (2017) 44:61–8. doi: 10.1016/j.coi.2017.03.010

24. Besnard AG, Guabiraba R, Niedbala W, Palomo J, Reverchon F, Shaw TN, et al. IL-33-mediated protection against experimental cerebral malaria is linked to induction of type 2 innate lymphoid cells, M2 macrophages and regulatory T cells. *PLoS Pathog.* (2015) 11:e1004607. doi: 10.1371/journal.ppat.1004607

25. Jones LA, Roberts F, Nickdel MB, Brombacher F, Mckenzie AN, Henriquez FL, et al. Il-33 Receptor (T1/St2) signalling is necessary to prevent the development of encephalitis in mice infected with *Toxoplasma Gondii.* *Eur J Immunol.* (2010) 40:426–36. doi: 10.1002/eji.200939705

26. Eberl G, Di Santo JP, Vivier E. The brave new world of innate lymphoid cells. *Nat Immunol.* (2015) 16:1–5. doi: 10.1038/ni.3059

27. Bal SM, Bernink JH, Nagasawa M, Groot J, Shikhagaie MM, Golebski K, et al. IL-1beta, IL-4 and IL-12 control the fate of group 2 innate lymphoid cells in human airway inflammation in the lungs. *Nat Immunol.* (2016) 17:636–45. doi: 10.1038/ni.3444

28. Lim AI, Menegatti S, Bustamante J, Le Bourhis L, Allez M, Rogge L, et al. Il-12 drives functional plasticity of human group 2 innate lymphoid cells. *J Exp Med.* (2016) 213:569–83. doi: 10.1084/jem.20151750

29. Ohne Y, Silver JS, Thompson-Snipes L, Collet MA, Blanck JP, Cantarel BL, et al. Il-1 is a critical regulator of group 2 innate lymphoid cell function and plasticity. *Nat Immunol.* (2016) 17:646–55. doi: 10.1038/ni.3447

30. Silver JS, Kearley J, Copenhaver AM, Sanden C, Mori A, Yu L, et al. Inflammatory triggers associated with exacerbations of copd orchestrate plasticity of group 2 innate lymphoid cells in the lungs. *Nat Immunol.* (2016) 17:626–35. doi: 10.1038/ni.3443

31. Wagage S, Harms Pritchard G, Dawson L, Buza EL, Sonnenberg GF, Hunter CA. The group 3 innate lymphoid cell defect in aryl hydrocarbon receptor deficient mice is associated with t cell hyperactivation during intestinal infection. *PloS ONE.* (2015) 10:E0128335. doi: 10.1371/journal.pone.0128335

32. Melo-Gonzalez F, Hepworth MR. Functional and phenotypic heterogeneity of group 3 innate lymphoid cells. *Immunology.* (2017) 150:265–75. doi: 10.1111/imm.12697

33. Bernink JH, Krabbendam L, Germar K, De Jong E, Gronke K, Kofoed-Nielsen M, et al. Interleukin-12 and−23 control plasticity of CD127(+)

34. Dunay IR, Diefenbach A. Group 1 innate lymphoid cells in *Toxoplasma gondii* infection. *Parasite Immunol.* (2018) 40:e12516. doi: 10.1111/pim.12516

35. Hauser WEJr, Sharma SD, Remington JS. Natural killer cells induced by acute and chronic toxoplasma infection. *Cell Immunol.* (1982) 69:330–46. doi: 10.1016/0008-8749(82)90076-4

36. Denkers EY, Gazzinelli RT, Martin D, Sher A. Emergence Of Nk1.1+ cells as effectors of ifn-gamma dependent immunity to *Toxoplasma gondii* in MHC class I-deficient mice. *J Exp Med.* (1993) 178:1465–72. doi: 10.1084/jem.178.5.1465

37. Gazzinelli RT, Hieny S, Wynn TA, Wolf S, Sher A. Interleukin 12 is required for the t-lymphocyte-independent induction of interferon gamma by an intracellular parasite and induces resistance in t-cell-deficient hosts. *Proc Natl Acad Sci USA.* (1993) 90:6115–9. doi: 10.1073/pnas.90.13.6115

38. Hunter CA, Subauste CS, Van Cleave VH, Remington JS. Production of gamma interferon by natural killer cells from toxoplasma gondii-infected scid mice: regulation by interleukin-10, interleukin-12, and tumor necrosis factor alpha. *Infect Immun.* (1994) 62:2818–24.

39. Cai G, Kastelein R, Hunter CA. Interleukin-18 (IL-18) enhances innate IL-12-mediated resistance to *Toxoplasma gondii.* *Infect Immun.* (2000) 68:6932–8. doi: 10.1128/IAI.68.12.6932-6938.2000

40. Hunter CA, Chizzonite R, Remington JS. Il-1 beta is required for Il-12 to induce production of Ifn-gamma by NK cells. A role for Il-1 beta in the T cell-independent mechanism of resistance against intracellular pathogens. *J Immunol.* (1995) 155:4347–54.

41. Ivanova DL, Fatima R, Gigley JP. Comparative analysis of conventional natural killer cell responses to acute infection with *Toxoplasma Gondii* strains of different virulence. *Front Immunol.* (2016) 7:347. doi: 10.3389/fimmu.2016.00347

42. Combe CL, Curiel TJ, Moretto MM, Khan IA. NK cells help to induce CD8(+)-T-cell immunity against *Toxoplasma gondii* in the absence of CD4(+) T cells. *Infect Immun.* (2005) 73:4913–21. doi: 10.1128/IAI.73.8.4913-4921.2005

43. Goldszmid RS, Bafica A, Jankovic D, Feng CG, Caspar P, Winkler-Pickett R, et al. Tap-1 indirectly regulates Cd4+ T cell priming in toxoplasma gondii infection by controlling NK cell ifn-gamma production. *J Exp Med.* (2007) 204:2591–602. doi: 10.1084/jem.20070634

44. Guan H, Moretto M, Bzik DJ, Gigley J, Khan IA. NK cells enhance dendritic cell response against parasite antigens via Nkg2d pathway. *J Immunol.* (2007) 179:590–6. doi: 10.4049/jimmunol.179.1.590

45. Goldszmid RS, Caspar P, Rivollier A, White S, Dzutsev A, Hieny S, et al. NK cell-derived interferon-gamma orchestrates cellular dynamics and the differentiation of monocytes into dendritic cells at the site of infection. *Immunity* (2012) 36:1047–59. doi: 10.1016/j.immuni.2012.03.026

46. Askenase MH, Han SJ, Byrd AL, Morais DA Fonseca D, Bouladoux N, et al. Bone-marrow-resident NK cells prime monocytes for regulatory function during infection. *Immunity* (2015) 42:1130–42. doi: 10.1016/j.immuni.2015.05.011

47. Petit-Jentreau L, Glover C, Coombes JL. Parasitized natural killer cells do not facilitate the spread of *Toxoplasma Gondii* to the brain. *Parasite Immunol.* (2018) 40:E12522. doi: 10.1111/pim.12522

48. Sultana MA, Du A, Carow B, Angbjar CM, Weidner JM, Kanatani S, et al. Downmodulation of effector functions in nk cells upon *Toxoplasma gondii* infection. *Infect Immun.* (2017) 85:e00069-17. doi: 10.1128/IAI.00069-17

49. Ueno N, Lodoen MB, Hickey GL, Robey EA, Coombes JL. *Toxoplasma gondii*-infected natural killer cells display a hypermotility phenotype *in vivo.* *Immunol Cell Biol.* (2015) 93:508–13. doi: 10.1038/icb.2014.106

50. Harms Pritchard G, Hall AO, Christian DA, Wagage S, Fang Q, Muallem G, et al. Diverse Roles For T-Bet in the effector responses required for resistance to infection. *J Immunol.* (2015) 194:1131–40. doi: 10.4049/jimmunol.1401617

51. Tong X, Lu F. Il-33/St2 involves the immunopathology of ocular toxoplasmosis in murine model. *Parasitol Res.* (2015) 114:1897–905. doi: 10.1007/s00436-015-4377-3

52. Kelly MN, Kolls JK, Happel K, Schwartzman JD, Schwarzenberger P, Combe C, et al. Interleukin-17/Interleukin-17 receptor-mediated signaling

is important for generation of an optimal polymorphonuclear response against *Toxoplasma gondii* infection. *Infect Immun.* (2005) 73:617–21. doi: 10.1128/IAI.73.1.617-621.2005

53. Guiton R, Vasseur V, Charron S, Arias MT, Van Langendonck N, Buzoni-Gatel D, et al. Interleukin 17 receptor signaling is deleterious during *Toxoplasma gondii* infection in susceptible Bl6 mice. *J Infect Dis.* (2010) 202:427–35. doi: 10.1086/653738

54. Schulthess J, Meresse B, Ramiro-Puig E, Montcuquet N, Darche S, Begue B, et al. Interleukin-15-dependent Nkp46+ innate lymphoid cells control intestinal inflammation by recruiting inflammatory monocytes. *Immunity* (2012) 37:108–21. doi: 10.1016/j.immuni.2012.05.013

55. Perona-Wright G, Mohrs K, Szaba FM, Kummer LW, Madan R, Karp CL, et al. Systemic but not local infections elicit immunosuppressive Il-10 production by natural killer cells. *Cell Host Microbe* (2009) 6:503–12. doi: 10.1016/j.chom.2009.11.003

56. Wagage S, John B, Krock BL, Hall AO, Randall LM, Karp CL, et al. The aryl hydrocarbon receptor promotes Il-10 production by NK cells. *J Immunol.* (2014) 192:1661–70. doi: 10.4049/jimmunol.1300497

57. Gazzinelli RT, Kalantari P, Fitzgerald KA, Golenbock DT. Innate sensing of malaria parasites. *Nat Rev Immunol.* (2014) 14:744–57. doi: 10.1038/nri3742

58. Palomo J, Quesniaux VFJ, Togbe D, Reverchon F, Ryffel B. Unravelling the roles of innate lymphoid cells in cerebral malaria pathogenesis. *Parasite Immunol.* (2018) 40:e12502. doi: 10.1111/pim.12502

59. Choudhury HR, Sheikh NA, Bancroft GJ, Katz DR, De Souza JB. Early nonspecific immune responses and immunity to blood-stage nonlethal *Plasmodium yoelii* malaria. *Infect Immun.* (2000) 68:6127–32. doi: 10.1128/IAI.68.11.6127-6132.2000

60. Mohan K, Moulin P, Stevenson MM. Natural killer cell cytokine production, not cytotoxicity, contributes to resistance against blood-stage *Plasmodium chabaudi* as infection. *J Immunol.* (1997) 159:4990–8.

61. Roland J, Soulard V, Sellier C, Drapier AM, Di Santo JP, Cazenave PA, et al. NK cell responses to plasmodium infection and control of intrahepatic parasite development. *J Immunol.* (2006) 177:1229–39. doi: 10.4049/jimmunol.177.2.1229

62. Miller JL, Sack BK, Baldwin M, Vaughan AM, Kappe SH. Interferon-mediated innate immune responses against malaria parasite liver stages. *Cell Rep.* (2014) 7:436–47. doi: 10.1016/j.celrep.2014.03.018

63. Agudelo O, Bueno J, Villa A, Maestre A. High IFN-gamma and TNF production by peripheral NK cells of Colombian patients with different clinical presentation of *Plasmodium falciparum*. *Malar J.* (2012) 11:38. doi: 10.1186/1475-2875-11-38

64. Teirlinck AC, Mccall MB, Roestenberg M, Scholzen A, Woestenenk R, De Mast Q, et al. Longevity and composition of cellular immune responses following experimental *Plasmodium falciparum* malaria infection in humans. *Plos Pathog.* (2011) 7:E1002389. doi: 10.1371/journal.ppat.1002389

65. Mccall MB, Roestenberg M, Ploemen I, Teirlinck A, Hopman J, De Mast Q, et al. Memory-like Ifn-gamma response by nk cells following malaria infection reveals the crucial role of t cells in NK cell activation by *P. falciparum*. *Eur J Immunol.* (2010) 40:3472–7. doi: 10.1002/eji.2010 40587

66. Artavanis-Tsakonas K, Riley EM. Innate immune response to malaria: rapid induction of IFN-gamma from human NK cells by live *Plasmodium falciparum*-infected erythrocytes. *J Immunol.* (2002) 169:2956–63. doi: 10.4049/jimmunol.169.6.2956

67. Hermsen CC, Konijnenberg Y, Mulder L, Loe C, Van Deuren M, Van Der Meer JW, et al. Circulating concentrations of soluble granzyme A and B increase during natural and experimental *Plasmodium falciparum* infections. *Clin Exp Immunol.* (2003) 132:467–72. doi: 10.1046/j.1365-2249.2003.02160.x

68. Orago AS, Facer CA. Cytotoxicity of human natural killer (Nk) cell subsets for *Plasmodium falciparum* erythrocytic schizonts: stimulation by cytokines and inhibition by neomycin. *Clin Exp Immunol.* (1991) 86:22–9. doi: 10.1111/j.1365-2249.1991.tb05768.x

69. Korbel DS, Newman KC, Almeida CR, Davis DM, Riley EM. Heterogeneous human NK cell responses to *Plasmodium falciparum*-infected erythrocytes. *J Immunol.* (2005) 175:7466–73. doi: 10.4049/jimmunol.175.11.7466

70. Baratin M, Roetynck S, Lepolard C, Falk C, Sawadogo S, Uematsu S, et al. Natural killer cell and macrophage cooperation in MyD88-dependent innate responses to *Plasmodium falciparum*. *Proc Natl Acad Sci USA* (2005) 102:14747–52. doi: 10.1073/pnas.0507355102

71. Chen Q, Amaladoss A, Ye W, Liu M, Dummler S, Kong F, et al. Human natural killer cells control *Plasmodium falciparum* infection by eliminating infected red blood cells. *Proc Natl Acad Sci USA.* (2014) 111:1479–84. doi: 10.1073/pnas.1323318111

72. Ing R, Stevenson MM. Dendritic cell and NK cell reciprocal cross talk promotes gamma interferon-dependent immunity to blood-stage *Plasmodium chabaudi* as infection in mice. *Infect Immun.* (2009) 77:770–82. doi: 10.1128/IAI.00994-08

73. Stegmann KA, De Souza JB, Riley EM. Il-18-induced expression of high-affinity Il-2r on murine NK cells is essential for NK-cell Ifn-gamma production during murine *Plasmodium yoelii* infection. *Eur J Immunol.* (2015) 45:3431–40. doi: 10.1002/eji.201546018

74. Horowitz A, Hafalla JC, King E, Lusingu J, Dekker D, Leach A, et al. Antigen-specific Il-2 secretion correlates with NK cell responses after immunization of tanzanian children with the Rts,S/As01 malaria vaccine. *J Immunol.* (2012) 188:5054–62. doi: 10.4049/jimmunol.1102710

75. Artavanis-Tsakonas K, Eleme K, Mcqueen KL, Cheng NW, Parham P, Davis DM, et al. Activation of a subset of human NK cells upon contact with *Plasmodium falciparum*-infected erythrocytes. *J Immunol.* (2003) 171:5396–405. doi: 10.4049/jimmunol.171.10.5396

76. Ing R, Gros P, Stevenson MM. Interleukin-15 enhances innate and adaptive immune responses to blood-stage malaria infection in mice. *Infect Immun.* (2005) 73:3172–7. doi: 10.1128/IAI.73.5.3172-3177.2005

77. Lieberman LA, Villegas EN, Hunter CA. Interleukin-15-deficient mice develop protective immunity to *Toxoplasma gondii*. *Infect Immun.* (2004) 72:6729–32. doi: 10.1128/IAI.72.11.6729-6732.2004

78. Newman KC, Korbel DS, Hafalla JC, Riley EM. Cross-talk with myeloid accessory cells regulates human natural killer cell interferon-gamma responses to malaria. *PLoS Pathog.* (2006) 2:E118. doi: 10.1371/journal.ppat.0020118

79. Baratin M, Roetynck S, Pouvelle B, Lemmers C, Viebig NK, Johansson S, et al. Dissection of the role of PfEMP1 and ICAM-1 in the sensing of *Plasmodium-falciparum*-infected erythrocytes by natural killer cells. *PLoS ONE.* (2007) 2:e228. doi: 10.1371/journal.pone.0000228

80. Mavoungou E, Held J, Mewono L, Kremsner PG. A duffy binding-like domain is involved in the Nkp30-mediated recognition of *Plasmodium falciparum*-parasitized erythrocytes by natural killer cells. *J Infect Dis.* (2007) 195:1521–31. doi: 10.1086/515579

81. Bottger E, Multhoff G, Kun JF, Esen M. *Plasmodium falciparum*-infected erythrocytes induce granzyme B by NK cells through expression of host-Hsp70. *PLoS ONE.* (2012) 7:e33774. doi: 10.1371/journal.pone.0033774

82. Ryg-Cornejo V, Nie CQ, Bernard NJ, Lundie RJ, Evans KJ, Crabb BS, et al. NK cells and conventional dendritic cells engage in reciprocal activation for the induction of inflammatory responses during *Plasmodium berghei* anka infection. *Immunobiology* (2013) 218:263–71. doi: 10.1016/j.imbio.2012.05.018

83. Oakley MS, Sahu BR, Lotspeich-Cole L, Solanki NR, Majam V, Pham PT, et al. The transcription factor T-bet regulates parasitemia and promotes pathogenesis during *Plasmodium berghei* anka murine malaria. *J Immunol.* (2013) 191:4699–708. doi: 10.4049/jimmunol.1300396

84. Spits H, Bernink JH, Lanier L. NK cells and type 1 innate lymphoid cells: partners in host defense. *Nat Immunol.* (2016) 17:758–64. doi: 10.1038/ni.3482

85. Ng SS, Souza-Fonseca-Guimaraes F, Rivera FL, Amante FH, Kumar R, Gao Y, et al. Rapid loss of group 1 innate lymphoid cells during blood stage plasmodium infection. *Clin Transl Immunol.* (2018) 7:E1003. doi: 10.1002/cti2.1003

86. Hansen DS, Bernard NJ, Nie CQ, Schofield L. NK cells stimulate recruitment of Cxcr3+ T cells to the brain during *Plasmodium berghei*-mediated cerebral malaria. *J Immunol.* (2007) 178:5779–88. doi: 10.4049/jimmunol.178.9.5779

87. Ishida H, Matsuzaki-Moriya C, Imai T, Yanagisawa K, Nojima Y, Suzue K, et al. Development of experimental cerebral malaria is independent Of Il-23 AND Il-17. *Biochem Biophys Res Commun.* (2010) 402:790–5. doi: 10.1016/j.bbrc.2010.10.114

88. Mastelic B, Do Rosario AP, Veldhoen M, Renauld JC, Jarra W, Sponaas AM, et al. Il-22 protects against liver pathology and lethality of an

experimental blood-stage malaria infection. *Front Immunol.* (2012) 3:85. doi: 10.3389/fimmu.2012.00085

89. Herbert F, Tchitchek N, Bansal D, Jacques J, Pathak S, Becavin C, et al. Evidence Of Il-17, Ip-10, and Il-10 involvement in multiple-organ dysfunction and Il-17 pathway in acute renal failure associated to *Plasmodium falciparum* malaria. *J Transl Med.* (2015) 13:369. doi: 10.1186/s12967-015-0731-6

90. Ishida H, Imai T, Suzue K, Hirai M, Taniguchi T, Yoshimura A, et al. Il-23 protection against *Plasmodium berghei* infection in mice is partially dependent on Il-17 from macrophages. *Eur J Immunol.* (2013) 43:2696–706. doi: 10.1002/eji.201343493

91. Brant F, Miranda AS, Esper L, Rodrigues DH, Kangussu LM, Bonaventura D, et al. Role of the aryl hydrocarbon receptor in the immune response profile and development of pathology during *Plasmodium berghei* anka infection. *Infect Immun.* (2014) 82:3127–40. doi: 10.1128/IAI.01733-14

92. Sellau J, Alvarado CF, Hoenow S, Mackroth MS, Kleinschmidt D, Huber S, et al. Il-22 dampens the T cell response in experimental malaria. *Sci Rep.* (2016) 6:28058. doi: 10.1038/srep28058

93. Burrack KS, Huggins MA, Taras E, Dougherty P, Henzler CM, Yang R, et al. Interleukin-15 complex treatment protects mice from cerebral malaria by inducing interleukin-10-producing natural killer cells. *Immunity* (2018) 48:e4. doi: 10.1016/j.immuni.2018.03.012

94. Ungar BL, Kao TC, Burris JA, Finkelman FD. Cryptosporidium infection in an adult mouse model. independent roles for Ifn-gamma and Cd4+ T lymphocytes in protective immunity. *J Immunol.* (1991) 147:1014–22.

95. Mcdonald V, Bancroft GJ. Mechanisms of innate and acquired resistance to *Cryptosporidium parvum* infection in scid mice. *Parasite Immunol.* (1994) 16:315–20. doi: 10.1111/j.1365-3024.1994.tb00354.x

96. Rohlman VC, Kuhls TL, Mosier DA, Crawford DL, Greenfield RA. *Cryptosporidium parvum* infection after abrogation of natural killer cell activity in normal and severe combined immunodeficiency mice. *J Parasitol.* (1993) 79:295–7. doi: 10.2307/3283525

97. Korbel DS, Barakat FM, Di Santo JP, Mcdonald V. Cd4+ T cells are not essential for control of early acute *Cryptosporidium parvum* infection in neonatal mice. *Infect Immun.* (2011) 79:1647–53. doi: 10.1128/IAI.00922-10

98. Choudhry N, Petry F, Van Rooijen N, Mcdonald V. A protective role for interleukin 18 in interferon gamma-mediated innate immunity to *Cryptosporidium parvum* that is independent of natural killer cells. *J Infect Dis.* (2012) 206:117–24. doi: 10.1093/infdis/jis300

99. Urban JF Jr, Fayer R, Chen SJ, Gause WC, Gately MK, Finkelman FD. Il-12 Protects immunocompetent and immunodeficient neonatal mice against infection with *Cryptosporidium parvum*. *J Immunol.* (1996) 156:263–8.

100. Takeda K, Omata Y, Koyama T, Ohtani M, Kobayashi Y, Furuoka H, et al. Increase Of Th1 type cytokine mRNA expression in peripheral blood lymphocytes of calves experimentally infected with *Cryptosporidium parvum*. *Vet Parasitol.* (2003) 113:327–31. doi: 10.1016/S0304-4017(03)00080-3

101. Dann SM, Wang HC, Gambarin KJ, Actor JK, Robinson P, Lewis DE, et al. Interleukin-15 activates human natural killer cells to clear the intestinal protozoan cryptosporidium. *J Infect Dis.* (2005) 192:1294–302. doi: 10.1086/444393

102. Olsen L, Akesson CP, Storset AK, Lacroix-Lamande S, Boysen P, Metton C, et al. The early intestinal immune response in experimental neonatal ovine cryptosporidiosis is characterized by an increased frequency of perforin expressing Ncr1(+) NK cells and by Ncr1(-) Cd8(+) cell recruitment. *Vet Res.* (2015) 46:28. doi: 10.1186/s13567-014-0136-1

103. Zhao GH, Cheng WY, Wang W, Jia YQ, Fang YQ, Du SZ, et al. The expression dynamics of Il-17 and Th17 response relative cytokines in the trachea and spleen of chickens after infection with *Cryptosporidium baileyi*. *Parasit Vectors* (2014) 7:212. doi: 10.1186/1756-3305-7-212

104. Zhao GH, Fang YQ, Ryan U, Guo YX, Wu F, Du SZ, et al. Dynamics Of Th17 associating cytokines in *Cryptosporidium parvum*-infected mice. *Parasitol Res.* (2016) 115:879–87. doi: 10.1007/s00436-015-4831-2

105. Lillehoj HS, Trout JM. Avian gut-associated lymphoid tissues and intestinal immune responses to eimeria parasites. *Clin Microbiol Rev.* (1996) 9:349–60. doi: 10.1128/CMR.9.3.349

106. Smith AL, Rose ME, Wakelin D. The role of natural killer cells in resistance to coccidiosis: investigations in a murine model. *Clin Exp Immunol.* (1994) 97:273–9. doi: 10.1111/j.1365-2249.1994.tb06080.x

107. Rose ME, Hesketh P, Wakelin D. Cytotoxic effects of natural killer cells have no significant role in controlling infection with the intracellular protozoon eimeria vermiformis. *Infect Immun.* (1995) 63:3711–4.

108. Schito ML, Barta JR. Nonspecific Immune responses and mechanisms of resistance to eimeria papillata infections in mice. *Infect Immun.* (1997) 65:3165–70.

109. Rosenberg B, Juckett DA, Aylsworth CF, Dimitrov NV, Ho SC, Judge JW, et al. Protein from intestinal eimeria protozoan stimulates Il-12 release from dendritic cells, exhibits antitumor properties *in vivo* and is correlated with low intestinal tumorigenicity. *Int J Cancer* (2005) 114:756–65. doi: 10.1002/ijc.20801

110. Stange J, Hepworth MR, Rausch S, Zajic L, Kuhl AA, Uyttenhove C, et al. Il-22 mediates host defense against an intestinal intracellular parasite in the absence of ifn-gamma at the cost of Th17-driven immunopathology. *J Immunol.* (2012) 188:2410–8. doi: 10.4049/jimmunol.1102062

111. Wood PR, Clark IA. Apparent irrelevance of NK cells to resolution of infections with *Babesia microti* And *Plasmodium vinckei* petteri in mice. *Parasite Immunol.* (1982) 4:319–27. doi: 10.1111/j.1365-3024.1982.tb00443.x

112. Igarashi I, Honda R, Shimada T, Miyahara K, Sakurai H, Saito A, et al. Changes of lymphocyte subpopulations and natural killer cells in mice sensitized with toxoplasma lysate antigen before and after babesia infection. *Nihon Juigaku Zasshi* (1990) 52:969–77. doi: 10.1292/jvms1939.52.969

113. Aguilar-Delfin I, Homer MJ, Wettstein PJ, Persing DH. Innate resistance to Babesia infection is influenced by genetic background and gender. *Infect Immun.* (2001) 69:7955–8. doi: 10.1128/IAI.69.12.7955-7958.2001

114. Aguilar-Delfin I, Wettstein PJ, Persing DH. Resistance to acute babesiosis is associated with interleukin-12- and gamma interferon-mediated responses and requires macrophages and natural killer cells. *Infect Immun.* (2003) 71:2002–8. doi: 10.1128/IAI.71.4.2002-2008.2003

115. Goff WL, Johnson WC, Horn RH, Barrington GM, Knowles DP. The innate immune response in calves to boophilus microplus tick transmitted *Babesia bovis* involves type-1 cytokine induction and NK-like cells in the spleen. *Parasite Immunol.* (2003) 25:185–8. doi: 10.1046/j.1365-3024.2003.00625.x

116. Goff WL, Storset AK, Johnson WC, Brown WC. Bovine splenic NK cells synthesize ifn-gamma in response To Il-12-containing supernatants from *Babesia bovis*-exposed monocyte cultures. *Parasite Immunol.* (2006) 28:221–8. doi: 10.1111/j.1365-3024.2006.00830.x

117. Bastos RG, Johnson WC, Mwangi W, Brown WC, Goff WL. Bovine NK cells acquire cytotoxic activity and produce IFN-gamma after stimulation by *Mycobacterium bovis* BCG- or *Babesia bovis*-exposed splenic dendritic cells. *Vet Immunol Immunopathol.* (2008) 124:302–12. doi: 10.1016/j.vetimm.2008.04.004

118. Sun JC, Ugolini S, Vivier E. Immunological memory within the innate immune system. *Embo J.* (2014) 33:1295–303. doi: 10.1002/embj.201387651

119. Kwong B, Rua R, Gao Y, Flickinger JJr, Wang Y, Kruhlak MJ, et al. T-bet-dependent Nkp46+ innate lymphoid cells regulate the onset of Th17-induced neuroinflammation. *Nat Immunol.* (2017) 18:1117–27. doi: 10.1038/ni.3816

120. Crome SQ, Nguyen LT, Lopez-verges S, Yang SY, Martin B, Yam JY, et al. A distinct innate lymphoid cell population regulates tumor-associated T cells. *Nat Med.* (2017) 23:368–75. doi: 10.1038/nm.4278

121. Rydyznski C, Daniels KA, Karmele EP, Brooks TR, Mahl SE, Moran MT, et al. Generation of cellular immune memory and B-cell immunity is impaired by natural killer cells. *Nat Commun.* (2015) 6:6375. doi: 10.1038/ncomms7375

122. Cook KD, Kline HC, Whitmire JK. NK cells inhibit humoral immunity by reducing the abundance of CD4+ T follicular helper cells during a chronic virus infection. *J Leukoc Biol.* (2015) 98:153–62. doi: 10.1189/jlb.4HI1214-594R

123. Crouse J, Xu HC, Lang PA, Oxenius A. NK cells regulating T cell responses: mechanisms and outcome. *Trends Immunol.* (2015) 36:49–58. doi: 10.1016/j.it.2014.11.001

124. Waggoner SN, Daniels KA, Welsh RM. Therapeutic depletion of natural killer cells controls persistent infection. *J Virol.* (2014) 88:1953–60. doi: 10.1128/JVI.03002-13

Innate Lymphoid Cells in Protection, Pathology and Adaptive Immunity During Apicomplexan...

91

125. Xu HC, Grusdat M, Pandyra AA, Polz R, Huang J, Sharma P, et al. Type I interferon protects antiviral Cd8+ T cells from NK cell cytotoxicity. *Immunity* (2014) 40:949–60. doi: 10.1016/j.immuni.2014.05.004

126. Schuster IS, Wikstrom ME, Brizard G, Coudert JD, Estcourt MJ, Manzur M, et al. Trail+ NK cells control Cd4+ T cell responses during chronic viral infection to limit autoimmunity. *Immunity* (2014) 41:646–56. doi: 10.1016/j.immuni.2014.09.013

127. Peppa D, Gill US, Reynolds G, Easom NJ, Pallett LJ, Schurich A, et al. Up-regulation of a death receptor renders antiviral t cells susceptible to NK cell-mediated deletion. *J Exp Med.* (2013) 210:99–114. doi: 10.1084/jem.20121172

128. Cook KD, Whitmire JK. The depletion of NK cells prevents T cell exhaustion to efficiently control disseminating virus infection. *J Immunol.* (2013) 190:641–9. doi: 10.4049/jimmunol.1202448

129. Lang PA, Lang KS, Xu HC, Grusdat M, Parish IA, Recher M, et al. Natural killer cell activation enhances immune pathology and promotes chronic infection by limiting Cd8+ T-cell immunity. *Proc Natl Acad Sci USA.* (2012) 109:1210–5. doi: 10.1073/pnas.11188 34109

8

CD100/Sema4D Increases Macrophage Infection by *Leishmania (Leishmania) amazonensis* in a CD72 Dependent Manner

Mariana K. Galuppo[1], Eloiza de Rezende[1], Fabio L. Forti[2], Mauro Cortez[1], Mario C. Cruz[3], Andre A. Teixeira[2], Ricardo J. Giordano[2] and Beatriz S. Stolf[1]*

[1] *Department of Parasitology, Institute of Biomedical Sciences, University of São Paulo, São Paulo, Brazil,* [2] *Department of Biochemistry, Institute of Chemistry, University of São Paulo, São Paulo, Brazil,* [3] *Department of Immunology, Institute of Biomedical Sciences, University of São Paulo, São Paulo, Brazil*

*Correspondence:
Beatriz S. Stolf
bstolf@usp.br

Leishmaniasis is caused by trypanosomatid protozoa of the genus *Leishmania*, which infect preferentially macrophages. The disease affects 12 million people worldwide, who may present cutaneous, mucocutaneous or visceral forms. Several factors influence the form and severity of the disease, and the main ones are the *Leishmania* species and the host immune response. CD100 is a membrane bound protein that can also be shed. It was first identified in T lymphocytes and latter shown to be induced in macrophages by inflammatory stimuli. The soluble CD100 (sCD100) reduces migration and expression of inflammatory cytokines in human monocytes and dendritic cells, as well as the intake of oxidized low-density lipoprotein (oxLDL) by human macrophages. Considering the importance of macrophages in *Leishmania* infection and the potential role of sCD100 in the modulation of macrophage phagocytosis and activation, we analyzed the expression and distribution of CD100 in murine macrophages and the effects of sCD100 on macrophage infection by *Leishmania (Leishmania) amazonensis*. Here we show that CD100 expression in murine macrophages increases after infection with *Leishmania*. sCD100 augments infection and phagocytosis of *Leishmania (L.) amazonensis* promastigotes by macrophages, an effect dependent on macrophage CD72 receptor. Besides, sCD100 enhances phagocytosis of zymosan particles and infection by *Trypanosoma cruzi*.

Keywords: CD100, *Leishmania amazonensis*, macrophages, phagocytosis, infection index, CD72

INTRODUCTION

Leishmaniasis is a complex of diseases caused by trypanosomatid protozoa of the genus *Leishmania*, which can be grouped into cutaneous or visceral forms (Alvar et al., 2012). Due to their considerable impact on global health, leishmaniasis are listed among the priority endemic diseases of the World Health Organization (WHO). It is estimated that 12 million people in the world are infected, and about 1.5 million new cases are reported every year (Alvar et al., 2012). The disease currently affects 98 countries, and in Brazil it has been observed an increase in the number of cases in recent years, accompanied by their geographical spread (WHO, 2015). Many species of *Leishmania* cause leishmaniasis in humans. The parasite species as well as the host immune response are the main determinants of the clinical form and the course of the disease (McMahon-Pratt and Alexander, 2004). The available treatment options for many *Leishmania* species and clinical forms are toxic and not always effective (McGwire and Satoskar, 2014). Thus, understanding the molecular basis of infection may be an important step toward the development of novel therapeutic approaches for this disease.

Leishmania is an intracellular parasite that infects mononuclear phagocytic cells of vertebrates. Macrophages are the main parasite host cells and their activation is crucial for the resolution of the infection (Iniesta et al., 2002, 2005). The general process of phagocytosis is an essential mechanism of the innate immune response by which phagocytes such as macrophages internalize microorganisms, dead or dying cells, and debris. It is an actin-dependent process triggered by the interaction between phagocyte's receptors and ligands of the particle to be engulfed (May and Machesky, 2001; Underhill and Goodridge, 2012).

The receptors most frequently involved in the phagocytosis of *Leishmania* are complement receptors 3 (CR3) and 1 (CR1), mannose receptor (MR), fibronectin receptor (FnR) and receptors Fc gamma (FcγRs) (Blackwell et al., 1985; Mosser and Edelson, 1985; Wyler et al., 1985; Da Silva et al., 1989; Guy and Belosevic, 1993). The receptors and internalization pathways may vary depending on the parasite stage (Ueno and Wilson, 2012). The actin cytoskeleton also plays important role in *Leishmania* binding and internalization, and was studied in more detail in *L. (Leishmania) donovani* (May et al., 2000; Roy et al., 2014; Podinovskaia and Descoteaux, 2015). The association of polymerized F-actin and parasite binding was also shown for *L. (Viannia) braziliensis* (Azevedo et al., 2012), *L. (L.) amazonensis*, and *L. (Leishmania) major* (Courret et al., 2002).

CD100, also known as Sema4D, belongs to class IV of semaphorins and was the first semaphorin described in the immune system (Bougeret et al., 1992; Mizui et al., 2009; Ch'ng and Kumanogoh, 2010). It exists as a membrane bound dimer or as a soluble protein originated by proteolytic cleavage (Elhabazi et al., 2003; Basile et al., 2007) that interacts with specific receptors, mainly plexin B1 (Basile et al., 2004; Conrotto et al., 2005; Nkyimbeng-Takwi and Chapoval, 2011) and CD72 (Kumanogoh et al., 2000; Ishida et al., 2003; Smith et al., 2011).

CD100 is expressed by the majority of the cells of the hematopoietic system, including B and T lymphocytes, natural killer and myeloid cells, and its expression usually increases upon activation (Elhabazi et al., 2003). Membrane CD100 is cleaved from the cell surface in an activation-dependent manner (Kikutani and Kumanogoh, 2003). In fact, sCD100 is shed by activated T and B cells, and sCD100 can be detected in sera of mice immunized with T-cell–dependent antigens or in sera of MRL/lpr mice with autoimmune disease (Wang et al., 2001). In mice, sCD100 increases proliferation, differentiation and IgG1 production by stimulated B cells (Kumanogoh et al., 2000; Shi et al., 2000). CD100 mediates DC-T cell interaction increasing activation, proliferation and differentiation of T cells (Shi et al., 2000; Kumanogoh et al., 2002; Mizui et al., 2009), and inducing DC maturation (Kumanogoh et al., 2002). In humans, sCD100 inhibits migration of B cells (Delaire et al., 2001), monocytes and immature DCs (Chabbert-de Ponnat et al., 2005). It also increases IL-10 secretion and reduces IL-6, IL-8 and TNF-α in monocytes and DCs (Chabbert-de Ponnat et al., 2005).

Although it is known that CD100 is expressed in macrophages (Kikutani and Kumanogoh, 2003; Nkyimbeng-Takwi and Chapoval, 2011), few studies have reported its effects on these cells. One of them analyzed the role of macrophage shed sCD100 in tumor angiogenesis (Sierra et al., 2008). Other showed that CD100 is also important in glomerular nephritis, enhancing T and B cell activation and the recruitment of macrophages (Li et al., 2009). We have shown that macrophages from human atherosclerotic plaques express CD100, and that sCD100 inhibits internalization of oxidized LDL (Luque et al., 2013). We have also shown that CD100 participates on the interaction between human monocyte and endothelial cell by binding to plexins B1 and B2 (Luque et al., 2015).

The effect of sCD100 on oxLDL phagocytosis by macrophage, the main *Leishmania* host cells, prompted us to study the expression of this molecule and its effects on the phagocytosis of this parasite. *Leishmania* lesions are characterized by intense inflammatory infiltrates, and thus sCD100 is probably shed by activated T and B cells near infected and non-infected macrophages. Here we show that sCD100 increases macrophage phagocytosis of *L. (L.) amazonensis* promastigotes, *Trypanosoma cruzi* trypomastigotes and zymosan particles. In addition, we demonstrated that sCD100 effects depend on macrophage CD72, a receptor for CD100. This is the first report of CD100 effect on a parasitic infection, and further studies should address the role of this molecule in animal models of leishmaniasis.

MATERIALS AND METHODS

Leishmania (Leishmania) amazonensis Promastigotes

Promastigotes of *L. (L.) amazonensis* LV79 strain (MPRO/BR/72/M1841) were cultured at 24°C in M199 medium supplemented with 10% fetal calf serum (FCS). Parasites were subcultured every 7 days at an initial inoculum of 2×10^6/mL.

When indicated, promastigotes were incubated for 2 h with 200 ng/ml sCD100 in M199 at 24°C, centrifuged at $2,500 \times g$ for 10 min and resuspended in RPMI 1640 medium supplemented with 10% FBS for subsequent infection of peritoneal macrophages.

Ethics Statement

All animals were used according to the Brazilian College of Animal Experimentation guidelines, and the protocols were approved by the Institutional Animal Care and Use Committee (CEUA) of the University of São Paulo (protocol number 001/2009).

Recombinant sCD100 Production

sCD100 protein fused to Fc portion of IgG was produced in HEK (human embryonic kidney) 293T cells transfected with CD100-Fc plasmid, kindly given byKumanogoh et al. (2000). Briefly, $7,5 \times 10^6$ HEK cells were plated in DMEM with 5% serum "low-IgG" (Life Technologies) supplemented with 2 mM L-glutamine, 1 mM sodium pyruvate and 1× antibiotic-antimycotic solution (Life Technologies). Ten micrograms of

CD100-Fc plasmid were mixed with 1 mL of a 150 mM NaCl solution and then with 100 μL of a polyethylenimine solution (PEI, Sigma) at 0.45 mg/mL. The total volume was added slowly to each dish, which was then incubated at 37°C with 5% CO_2 for 7 days. After this period, supernatants of cell cultures were collected, filtered through a 0.22 μm membrane and centrifuged at 7,500 × g for 10 min. PMSF to 100 μM was added to the supernatant and proteins were precipitated with 60% w/v ammonium sulfate under slow stirring at 4°C for 24 h. Two successive centrifugations at 10,000 × g for 45 min were performed, precipitates were resuspended in PBS and centrifuged. The supernatant was incubated with protein G beads (1 mL Protein G Sepharose 4FF GE beads/50 mL supernatant) under rotation at 4°C for 24 h. The suspension was then centrifuged at 800 × g for 5 min and the beads were transferred to a chromatography column (Bio-Rad). The column was washed twice with 5 mL ice cold PBS and protein was eluted in aliquots of 500 μL using 0.1 M glycine buffer, pH 3.0, neutralized by 50 μl 1 M Tris buffer pH 8.0. Protein concentrations were determined by Bradford (Bio-Rad) and sCD100 was analyzed by SDS–PAGE and Western blot.

Macrophage Infection With *Leishmania* and Phagocytosis of Zymosan

Peritoneal macrophages were isolated as previously described (Velasquez et al., 2016). We then transferred 8 × 10^5 cells in RPMI 1640 pH 7.2 to each well of 24 well plates laid with 13 mm circular coverslips. After 2 h of incubation at 37°C in 5% CO_2, the medium was changed to RPMI with 10% FCS with or without 100 or 200 ng/mL sCD100 and cells were incubated until the next day. Infection was performed with *L. (L.) amazonensis* promastigotes at the beginning of stationary phase (day four) using a multiplicity of infection (MOI) of 5:1 for 4 h. After removing the non-internalized parasites, cells were further incubated for 24, 48, and 72 h with or without (control) sCD100. Control experiments for the effect of sCD100 Fc portion on *Leishmania* infection were performed using recombinant IgG1 and FcR blocker, and are described latter. Zymosan particles were incubated with macrophages at a ratio of 1:1 for 1 h to analyze the phagocytosis index. In *Leishmania* and zymosan experiments cells were fixed with methanol, stained with Giemsa and mounted with Entellan (Merck). One hundred macrophages were analyzed per glass slide to determine the proportion of infected cells (IM), the total number of amastigotes (AMA), amastigotes/infected macrophage and Infection Index or Phagocytosis Index (II = IM x AMA). Three coverslips were prepared for each condition.

Cell Infection by *Trypanosoma cruzi*

Experimental procedures were carried as previously described (Teixeira A. A. et al., 2015). Briefly, peritoneal macrophages were seeded in 24 well plates laid with 13 mm circular coverslips as described above, with or without 200 ng/mL sCD100. Cells were then infected with tissue culture-derived trypomastigotes (Y strain) at MOI = 10 with or without 200 ng/mL CD100 (N = 3 for each condition) for 2 h at 37°C. The cells were then washed 10 times with PBS and further cultivated for 24 h to allow parasite differentiation. Macrophages were fixed with 4% paraformaldehyde, stained with anti-*T. cruzi* polyclonal antibody and propidium iodide and photographed with an epifluorescence microscope. Quantification was performed by counting the number of total and infected cells in at least 4 different fields (20 × magnification) for each replicate.

Macrophage Infections With sCD100 and Fc Receptor Blocker, Human Recombinant IgG1, or Anti-CD72

To monitor the effect of sCD100 Fc portion on *Leishmania* infection, incubations with *L. (L.) amazonensis* were performed in the presence of sCD100 and FcR blocker, and in the presence of human recombinant Fc portion of IgG1. To evaluate the role of CD72 in sCD100 effects, infections were done in the presence of anti-CD72. For FcR blocking: macrophages were plated and incubated with Fc receptor blockers (CD16 and CD32-BD Biosciences) at 0.1 ug/mL for 10 min, and then 200 ng/mL of sCD100 was added. *Leishmania* was added in the following day in the presence of FcR blocker and sCD100 for 4 and 24 h. For IgG1, macrophages were plated and incubated with 70 ng/mL of human recombinant IgG1 Fc (R&D Systems) and 200 ng/mL sCD100, and infected in the following day in the presence of the same proteins. For anti-CD72, plated macrophages were incubated with 10 μg/mL of anti-CD72 H-96 (Santa Cruz Biotechnology) and 1 h later sCD100 was added to 200 ng/mL. Infection was performed in the following day in the presence of both proteins. Control conditions included incubation only with sCD100 and with each treatment (Fc blocker or Fc-IgG1) separately, as well as untreated infected macrophages. The analysis and comparisons were based on infection rates.

Immunofluorescence for Phagocytosis and for F-Actin, CD100, and CD72 Labeling

Resident peritoneal macrophages from BALB/c mice were plated on glass slides as described and incubated with no stimulus or with 100 or 200 ng/mL of sCD100, or 100 or 200 ng/mL of BSA overnight.

For phagocytosis and for F-actin and CD100 labeling: Promastigotes of *L. (L.) amazonensis* were added in the proportion of 10 parasites per cell in the presence or absence of sCD100 or BSA and the plate was kept on ice for 2 h, and at 33°C with 5% CO_2 for different periods. After washing, macrophages were fixed with 4% paraformaldehyde for 10 min, washed with PBS 1X with 2% FBS, incubated for 30 min in 50 mM ammonium chloride and washed in PBS 1X with 2% FBS.

For labeling of CD100 and actin, cells were permeabilized with TBS containing 1% BSA and 0.1% Triton for 10 min. Slides were washed and incubated overnight with anti-CD100 (eBioscience) at 1:50 dilution, and after washing were incubated with anti-Rat IgG Alexa Fluor 568 (Thermo Scientific) diluted 1: 1000 and DAPI 1: 600 for 1 h. Alternatively, cells were incubated with phalloidin Texas Red (Molecular Probes) 1: 500 and DAPI 1: 600 for 1 h. In both cases, coverslips were washed five times with PBS and mounted in ProLong (Molecular Probes).

For analysis of phagocytosis glass slides were incubated overnight with anti-*Leishmania* serum diluted 1:75 in PBS 1X, washed five times with PBS and incubated for 1 h with a mix containing anti-mouse IgG Alexa Fluor 488 (Thermo Scientific) 1: 1000. After washing, permeabilization with TBS containing 1% BSA and 0.1% Triton for 10 min and further washing, phalloidin Texas Red (Molecular Probes) 1: 500 and DAPI 1: 600 were added for 1 h. After five washes, cells were mounted in ProLong (Molecular Probes). For calculation of the phagocytosis index, 500 macrophages were analyzed and promastigotes were quantified as attached (labeled in green and blue) or internalized (labeled only with blue-DAPI).

For CD72 labeling, slides containing non-infected macrophages were fixed as described. After washing they were incubated with anti-CD72 antibody M-96 (Santa Cruz Biotechnologies) 1:75 overnight, washed and incubated for 2 h

with DAPI at 1: 600 and anti-rabbit Alexa Fluor 488 (Thermo Scientific) 1: 100. After labeling, coverslips were washed three times in PBS 1X with 2% FBS and cells were mounted in ProLong (Molecular Probes).

For CD100 quantification, images were acquired in a DMI6000B/AF6000 (Leica) fluorescence microscope coupled to a digital camera system (DFC 365 FX) and analyzed with the Image J program.

For actin and CD72 labeling and for the phagocytosis assay, images were captured using a Zeiss LSM 780 confocal laser scanning inverted microscope (Carl Zeiss, Germany) in a 1024 × 1024 pixel format. Image stacks comprised 8 images captured with a Plan-Apochromat 63×/1.4 DIC Oil M27 objective (Zeiss), applying a zoom factor of 1.0. Step intervals along the Z-axis ranged from 450 nm. Image acquisition and processing were performed using the Zen 2011 software (Zeiss, version 11.00.190).

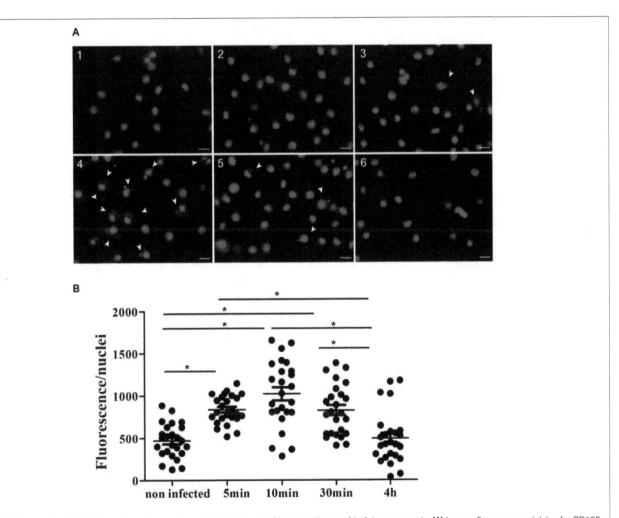

FIGURE 1 | Expression of CD100 in peritoneal macrophages infected or not with promastigotes of *L. (L.) amazonensis*. **(A)** Immunofluorescence staining for CD100 on infected and non-infected macrophages. Peritoneal macrophages from BALB/c mice non-infected (1 and 2), infected with promastigotes of *L. (L.) amazonensis* at MOI of 10:1 for 5 min (3), 10 min (4), 30 min (5), and 4 h (6). Staining with anti-CD100 antibody and secondary anti-rat Alexa Fluor 568 (red) and DAPI (blue nucleus). Control: DAPI (1) and secondary anti-rat Alexa Fluor 568 + DAPI (2). Images were captured in a DMI6000B/AF6000 (Leica) fluorescence microscope coupled to a digital camera system (DFC 365 FX). White bars correspond to 10 μm. **(B)** Quantification of red fluorescence/nuclei in 25 fields for each condition. Statistical analysis by ANOVA with Tukey's post-test, significant differences are labeled as *$p \leq 0.05$.

SDS–PAGE and Western Blot

SDS–PAGE (running gels with 10% acrylamide: bisacrylamide) and Western blots were performed as we previously described (Teixeira P. C. et al., 2015), using the following antibodies and incubation conditions: anti β-actin (Imuny, Brazil) 1: 1000 overnight and anti-rabbit IgG (H + L) (Imuny, Brazil) 1: 2000 for 1 h; anti-CD72 H-96 (Santa Cruz Biotechnology) 1: 200 overnight and anti-rabbit HRP (Imuny) 1: 1000 for 1 h, anti-GAPDH (Sigma-Aldrich) 1: 10000 overnight and anti-rabbit HRP (Imuny) 1: 1000 for 1 h. Normalizations for CD72 were done using anti-GAPDH while actin polymerization was estimated by F/G ratio.

Statistical Analysis

Statistical analyses were done using t-test or one-way ANOVA followed by Tukey's multiple comparison test, depending on the number of samples. Data were considered statistically different (*) when $p < 0.05$.

RESULTS

CD100 Expression Increases in Macrophages During Infection With Leishmania (L.) amazonensis

Although CD100 expression in macrophages has already been documented (Kikutani and Kumanogoh, 2003; Nkyimbeng-Takwi and Chapoval, 2011), its expression and effects during parasitic infection were never explored. Thus, we have performed labeling and quantification of CD100 protein in peritoneal BALB/c macrophages under controlled conditions and at different time points following infection with L. (L.) amazonensis promastigotes at a MOI (multiplicity of infection) of 10 parasites per macrophage. We observed that CD100 protein levels are altered following infection in a time dependent manner (**Figure 1A**): intracellular CD100 increases between 5 and 30 min after infection and then returns to basal levels within 4 h (**Figure 1B**).

Soluble CD100 Increases Infection of Macrophages by Leishmania (L.) amazonensis

After demonstrating that Leishmania infection increases macrophage CD100 endogenous levels, we evaluated whether the host cell infection by the parasite was affected by soluble CD100 (sCD100) added to the media. In the Leishmania lesion environment, sCD100 may be shed by macrophages, which express low levels of the protein (Sierra et al., 2008; Li et al., 2009; Luque et al., 2013), or by other cells, mainly activated T cells, which are known to release sCD100 (Wang et al., 2001). We thus analyzed the role of exogenous sCD100 on macrophage infection by Leishmania. We produced sCD100-Fc recombinant protein (from now on named as sCD100) in HEK293T and incubated macrophages with sCD100 before and together with L. (L.) amazonensis for different times.

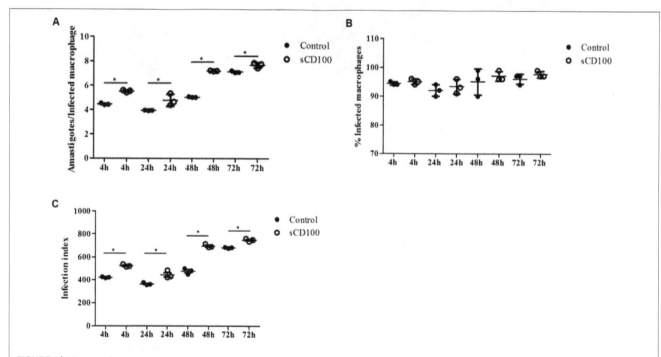

FIGURE 2 | Effects of sCD100 on infection of macrophages. Macrophages from BALB/c mice were infected with L. (L.) amazonensis promastigotes at a MOI of 5 per 4, 24, 48, or 72 h in the presence or not of 100 ng/mL sCD100. **(A)** Amastigotes per infected cell. **(B)** Percentage of infected macrophages. **(C)** Infection index. Statistical analysis was performed by ANOVA with Tukey's post-test, and significant differences are labeled as *$p \leq 0.05$. Results of a representative experiment of three with similar profiles.

Our results show that the number of amastigotes per cell (**Figure 2A**), and consequently infection rates (calculated as a product of the proportion of infected cells and the number of amastigotes) (**Figure 2C**), increase significantly in the presence of sCD100 in 4, 24, 48, and 72 h of infection. On the other hand, the percentages of infected macrophages (**Figure 2B**) do not change significantly over time with or without sCD100.

Pre-incubation of Promastigotes With sCD100 Does Not Increase Infection of Macrophages

A possible explanation for the increase of infection by L. (L.) amazonensis induced by sCD100 could be the binding of this molecule to the parasite, promoting its adhesion to a CD100 receptor present on the macrophage or to Fc receptors, as sCD100 protein is fused to human Fc region of IgG1 (Kumanogoh et al., 2000). To verify the first hypothesis, we pre-incubated promastigotes with sCD100 prior to macrophage infection. Again, infection was performed for 4, 24, 28, and 72 h. No significant difference in the number of macrophages infected with L. (L.) amazonensis or in the number of amastigote forms inside individual infected cells was observed by pre-incubation with sCD100 relative to controls at all time points (**Figure 3**). These

data indicate that sCD100 does not increase infection by direct contact/interaction with the parasite. On the other hand, when macrophages are pre-incubated with sCD100, the infection rate increases significantly (**Figures 3A–D**, control vs. sCD100).

Because the recombinant sCD100 that we used is produced as fusion between sCD100 and the Fc portion of IgG1, we next analyzed whether its effect on phagocytosis could be due to an interaction of the Fc IgG1 portion with the macrophage Fc receptor (FcR). To evaluate this possibility, macrophage infection assays were repeated in the presence of recombinant Fc region of human IgG1. The same control protein has been used in different studies, including one with Leishmania infection (Cortez et al., 2011). As expected, sCD100 alone increased macrophage infection by L. (L.) amazonensis while soluble IgG1 had no effect (**Figure 4**). Similar results were obtained when we blocked Fc receptor using the commercial blockers CD16 and CD32 (Supplementary Figure 1). Taken together, these results demonstrate that the increase in infection is directly mediated by sCD100.

CD72 Is Expressed in Macrophages and Mediates sCD100 Effects on Infection

CD72 is considered the main receptor for CD100 in macrophages (Kumanogoh et al., 2000; Ishida et al., 2003; Smith et al., 2011),

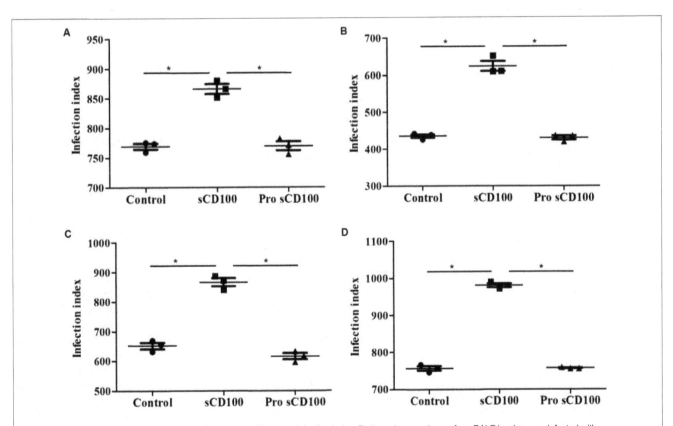

FIGURE 3 | Effects of preincubation of promastigotes with sCD100 on infection index. Peritoneal macrophages from BALB/c mice were infected with L. (L.) amazonensis at a MOI of 5 for 4 **(A)**, 24 **(B)**, 48 **(C)**, or 72 **(D)** hours at different conditions: macrophages and parasites without sCD100 (control), promastigotes preincubated with sCD100 at a concentration of 200 ng/mL (promastigote+sCD100), macrophages and promastigotes in the continuous presence of sCD100 at a concentration of 200 ng/mL (sCD100). Statistical analysis was performed by ANOVA with Tukey's post-test, and significant differences are labeled as *$p \leq 0.05$. Results of a representative experiment of three.

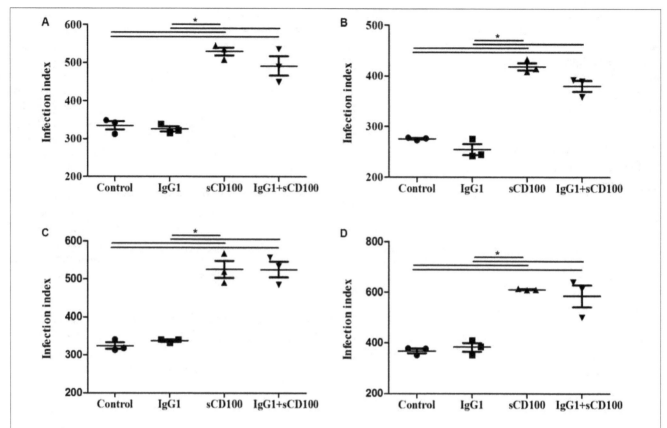

FIGURE 4 | Effects of IgG1 competition on infection index. Peritoneal macrophages from BALB/c mice were infected with *L. (L.) amazonensis* at a MOI of 5 for 4 **(A)**, 24 **(B)**, 48 **(C)**, and 72 **(D)** hours in the absence of stimulus (control), in the presence of 200 ng/mL of sCD100, 70 ng/mL of human IgG1 or IgG1+sCD100. Statistical analysis was performed by ANOVA with Tukey's post-test, and significant differences are labeled as *$p \leq 0.05$. Results of a representative experiment of three.

but its expression has not been analyzed in murine peritoneal macrophages. We thus verified the expression of this receptor in these cells. By Western blot we observed the reactivity of CD72 immunospecific antibodies with a 45 kDa protein, the expected molecular weight for this receptor (**Figure 5A**, lane 1). Its expression is not altered upon incubation of the macrophages with sCD100, since we observed similar levels (ratios of CD72/GAPDH, the endogenous control used) in macrophages plated in the presence or not of sCD100 (**Figure 5A**, lane 2). An unrelated cell line (L929 fibroblast), which does not express CD72, was used as negative control (**Figure 5A**, lane 3). By immunofluorescence, we observed CD72 labeling in peritoneal macrophages (**Figure 5B**), confirming the presence of the receptor in these cells.

Next, we evaluated whether blockage of CD72 would affect sCD100-induced increase in macrophage infection. Macrophages were preincubated with anti-CD72 antibodies and infected with *Leishmania*. We observed that anti-CD72 antibodies alone have no effect on macrophage infection (**Figure 5C**, lane 2), as the number of infected cells is similar to control, and that sCD100 increases macrophage infection, as expected. However, when anti-CD72 antibody is added before sCD100, infection levels returned to basal levels (**Figure 5C**). These results indicate that sCD100 increases *L. (L.) amazonensis* infection in a CD72 dependent manner.

sCD100 Increases Phagocytosis of *L. (L.) amazonensis* and Zymosan Particles

We have shown that sCD100 increases infection of macrophages after 4 h of incubation with *Leishmania*, suggesting that the molecule could participate in the initial steps of phagocytosis. To test this hypothesis, we performed a phagocytosis assay in which macrophages were plated (overnight) in the presence or absence of sCD100 and then incubated with promastigotes in the presence or absence of sCD100 for only 5 min. Promastigotes attached to the host cell were visualized by fluorescent microscopy in green and blue (anti-*Leishmania* and DAPI, respectively), while internalized parasites were labeled only in blue (DAPI) (Supplementary Figure 2). Phagocytosis of *Leishmania* was assessed quantitatively by the percentage of infected macrophages and the total number of promastigotes phagocytosed. Phagocytosis of zymosan was also analyzed. An increase in infected macrophages and internalized promastigotes (**Figures 6A,B**) was observed in the presence of sCD100, indicating that it affects the initial steps of phagocytosis. Besides, there was a significant increase in the phagocytosis of zymosan (represented by the phagocytosis index) at both sCD100 concentrations tested (**Figure 6C**), indicating that this protein augments phagocytosis in general and not specifically of *Leishmania* parasites.

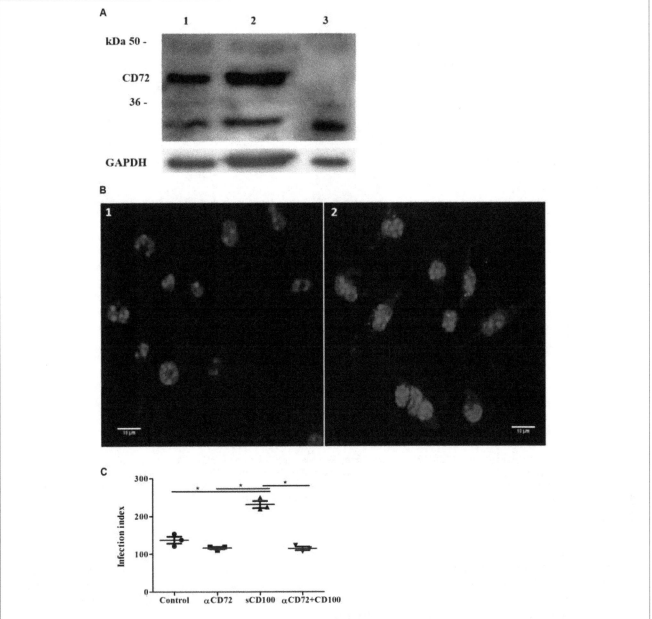

FIGURE 5 | Expression of CD72 and its role in sCD100 effects on macrophages. **(A)** Western blot showing expression of CD72 and GAPDH in peritoneal macrophages from BALB/c mice (lane 1), macrophage incubated with 200 ng/mL of sCD100 for 48 h (lane 2) and L929 cells (negative control - lane 3). Thirty micrograms of protein extracts were analyzed in 10% SDS–PAGE. **(B)** Immunofluorescence staining for CD72 in peritoneal macrophages from BALB/c mice: control incubated with anti-rabbit Alexa Fluor 488 secondary antibody and DAPI (image 1), macrophages incubated with anti-CD72, anti-rabbit Alexa Fluor 488 secondary antibody and DAPI (image 2). Images were captured in Zeiss LSM 780-NLO confocal microscope, magnifying 63 ×, 1.0 zoom. **(C)** Infection index of macrophages from BALB/c mice in the presence or absence of sCD100, preincubated or not with anti-CD72 for 48 h. Data represent means and standard deviations of one experiment with triplicates. Statistical analysis was performed by ANOVA followed by Tukey's post-test, and significant differences are labeled as *$p \leq 0.05$.

sCD100 Does Not Affect Actin Polymerization

Since *Leishmania* is internalized in an actin-dependent process, we analyzed whether sCD100 modulated actin polymerization. Actin was analyzed in macrophages plated in the presence or abscence of sCD100 and infected with promastigotes in the presence or abscence of sCD100 for different periods. **Figure 7A** shows representative confocal images of immunofluorescence of

macrophages incubated with sCD100 and infected for 30 min and 4 h, as well as the same conditions with no sCD100. The analysis of multiple fields at 4 h of infection showed that F-actin (polymerized actin, labeled with Texas Red Phalloidin) has a different organization in macrophages stimulated with sCD100. In fact, while a cortical distribution (arrowhead) of F-actin is shown in the absence of sCD100 (**Figure 7A**, image 3), the presence of sCD100 leads to a more heterogeneous

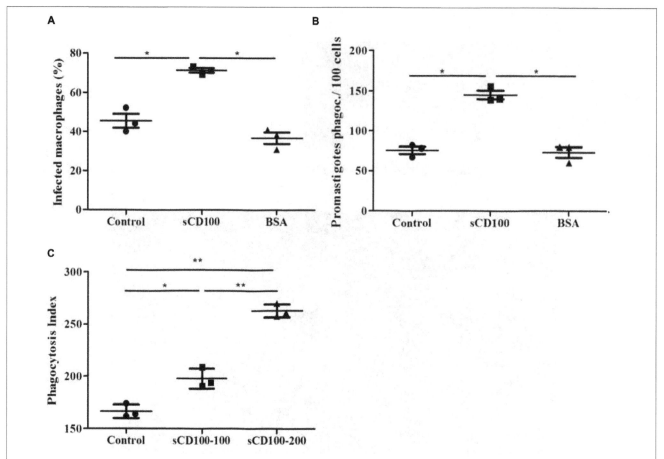

FIGURE 6 | Effect of sCD100 on phagocytosis of *Leishmania* and zymosan by peritoneal macrophages from BALB/c. **(A)** Percentage of infected macrophages and **(B)** promastigotes phagocytosed by 100 macrophages in the continuous presence of 100 ng/mL sCD100 or BSA or with no stimulus (control), analyzed by immunofluorescence. Data represent means and standard deviations of three independent experiments. **(C)** Phagocytosis index of zymosan using 1 particle per macrophage for 1 h in the continuous presence of 100 or 200 ng/mL sCD100 or with no stimulus (control). Results of a representative experiment out of three with similar values. Statistical analysis was performed by ANOVA followed by Tukey's post-test, and significant differences are labeled as *$p \leq 0.05$.

and cytoplasmic distribution of polymerized actin (**Figure 7A,** image 4). A cytoplasmic pattern of F-actin was also visualized at 30 min of infection, in both conditions (**Figure 7A,** images 1, 2). Confirming our previous results, the presence of sCD100 at 4 h of infection increased the number of promastigotes attached (arrows) and internalized by macrophages (**Figure 7A,** images 6,5, respectively), suggesting a correlation between the effect of sCD100 on F-actin dynamics and *Leishmania* infection.

Since small differences in F-actin polymerization may not be perceived by immunofluorescence, we evaluated actin polymerization in control macrophages and in macrophages treated with sCD100, infected or not with *L. (L.) amazonensis* by Western blot (**Figure 7B**). The experiment was based on the separation of F-actin (insoluble) and G-actin (soluble) by ultracentrifugation, followed by blotting for actin in the two fractions. As a technical control, we employed extracts of macrophages treated with Latrunculin A, which blocks actin polymerization (Oliveira et al., 1996). Under all conditions F-actin band is about two times more intense than G-actin band, irrespective of sCD100 stimulus or infection by *L. (L.) amazonensis* (**Figure 7B,** representative experiment). Thus, no

clear correlation between sCD100 and actin polymerization can be drawn. The control with Latrunculin A shows a clear decrease in the F-actin band, indicating that the separation of soluble and insoluble actin was efficient using this method.

Soluble CD100 Increases Infection of Macrophages by *Trypanosoma cruzi*

We have here shown that sCD100 binds to macrophage CD72 and increases *Leishmania* phagocytosis. We have also shown that treatment of macrophages with sCD100 increases phagocytosis of zymosan, indicating that this effect is not specific for *Leishmania*. Therefore, we decided to investigate whether cCD100 could modulate infection of macrophage by other parasites.

Trypanosoma cruzi has several developmental stages, and the infective trypomastigotes can enter almost all nucleated cells of the vertebrate host, phagocytic or non-phagocytic. Tissue resident macrophages are important targets for early infection, and parasite entry into these cells can occur by a phagocytic-like or a non-phagocytic mechanism (Epting et al., 2010; Barrias et al., 2013). We thus analyzed whether sCD100 could

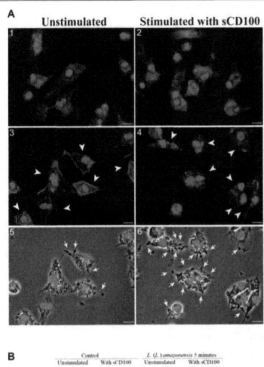

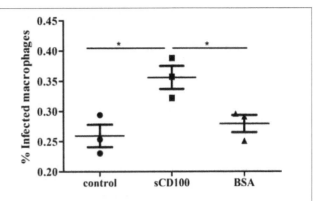

FIGURE 8 | Effects of sCD100 on infection of macrophages by Trypanosoma cruzi. Macrophages from BALB/c mice were infected with *T. cruzi* trypomastigotes at a MOI of 10 for 24 h in the presence or not of 200 ng/mL sCD100. Statistical analysis was performed by ANOVA with Tukey's post-test, and significant differences are labeled as *$p \leq 0.05$. Results of one experiment representative of two with similar profile.

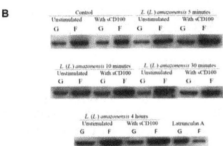

FIGURE 7 | Effect of sCD100 on actin polymerization in infected and non-infected macrophages. **(A)** Peritoneal macrophages from BALB/c mice unstimulated (1, 3, 5) or stimulated with 200 ng/mL of sCD100 (2, 4, 6) were infected with *L. (L.) amazonensis* at MOI of 10 for 30 min (1, 2) or 4 h (3, 4), followed by staining with phalloidin Red: Actin (labeled with phalloidin-Texas Red), Blue: nuclear DNA and kinetoplast (DAPI). Images were captured in DMI6000B/AF6000 (Leica) fluorescence microscope coupled to a digital camera system (DFC 365 FX). White bars correspond to 10 μm. The arrowheads point to macrophages presenting cortical (white) or cytoplasmic (yellow) organization of F-actin. Contrast phase of the samples at 4 h from unstimulated and stimulated with sCD100 (5, 6). The arrows point to parasites attached to macrophages. The images are representative of two independent experiments. **(B)** Western blot for actin in soluble and insoluble fractions of bone marrow macrophages incubated with or without sCD100, infected or not for 5, 10, 30 min or 4 h. This representative image shows soluble actin (supernatant, G-actin), and polymerized actin (pellet, F-actin) bands, and the graph shows F/G actin ratio after densitometry. Results of a representative experiment of three with the same profile.

also affect macrophage infection by *T. cruzi* trypomastigotes. Trypomastigotes were incubated with macrophages in the presence or absence of sCD100 and the percentage of infected cells was quantified. Similar to *Leishmania*, we observed that sCD100 promoted a significant increase in cell infection by *T. cruzi* (**Figure 8**). These results suggest that CD100 may play an important role in macrophage infection by different trypanosomatid parasites.

DISCUSSION

Monocytes and the mature macrophage cells are key elements in immunity, and their role in parasitic infection has been clearly demonstrated for trypanosomatids (Dos-Santos et al., 2016). Understanding the molecular mechanisms of parasite phagocytosis by these cells is an important step toward the development of novel therapeutic options for infected patients, in particular for visceral leishmaniasis, for which treatment is necessary but therapeutic options are usually toxic and with poor efficacy (McGwire and Satoskar, 2014). CD100 is an important molecule involved in the communication between immune cells (Kumanogoh et al., 2000; Shi et al., 2000; Mizui et al., 2009), but its role in macrophage functions has been poorly studied. In fact, the only report concerning CD100 and phagocytosis by these cells is a previous paper from our group showing that soluble CD100 (sCD100) decreases internalization of oxidized LDL by human macrophages by inhibiting the expression of the scavenger receptor CD36 (Luque et al., 2015).

Apart from their role in immune response, macrophages are the main host cells for *Leishmania*. We here showed that these cells respond to sCD100 by increasing phagocytosis of *Leishmania*, *Trypanosoma cruzi* and zymosan. Zymosan is a β-glucan rich particle derived from the yeast *Saccharomyces cerevisiae*, frequently used as a model for phagocytosis. Non-opsonized zymosan is mainly recognized by macrophage dectin-1 receptor (Brown et al., 2002), which is not involved in *Leishmania* phagocytosis. *T. cruzi* is internalized by host cells via multiple endocytic pathways. Entry into macrophages occurs mainly but not only by phagocytosis (Epting et al., 2010; Barrias et al., 2013), and involves several macrophage receptors, some of them different from the ones used for *Leishmania* internalization. Thus, the effect of sCD100 on phagocytosis probably does not depend on a specific phagocytic receptor of macrophages.

The increase in *Leishmania* infection promoted by sCD100 depends on its interaction with CD72 receptor. The effects of sCD100 on phagocytosis may differ in murine and human macrophages. In fact, CD72 is the main CD100 receptor in murine macrophages (Tamagnone et al., 1999; Kumanogoh et al., 2000), while we have shown that plexin B2 is an effective CD100 receptor in human monocytes and macrophages (Luque et al., 2015). CD72 was shown to be expressed in bronchial epithelial cells, alveolar macrophages, B cells, dendritic cells, fibroblasts, basophils (Kikutani and Kumanogoh, 2003; Mizui et al., 2009; Smith et al., 2011), and we here show its expression also in murine resident peritoneal macrophages. CD72 belongs to the superfamily of C-type lectins, which contain a cytoplasmic domain with two tyrosine inhibitory motifs (ITIMs) that when phosphorylated bind to the protein tyrosine phosphatase 1 (SHP-1) and the adapter protein Grb2 (Wu and Bondada, 2009; Nkyimbeng-Takwi and Chapoval, 2011). No study has ever analyzed CD72 signaling in macrophages, but most studies show that binding of CD100 to CD72 in B cell reverse the inhibitory potential of CD72 to cause dephosphorylation ITIM and release of SHP-1 (Wu and Bondada, 2009). It will be interesting to analyze whether sCD100 binding to macrophage affects not only parasite entry, as we demonstrated here, but also further signaling events such as ITIM phosphorylation and SHP1 release from the CD72 cytoplasmic tail. Infection in the presence of sCD100 led to changes in F-actin organization. Indeed, the cortical distribution of F-actin observed in macrophages at 4 h of infection changed to a heterogeneous and cytoplasmic pattern in the presence of sCD100. Similar changes in actin organization have already been reported in medullary macrophages when infected with *Leishmania amazonensis* (de Menezes et al., 2017) and in cultured chromaffin cells compared

to cells in adrenomedullary tissue (Gimenez-Molina et al., 2017).

This work is the first to report the role of CD100 in parasitic infection. Further studies must be performed to unravel how CD100 binding to macrophage CD72 increases phagocytosis of zymosan, *Leishmania* and *T. cruzi*, which interact with different surface receptors. Further studies should also address the role of sCD100 in *in vivo* models of leishmaniasis, and on *Leishmania* phagocytosis by human macrophages.

AUTHOR CONTRIBUTIONS

MG was the student responsible for the project, who performed most experiments, wrote the paper, and prepared most figures. ER performed immunofluorescence for CD100, prepared the corresponding figure, and revised the paper. FF helped in experimental design and phosphatase experiment (not included) and revised the paper. MC contributed with actin separation and immunofluorescence experiments and revised the paper. MCC performed confocal microscopy. AT and RG designed and performed *T. cruzi* infection experiments and revised the paper. BS designed and supervised the project, wrote the paper, and was responsible for the funding.

ACKNOWLEDGMENTS

We thank Atsushi Kumanogoh for CD100-Fc plasmid, Silvia Boscardin for help with protein production, Ana Paula Lepique for FcR blocker, and Silvia Uliana for important discussions during this project. We also thank CEFAP (Centro de Facilidades de Apoio a Pesquisa) -USP for confocal microscopy facility.

REFERENCES

1. Alvar, J., Velez, I. D., Bern, C., Herrero, M., Desjeux, P., Cano, J., et al. (2012). Leishmaniasis worldwide and global estimates of its incidence. *PLoS One* 7:e35671. doi: 10.1371/journal.pone.0035671
2. Azevedo, E., Oliveira, L. T., Castro Lima, A. K., Terra, R., Dutra, P. M., and Salerno, V. P. (2012). Interactions between *Leishmania braziliensis* and macrophages are dependent on the cytoskeleton and Myosin Va. *J. Parasitol. Res.* 2012:275436. doi: 10.1155/2012/275436
3. Barrias, E. S., de Carvalho, T. M., and De Souza, W. (2013). *Trypanosoma cruzi*: entry into Mammalian host cells and parasitophorous vacuole formation. *Front. Immunol.* 4:186. doi: 10.3389/fimmu.2013.00186
4. Basile, J. R., Barac, A., Zhu, T., Guan, K. L., and Gutkind, J. S. (2004). Class IV semaphorins promote angiogenesis by stimulating Rho-initiated pathways through plexin-B. *Cancer Res.* 64, 5212–5224. doi: 10.1158/0008-5472.CAN-04-0126
5. Basile, J. R., Holmbeck, K., Bugge, T. H., and Gutkind, J. S. (2007). MT1-MMP controls tumor-induced angiogenesis through the release of semaphorin 4D. *J. Biol. Chem.* 282, 6899–6905. doi: 10.1074/jbc.M6095 70200
6. Blackwell, J. M., Ezekowitz, R. A., Roberts, M. B., Channon, J. Y., Sim, R. B., and Gordon, S. (1985). Macrophage complement and lectin-like receptors bind *Leishmania* in the absence of serum. *J. Exp. Med.* 162, 324–331. doi: 10.1084/jem.162.1.324
7. Bougeret, C., Mansur, I. G., Dastot, H., Schmid, M., Mahouy, G., Bensussan, A., et al. (1992). Increased surface expression of a newly identified 150-kDa dimer early after human T lymphocyte activation. *J. Immunol.* 148, 318–323.
8. Brown, G. D., Taylor, P. R., Reid, D. M., Willment, J. A., Williams, D. L.,

Martinez-Pomares, L., et al. (2002). Dectin-1 is a major beta-glucan receptor on macrophages. *J. Exp. Med.* 196, 407–412. doi: 10.1084/jem.20020470
9. Chabbert-de Ponnat, I., Marie-Cardine, A., Pasterkamp, R. J., Schiavon, V., Tamagnone, L., Thomasset, N., et al. (2005). Soluble CD100 functions on human monocytes and immature dendritic cells require plexin C1 and plexin B1, respectively. *Int. Immunol.* 17, 439–447. doi: 10.1093/intimm/dxh224
10. Ch'ng, E. S., and Kumanogoh, A. (2010). Roles of Sema4D and Plexin-B1 in tumor progression. *Mol. Cancer* 9:251. doi: 10.1186/1476-4598-9-251
11. Conrotto, P., Valdembri, D., Corso, S., Serini, G., Tamagnone, L., Comoglio, P. M., et al. (2005). Sema4D induces angiogenesis through Met recruitment by Plexin B1. *Blood* 105, 4321–4329. doi: 10.1182/blood-2004-07-2885
12. Cortez, M., Huynh, C., Fernandes, M. C., Kennedy, K. A., Aderem, A., and Andrews, N. W. (2011). *Leishmania* promotes its own virulence by inducing expression of the host immune inhibitory ligand CD200. *Cell Host Microbe* 9, 463–471. doi: 10.1016/j.chom.2011.04.014
13. Courret, N., Frehel, C., Gouhier, N., Pouchelet, M., Prina, E., Roux, P., et al. (2002). Biogenesis of *Leishmania*-harbouring parasitophorous vacuoles following phagocytosis of the metacyclic promastigote or amastigote stages of the parasites. *J. Cell Sci.* 115(Pt 11), 2303–2316.
14. Da Silva, R. P., Hall, B. F., Joiner, K. A., and Sacks, D. L. (1989). CR1, the C3b receptor, mediates binding of infective Leishmania major metacyclic promastigotes to human macrophages. *J. Immunol.* 143, 617–622.
15. de Menezes, J. P., Koushik, A., Das, S., Guven, C., Siegel, A., Laranjeira-Silva, M. F., et al. (2017). *Leishmania* infection inhibits macrophage motility by altering F-actin dynamics and the expression of adhesion complex proteins. *Cell Microbiol.* 19:3. doi: 10.1111/cmi.12668

16. Delaire, S., Billard, C., Tordjman, R., Chedotal, A., Elhabazi, A., Bensussan, A., et al. (2001). Biological activity of soluble CD100. II. Soluble CD100, similarly to H-SemaIII, inhibits immune cell migration. *J. Immunol.* 166, 4348–4354. doi: 10.4049/jimmunol.166.7.4348

17. Dos-Santos, A. L., Carvalho-Kelly, L. F., Dick, C. F., and Meyer-Fernandes, J. R. (2016). Innate immunomodulation to trypanosomatid parasite infections. *Exp. Parasitol.* 167, 67–75. doi: 10.1016/j.exppara.2016.05.005

18. Elhabazi, A., Marie-Cardine, A., Chabbert-de Ponnat, I., Bensussan, A., and Boumsell, L. (2003). Structure and function of the immune semaphorin CD100/SEMA4D. *Crit. Rev. Immunol.* 23, 65–81. doi: 10.1615/CritRevImmunol.v23.i12.40

19. Epting, C. L., Coates, B. M., and Engman, D. M. (2010). Molecular mechanisms of host cell invasion by *Trypanosoma cruzi*. *Exp. Parasitol.* 126, 283–291. doi: 10.1016/j.exppara.2010.06.023

20. Gimenez-Molina, Y., Villanueva, J., Nanclares, C., Lopez-Font, I., Viniegra, S., Frances, M. D. M., et al. (2017). The differential organization of f-actin alters the distribution of organelles in cultured when compared to native Chromaffin cells. *Front. Cell. Neurosci.* 11:135. doi: 10.3389/fncel.2017.00135

21. Guy, R. A., and Belosevic, M. (1993). Comparison of receptors required for entry of *Leishmania* major amastigotes into macrophages. *Infect Immun.* 61, 1553–1558. Iniesta, V., Carcelen, J., Molano, I., Peixoto, P. M., Redondo, E., Parra, P., et al. (2005). Arginase I induction during *Leishmania* major infection mediates the development of disease. *Infect Immun.* 73, 6085–6090. doi: 10.1128/IAI.73.9. 6085-6090.2005

22. Iniesta, V., Gomez-Nieto, L. C., Molano, I., Mohedano, A., Carcelen, J., Miron, C., et al. (2002). Arginase I induction in macrophages, triggered by Th2-type cytokines, supports the growth of intracellular *Leishmania* parasites. *Parasite Immunol.* 24, 113–118. doi: 10.1046/j.1365-3024.2002.00444.x

23. Ishida, I., Kumanogoh, A., Suzuki, K., Akahani, S., Noda, K., and Kikutani, H. (2003). Involvement of CD100, a lymphocyte semaphorin, in the activation of the human immune system via CD72: implications for the regulation of immune and inflammatory responses. *Int. Immunol.* 15, 1027–1034. doi: 10.1093/intimm/dxg098

24. Kikutani, H., and Kumanogoh, A. (2003). Semaphorins in interactions between T cells and antigen-presenting cells. *Nat. Rev. Immunol.* 3, 159–167. doi: 10.1038/ nri1003

25. Kumanogoh, A., Suzuki, K., Ch'ng, E., Watanabe, C., Marukawa, S., Takegahara, N., et al. (2002). Requirement for the lymphocyte semaphorin, CD100, in the induction of antigen-specific T cells and the maturation of dendritic cells. *J. Immunol.* 169, 1175–1181. doi: 10.4049/jimmunol.169.3.1175

26. Kumanogoh, A., Watanabe, C., Lee, I., Wang, X., Shi, W., Araki, H., et al. (2000). Identification of CD72 as a lymphocyte receptor for the class IV semaphorin CD100: a novel mechanism for regulating B cell signaling. *Immunity* 13, 621–631. doi: 10.1016/S1074-7613(00)00062-5

27. Li, M., O'Sullivan, K. M., Jones, L. K., Lo, C., Semple, T., Kumanogoh, A., et al. (2009). Endogenous CD100 promotes glomerular injury and macrophage recruitment in experimental crescentic glomerulonephritis. *Immunology* 128, 114–122. doi: 10.1111/j.1365-2567.2009.03098.x

28. Luque, M. C., Gutierrez, P. S., Debbas, V., Kalil, J., and Stolf, B. S. (2015). CD100 and plexins B2 and B1 mediate monocyte-endothelial cell adhesion and might take part in atherogenesis. *Mol. Immunol.* 67, 559–567. doi: 10.1016/j.molimm. 2015.07.028

29. Luque, M. C., Gutierrez, P. S., Debbas, V., Martins, W. K., Puech-Leao, P., Porto, G., et al. (2013). Phage display identification of CD100 in Human atherosclerotic plaque macrophages and foam cells. *PLoS One* 8:e75772. doi: 10.1371/journal.pone.0075772

30. May, R. C., Caron, E., Hall, A., and Machesky, L. M. (2000). Involvement of the Arp2/3 complex in phagocytosis mediated by FcgammaR or CR3. *Nat. Cell Biol.* 2, 246–248. doi: 10.1038/35008673

31. May, R. C., and Machesky, L. M. (2001). Phagocytosis and the actin cytoskeleton. *J. Cell Sci.* 114(Pt 6), 1061–1077.

32. McGwire, B. S., and Satoskar, A. R. (2014). Leishmaniasis: clinical syndromes and treatment. *QJM* 107, 7–14. doi: 10.1093/qjmed/hct116

33. McMahon-Pratt, D., and Alexander, J. (2004). Does the *Leishmania* major paradigm of pathogenesis and protection hold for New World cutaneous Leishmaniases or the visceral disease? *Immunol. Rev.* 201, 206–224.

34. Mizui, M., Kumanogoh, A., and Kikutani, H. (2009). Immune semaphorins: novel features of neural guidance molecules. *J. Clin. Immunol.* 29, 1–11. doi: 10.1007/ s10875-008-9263-7

35. Mosser, D. M., and Edelson, P. J. (1985). The mouse macrophage receptor for C3bi (CR3) is a major mechanism in the phagocytosis of Leishmania promastigotes. *J. Immunol.* 135, 2785–2789.

36. Nkyimbeng-Takwi, E., and Chapoval, S. P. (2011). Biology and function of neuroimmune semaphorins 4A and 4D. *Immunol. Res.* 50, 10–21. doi: 10.1007/ s12026-010-8201-y

37. Oliveira, C. A., Kashman, Y., and Mantovani, B. (1996). Effects of latrunculin A on immunological phagocytosis and macrophage spreading-associated changes in the F-actin/G-actin content of the cells. *Chem. Biol. Interact.* 100, 141–153. doi: 10.1016/0009-2797(96)03695-2

38. Podinovskaia, M., and Descoteaux, A. (2015). *Leishmania* and the macrophage: a multifaceted interaction. *Fut. Microbiol.* 10, 111–129. doi: 10.2217/fmb. 14.103

39. Roy, S., Kumar, G. A., Jafurulla, M., Mandal, C., and Chattopadhyay, A. (2014). Integrity of the actin cytoskeleton of host macrophages is essential for *Leishmania donovani* infection. *Biochim. Biophys. Acta* 1838, 2011–2018. doi: 10.1016/j.bbamem.2014.04.017

40. Shi, W., Kumanogoh, A., Watanabe, C., Uchida, J., Wang, X., Yasui, T., et al. (2000). The class IV semaphorin CD100 plays nonredundant roles in the immune system: defective B and T cell activation in CD100-deficient mice. *Immunity* 13, 633–642. doi: 10.1016/S1074-7613(00)00063-7

41. Sierra, J. R., Corso, S., Caione, L., Cepero, V., Conrotto, P., Cignetti, A., et al. (2008). Tumor angiogenesis and progression are enhanced by Sema4D produced by tumor-associated macrophages. *J. Exp. Med.* 205, 1673–1685. doi: 10.1084/jem. 20072602

42. Smith, E. P., Shanks, K., Lipsky, M. M., DeTolla, L. J., Keegan, A. D., and Chapoval, S. P. (2011). Expression of neuroimmune semaphorins 4A and 4D and their receptors in the lung is enhanced by allergen and vascular endothelial growth factor. *BMC Immunol.* 12:30. doi: 10.1186/1471-2172- 12-30

43. Tamagnone, L., Artigiani, S., Chen, H., He, Z., Ming, G. I., Song, H., et al. (1999). Plexins are a large family of receptors for transmembrane, secreted, and GPI-anchored semaphorins in vertebrates. *Cell* 99, 71–80. doi: 10.1016/ S0092- 8674(00)80063-X

44. Teixeira, A. A., de Vasconcelos Vde, C., Colli, W., Alves, M. J., and Giordano, R. J. (2015). *Trypanosoma cruzi* binds to Cytokeratin through conserved peptide motifs found in the laminin-G-like domain of the gp85/Trans-sialidase proteins. *PLoS Negl. Trop. Dis.* 9:e0004099. doi: 10.1371/journal.pntd.00 04099

45. Teixeira, P. C., Velasquez, L. G., Lepique, A. P., de Rezende, E., Bonatto, J. M., Barcinski, M. A., et al. (2015). Regulation of *Leishmania* (L.) amazonensis protein expression by host T cell dependent responses: differential expression of oligopeptidase B, tryparedoxin peroxidase and HSP70 isoforms in amastigotes isolated from BALB/c and BALB/c nude mice. *PLoS Negl. Trop. Dis.* 9:e0003411. doi: 10.1371/journal.pntd.0003411

46. Ueno, N., and Wilson, M. E. (2012). Receptor-mediated phagocytosis of *Leishmania*: implications for intracellular survival. *Trends Parasitol.* 28, 335–344. doi: 10.1016/j.pt.2012.05.002

47. Underhill, D. M., and Goodridge, H. S. (2012). Information processing during phagocytosis. *Nat. Rev. Immunol.* 12, 492–502. doi: 10.1038/nri3244

48. Velasquez, L. G., Galuppo, M. K., De Rezende, E., Brandao, W. N., Peron, J. P., Uliana, S. R., et al. (2016). Distinct courses of infection with Leishmania (L.) amazonensis are observed in BALB/c, BALB/c nude and C57BL/6 mice. *Parasitology* 143, 692–703. doi: 10.1017/S003118201600024X

49. Wang, X., Kumanogoh, A., Watanabe, C., Shi, W., Yoshida, K., and Kikutani, H. (2001). Functional soluble CD100/Sema4D released from activated lymphocytes: possible role in normal and pathologic immune responses. *Blood* 97, 3498–3504. doi: 10.1182/blood.V97.11.3498

50. Wu, H. J., and Bondada, S. (2009). CD72, a coreceptor with both positive and negative effects on B lymphocyte development and function. *J. Clin. Immunol.* 29, 12–21. doi: 10.1007/s10875-008-9264-6

51. WHO (2015). *World Health Statistics*. Available at: http://www.who.int/gho/publications/world_health_statistics/2015/en/

52. Wyler, D. J., Sypek, J. P., and McDonald, J. A. (1985). In vitro parasite-monocyte interactions in human Leishmaniasis: possible role of fibronectin in parasite attachment. *Infect Immun.* 49, 305–311.

9

Immunomodulation by Helminths: Intracellular Pathways and Extracellular Vesicles

Amin Zakeri[1]*, Eline P. Hansen[2], Sidsel D. Andersen[1], Andrew R. Williams[2] and Peter Nejsum[1]*

[1] Department of Clinical Medicine, Faculty of Health, Aarhus University, Aarhus, Denmark, [2] Department of Veterinary and Animal Sciences, Faculty of Health and Medical Sciences, University of Copenhagen, Frederiksberg, Denmark

*Correspondence:
Amin Zakeri
amin.zakeri@clin.au.dk
Peter Nejsum
pn@clin.au.dk

Helminth parasites are masters at manipulating host immune responses, using an array of sophisticated mechanisms. One of the major mechanisms enabling helminths to establish chronic infections is the targeting of pattern recognition receptors (PRRs) including toll-like receptors, C-type lectin receptors, and the inflammasome. Given the critical role of these receptors and their intracellular pathways in regulating innate inflammatory responses, and also directing adaptive immunity toward Th1 and Th2 responses, recognition of the pathways triggered and/or modulated by helminths and their products will provide detailed insights about how helminths are able to establish an immunoregulatory environment. However, helminths also target PRRs-independent mechanisms (and most likely other yet unknown mechanisms and pathways) underpinning the battery of different molecules helminths produce. Herein, the current knowledge on intracellular pathways in antigen presenting cells activated by helminth-derived biomolecules is reviewed. Furthermore, we discuss the importance of helminth-derived vesicles as a less-appreciated components released during infection, their role in activating these host intracellular pathways, and their implication in the development of new therapeutic approaches for inflammatory diseases and the possibility of designing a new generation of vaccines.

Keywords: extracellular vesicle, helminths, immunosuppression, intracellular pathways, pattern recognition receptors

INTRODUCTION

Host-Parasite Interactions (Live Infection, Excretory Secretory Molecules, and Extracellular Vesicle)

Parasitic worms (helminths) constitute a very successful group of pathogens that have evolved a number of unique host adaptations (1). Despite their large size, and local or systemic migration throughout the host body, the worms only elicit limited inflammation in invaded tissues and install an immunoregulatory environment which ensures their survival (1). Such a masterful adaption is ascribed to their long coevolution with the hosts enabling them to perform an effective modulation of the immune system (2). Of note, this mutual relationship between worm and host evolves to reciprocal beneficial outcomes, as deworming can result in the emergence of immune-related disorders along with clinical manifestations (3). Various mechanisms have been identified by which helminths restrain host immune responses including expansion of regulatory cells (4), induction of apoptosis in immune cells (5), manipulation of pattern recognition receptors (PRRs) and downstream signaling (6), and suppression of Th1/Th2 cells and associated cytokines (7). However, there are likely to still be complex and unknown aspects of the strategies underpinning this sophisticated interface which are yet to be investigated (8).

In recent years, the regulatory functions of helminths and their potential ability to ameliorate inflammatory diseases have received much interest (8). Seminal research in this area mostly derives from the hypothesis of Strachan et al. who suggested an inverse relationship between sanitation and prevalence of allergy in different societies, the so-called "hygiene hypothesis" (9, 10). Based on this hypothesis, changes in or eradication of infections can lead to dysregulation of host immune responses, paving the way for allergic and autoimmune disorders (11).

A number of animal models along with some human pilot studies have evaluated the effects of live helminth infections on various inflammatory and autoimmune diseases, such as experimental autoimmune encephalomyelitis (12), asthma (13, 14), anaphylaxis (15) and inflammatory bowel disease (IBD) (16, 17). These experimental studies provided promising results concerning the beneficial effects of helminth infections on allergic and autoimmune diseases through stimulation of Treg cells, activation of toll-like receptor (TLRs), and induction of anti-inflammatory cytokines, such as TGFβ and IL-10 (18). Promising results obtained in both human and animal studies prompted clinical evaluations (16), but due to potential deleterious consequences and side effects which live worms may cause for humans, investigations have also focused on characterizing and recognition of helminth-derived products (HDPs) via exploiting high-throughput assays and omics-based techniques, such as proteomics (19, 20).

There are a number of studies indicating that many HDPs possess immunoregulatory properties. For example, the tapeworm, *Echinococcus granulosus* is able to bypass host immunosurveillance and polarize immune response toward the regulatory state (21). Antigen B (AgB) and sheep hydatid fluid (SHF) are two major components by which *E. granulosus* suppresses dendritic cell (DC) maturation and monocyte differentiation, resulting in reduced anti-parasite responses (21). Likewise, a well-known compound with remarkable regulatory functions is the phosphorylcholine-containing glycoprotein, ES-62 released by the filarial worm, *Acanthocheilonema viteae*, which has widely been investigated by Harnett and collogues (22). In addition, glycan-based compounds, such as Lacto-N-fucopentaose III /LewisX from helminths have been found to be central molecules eliciting Th2 responses and orchestration of immunoregulation through the involvement of C-type lectin receptors (23). Interestingly, some worms, such as the whipworm, *Trichuris suis* can forestall pro-inflammatory responses in human DCs (24). *T. suis* has been found to possess a high level of lipid-based biomolecules, such as prostaglandin (PGE2) which impairs TLR4-associated myeloid differentiation primary response protein 88 (MyD88) and the TIR-domain-containing adaptor-inducing interferon-β (TRIF) signaling (25, 26). Similarly, there is evidence showing that helminth defense molecules contribute to immunomodulatory

outcomes of parasitic infections via targeting innate immunity (27). However, the study of HDPs is still a major research area and fractionating HDPs and subsequent detailed studies have opened a new avenue for ongoing investigations.

Recently, extracellular vesicles (EVs) have emerged as a previously unappreciated entity of HDPs which may play a crucial role in parasite immunomodulation. These "magic bullets" have encouraged investigators to unravel their role in pathogenicity, invasion, and longevity of parasitic infections (28). Currently, EVs have shown that may be central in the host-parasite interplay and intracellular communication (29). During infection, the immune system is constantly interacting with a wide range of helminth-derived products including EVs which eventually results in either immune stimulation or immunoregulation. For example, it has recently been documented that parasite EVs can manipulate macrophage activation and regulate inflammatory responses (30, 31). The intercellular delivery of EV-associated RNAs, such as microRNAs, has identified them as important means for inducing epigenetic modifications in intracellular signaling and post-transcriptional regulation of gene expression (30, 32).

In this review, we aim to elaborate modulation of intracellular pathways, mainly in antigen presenting cells (APCs), by which HDPs polarize and suppress host immunity. Moreover, we suggest that understanding the intracellular outcomes upon interaction with HDPs will provide a broad insight into the possible interactions between EVs (as an important component of HDPs) and host intracellular machinery. The putative pathways enabling EVs to impose immunomodulatory effects on host immunity are highlighted. Furthermore, the implication of these vehicles in the development of new therapeutic approaches against inflammatory responses and possibilities of designing a new generation of vaccines based on EVs are discussed.

HELMINTH-DERIVED PRODUCTS (HDPS) AS POTENT IMMUNOMODULATORS

How HDPs Polarize Immune Responses by Targeting Intracellular Pathways

Helminths have evolved sophisticated mechanisms to target intracellular machinery in host cells (33). They have shown a remarkable ability to induce a tolerogenic immune microenvironment by releasing an array of bioactive materials (33). A large body of literature has identified HDPs as powerful modulators of inflammatory signals comprising an impressive range of molecular pathways elicited against parasites (33). HDPs, in total and as individual compounds, play a central role establishing a beneficial niche for the parasite via an effective manipulation of the host immunity to engage a receptor, degrade intracellular molecules, and interfering with essential signals (34). However, the majority of intracellular pathways targeted by these biomolecules are poorly described, but in the following, we focus on innate receptors as important sensors which are targeted by HDPs.

Pattern recognition receptors (PRRs) are one of the most important immune receptors, and their signaling is now becoming more apparent in regulation of immune responses (35). PRRs are a family of highly sensitive extra and intracellular sensors including Toll-like receptors (TLRs), nucleotide-binding oligomerization domain (NODs)-like receptors (NLRs), retinoic acid-inducible gene-like receptors (RIG-like receptors), and C-type lectin receptors (CLRs) (35). They are widely expressed by immune cells, in particular, those responsible for immunosurveillance, such as DCs and macrophages. PRRs are able to trigger a complex of intracellular crosstalk resulting in DC maturation and T cell priming (36).

Since HDPs are mostly rich in glycan-based products, such as glycoprotein along with lipid structures, TLRs and CLRs have been found to be predominantly targeted by these antigens during immunomodulation and hyporesponsiveness (37). HDPs not only alter the expression of TLRs but also masterfully manipulate their intracellular signaling, reflecting a strict control over host immunity by helminths (6). Interfering with these intracellular pathways, which are main drivers for priming inflammatory responses, suggests that these extracellular parasites can release substances modulating early responding cells in innate immunity (38). Despite the general view that microbial components can engage PRRs and thereby activate DCs, it is well-known that DCs exposed concurrently to HDPs and TLR agonists, such as viral or bacterial products do often not express markers associated with classical maturation (39, 40). For instance, murine DCs treated with soluble SEA fail to express MHC-II, costimulatory molecules, and proinflammatory cytokines in response to LPS (40). In the same way, the release of antigen B (AgB) (a hydatid cyst-derived antigen) by *E. granulosus* prevents upregulation of LPS-induced CD80, CD86, and TNFα in DCs (21), monocytes, and macrophages via an IL-10 independent manner (41).

Intriguingly, HDPs can also modulate TLRs signaling to prime a tolerogenic phenotype of DCs that produce anti-inflammatory cytokines (42). *Schistosoma mansoni* and released eggs can produce bioactive antigens, such as lysophosphatidylserine, lacto-N-fucopentaose III (LNFPIII), and double-stranded RNA (dsRNA) which attenuate inflammatory responses by targeting TLRs. LNFPIII has also been reported to induce DCs maturation and Th2 response polarization through CLRs (23). Another biomolecule that interacts with TLRs is ES-62 released by *A. viteae* which targets TLR4 on host immune cells. ES-62 is able to interfere with the downstream signalings mediated by TLR4, and through which diminishes the production of inflammatory mediators (22).

Likewise, many other HDPs, such as body fluid from adult *Ascaris suum,* have also been documented to induce hyporesponsiveness in human APCs treated with LPS and modulate different human macrophage phenotypes (43, 44). Although HDPs mainly seem to impair TLR4-associated inflammatory responses, it appears that these components tend to target manifold pathways in TLRs and CLRs signaling. Recent bioinformatics-based data has suggested that HDPs constitute a myriad of molecules with complex structures (20). Thus, recognition of a target on DCs would be essential to dissect and identify the major immunosuppressive functions. Here we focus on the main PRR-associated intracellular machinery that is

altered by HDPs to favor helminth survival and persistence in the host (**Figure 1**).

TLR Signaling (Map Kinases and Nf-κ B Cascade)

Mitogen-activated protein kinases (MAPKs) are a group of highly important molecules orchestrating the production of different cytokines via involving various downstream accessory proteins in DCs (45). The MAPK pathway is one of the main signaling cascades induced as a result of TLRs stimulation (45). Different kinases contribute to MAPK signaling including the extracellular signal-related kinases 1 and 2 (ERK 1/2), c-jun NH2-terminal kinase (JNK), and p38 MAPK. Activation of these molecules results in DC maturation, cytokine production, and gene expression via stimulation of transcription factors, such as activating protein 1 (AP-1), nuclear factor-κB (NF-κB), and IFN regulatory factors (IRFs) (45). ERK1/2 signaling mostly mediates Th2 response and DCs hyporesponsiveness due to stabilization of the c-fos transcription factor which suppresses IL-12 production (46, 47), whereas JNK and p38 are mostly associated with Th1 responses and DCs activation (47). In support of this, blocking ERK1/2 pathway by the specific inhibitor U0126 up-regulates IL-12 and suppresses TLR2-induced IL-10 production (47). Furthermore, it has been reported that ERK1 knockout mice spontaneously develop autoimmunity (48). On the other hand, two important adaptor molecules associated with TLRs signaling are MyD88 and TRIF, and TLR-induced activation of these molecules is responsible for the expression of genes encoding inflammatory mediators, such as IL-12 and TNFα (36). A number of helminths release molecules that are capable of triggering anti-inflammatory responses via interference with these downstream pathways (38, 49, 50). For example, soluble products of *T. suis* not only suppress transcription of essential molecules orchestrating both MyD88 and TRIF pathways in LPS-treated DCs, but also restrain TLR4 expression preventing DC maturation (26). The precise mechanisms by which HDPs influence these intracellular events are currently the subject of intense investigation. However, interesting data is becoming available regarding inhibitory effects of some HDPs, such as ES-62 and LNFPIII on key molecules involved in these inflammatory pathways.

One of the most important molecules that is targeted by HDPs to subvert TLRs signaling is ERK1/2. This intracellular component plays an essential role in mediation of anti-inflammatory functions of ES-62 and LNFPIII. In fact, both LNFP-III and ES-62, through engagement of TLR4 on DCs, induce Th2 responses (38, 49, 50). Although the capacity of TLR4 in skewing immune response toward Th2 seems surprising, various mechanisms might be at play and might explain the strikingly different response to LPS and some HDPs (51). The main explanations for this phenomenon are selective stimulation of ERK1/2 signaling and involvement of different co-receptors by HDPs which eventually interfere with TLR4-induced inflammatory signals in DCs (38, 51). In addition, it should be noted that TLR4 signaling can be conducted by two distinct of adaptor molecule pathways (TRIF and MyD88), however, it is still obscure which adaptor molecule is responsible for induction of immunoregulatory signals and how it is selectively activated by HDPs (38).

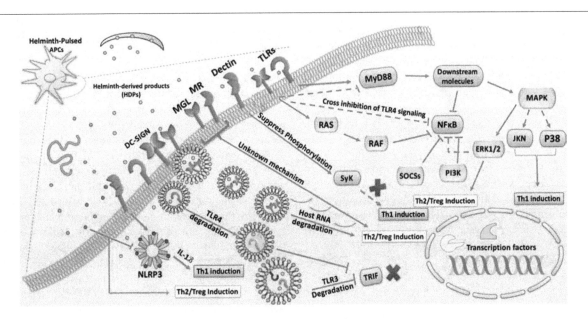

FIGURE 1 | Involvement of TLRs and CLRs during interaction with HDPs. TLRs and CLRs are widely targeted by HDPs during induction of immunomodulation and hyporesponsiveness in APCs. HDPs not only alter the expression of TLRs and CLRs in APCs but also masterfully manipulate their intracellular signaling. Some HDPs are able to redirect TLR4 signaling toward MAPK pathway and ERK1/2 activation supporting Treg/Th2 induction. In addition, co-engagement of DC-SIGN along with TLR4 enables HDPs to trigger unknown intracellular pathways which cross-inhibit MyD88 and NFκB activation. HDPs can further restrain NFκB activity via DC-SIGN-mediated RAF signaling along with upregulation of negative regulators of TLRs signaling, such as SOCSs and PI3K. Obviously, strict inhibition of NFκB as the main transcription factor supporting inflammation results in prevention of priming Th1 cells. Other CLRs have been reported to participate in priming Treg/Th2 cells upon stimulation by HDPs. For example, some HDPs suppress phosphorylation of Dectin1/2-induced Syk molecule and through which inhibit deviation of immune response toward Th1. On the other hand, MR and MGL upon activation by HDPs through an unknown mechanism support Treg/Th2 differentiation. Degrading host key intracellular molecules is another strategy that HDPs exploit to reprogram host immunity. Omega-1, ES-62, and FheCL1 by degrading host mRNA, endosomal TLR4, and TLR3, respectively, not only strengthen Treg/Th2 responses but also forestall anti-parasite immunity. NLRP3 also has been revealed to be targeted by some HDPs to modulate inflammatory responses. However, there has been reported that some HDPs are able to fight anti-worm immunity by stimulation of NLRP3 leading to release of IL-1B and Th1 amplification.

There is strong evidence that activation of ERK1/2 signaling inhibits a Th1 response and instead polarizes immune responses toward anti-inflammatory and Th2 response both *in vivo* and *in vitro* (45, 52). LNF-PIII is one the most powerful HDPs in supporting ERK signaling which significantly induces phosphorylation of ERK and TLR4-dependent differentiation of naive DCs to a DC2 phenotype (50). It seems that such a dysregulation of TLR signaling with a bias toward ERK1/2 is an effective strategy employed by the parasite to suppress Th1 responses and polarization of host immunity. In addition, *Trichinella spiralis* muscle larvae secrete bioactive components which strongly induce transient ERK1/2 signaling, thereby priming Th2/Treg-inducing DCs (53). However, different stages of this nematode have also been shown to arrest NF-κB translocation and the phosphorylation of p38 and ERK1/2 in LPS-treated J774A.1 murine macrophage cell line (54).

To further explore the mechanism of these biomolecules on immune cells, it is necessary to compare the signaling pathway(s) triggered by these antigens and LPS (38). First, stimulation of TLR4 by LPS results in triggering three different aforementioned MAPK cascades (ERK1/2, JNK, and p38 MAP kinases) along with NF-κB pathway activation which ultimately leads to the release of pro-inflammatory mediators (55). In contrast to the response to LPS, it has been shown that LNFPIII and ES-62 are able to induce mainly ERK1/2 signaling without significant stimulation of p38

and JNK. Second, further molecular dissection revealed that these HDPs not only slightly activate NF-κB signaling relative to LPS, but also shorten NF-κB longevity by stabilizing its inhibitor (50, 56). Third, the suppressive functions of ES-62 have been ascribed to inhibition of p38 and JNK, which play a central role in the production of Th1-associated cytokines, such as IL-12, IL-6, and TNFα (56, 57). Fourth, it should be noted that another explanation for such a difference in signal transduction between LPS and ES-62 might be due to the discrepancy in ubiquitylation of TLR4 and/or downstream signaling complexes (57). These data support the notion that some HDPs can elicit Th2 response by TLR4 stimulation in a manner distinct from customary agonists like LPS, which is a strong Th1 inducer.

The modulatory effects of ES-62 are not restricted only to the skewing of TLR4 signaling toward ERK1/2. Melendez et al. showed that ES-62 can also degrade key molecules involved in FcεRI signaling on mast cells via TLR4 engagement (58). Multiple downstream molecules are activated upon binding IgE to FcεRI, such as protein kinase Cα (PKCα), phospholipase D-coupled, and sphingosine kinase 1 (SPHK1) which subsequently trigger NF-κB signaling. In comparison to LPS, which strengthens (FcεRI)-mediated signaling, ES-62 directs PKCα toward degradation via a TLR4-dependent and proteasome-independent manner, suppressing mast cell activation in response to IgE stimulation (58). Importantly, other members of the PKC family (PKCβ,

PKCδ, PKCι, and PKCζ) can also be degraded by ES-62 (58, 59). Among them, PKCδ is regarded as a TLR4-mediated pathway molecule, which plays an important role in full activation of LPS-induced inflammation (60). Eason et al. have recently reported that despite LPS, ES-62 can exert downregulation and autophagolysosomal degradation of PKCδ in DCs to undergo autophagy (60).

Finally, a significant discrepancy between LPS and ES-62 stimulation of TLR4 relates to intracellular trafficking of this receptor. It has been shown that ES-62 can trigger TLR4 trafficking to a distinct caveolae lipid raft route leading to TLR4 degradation, whereas the route through which LPS induces TLR4 trafficking is associated with the promotion of Th1 and inflammatory responses (58) . Owing to promising results achieved from ES-62, analog molecules of ES-62 termed 11a, 11e, 11i, and 12b have been synthesized by Harnett and colleagues. These synthetic structures could experimentally suppress collagen-induced arthritis (CIA) by downregulation of key adaptor molecules in TLRs signaling, such as MyD88 and NF-κB (61–63).

Of note, other helminthes, such as S. mansoni and Ascaris lumbricoides can induce an imbalance in the intracellular signaling of LPS-treated human DCs via engagement of TLR2 and high stimulation of the ERK pathway. Given the fact that ERK1/2 signaling can increase c-Fos stabilization and IL-12 inhibition (47), it has been demonstrated that S. mansoni and A. lumbricoides-derived phospholipids support Th2 polarization via induction of imbalance in TLR2 signaling by strengthening ERK pathway in human monocyte-derived DCs (64). Interestingly, soluble SEA through TLR2 signaling induces a crosslink manipulation on the expression of co-inhibitory-associated genes, such as programmed death-ligand 1 (PD-1) and PD-L2 on murine BMDCs and CD4+ T cells, respectively. Upregulation of PD-1 and PD-L2 expression by egg antigens is a TLR2-dependent mechanism leading to anergy and hyporesponsiveness during interaction between macrophages and CD4+ T cells (65).

In addition, Correale et al. have suggested that SEA can activate several genes associated with retinoic acid synthesis, such as SOCS3 and IL-10R in DCs, via engagement of TLR2 and activation of ERK1/2 signaling (66). Importantly, egg antigen-treated DCs have been shown to strongly prime Tregs and suppress production of inflammatory cytokines, indicating a clear polarization by targeting TLR signaling. Mechanistically, Agrawal et al. suggested that immunoregulatory function of egg antigen is mediated via ERK1/2-induced c-Fos phosphorylation, as in the absence of c-Fos immune response were redirected toward Th1 (47).

Moreover, some HDPs, such as egg antigens condition DCs to prime Foxp3 Tregs via TLR2-dependent ERK1/2 signaling. This effect can also be observed with the antigen SJMHE1 from S. japonicum which increases proliferation and suppressive functions of Tregs by activating TLR2 (67–69). However, it is unknown how HDPs modify TLRs on Tregs to optimize their lifespan and suppressive activity, so further research is required to document the underlying molecular mechanism. Generally, TLRs signaling is mediated through two distinct pathways known as MAPK and NF-κB cascade. NF-κB signaling also plays an essential role in priming Th2 response, since the lack of NF-κB in DCs has been shown to result in Th2 impairment in the presence of egg antigens and LNFPIII (70, 71).

SOCSs, JAK/STAT, and PI3K

There is evidence suggesting that some HDPs can directly manipulate molecules controlling TLRs signaling, such as suppressor of cytokine signaling 3 (SOCS3) (66, 72). In this regard, it has been shown that F. hepatica produces biomolecules, such as tegumental coat antigens (FhTeg) and cathepsin L1 cysteine protease (FheCL1) which are capable of interfering with both the NF-κB and ERK/MAPK pathways in a manner distinct from other HDPs (72, 73). For instance, FhTeg can diminish the expression of inflammatory mediators in LPS-treated DCs via upregulation of a negative regulator of the TLRs pathway known as SOCS3 (72). On the other hand, FheCL1 is involved in neutralizing TLR3 signaling, as a TLR utilizing TRIF adaptor as an activator of downstream molecules. In fact, Donnelly et al. indicated that TRIF-dependent MyD88-independent signaling pathway is impaired by FheCL1 via degradation of TLR3 (73). Similar to FheCL1, SmCB-1 from S. mansoni has been found to enter the endosome and degrade TLR3. The protective effects of these antigens (FheCL1 and SmCB-1) against LPS-induced lethality were found to be mediated through MyD88-independent and TRIF-dependent pathways shared by both TLR4 and TLR3, suggesting the potential of HDPs as druggable targets due to their ability to disrupt intracellular pathways activated during inflammation (73). The TRIF-dependent pathway of TLR4 signaling can also be inhibited by T. spiralis-derived antigens as a mechanism to orchestrate regulatory responses (74). Brugia malayi has also been shown to produce a component known as abundant larval transcript (ALT-2) which promotes type 2 immune response and attenuates IFN-dependent signals via activation of GATA-3 and SOCS-1 in macrophages (75). SOCS-1 has also been reported to be upregulated by SEA in human DCs exposed to LPS which was associated with inhibition of pro-inflammatory cytokines (76).

Apart from ES-62, another well-known and highly bioactive component from A. viteae with significant intracellular activity is AvCystatin (77). Generally, cystatins are regarded as protease inhibitors which have been detected in excretory-secretory products of most filarial nematodes (78). Macrophages and IL-10 have been found to be central in the immunoregulatory effects of AvCystatin on experimental models of colitis and asthma (77, 79). AvCystatin is able to induce regulatory macrophages (Mreg) representing remarkable suppressive effects on DCs via IL-10 dependent and cell-contact independent mechanism (79). Klotz et al. identified the molecular mechanism by which AvCystatin can reprogram the macrophage phenotype and suppresses inflammation. They suggest that AvCystatin is taken up by macrophages and through stimulation of dual specificity phosphatases (DUSPs), which are negative regulators of MAPK signaling and IL-10 expression, targets ERK1/2 and p38 to modulate downstream signals inducing regulatory responses (77). Through this mechanism, the immunoregulatory effects of AvCystatin are mediated via the phosphorylation of the CREB and STAT3 (77). In addition, some HDPs, such as dsRNA derived from *S. mansoni* egg can also modulate STAT1 signaling (80). This dsRNA is able to engage TLR3 and phosphorylate STAT1 in DCs supporting signaling pathway associated with type I IFN expression (80). Yang et al. have recently provided evidence suggesting that the immunomodulatory activity of *S. mansoni* egg antigens (SEA) and *S. japonicum* worm antigen (SWA) in myeloid-derived suppressor cells (MDSCs) is mediated through the Janus kinase/signal transducers and activators of transcription 3 (JAK/STAT3) pathway (81). They corroborated their findings by application of a JAK inhibitor (JSI-124) which abrogated immunomodulatory functions of SEA and SWA (81). Besides STAT1 and 3, STAT6 signaling has also been found to be manipulated by some HDPs, such as *T. spiralis*-derived cathepsin B-like protein (82). Liu et al. indicated that the recombinant form of this antigen (rTsCPB) can significantly restrain intestinal ischemia/reperfusion injury in mice by active reprogramming macrophages from an inflammatory (M1) to an alternative phenotype (M2) (82). One of the main intracellular signalings for such a phenotypic alteration is activation of STAT6 in M1 macrophages (82). Mechanistically, rTsCPB was shown to support upregulation of M2-associated markers and subsequently transition of M1 to M2 macrophage via STAT6-dependent manner, as inhibition of STAT6 restored disease severity and M1 domination (82).

Some parasites tend to target another pathway in TLR signaling known as phosphoinositide 3-kinase (PI3K) which is a strong inhibitor of TLR-induced IL-12 production and DCs maturation (77, 83, 84). Accordingly, this pathway has been revealed to shape immune response toward Th2 and IL-10 production. For instance, some protozoan parasites, such as *Giardia lamblia* and *Leshmania major*, along with *A. vitae*, are able to interfere with TLR-mediated DCmaturation via stimulation of PI3K signaling maturation (77, 83, 84). Importantly, both CLRs and TLRs can share ERK and PI3K signaling to redirect immune response toward Th2 during infection with helminths (85).

These data show how HDPs may impact TLR signaling, thereby bypassing inflammatory responses. The predominant pathway triggered by HDPs is ERK1/2 signaling which supports phosphorylation of the transcription factor c-Fos inducing modified Th2 and/or anti-inflammatory responses (46, 50, 56). Generally, it seems that one of the main mechanisms by which helminths minimize host tissue injury is suppression of innate immunity via modification of TLR signaling (6, 85).

C-Type Lectins Receptor (CLRs) Signaling

There is evidence suggesting the commencement of Th2 response can be initiated independent of the two adaptor proteins MyD88 and TRIF (86). In this case, it is expected that other PRRs beside TLRs also can initiate the Th2 response (37). As mentioned above, APCs express an array of receptors known as CLRs specialized in the recognition of glycans (87). CLRs can mediate different immunological processes including antigen uptake, intracellular trafficking, and priming innate immunity (87). Various types of CLRs are expressed by APCs including DC-specific ICAM-3 grabbing nonintegrin (DC-SIGN), macrophage galactose binding lectin

receptor (MGL), mannose receptor (MR), and Dectin-1. DC-SIGN is involved in recognition of high mannose glycans and is able to stimulate TLR signaling (87). MGL and MR detect pathogens-associated mannose-containing glycans with high sensitivity (87). Recently, surfactant protein (SP)-D, collectin related to the family of C-type lectins, has also been reported to interact with carbohydrate-based compartments of worms, such as *Nippostrongylus brasiliensis* in the lung (88). Thawer et al. demonstrated that SP-D KO mice are unable to control *N. brasiliensis* in the lung, as this protein plays a key role in stimulation of Th2 responses and alternative activation of alveolar macrophages (alvM) which is essential for binding to and killing L4 parasites (88).

Importantly, CLRs play an important role in host-parasite interaction through recognition of glycan-based components in helminth-derived antigens (89). These parasite-derived glycans constitute versatile glycoconjugates with highly various structures targeting CLRs, and in turn skew adaptive immunity (90). For instance, N-linked glycoconjugates from *A. suum* extract engage DC-SIGN and MR to suppress LPS-induced DCs maturation and triggering inflammatory signals (89). Similarly, it has been shown that DC-SIGN, MR, and MGL can be involved in capturing and internalization of SEA (91–93). Also, some HDPs are quite similar to host glycans which, during interplay with CLRs of DCs, induce both Th2 suppression and Treg proliferation, establishing a tolerogenic state in host immune function (94). In this way, this mechanism can create a balance between Th1 and Th2 responses through the involvement of CLRs on DCs (37, 95). Unfortunately, limited data are available on the parasite components inducing immunological bias via the involvement of CLRs.

One of the main pathways shared by most CLRs to trigger downstream signaling is the spleen tyrosine kinase (Syk) pathway, which has been shown to contribute to DC priming and elicitation of inflammatory responses (96). Interestingly, *Heligmosomoides polygyrus* and its products elicit a strong downregulation of different CLRs including CLEC7A, 9A, 12A, and 4N along with suppression of Syk phosphorylation (96). In fact, it is suggested that the inhibitory effects of this worm on CLRs and Syk expression leading to induction of regulatory DCs in intestine and mitigation of colitis in infected mice (96). In another way, excretory-secretory products of *Taenia crassiceps* (TcES) have been found to inhibit DCs maturation in response to TLR4 and TLR9 agonist (97). Molecular dissections revealed that TcES are able to interfere with TLR signaling and induce tolerogenic DCs. Terrazas et al. delineated that TcES support Th2 response by activation of MGL, MR, and TLR2 (97). The reported that the major intracellular mechanism by which TcES prevent TLR4-mediate DCs maturation is by targeting c-RAF, which is a MAP3K acting on downstream pathways of the Ras family (97). Indeed, TcES significantly suppress downstream molecules, such as p38 and NF-κB by phosphorylation of c-RAF and consequently polarize immune responses toward a Th2 phenotype (97). It has also recently been observed that *T. crassiceps*-induced Ly6C^hi monocyte-derived alternatively activated macrophages (AAMs) express a high level of MR (CD206), PD-L2, and CCR2/CX3CR1 enabling them to prime Tregs and suppress experimental autoimmune encephalomyelitis in mice (98).

CLRs have also been suggested to associate with induction of Th2 responses by *Toxocara*-derived antigens (99). Among them, DC-SIGN is one of the most important receptors in recognition of *T. canis*, *F. hepatica*, and *B. malayi*-derived glycan products shaping the immune response toward a Th2/regulatory state (100–102). Rodríguez and colleagues have recently found that DC-SIGN plays a central role in priming Treg upon interaction with *F. hepatica*-derived glycans (102). The presence of mannose and fucose residues in *F. hepatica*-glycoconjugates can facilitate DC-SIGN stimulation and trigger intracellular pathway enabling DCs to prime Treg and inhibit proliferation of allogeneic T cells (102). Surprisingly, stimulation of DC-SIGN with *F. hepatica*-glycoconjugates activates a pathway in DCs which, during intracellular crosstalk with TLR-mediated signaling, induces IL-10 and IL-27 secretion in support of Treg expansion (102). A similar mechanism has been reported for immunoregulatory effects of *F. hepatica*-derived glycans upon engagement of MGL on both human monocyte-derived DCs (mo-DCs) and mMgl2$^+$ CD11$^+$ cells in mice (103). In this study, the authors suggest that a cross regulation between pathways due to co-stimulation of MGL and TLR4 with *F. hepatica*-derived glycans and LPS, respectively, which enables DCs to produce immunoregulatory cytokines and support Th2/Treg proliferation (103). MR can recognize *F. hepatica* tegumental antigens (FhTeg) and condition DCs to induce anergy in CD4$^+$ T cells (104). In addition, this receptor is able to suppress DCs maturation or Th2 induction in response to *F. hepatica* total extract (105, 106). However, it is believed that MR is not solely involved in conduction of immunosuppressive function of FhTeg and other CLRs most likely also contribute to these interactions (107). In support of this, *F. hepatica* excretory-secretory products (FhESP) have been demonstrated to suppress T cell activation via Dectin-1 dependent upregulation of PD-L2 and IL-10 in macrophages (108). Also, the strong suppressive activity of FhESP has been ascribed to co-activation of MR and Dectine-1 in macrophages underpinned by high levels of TGF-β and IL-10 production (109).

SEA possesses an array of complex glycan-based products which are predominantly recognized and taken up by surface CLRs on DC including MR, MGL, DC-SIGN, and Dectin1, triggering SYK-mediated intracellular pathways (91–93, 110). Endocytosis of egg-derived antigens results in interference with TLR signaling in DCs (93). The most well-known antigens of *schistosoma* egg which stimulate CLRs are LEX-containing glycans, omega-1, lacto-N-fucopentaose III and lacto-N-neotetraose. LEX-containing glycans involve DC-SIGN on DCs and trigger intracellular signaling, thereby promoting Th2 responses (111). Moreover, plant-based reconstruction of omega-1 has recently been reported to provoke Th2 responses by engaging DC-SIGN (51). Omega-1 is a Lex-containing glycoprotein structure representing T2 ribonuclease (RNase) activity. The MR has also been displayed to capture and internalize omega-1 leading to Th2 polarization along with interfering protein synthesis via degrading host cell RNAs (112, 113). LNFPIII and lacto-N-neotetraose are potent suppressors of

T cell proliferation and DCs activation through stimulation of IL-10 production (114). Interestingly, it has been indicated that the immunoregulatory functions of these glycan-based biomolecules are mediated via the MR and DC-SIGN (38, 49, 115). Of interest is a recent study by Kooij et al. which highlighted a critical role of MR in polarization of human classical monocytes toward regulatory phenotype (expressing SOCS1, IL-10, and TGFβ) upon interaction with soluble products of *T. suis* (TsSP) (116). In this study, MR was found to respond to TsSP and triggers a PKC-mediated signaling (mainly PKCδ) responsible for induction of anti-inflammatory monocytes (116). Also, glycan compounds in *T. spiralis* muscle larvae excretory-secretory antigens (ES L1) have been reported to be able to polarize host immunity toward Th2/Treg via corroboration of ERK1/2 signaling in DCs and production of IL-10 and TGFβ (117). However, the major receptor responsible for such modulation is obscure and possible candidates need to be investigated (117).

These data suggest that CLRs can strongly react to HDPs and condition DCs to redirect immune response toward Th2 immunity and/or an anti-inflammatory response (118). However, the precise shared pathway by TLRs and CLRs upon simultaneous activation leading to release of regulatory cytokines remains enigmatic. In the following, we discuss this topic, to which less attention has been given.

Co-involvement of TLRs and CLRs by HDPs

Interestingly, recent data suggest that the immunomodulatory functions of some HDPs are mediated via simultaneous involvement of TLRs and CLRs. In fact, signaling pathways of CLRs have shown to co-operate with TLRs which strengthen effective immunomodulation. For example, *S. mansoni* secretes glycolipids which co-involve DC-SIGN and TLR4 in human DCs (119). Regarding intracellular crosstalk, Meyer-Wentrup et al. suggested that TLR8-mediated production of inflammatory cytokines, such as IL-12 and TNFα can be forestalled by dendritic cell immunoreceptor (DCIR) as a C-type lectin receptor (120).

This complex mechanism suggests an intricate intracellular crosstalk between two distinct receptors which results in hyporesponsiveness and immunosuppression. Activation of CLR signaling can modify inflammatory responses via manipulation of TLRs signaling (121, 122). For instance, SEA and LNFPIII are among the well-known schistosome-associated antigens which have been reported to co-involve TLRs and CLRs in host DCs. Egg antigens can regulate TLR2, TLR3, and TLR4 signaling through stimulation of β-galactoside-binding lectin galectin 3 (40, 80, 123–125), while LNFPIII via interaction with DC-SIGN and MGL1(23, 126), cross-inhibits the TLR4 pathway (101). DC-SIGN also strongly directs the immune response toward Th2, Treg, and modulation of inflammatory reactions. In this regard, Geijtenbeek et al. showed that mannosylated components of Mycobacterial cell walls diminish TLR4-associated inflammation via DC-SIGN (122). Similarly, other pathogens seem to modify TLR-mediated inflammatory consequences through stimulating DC-SIGN-associated Raf-1 signaling (127).

Likewise, other glycan-based compounds released by *S. mansoni* are expected to modify inflammatory responses via co-involvement (128). The immunoregulatory activity of schistosome-derived lysoPS may be similar to zymosan, which co-engages TLR2 and Dectin-1 (a type of CLRs) on DCs and induces Treg priming along with IL-10 production (129). Stimulation of Dectin-2 by whole extracts of *S. mansoni* eggs was reported to trigger Syk and inflammasome signaling and thereby enable inhibition of TLR signaling (110). Apart from intracellular crosstalk, physical interaction between CLRs and other surface receptors is believed to affect their intracellular signaling leading to a significant modification in immune response (128). Generally, it seems that glycan-based materials released by helminths can modulate host immunity through manifold signaling stemming from different receptors, such as TLRs, CLRs, and likely other PRRs provoking both Th2 and regulatory responses (23, 130). Tracking the mechanisms through which HDPs induce Th2 and/or regulatory responses will provide new insight into recognition of molecules and targets that selectively stimulate ERK signaling, which may be beneficial in development of new generations of vaccines and therapeutics against inflammatory diseases.

Inflammasome

Inflammasomes constitute an intracellular platform possessing NOD-like receptor (NLR) family proteins which are highly sensitive to various PAMPs and DAMPs (131). These cytosolic sensors include different family of NLRPs and absent in melanoma 2 (AIM2) which play a key role in triggering inflammatory signals in most immune cells, but mainly in APCs (131). Stimulation of inflammasomes results in activation of a cascade signaling supporting active release of IL-1β and IL-18 (131). However, limited data is available on the interaction of helminths with inflammasome, but some studies have provided interesting results in this regard. For example, Rzepecka et al. reported that a synthetic analog of ES-62 known as SMA-12b is able to suppress arthritis in mice by prevention of inflammasome activation (132). Further in-depth molecular dissection on murine macrophages revealed the underlying mechanisms are mediated through downregulation of IL-1β and inflammasome-associated signals which strongly counters inflammasome-induced responses supporting arthritis (132). Some helminth infections and their products are able to activate inflammasome in order to restrict production of early released innate cytokines, such as IL-25 and IL-33 (133). For example, *H. polygyrus* has been found to instigate NLRP3 in intestinal lamina propria cells inducing IL-1β secretion and by this mechanism prevents Th2 response initiation, ILC2 expansion, and eventually helminth expulsion (133). The same scenario has recently been reported for *T. muris* as Alhallaf et al. unraveled a novel mechanism by which *T. muris* exosomes and ESP suppress anti-parasite immunity by targeting NLRP3 (134). This study showed that this worm and its released compounds actively counter Th2 response and worm expulsion by increasing NLRP3-mediated IL-18 both *in vivo* and *in vitro* (134). Thus, this intracellular sensor may be targeted by helminths to suppress Th2 responses via IL-1β and IL-18 (133, 134).

Likewise, a well-known component from *S. mansoni* called omega-1 has also shown to be able to activate NLRP3 via co-involvement of Dectin-1 in macrophages (135). However,

it is unknown how modulating the inflammasome can facilitate infection. In the same line, Ritter et al. studied the inflammasome-associated activity of SEA (110). They suggested that egg antigens can simultaneously suppress TLR signaling and activate NLRP3. Mechanistically, egg antigens were found to require co-activation of Dectin-1/FcγR and downstream signaling (Syk kinase signaling) to irritate NLRP3 via activation of reactive oxygen species and potassium efflux leading to IL-1β secretion in BMDCs (100).

Targeting Non-PRR Signaling

Generally, no precise pattern of intra- and extracellular sensors along with downstream signaling has been fully recognized by which HDPs exert immunomodulation. Indeed, helminths have shown to be able to exploit an array of highly complex strategies beyond the manipulation of canonical PRRs signaling to restore aberrant immune responses (136). In the following section, immunosuppressive functions of some HDPs through a PRR-independent manner will be discussed (**Figure 2**).

Impairment in antigen presentation, T cell receptor (TCR), and B cell receptor (BCR) signaling

Given the myriad biomolecules released by helminths, it is not surprising that some HDPs manipulate host immune cells via receptor-independent manner, such as enzymatic activity. For instance, *B. malayi* cystatins, such as Bm-CPI-1 (produced by the L2 and L3 stage of *B. malayi*) and Bm-CPI-2 are able to impede antigen presentation in APCs via interference with host cysteine protease function, reducing T cell priming (136, 137). In this way, Bm-CPI-2 was reported to inhibit human B cells to present tetanus toxoid associated peptide. Bm-CPI-2 was shown to possess two inhibitory sites enabling it to hinder host cysteine proteases and asparaginyl endopeptidase (AEP) (136–138). Likewise, *Onchocerca volvulus* was shown to diminish HLA-DR expression by release of onchocystatin (139, 140). Other worms, such as *Nippostrongylus brasiliensis* and *Litomosoides sigmodontis* produce cystatins enabling these worms to block B cell-associated endosomal proteases and T cell proliferation via IL-10 induction, respectively (140–143). However, the main mechanism through which helminth-derived cystatins affect host cells is unknown, but there is evidence suggesting the involvement of scavenger receptors and the transforming growth factor-β receptor (TGFβ R) pathways in particular by Avcystatin (*A. viteae*-derived recombinant cystatin) and calreticulin (a protein secreted by *H. polygyrus*), thereby polarizing Th2 responses (144, 145). In support of the critical role of helminth cystatins in promoting worm longevity, it has been suggested that presence of anti-cystatin circulating antibodies in mice can confine infection, suggesting that cystatins restrict the process of antigen loading and presentation by MHCII in APCs (141).

TCR signaling can also be affected by some HDPs in favor of shaping immune response toward immunoregulation (146–148). A well-known component of SEA known as omega-1 is the best example of HDPs which directs host immunity toward Th2 response through an intriguing mechanism. Mechanistically, omega-1 has been found to target cytoskeletal compartments to

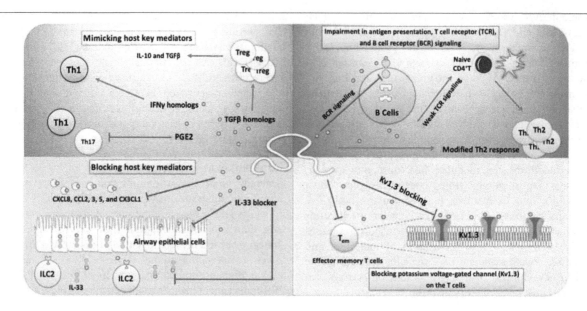

FIGURE 2 | Some HDPs has been shown to target non-PRRs sensors including Kv1.3 and TCRs on T cells. Blocking Kv1.3 can significantly decrease Th1 cell activity and proliferation. Also, presenting HDPs on the MHCII leads to induction a weak TCR signaling in naïve CD4 T cells which corroborates Th2 differentiation. Of note, the main phenotype of Th2 response elicited by helminths and their products is "modified Th2" immunity in which IL-5, IL-13, eosinophilia, and IgE are all downregulated, while IL-4, TGFβ, and IL-10 are increased. BCR signaling has also been shown to be impaired by some HDPs which prevent B cell activation. HDPs have recently been more considered as magic components which are able to mimic or block several host key mediators which play an important role in immunosuppression and Th2 amplification, respectively.

confine the formation of a stable DC-CD4$^+$ T cell interplay, leading to suppression of TCR signaling strength and eventually Th2 cell differentiation. Since it has been documented that low dose antigens, which induce a weak TCR signaling, can prime Th2 response, the Th2-inducing property of omega-1 has also been ascribed to this hypothesis (149). Although omega-1 is able to inhibit TLR4-mediated DC stimulation independent of TLR-, MyD88- and TRIF, the main receptor targeted by omega-1 is still unknown, and it is thought that its enzymatic activity (T2 ribonuclease) likely contributes to such effects (86, 146). More investigations are required to identify whether other *S. mansoni* egg-derived antigens deviate immune responses toward Th2 by targeting TCR signaling (147). In support of helminth-mediated TCR signaling manipulation, Appleby et al. recently reported that in schistosome-endemic area of rural Zimbabwe, patients infected with *S. haematobium* had lower expression of CD3ζ (an integral part of TCR signaling) on peripheral blood mononuclear cells (PBMCs) than non-infected individuals, suggesting a possible TCR-targeted mechanism for hyporesponsiveness and immunosuppression (150).

In comparison to omega-1, the precise interruptive effects of ES-62 on TCR and BCR signaling have widely been determined (148). In fact, ES-62 by degradation of key components of downstream TCR and BCR signaling induces desensitization and in turn restrains cell proliferation and antibody production (151). Protein kinase C (PKC) and its different isoforms are one group of the major molecules that play a central role in orchestration of downstream cascade in TCR and BCR signaling for activation of transcription factors (152). It has been documented that ES-62 not only targets PKCs to be degraded/down-regulated

in B and T cells but also up-regulates negative regulators of MAPKs signaling, such as RasGAP to suppress this pathway in Jurkat T cells (153). In addition, exposure of activated Th17 cells to LPS in the presence of ES-62 resulted in down-regulation of MyD88 and inhibition of LPS-mediated IL-17 production (154).

IgE signaling

Some HDPs, such as *Dirofilaria immitis*-derived antigen (DiAg) and *Clonorchis sinensis*-derived components called venom allergen-like proteins (CsVAL) are able to impair IgE-mediated degranulation followed by downstream signaling (155, 156). In this way, DiAg has been demonstrated to suppress type 1 diabetes in non-obese diabetic mice via Th1 inhibition and IL-10 induction (157). Interestingly, application of recombinant DiAg was associated with induction of nonspecific IgE by involving CD40 on B cells and saturation of FcεRI on mast cells, representing protective function against passive cutaneous anaphylaxis in rats (155). CsVAL has also displayed inhibitory activity on IgE-mediated degranulation of mast cells via targeting downstream pathways (156). Prevention of IgE receptor signaling has also been observed during exposure of human PBMCs to *S. mansoni* (158). It was revealed that the worm is able to secrete a component termed as schistosome-generated (SG) sCD23 which not only functions as a soluble decoy for the IgE receptor but also decreases the expression of this receptor (158). In addition, one of the well-characterized HDPs with interruptive effects on IgE signaling is ES-62. Collectively, these molecules might be considered as a potential therapeutic candidate in allergic disorders.

Mimicking and blocking host key mediators

TGFβ is one of the most powerful cytokines with immunoregulatory activity, which stimulates naïve T cells into regulatory T and B cells inducing immunobalance and tolerance in mucosal tissues, such as the intestine (159). This immunosuppressive cytokine and its receptor pathway have been reported to be mimicked and manipulated by helminths (159). Up to now, various components from nematodes like *A. caninum*, *B. malayi*, *H. polygyrus*, and trematodes, such as *F. hepatica* and the *Schistosoma* species have shown to produce TGFβ homologs (159). Bm-tgh-1 and Bm-tgh-2 from Brugia species and SmRK-1, 2, a TGF-β receptor homolog, from *S. mansoni* are well-known examples of HDPs with immunoregulatory activity due to mimicking TGFβ-induced mechanism (159). *H. polygyrus* is also able to stimulate naive T cells to express Treg-associated markers, such as Foxp3 amplifying immunoregulation via an unknown mechanism (160). Recently, Johnston et al. have characterized an important component from this worm known as *H. polygyrus* TGF-β mimic (Hp-TGM) which is structurally similar to a member of the complement control protein superfamily (161). Interestingly, Hp-TGM is functionally able to ligand mammalian TGFβR and mimic properties of TGFβ in induction of both mouse and human Foxp3$^+$ Treg cells (161).

Furthermore, Sulaiman et al. have recently suggested that juvenile stages of *F. hepatica* release a TGF-like molecule known as FhTLM, engaging host TGF-β receptors and triggers Smad2/3 signaling in leukocytes (162). They showed that TGF-β RII is the main target of this component through which FhTLM increases the production of IL-10 and PD-L1 and the mannose receptor expression which eventually facilitate the early evasion of juvenile by suppression host immune activation (162).

Another class of host mediators which are masterfully mimicked by some helminths, such as *S. mansoni* (163), *Taenia taeniaeformis*, and *B. malayi* are prostaglandins (PGs) (164). Among various PGs, the immunoregulatory properties of PGE2 have widely been documented (165), and it is known that it can modulate DC function to polarize immune response from Th1 toward Th2 (166). Laan et al. have recently found that *T. suis* releases high levels of PGE2 in its excretory-secretory products which are likely responsible for inhibition of LPS-induced production of inflammatory cytokines from human DCs (25). By contrast, *T. muris* may expedite Th1 response by production of IFNγ homologs to engage IFNγ receptors leading to Th1 amplification and suppression of IL-4 mediated responses against the worm (167, 168). Of note, the immune response depends on the host genotype and the infection levels, for example, resistant genotypes display Th2 response while susceptible hosts represent Th1 response. Also, low infection levels of *T. muris* elicit a Th1 and high infection induces a Th2 response (168).

Another strategy whereby helminths attenuate inflammatory signals is production of bioactive blockers to occupy receptors and entrap mediators triggering inflammatory responses, such as chemokines (169). For instance, a well-known chemokine blocker is a chemokine-binding protein which is released by SEA called smCKBP (169). This component has been found to be able to bind several chemokine ligands including CXCL8, CCL2, 3, 5, and CX3CL1 resulting in suppression of both inflammatory signals and recruitment of inflammatory cells at the site of insult (169). Relevant to helminth-derived blocking compounds, a very recent study by Osbourn et al. recognized a potent IL-33 blocking component called *H. polygyrus* Alarmin Release Inhibitor (HpARI) (170). Mechanistically, HpARI binds to both nuclear DNA and mature IL-33, preventing its release and interaction with IL-33R on airway epithelial cells and ILC2. Further experiments in mice confirmed the suppression ability of HpARI on IL-33 and subsequent airway allergic responses, involving eosinophilia and IL-5 and−13 (170). These authors revealed a novel mechanism of suppressing Th2 response onset via inhibition of IL-33 released from necrotic epithelial cells which are insulted during helminth infection and exposure to airway allergens (170).

Blocking potassium voltage-gated channel (Kv1.3) on the T cells

It has recently been shown that some HDPs can control the function of T cells by blocking potassium voltage-gated channel (Kv1.3) (171). AcK1 and BmK1 are a large family of Stichodactyla helianthus toxin (ShK) composed of peptide structures secreted by *A. ceylanicum* and *B. malayi*, respectively. These compounds are able to block Kv1.3 channels on T cells by engaging the outer vestibule of the channel (171). Kv1.3 channels have been proved to widely be expressed and involved in activation of human T cells (172). Since there are an immense number of myelin-reactive T cells (autoreactive) resembling Kv1.3^{high} phenotype in multiple sclerosis (MS) forestalling these cells by targeting Kv1.3 channels would be of great interest (173, 174). In accordance with this, some clinical trial studies have been launched to evaluate the efficacy of AcK1 and BmK1 in attenuation of inflammation (NCT02446340; NCT02435342).

Taken together, these data show that a complex of diverse intracellular pathways is triggered by HDPs which ultimately converge host immunity toward hyporesponsiveness and immunological tolerance via manipulation of PRR-dependent and independent strategies. Up to now, we have briefly reviewed the intracellular interferences of HDPs as a foundation to provide novel insights into the possible mechanisms of extracellular vesicles (EVs) as an important component of HDPs. In the following section, we aim to discuss the recognized pathways utilized by EVs released during helminth infections to bypass host immunity with the aim of proposing other unknown mechanisms.

EXTRACELLULAR VESICLES

Biogenesis, Content, and Morphological Properties

Various types of extracellular vesicles exist, but the structures that are most often referred to are called exosomes, which are 30–100 nm in diameter, or microvesicles, which measure about 100–1,000 nm in diameter (175). In terms of morphological properties and contents, exosomes are endocytic vesicles with a spherical shape surrounded by a bilamellar membrane. Their contents constitute a wide variety of biomolecules including glycans, proteins, lipids, and nucleic acids (176). Exosomes are originally derived from endosomes via budding from their wall, and then aggregated in a large body known as the multivesicular body (MVB). Exosomes are unleashed in extracellular environment upon exocytosis of MVB through fusion with the plasma membrane (176). Apart from exosomes, other distinct vesicles with similar function and properties can be detected in extracellular space including microvesicles (plasma membrane-derived microparticle) and apoptotic bodies, which can be distinguished from exosomes in terms of biogenesis, size, protein contents, density, and isolation technique (176). Also, the formation of microvesicles is simpler and happens through an outward budding of the plasma membrane (177). Generally, all of them are considered as EV and exosomes are the smallest EV with the lowest density (176). Apoptotic bodies are not the subjects of this review and beyond our discussion.

Uptake in Recipient Cells

EVs have been acknowledged as important elements of cell-cell communication due to their role as vehicles for molecules and biological signals to be shuttled from one cell to another (178). Transfer of molecules, such as protein and miRNA can completely change the physiology of the receiving target cell and can in this way control both normal biological processes as well as distinct pathological processes (178).

EVs recognize and attach to their target cells through surface proteins, such as integrins, tetraspannins, proteoglycans, lectins, and immunoglobulins (179). The transfer of the EV content occurs as the EVs fuse with the target cells, which can be facilitated by various endocytic internalization pathways and the fusion can appear as rapidly as 15 min after exposure (180). Macropinocytosis is one such mechanism where EVs are captured and enclosed during the invagination of ruffled extensions from the plasma membrane (179). Another mechanism is phagocytosis, which is exploited by bacteria and viruses as well as DCs and macrophages and is facilitated by absorbing EVs by extended pseudopodia (180). Alternatively, EVs can be taken up by clathrin-mediated endocytosis, which involves the deformation of the target cell membrane by clathrin on the EV surface creating an inward bud that encloses the EVs, which can then pinch off and fuse with the endosome (181). Calveolin-dependent endocytosis is yet another mechanism for EV uptake where EVs oligomerize calveolin proteins on the membrane of the target cells facilitating the formation of intracellular calveolin-rich vesicles which then transports the EV contents to the target site (182). Finally, under specific conditions, EVs can fuse directly with the cell surface membrane (183).

Parasites use this remarkable ability of EVs to communicate with other parasite cells (parasite-parasite communication) (184) and host cells (host-parasite communication) (185). Strong evidence of the uptake of EVs by host cells has been obtained for a range of parasite species, including *Giardia duodenalis* (186), *Leishmania major* (187), *Plasmodium falciparum* (184), *Trichomonas vaginalis* (188), *Trypanosoma brucei* (189), *T. cruzi* (190), *Echinostoma caproni* (191), *F. hepatica* (28), *H. polygyrus*

(30), *S. mansoni* (192), *A. suum*, *O. Dentatum*, and *T. suis* (Hansen et al., unpublished). Interestingly, Eichenberger et al. have recently employed organoids from murine colonic crypts to explore uptake of *T. muris*-derived EVs (193). These authors showed that when labeled EVs are delivered into the central lumen of organoids, they are internalized within 3 h and this process can be inhibited upon prevention of endocytosis (193). Furthermore, in this study transcriptomic and proteomic profile of *T. muris* EVs were characterized in which a number of miRNA with potential immunoregulatory effects on host immunity were identified (193). Upon fusion, specifically loaded compounds and biological signals in the EVs are transferred, which then can exert its function in the target cell. These events are responsible for the EV-related host immune manipulation (30, 194, 195), pathogenesis (196, 197) and parasite development (198), that have been reported for many parasitological diseases as described previously.

EVs FOR THE HOST IMMUNE SYSTEM
EV-Mediated Delivery of Message by Helminths

A number of parasites have shown to release EVs and they have received great interest due to their remarkable immunomodulatory properties including suppression of IL-6, TNFα, and IL-17A in mice (191, 199, 200). Various potential mechanisms have been suggested through which these vesicles might affect host cells (201). In fact, they have unique biological properties mediating cell-cell interaction both via direct contact and/or delivering biomaterial contents affecting intracellular crosstalk (202). However, the specific intracellular mechanisms that are targeted remain unknown or only partially characterized.

In recent years, helminth-associated EVs have shown to be essential mediators that contain bioactive cargo that contribute to establishing a permissive infection (30, 202). Apart from helminths, other microbes including fungi, bacteria, and protozoa are able to produce EVs and mediate active interaction with their host immunity to achieve a suitable niche (203). The release of such a protected package can undoubtedly optimize the integrity of contents, which in turn improve their efficacy in genetic exchange and secure delivery to modulate host immunity (203). Indeed, several studies have shown that powerful biomolecules are present in the helminth-derived EVs, which can offer potential and druggable candidates against inflammatory diseases (204). In addition, omics-based approaches, such as proteomics and transcriptomics have provided a plethora of valuable data facilitating recognition of major components mediating host immunosuppression. Such explorations provide novel insight into previously unknown strategies by which worms send messages to host cells to manipulate the host immune system and may therefore also pave the way to new ways to control infections (204–206).

Given interesting results achieved from EVs investigation, a surge of interest has been paid to focus on their contents. In the following, the most important biomolecules represented by helminth EVs along with their potential implications are discussed.

miRNAs as an Important Player for Intracellular Communication

One important component of EVs is miRNA, which is an evolutionary conserved class of short non-coding RNA, of 19–24 nucleotides in length, which plays an essential role in post-transcriptional gene regulation and is involved in the fine-tuning of a range of cellular processes. miRNA has been discovered in all types of human body fluids (207) and in various different species (208), including parasitic organisms (209, 210).

miRNA has been shown to take part in the regulation of any kind of biological process, here among embryonic development (211), cell differentiation and apoptosis (212–214) but also various immunological processes (215). In fact, miRNA seems to be involved in basically all aspects of immunological events of both innate and adaptive character. That being differential and activation of macrophages (216), dendritic cells (217), granulocytes (218), NK cells (219), and other innate immune cells (220) as well as development and function of B cells (221, 222) and T cells (223, 224).

Recent investigations suggest that helminth EVs also contain various RNA molecules including miRNA which may participate to the manipulating signaling pathways which orchestrating inflammatory responses (193). This mechanism may enable worms to directly interfere with host gene translation and thereby immunity to facilitate parasite survive (29, 30, 225). In support of this, an *in vitro* study showed that *E. multilocularis* produces a type of miRNA (emu-miR-71) which is able to suppress NO production and inflammation-associated miRNAs in LPS/IFN-treated murine macrophage RAW264.7 (29). By contrast, the effects of *S. japonicum*-derived exosomes on the same cell line of macrophages showed an increase of iNOS and TNF-α, supporting M1-type macrophage development (226). The steadily growing body of literature is supporting the critical role of exosome-associated miRNA as an important player involved in suppression or stimulation of target cells (30). One of this miRNA-mediated mechanism which has been recently suggested by Buck et al. is genetically blocking or targeting host mRNA for degradation, causing a severe defect in host immune response to confine worm expulsion. Molecular digestion showed that this miRNA is able to target 3′ untranslated region of the mRNA encoding Th2-associated cytokines, such as IL-33 which in turn prevents the ILC2 expansion and eliciting a strong Th2 response (30). Thus, it seems that helminths possess EVs with bioactive compounds, such as miRNAs that are able to effectively neutralize host immunity and polarize immune responses toward the way supporting their survival.

Gu et al. also suggest that some helminth miRNAs only might target host genes and that their release is a selective process as the profile of released miRNAs in the excretory-secretory products differed from that of adult extracts of *Haemonchus contortus* (227).

In addition to miRNA, other RNA molecules have been identified within helminth EVs, such as mRNA and tsRNA (193, 228) but their potential function and role in host-parasite interaction still need to be elucidated.

Proteins and Lipids in EVs

In addition to nucleic acid, EVs do also contain a diverse collection of molecules including lipids and proteins (229, 230). The protein composition has been characterized in excretory-secretory products from several parasite species using proteomic approaches based on mass spectrometry and has shown that it contains a suite of immunomodulatory proteins with immune suppressive effects e.g., on type 1 and type 2 effector molecules (30, 231–233).

Proteins identified in EVs comprise several peptidases, proteases, cytoskeletal proteins, nuclear proteins, calcium-binding proteins as well as stress-related proteins (28, 234, 235). Importantly, Coakley et al. demonstrated that *H. polygyrus* secretes EVs containing Argonaute protein, which is a central protein in the RNA-induced silencing complex (RISC) and is a powerful mechanism of gene silencing (229, 236). Furthermore, EVs are expected to be an important part of the secretome and it has been shown that the secreotomes of many helminths contain a variety of highly-abundant leaderless proteins, which is homolog to damage-associated molecular pattern molecules (DAMPs) in the host (28, 197). These DAMPs can, just like the host's DAMPs, modulate the host innate cells, such as stimulation of cytokine secretion in macrophages and lymphocytes. This could indicate that helminths have evolved mechanisms that are similar to their hosts in order to avoid elimination by the immune response of the hosts (182, 237).

Interestingly, besides parasite proteins, EVs have also been shown to contain host-derived proteins. Marcilla et al. identified 36 different host proteins in vesicles from the trematode *E. caproni*, which mainly corresponded to histones, partial sequences of mucins, metabolic enzymes, and immunoglobulins (28). Their study suggests that EVs might be an important part of the host-parasite communication as host proteins were identified in the parasite EVs and as the vesicles were taken up by host cells. These findings are interesting, however further studies are needed to confirm the role of the vesicles for the establishment of the infection (28). Very recently a similar study has been conducted by Eichenberger et al. in which proteomic profile of *T. muris*-derived EVs also identified a number of proteins of importance in host-parasite interaction. Of interest, among the common most proteins were predicted not to have a signal peptide supporting the idea that EVs constitute an important mechanism by which molecules are transferred to the host (193).

Surprisingly, several studies have shown that a significant proportion of the EV proteins are lacking an N-terminal presequence, also referred to as transit peptide. The transit peptide is required for protein transport across relevant membranes and indicates a protein transport through a classical sorting pathway via ER/Golgi pathway (238). Since a significant proportion of the parasite proteins are lacking the transit peptide, this suggests that EVs may be an important mechanism for transport of proteins host cells (28, 185, 239).

Lipids are a major component of EVs and play an important role in the function, stability, rigidity, and uptake of EVs, as they are directly exposed to the environment. Most of the lipidomic studies have been performed in cancer cells and these studies have indicated that EVs may have a function as lipid carriers where they carry bioactive lipids to recipient cells. In the context of the tumor microenvironment, this transport may have an effect on the enrichment of tumor progression and immunosuppressive lipids, such as prostaglandins that enhance tumor growth (240, 241). Even though lipids are central to EV trafficking, only a few studies have yet explored the lipid content of EVs in parasites and their specific role remain to be elucidated (242, 243).

EVs AS NOVEL VACCINES

Even though helminth parasites infect over 25% of the world's population and are highly prevalent in livestock worldwide, these infections are one of the most "neglected" tropical diseases with no effective vaccines available for humans and only a few for animals (244, 245). The use of EVs as vaccines is an area of growing interest due to their immunomodulation role and EVs ability to generate specific antibodies (30, 191, 202).

Using EVs purified from *Echinostoma caproni*, Trelis et al. found that subcutaneous injection could reduce symptom severity and mortality of subsequent experimental infection in mice (191). Likewise, EV vaccination in mice generates specific antibodies and was sufficient to confer protective immunity against *H. polygyrus* challenge (202). *T. muris*-derived EVs has also recently been found to confer protection against subsequent infection (246). Several proteins were identified in the *T. muris* EVs and some proposed to be potential candidates for vaccine (246).

However, further studies are needed to further explore the potential of parasite-derived EVs as novel vaccine candidates (206). In another approach, DCs have been stimulated or infected with protozoan parasites following isolation of EVs, which then have been tested as vaccines. In this way, DC-derived EVs have shown to confer protective immunity against *Toxoplasma gondii* (247), *Leishmania major* (248).

Sotillo et al. observed that 31% of the identified proteins in EVs secreted from *S. mansoni* are homolog to previous describes vaccine candidates, where several of these proteins are common throughout the life cycle of the parasite. This indicates that a vaccine based on EVs could target different life stages of the parasite and may be effective against *S. mansoni* infection (249). However, EVs are biological complex and virtually nothing is known about their specific mechanisms and how they engage with the immune system. However, it was recently demonstrated that EVs from *H. polygyrus* are able to suppress both the activation of macrophages and target the Il-33 pathway, which is known to be essential for worm expulsion (202). Taken together, all these observations indicate that EVs hold a great potential for future vaccine development, and thereby pave the way for novel treatment options against parasite infection (206).

EVs AS NOVEL GENERATION OF BIOMARKERS: POSSIBILITIES AND POTENTIALS FOR EARLY DIAGNOSIS OF PARASITIC INFECTIONS

EVs have shown to contain a rich source of molecules and as these are protected from the environment by a membrane they are stable over time (250). In addition, as EVs are distributed in various body fluids and organs, they have received great interest for biomarker-based diagnosis (250). Indeed, the potential of EVs as a biomarker has widely been investigated in the field of cancers and the contents of exosomes derived from ovarian cancer patients have shown to differ from that of healthy individuals (250). Interestingly, some cancer types are associated with specific miRNA signatures in the exosomes and may, therefore, serve as a novel way of diagnosis and monitoring progression of treatment (251, 252). In infectious diseases, EVs isolated from serum samples have also shown potential in diagnostics (253). However, the physical location of the pathogen may affect the applicability of this method or at least the way samples should be collected. Buck et al. found that miRNA of *Litomosoides sigmodontis*, which is located in the pleural cavity, could be identified in the host serum whereas no miRNA of *H. polygyrus*, which resides in the gut lumen could be detected (30).

With the advent of high throughput assays, which now also includes EV array (254), a profound understanding is being established regarding host-parasite interplay and the main pathway by which EVs target host immune cells. Proteomics analysis on the HDPs concentrated in EVs has provided invaluable data to identify and purify the central candidate components for biomarkers, diagnostic tools, and vaccine development (255, 256). Likewise, HDPs merely have shown an acceptable potential to be considered as an approach to early infection diagnosis (257). For instance, cathepsin B1 from *Opisthorchis viverrini* has shown a potential candidate for further consideration as a biomarker in sera (258).

Altogether, the release of EVs might be a reciprocal beneficial interaction for both host and helminths. Eliciting an effective immune response against EVs is an obvious reason for the presence of highly immunogenic components which may offer possible biomarker candidate. On the other hand, helminths constantly explore a way to defeat host immunity and set up a permissive infection which production of EVs containing various types of material is might be a strong strategy (**Figure 3**).

PERSPECTIVES

Until now, many different and highly complex mechanisms have been suggested for immunosuppressive functions of HDPs. But, given the advances in recognition of EVs and their importance as an effective tool in manipulation of host immune cells, it makes sense to suppose the possible involvement of EVs in most HDPs-mediated immunomodulation.

Main intracellular pathways manipulated by HDPs were reviewed, but limited information has been provided regarding interaction between helminth-derived EVs and immune cells. Although several investigations have recently reported the potential intracellular functions of EVs, they are only partially characterized. Given the different mechanisms by which EVs are taken up by recipient cells (discussed in EV section), future investigations should focus on the intracellular mechanisms and pathways responsible for immunosuppression.

We believe that most mechanistic pathways which have been reported for HDPs can be tracked for EVs and their contents. Most biomolecules form contents of EVs require to reach into

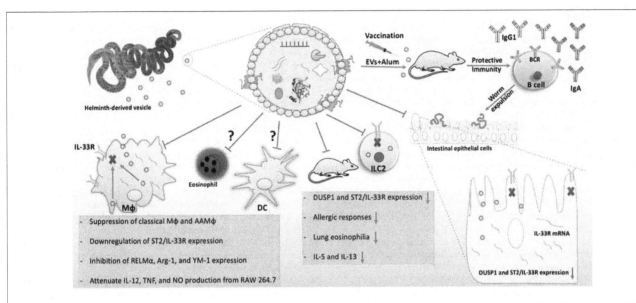

FIGURE 3 | Schematic illustration of known effects imposed by helminth-derived EVs during interaction with host immunity. As illustrated here, EVs can affect different host cells including immune cells and intestinal epithelial cells (IECs). Also, they can potentially be used to develop new vaccines against helminths. EVs deliver cargo containing various biomolecules to host cells which can interfere with host cell gene transcription. EVs are internalized by macrophages and IECs via unknown mechanism and target IL-33R and DUSP1 expression reducing signal transmission and leads to inhibition of helminth expulsion. EVs have also shown great potential in priming host immunity along with Alum as a vaccine complex against helminth infections. Effective suppression of both classical Mϕ and AAMϕ have also been reported, implying EVs are well-equipped with a wide range of active components. In addition to *in vitro* studies, immunomodulatory functions of EVs have also been monitored in *in vivo* model in which allergic responses, associated cytokines, ILC2, and eosinophilia are down-regulated in Alternaria-exposed mice.

the recipient cells to show their functions. The intracellular and PRR-targeting mechanisms of HDPs which were discussed in this review provide a framework to explore the possible interaction between EVs contents and intracellular components. In this regard, study on the PRRs-EV interplay would be of great interest to address some of the intracellular effects mediated by EVs. Release of EVs cargo in host immune cells can be associated with various outcomes, so determining the potential interaction between EVs cargo and PRRs downstream signaling would be valuable. For instance, Kojima et al. (259) showed that mesenteric lymph is able to exacerbate inflammatory responses via activation of TLR4 on macrophages without uptake through this receptor. They also showed that TLR4 signaling pathway is essential for exosome-induced macrophage activation (259).

EVs have recently been considered as a promising option to tune immune responses, as well as reprogram aberrant reactions to innocuous antigens. With respect to this, unraveling the main components of helminth-derived EVs, which are responsible for host immunomodulation may offer personalized therapeutic approaches in translational medicine.

Also, from a diagnostic point of view, EVs released by helminths may pave the way for developing a rapid diagnostic test that also can detect early parasitic infection. In addition, recognition and targeting main players in the biogenesis of helminth-derived EVs will be associated with novel insights into control of parasitic infections. Obviously, suppression of EVs synthesis containing a wide array of bioactive components will neutralize one of the central mechanism of helminths to

overcome host immunity. Interestingly, interfering with EVs biogenesis with exploiting selective inhibitors has provided promising results in the field of cancer therapy (260), but the applicability of this approach to combat helminth infections remains elusive. However, several investigations have been conducted to assess the potential of protozoan EVs for vaccine development against toxoplasmosis and leishmaniasis (248, 261). In these studies, exosomes derived from DCs exposed to parasite antigens have shown to be able to protect against infection in experimental models. Collectively, it seems that the importance of EVs and their relevance in establishment of a chronic infection are less-known and eagerly awaited to precisely be unraveled in the near future.

AUTHOR CONTRIBUTIONS

AZ was the major contributor in conception, design, illustrations, and writing of the manuscript. EH and SA wrote the EV section. PN and AW edited the manuscript and provided critical comments, suggestions, and insightful revisions. This work was supervised by PN.

ACKNOWLEDGMENTS

All the authors thank their respective Institutes and Universities.

REFERENCES

1. Allen JE, Maizels RM. Diversity and dialogue in immunity to helminths. *Nat Rev Immunol.* (2011) 11:375–88. doi: 10.1038/nri2992

2. Jackson JA, Friberg IM, Little S, Bradley JE. Review series on helminths, immune modulation and the hygiene hypothesis: immunity against helminths and immunological phenomena in modern human populations: coevolutionary legacies? *Immunology* (2009) 126:18–27. doi: 10.1111/j.1365-2567.2008.03010.x

3. Wammes LJ, Mpairwe H, Elliott AM, Yazdanbakhsh M. Helminth therapy or elimination: epidemiological, immunological, and clinical considerations. *Lancet Infect Dis.* (2014) 14:1150–62. doi: 10.1016/S1473-3099(14)70771-6

4. Finlay CM, Walsh KP, Mills KH. Induction of regulatory cells by helminth parasites: exploitation for the treatment of inflammatory diseases. *Immunol Rev.* (2014) 259:206–30. doi: 10.1111/imr.12164

5. Zakeri A. Helminth-induced apoptosis: a silent strategy for immunosuppression. *Parasitology* (2017) 144:1663–76. doi: 10.1017/S0031182017000841

6. Zakeri A, Borji H, Haghparast A. Interaction between helminths and toll-like receptors: possibilities and potentials for asthma therapy. *Int Rev Immunol.* (2016) 35:219–48. doi: 10.3109/08830185.2015.1096936

7. Oliveira SC, Figueiredo BC, Cardoso LS, Carvalho EM. A double edged sword: *Schistosoma mansoni* Sm29 regulates both Th1 and Th2 responses in inflammatory mucosal diseases. *Mucosal Immunol.* (2016) 9:1366–71. doi: 10.1038/mi.2016.69

8. Harris NL, Loke P. Recent advances in Type-2-cell-mediated immunity: insights from helminth infection. *Immunity* (2017) 47:1024–36. doi: 10.1016/j.immuni.2017.11.015

9. Yazdanbakhsh M, Kremsner PG, van Ree R. Allergy, parasites, and the hygiene hypothesis. *Science* (2002) 296:490–4. doi: 10.1126/science.296.5567.490

10. Strachan DP. Hay fever, hygiene, and household size. *BMJ* (1989) 299:1259–60. doi: 10.1136/bmj.299.6710.1259

11. Bach JF. The hygiene hypothesis in autoimmunity: the role of pathogens and commensals. *Nat Rev Immunol.* (2018) 18:105–20. doi: 10.1038/nri.2017.111

12. La Flamme AC, Ruddenklau K, Backstrom BT. Schistosomiasis decreases central nervous system inflammation and alters the progression of experimental autoimmune encephalomyelitis. *Infect Immun.* (2003) 71:4996–004. doi: 10.1128/IAI.71.9.4996-5004.2003

13. Wilson MS, Taylor MD, Balic A, Finney CA, Lamb JR, Maizels RM. Suppression of allergic airway inflammation by helminth-induced regulatory T cells. *J Exp Med.* (2005) 202:1199–212. doi: 10.1084/jem.20042572

14. Schwartz C, Hams E, Fallon PG. Helminth modulation of lung inflammation. *Trends Parasitol.* (2018) 34:388–403. doi: 10.1016/j.pt.2017.12.007

15. Mangan NE, Fallon RE, Smith P, van Rooijen N, McKenzie AN, Fallon PG. Helminth infection protects mice from anaphylaxis via IL-10-producing B cells. *J Immunol.* (2004) 173:6346–56. doi: 10.4049/jimmunol.173.10.6346

16. Summers RW, Elliott DE, Urban JF, Jr., Thompson R, Weinstock JV. *Trichuris suis* therapy in Crohn's disease. *Gut* (2005) 54:87–90. doi: 10.1136/gut.2004.041749

17. Smith P, Mangan NE, Walsh CM, Fallon RE, McKenzie AN, van Rooijen N, et al. Infection with a helminth parasite prevents experimental colitis via a macrophage-mediated mechanism. *J Immunol.* (2007) 178:4557–66. doi: 10.4049/jimmunol.178.7.4557

18. Weinstock JV, Elliott DE. Helminth infections decrease host susceptibility to immune-mediated diseases. *J Immunol.* (2014) 193:3239–47. doi: 10.4049/jimmunol.1400927

19. Hepworth MR, Hartmann S. Worming our way closer to the clinic. *Int J Parasitol Drugs Drug Resist.* (2012) 2:187–90. doi: 10.1016/j.ijpddr.2012.07.001

20. Sotillo J, Toledo R, Mulvenna J, Loukas A. Exploiting helminth-host interactomes through big data. *Trends Parasitol.* (2017) 33:875–88. doi: 10.1016/j.pt.2017.06.011

21. Rigano R, Buttari B, Profumo E, Ortona E, Delunardo F, Margutti P, et al. *Echinococcus granulosus* antigen B impairs human dendritic cell differentiation and polarizes immature dendritic cell maturation towards a Th2 cell response. *Infect Immun.* (2007) 75:1667–78. doi: 10.1128/IAI.01156-06

22. Pineda MA, Eason RJ, Harnett MM, Harnett W. From the worm to the pill, the parasitic worm product ES-62 raises new horizons in the treatment of rheumatoid arthritis. *Lupus* (2015) 24:400–11. doi: 10.1177/0961203314560004

23. Harn DA, McDonald J, Atochina O, Da'dara AA. Modulation of host immune responses by helminth glycans. *Immunol Rev.* (2009) 230:247–57. doi: 10.1111/j.1600-065X.2009.00799.x

24. Summan A, Nejsum P, Williams AR. Modulation of human dendritic cell activity by Giardia and helminth antigens. *Parasite Immunol.* (2018) 40:e12525. doi: 10.1111/pim.12525

25. Laan LC, Williams AR, Stavenhagen K, Giera M, Kooij G, Vlasakov I, et al. The whipworm (*Trichuris suis*) secretes prostaglandin E2 to suppress proinflammatory properties in human dendritic cells. *FASEB J.* (2017) 31:719–31. doi: 10.1096/fj.201600841R

26. Klaver EJ, van der Pouw Kraan TC, Laan LC, Kringel H, Cummings RD, Bouma G, et al. *Trichuris suis* soluble products induce Rab7b expression and limit TLR4 responses in human dendritic cells. *Genes Immun.* (2015) 16:378–87. doi: 10.1038/gene.2015.18

27. Robinson MW, Donnelly S, Dalton JP. Helminth defence molecules-immunomodulators designed by parasites! *Front Microbiol.* (2013) 4:296. doi: 10.3389/fmicb.2013.00296

28. Marcilla A, Trelis M, Cortes A, Sotillo J, Cantalapiedra F, Minguez MT, et al. Extracellular vesicles from parasitic helminths contain specific excretory/secretory proteins and are internalized in intestinal host cells. *PLoS ONE* (2012) 7:e45974. doi: 10.1371/journal.pone.0045974

29. Zheng Y, Guo X, He W, Shao Z, Zhang X, Yang J, et al. Effects of *Echinococcus multilocularis* miR-71 mimics on murine macrophage RAW264.7 cells. *Int Immunopharmacol.* (2016) 34:259–62. doi: 10.1016/j.intimp.2016.03.015

30. Buck AH, Coakley G, Simbari F, McSorley HJ, Quintana JF, Le Bihan T, et al. Exosomes secreted by nematode parasites transfer small RNAs to mammalian cells and modulate innate immunity. *Nat Commun.* (2014) 5:5488. doi: 10.1038/ncomms6488

31. Nazimek K, Bryniarski K, Askenase PW. Functions of exosomes and microbial extracellular vesicles in allergy and contact and delayed-type hypersensitivity. *Int Arch Allergy Immunol.* (2016) 171:1–26. doi: 10.1159/000449249

32. Ung TH, Madsen HJ, Hellwinkel JE, Lencioni AM, Graner MW. Exosome proteomics reveals transcriptional regulator proteins with potential to mediate downstream pathways. *Cancer Sci.* (2014) 105:1384–92. doi: 10.1111/cas.12534

33. Loukas A, Hotez PJ, Diemert D, Yazdanbakhsh M, McCarthy JS, Correa-Oliveira R, et al. Hookworm infection. *Nat Rev Dis Primers.* (2016) 2:16088. doi: 10.1038/nrdp.2016.88

34. Shepherd C, Navarro S, Wangchuk P, Wilson D, Daly NL, Loukas A. Identifying the immunomodulatory components of helminths. *Parasite Immunol.* (2015) 37:293–303. doi: 10.1111/pim.12192

35. Lee MS, Kim YJ. Signaling pathways downstream of pattern-recognition receptors and their cross talk. *Annu Rev Biochem.* (2007) 76:447–80. doi: 10.1146/annurev.biochem.76.060605.122847

36. De Nardo D. Toll-like receptors: activation, signalling and transcriptional modulation. *Cytokine* (2015) 74:181–9. doi: 10.1016/j.cyto.2015.02.025

37. Maizels RM, Hewitson JP. "Immune Recognition of Parasite Glycans," In: Kosma P, Müller-Loennies S. editors *Anticarbohydrate Antibodies.* Vienna: Springer (2012).

38. Harnett W, Harnett MM. Helminth-derived immunomodulators: can understanding the worm produce the pill? *Nat Rev Immunol.* (2010) 10:278–84. doi: 10.1038/nri2730

39. Falcon C, Carranza F, Martinez FF, Knubel CP, Masih DT, Motran CC, et al. Excretory-secretory products (ESP) from *Fasciola hepatica* induce tolerogenic properties in myeloid dendritic cells. *Vet Immunol Immunopathol.* (2010) 137:36–46. doi: 10.1016/j.vetimm.2010.04.007

40. Kane CM, Cervi L, Sun J, McKee AS, Masek KS, Shapira S, et al. Helminth antigens modulate TLR-initiated dendritic cell activation. *J Immunol.* (2004) 173:7454–61. doi: 10.4049/jimmunol.173.12.7454

41. Silva-Alvarez V, Folle AM, Ramos AL, Kitano ES, Iwai LK, Corraliza I, et al. *Echinococcus granulosus* Antigen B binds to monocytes and macrophages modulating cell response to inflammation. *Parasit Vectors* (2016) 9:69. doi: 10.1186/s13071-016-1350-7

42. Nono JK, Pletinckx K, Lutz MB, Brehm K. Excretory/secretory-products of *Echinococcus multilocularis* larvae induce apoptosis and tolerogenic properties in dendritic cells *in vitro*. *PLoS Negl Trop Dis*. (2012) 6:e1516. doi: 10.1371/journal.pntd.0001516

43. Midttun HLE, Acevedo N, Skallerup P, Almeida S, Skovgaard K, Andresen L, et al. *Ascaris Suum* infection downregulates inflammatory pathways in the pig intestine *in vivo* and in human dendritic cells *in vitro*. *J Infect Dis*. (2018) 217:310–19. doi: 10.1093/infdis/jix585

44. Almeida S, Nejsum P, Williams AR. Modulation of human macrophage activity by Ascaris antigens is dependent on macrophage polarization state. *Immunobiology* (2018) 223:405–12. doi: 10.1016/j.imbio.2017.11.003

45. Arthur JS, Ley SC. Mitogen-activated protein kinases in innate immunity. *Nat Rev Immunol*. (2013) 13:679–92. doi: 10.1038/nri3495

46. Dunand-Sauthier I, Santiago-Raber ML, Capponi L, Vejnar CE, Schaad O, Irla M, et al. Silencing of c-Fos expression by microRNA-155 is critical for dendritic cell maturation and function. *Blood* (2011) 117:4490–500. doi: 10.1182/blood-2010-09-308064

47. Agrawal S, Agrawal A, Doughty B, Gerwitz A, Blenis J, Van Dyke T, et al. Cutting edge: different Toll-like receptor agonists instruct dendritic cells to induce distinct Th responses via differential modulation of extracellular signal-regulated kinase-mitogen-activated protein kinase and c-Fos. *J Immunol*. (2003) 171:4984–9. doi: 10.4049/jimmunol.171.10.4984

48. Nekrasova T, Shive C, Gao Y, Kawamura K, Guardia R, Landreth G, et al. ERK1-deficient mice show normal T cell effector function and are highly susceptible to experimental autoimmune encephalomyelitis. *J Immunol*. (2005) 175:2374–80. doi: 10.4049/jimmunol.175.4.2374

49. White RR, Artavanis-Tsakonas K. How helminths use excretory secretory fractions to modulate dendritic cells. *Virulence* (2012) 3:668–77. doi: 10.4161/viru.22832

50. Thomas PG, Carter MR, Atochina O, Da'Dara AA, Piskorska D, McGuire E, et al. Maturation of dendritic cell 2 phenotype by a helminth glycan uses a Toll-like receptor 4-dependent mechanism. *J Immunol*. (2003) 171:5837–41. doi: 10.4049/jimmunol.171.11.5837

51. Wilbers RH, Westerhof LB, van Noort K, Obieglo K, Driessen NN, Everts B, et al. Production and glyco-engineering of immunomodulatory helminth glycoproteins in plants. *Sci Rep*. (2017) 7:45910. doi: 10.1038/srep45910

52. Tripathi P, Sahoo N, Ullah U, Kallionpaa H, Suneja A, Lahesmaa R, et al. A novel mechanism for ERK-dependent regulation of IL4 transcription during human Th2-cell differentiation. *Immunol Cell Biol*. (2012) 90:676–87. doi: 10.1038/icb.2011.87

53. Cvetkovic J, Sofronic-Milosavljevic L, Ilic N, Gnjatovic M, Nagano I, Gruden-Movsesijan A. Immunomodulatory potential of particular Trichinella spiralis muscle larvae excretory-secretory components. *Int J Parasitol*. (2016) 46:833–42. doi: 10.1016/j.ijpara.2016.07.008

54. Bai X, Wu X, Wang X, Guan Z, Gao F, Yu J, et al. Regulation of cytokine expression in murine macrophages stimulated by excretory/secretory products from *Trichinella spiralis in vitro*. *Mol Cell Biochem*. (2012) 360:79–88. doi: 10.1007/s11010-011-1046-4

55. Rosadini CV, Kagan JC. Early innate immune responses to bacterial LPS. *Curr Opin Immunol*. (2017) 44:14–9. doi: 10.1016/j.coi.2016.10.005

56. Goodridge HS, Marshall FA, Else KJ, Houston KM, Egan C, Al-Riyami L, et al. Immunomodulation via novel use of TLR4 by the filarial nematode phosphorylcholine-containing secreted product, ES-62. *J Immunol*. (2005) 174:284–93. doi: 10.4049/jimmunol.174.1.284

57. Goodridge HS, Deehan MR, Harnett W, Harnett MM. Subversion of immunological signalling by a filarial nematode phosphorylcholine-containing secreted product. *Cell Signal*. (2005) 17:11–6. doi: 10.1016/j.cellsig.2004.05.014

58. Melendez AJ, Harnett MM, Pushparaj PN, Wong WS, Tay HK, McSharry CP, et al. Inhibition of Fc epsilon RI-mediated mast cell responses by ES-62, a product of parasitic filarial nematodes. *Nat Med*. (2007) 13:1375–81. doi: 10.1038/nm1654

59. Bell KS, Al-Riyami L, Lumb FE, Britton GJ, Poole AW, Williams CM, et al. The role of individual protein kinase C isoforms in mouse mast cell function and their targeting by the immunomodulatory parasitic worm product, ES-62. *Immunol Lett*. (2015) 168:31–40. doi: 10.1016/j.imlet.2015.09.001

60. Eason RJ, Bell KS, Marshall FA, Rodgers DT, Pineda MA, Steiger CN, et al. The helminth product, ES-62 modulates dendritic cell responses by

61. inducing the selective autophagolysosomal degradation of TLR-transducers, as exemplified by PKCdelta. *Sci Rep*. (2016) 6:37276. doi: 10.1038/srep37276

61. Al-Riyami L, Pineda MA, Rzepecka J, Huggan JK, Khalaf AI, Suckling CJ, et al. Designing anti-inflammatory drugs from parasitic worms: a synthetic small molecule analogue of the Acanthocheilonema viteae product ES-62 prevents development of collagen-induced arthritis. *J Med Chem*. (2013) 56:9982–10002. doi: 10.1021/jm401251p

62. Lumb FE, Doonan J, Bell KS, Pineda MA, Corbet M, Suckling CJ, et al. Dendritic cells provide a therapeutic target for synthetic small molecule analogues of the parasitic worm product, ES-62. *Sci Rep*. (2017) 7:1704. doi: 10.1038/s41598-017-01651-1

63. Doonan J, Lumb FE, Pineda MA, Tarafdar A, Crowe J, Khan AM, et al. Protection against arthritis by the parasitic worm product ES-62, and its drug-like small molecule analogues, is associated with inhibition of osteoclastogenesis. *Front Immunol*. (2018) 9:1016. doi: 10.3389/fimmu.2018.01016

64. van Riet E, Everts B, Retra K, Phylipsen M, van Hellemond JJ, Tielens AG, et al. Combined TLR2 and TLR4 ligation in the context of bacterial or helminth extracts in human monocyte derived dendritic cells: molecular correlates for Th1/Th2 polarization. *BMC Immunol*. (2009) 10:9. doi: 10.1186/1471-2172-10-9

65. Gao Y, Chen L, Hou M, Chen Y, Ji M, Wu H, et al. TLR2 directing PD-L2 expression inhibit T cells response in Schistosoma japonicum infection. *PLoS ONE* (2013) 8:e82480 doi: 10.1371/journal.pone.0082480

66. Correale J, Farez MF. Parasite infections in multiple sclerosis modulate immune responses through a retinoic acid-dependent pathway. *J Immunol*. (2013) 191:3827–37. doi: 10.4049/jimmunol.1301110

67. van der Kleij D, Latz E, Brouwers JF, Kruize YC, Schmitz M, Kurt-Jones EA, et al. A novel host-parasite lipid cross-talk. Schistosomal lyso-phosphatidylserine activates toll-like receptor 2 and affects immune polarization. *J Biol Chem*. (2002) 277:48122–9. doi: 10.1074/jbc.M206941200

68. Layland LE, Rad R, Wagner H, da Costa CU. Immunopathology in schistosomiasis is controlled by antigen-specific regulatory T cells primed in the presence of TLR2. *Eur J Immunol*. (2007) 37:2174–84. doi: 10.1002/eji.200737063

69. Wang X, Zhou S, Chi Y, Wen X, Hoellwarth J, He L, et al. CD4+CD25+ Treg induction by an HSP60-derived peptide SJMHE1 from *Schistosoma japonicum* is TLR2 dependent. *Eur J Immunol*. (2009) 39:3052–65. doi:10.1002/eji.200939335

70. Thomas PG, Carter MR, Da'dara AA, DeSimone TM, Harn DA. A helminth glycan induces APC maturation via alternative NF-kappa B activation independent of I kappa B alpha degradation. *J Immunol*. (2005) 175:2082–90. doi: 10.4049/jimmunol.175.4.2082

71. Artis D, Kane CM, Fiore J, Zaph C, Shapira S, Joyce K, et al. Dendritic cell-intrinsic expression of NF-kappa B1 is required to promote optimal Th2 cell differentiation. *J Immunol*. (2005) 174:7154–9. doi: 10.4049/jimmunol.174.11.7154

72. Vukman KV, Adams PN, O'Neill SM. Fasciola hepatica tegumental coat antigen suppresses MAPK signalling in dendritic cells and up-regulates the expression of SOCS3. *Parasite Immunol*. (2013) 35:234–8. doi: 10.1111/pim.12033

73. Donnelly S, O'Neill SM, Stack CM, Robinson MW, Turnbull L, Whitchurch C, et al. Helminth cysteine proteases inhibit TRIF-dependent activation of macrophages via degradation of TLR3. *J Biol Chem*. (2010) 285:3383–92. doi: 10.1074/jbc.M109.060368

74. Yu YR, Deng MJ, Lu WW, Jia MZ, Wu W, Qi YF. Systemic cytokine profiles and splenic toll-like receptor expression during *Trichinella spiralis* infection. *Exp Parasitol*. (2013) 134:92–101. doi: 10.1016/j.exppara.2013.02.014

75. Gomez-Escobar N, Bennett C, Prieto-Lafuente L, Aebischer T, Blackburn CC, Maizels RM. Heterologous expression of the filarial nematode alt gene products reveals their potential to inhibit immune function. *BMC Biol*. (2005) 3:8. doi: 10.1186/1741-7007-3-8

76. Klaver EJ, Kuijk LM, Lindhorst TK, Cummings RD, van Die I. *Schistosoma mansoni* soluble egg antigens induce expression of the negative regulators SOCS1 and SHP1 in human dendritic cells via interaction with the mannose receptor. *PLoS ONE* (2015) 10:e0124089. doi: 10.1371/journal.pone.0124089

77. Klotz C, Ziegler T, Figueiredo AS, Rausch S, Hepworth MR, Obsivac N, et al. A helminth immunomodulator exploits host signaling events to regulate

cytokine production in macrophages. *PLoS Pathog.* (2011) 7:e1001248. doi: 10.1371/journal.ppat.1001248

78. Schierack P, Lucius R, Sonnenburg B, Schilling K, Hartmann S. Parasite-specific immunomodulatory functions of filarial cystatin. *Infect Immun.* (2003) 71:2422–9. doi: 10.1128/IAI.71.5.2422-2429.2003

79. Ziegler T, Rausch S, Steinfelder S, Klotz C, Hepworth MR, Kuhl AA, et al. A novel regulatory macrophage induced by a helminth molecule instructs IL-10 in CD4[+] T cells and protects against mucosal inflammation. *J Immunol.* (2015) 194:1555–64. doi: 10.4049/jimmunol.1401217

80. Aksoy E, Zouain CS, Vanhoutte F, Fontaine J, Pavelka N, Thieblemont N, et al. Double-stranded RNAs from the helminth parasite Schistosoma activate TLR3 in dendritic cells. *J Biol Chem.* (2005) 280:277–83. doi: 10.1074/jbc.M411223200

81. Yang Q, Qiu H, Xie H, Qi Y, Cha H, Qu J, et al. A *Schistosoma japonicum* infection promotes the expansion of myeloid-derived suppressor cells by activating the JAK/STAT3 Pathway. *J Immunol.* (2017) 198:4716–27. doi: 10.4049/jimmunol.1601860

82. Liu WF, Wen SH, Zhan JH, Li YS, Shen JT, Yang WJ, et al. Treatment with recombinant *Trichinella spiralis* cathepsin B-like protein ameliorates intestinal ischemia/reperfusion injury in mice by promoting a switch from M1 to M2 macrophages. *J Immunol.* (2015) 195:317–28. doi: 10.4049/jimmunol.1401864

83. Fukao T, Tanabe M, Terauchi Y, Ota T, Matsuda S, Asano T, et al. PI3K-mediated negative feedback regulation of IL-12 production in DCs. *Nat Immunol.* (2002) 3:875–81. doi: 10.1038/ni825

84. Kamda JD, Singer SM. Phosphoinositide 3-kinase-dependent inhibition of dendritic cell interleukin-12 production by *Giardia lamblia. Infect Immun.* (2009) 77:685–93. doi: 10.1128/IAI.00718-08

85. Motran CC, Ambrosio LF, Volpini X, Celias DP, Cervi L. Dendritic cells and parasites: from recognition and activation to immune response instruction. *Semin Immunopathol.* (2017) 39:199–213. doi: 10.1007/s00281-016-0588-7

86. Steinfelder S, Andersen JF, Cannons JL, Feng CG, Joshi M, Dwyer D, et al. The major component in schistosome eggs responsible for conditioning dendritic cells for Th2 polarization is a T2 ribonuclease (omega-1). *J Exp Med.* (2009) 206:1681–90. doi: 10.1084/jem.20082462

87. Brown GD, Willment JA, Whitehead L. C-type lectins in immunity and homeostasis. *Nat Rev Immunol.* (2018) 18:374–89. doi: 10.1038/s41577-018-0004-8

88. Thawer S, Auret J, Schnoeller C, Chetty A, Smith K, Darby M, et al. Surfactant protein-D is essential for immunity to helminth infection. *PLoS Pathog.* (2016) 2:e1005461. doi: 10.1371/journal.ppat.1005461

89. Favoretto BC, Casabuono AAC, Portes-Junior JA, Jacysyn JF, Couto AS, Faquim-Mauro EL. High molecular weight components containing N-linked oligosaccharides of Ascaris suum extract inhibit the dendritic cells activation through DC-SIGN and MR. *Mol Immunol.* (2017) 87:33–46. doi: 10.1016/j.molimm.2017.03.015

90. Tundup S, Srivastava L, Harn DA, Jr. Polarization of host immune responses by helminth-expressed glycans. *Ann NY Acad Sci.* (2012) 1253:1–13. doi: 10.1111/j.1749-6632.2012.06618.x

91. van Liempt E, Bank CM, Mehta P, Garcia-Vallejo JJ, Kawar ZS, Geyer R, et al. Specificity of DC-SIGN for mannose- and fucose-containing glycans. *FEBS Lett.* (2006) 580:6123–31. doi: 10.1016/j.febslet.2006.10.009

92. van Die I, van Vliet SJ, Nyame AK, Cummings RD, Bank CM, Appelmelk B, et al. The dendritic cell-specific C-type lectin DC-SIGN is a receptor for Schistosoma mansoni egg antigens and recognizes the glycan antigen Lewis x. *Glycobiology* (2003) 13:471–8. doi: 10.1093/glycob/cwg052

93. van Liempt E, van Vliet SJ, Engering A, Garcia Vallejo JJ, Bank CM, Sanchez-Hernandez M, et al. Schistosoma mansoni soluble egg antigens are internalized by human dendritic cells through multiple C-type lectins and suppress TLR-induced dendritic cell activation. *Mol Immunol.* (2007) 44:2605–15. doi: 10.1016/j.molimm.2006.12.012

94. van Die I, Cummings RD. Glycan gimmickry by parasitic helminths: a strategy for modulating the host immune response? *Glycobiology* (2010) 20:2–12. doi: 10.1093/glycob/cwp140

95. Paveley RA, Aynsley SA, Turner JD, Bourke CD, Jenkins SJ, Cook PC, et al. The Mannose Receptor (CD206) is an important pattern recognition receptor (PRR) in the detection of the infective stage of the helminth

96. Hang L, Blum AM, Kumar S, Urban JF, Jr., Mitreva M, Geary TG, et al. Downregulation of the syk signaling pathway in intestinal dendritic cells is sufficient to induce dendritic cells that inhibit colitis. *J Immunol.* (2016) 197:2948–57. doi: 10.4049/jimmunol.1600063

97. Terrazas CA, Alcantara-Hernandez M, Bonifaz L, Terrazas LI, Satoskar AR Helminth-excreted/secreted products are recognized by multiple receptors on DCs to block the TLR response and bias Th2 polarization in a cRAF dependent pathway. *FASEB J.* (2013) 27:4547–60. doi: 10.1096/fj.13-228932

98. Terrazas C, de Dios Ruiz-Rosado J, Amici SA, Jablonski KA, Martinez-Saucedo D, Webb LM, et al. Helminth-induced Ly6C(hi) monocyte-derived alternatively activated macrophages suppress experimental autoimmune encephalomyelitis. *Sci Rep.* (2017) 7:40814. doi: 10.1038/srep40814

99. Loukas A, Maizels RM. Helminth C-type lectins and host-parasite interactions. *Parasitol Today* (2000) 16:333–9. doi: 10.1016/S0169-4758(00)01704-X

100. Schabussova I, Amer H, van Die I, Kosma P, Maizels RM. O-methylated glycans from toxocara are specific targets for antibody binding in human and animal infections. *Int J Parasitol.* (2007) 37:97–109. doi: 10.1016/j.ijpara.2006.09.006

101. Tawill S, Le Goff L, Ali F, Blaxter M, Allen JE. Both free-living and parasitic nematodes induce a characteristic Th2 response that is dependent on the presence of intact glycans. *Infect Immun.* (2004) 72:398–407. doi: 10.1128/IAI.72.1.398-407.2004

102. Rodriguez E, Kalay H, Noya V, Brossard N, Giacomini C, van Kooyk Y, et al. *Fasciola hepatica* glycoconjugates immuneregulate dendritic cells through the dendritic cell-specific intercellular adhesion molecule-3-Grabbing Non-integrin inducing T cell anergy. *Sci Rep.* (2017) 7:46748 doi: 10.1038/srep46748

103. Rodriguez E, Carasi P, Frigerio S, da Costa V, van Vliet S, Noya V, et al. *Fasciola hepatica* immune regulates CD11c(+) cells by interacting with the macrophage Gal/GalNAc Lectin. *Front Immunol.* (2017) 8:264. doi: 10.3389/fimmu.2017.00264

104. Ravida A, Cwiklinski K, Aldridge AM, Clarke P, Thompson R, Gerlach JQ, et al. *Fasciola hepatica* surface tegument: glycoproteins at the interface of parasite and host. *Mol Cell Proteomics* (2016) 15:3139–53. doi: 10.1074/mcp.M116.059774

105. Aldridge A, O'Neill SM. *Fasciola hepatica* tegumental antigens induce anergic-like T cells via dendritic cells in a mannose receptor-dependent manner. *Eur J Immunol.* (2016) 46:1180–92. doi: 10.1002/eji.201545905

106. Rodriguez E, Noya V, Cervi L, Chiribao ML, Brossard N, Chiale C, et al. Glycans from *Fasciola hepatica* modulate the host immune response and TLR-induced maturation of dendritic cells. *PLoS Negl Trop Dis.* (2015) 9:e0004234. doi: 10.1371/journal.pntd.0004234

107. Ravida A, Aldridge AM, Driessen NN, Heus FA, Hokke CH, O'Neill SM. *Fasciola hepatica* surface coat glycoproteins contain mannosylated and phosphorylated N-glycans and exhibit immune modulatory properties independent of the mannose receptor. *PLoS Negl Trop Dis.* (2016) 10:e0004601. doi: 10.1371/journal.pntd.0004601

108. Guasconi L, Chiapello LS, Masih DT. *Fasciola hepatica* excretory-secretory products induce CD4[+]T cell anergy via selective up-regulation of PD-L2 expression on macrophages in a Dectin-1 dependent way. *Immunobiology* (2015) 220:934–9. doi: 10.1016/j.imbio.2015.02.001

109. Guasconi L, Serradell MC, Garro AP, Iacobelli L, Masih DT. C-type lectins on macrophages participate in the immunomodulatory response to *Fasciola hepatica* products. *Immunology* (2011) 133:386–96. doi: 10.1111/j.1365-2567.2011.03449.x

110. Ritter M, Gross O, Kays S, Ruland J, Nimmerjahn F, Saijo S, et al. Schistosoma mansoni triggers Dectin-2, which activates the Nlrp3 inflammasome and alters adaptive immune responses. *Proc Natl Acad Sci USA.* (2010) 107:20459–64. doi: 10.1073/pnas.1010337107

111. Aranzamendi C, Tefsen B, Jansen M, Chiumiento L, Bruschi F, Kortbeek T, et al. Glycan microarray profiling of parasite infection sera identifies the LDNF glycan as a potential antigen for serodiagnosis of trichinellosis. *Exp Parasitol.* (2011) 129:221–6. doi: 10.1016/j.exppara.2011.08.015

112. Everts B, Hussaarts L, Driessen NN, Meevissen MH, Schramm G, van der Ham AJ, et al. Schistosome-derived omega-1 drives Th2 polarization

96. Hang L, Blum AM, Kumar S, Urban JF, Jr., Mitreva M, Geary TG, et al.

by suppressing protein synthesis following internalization by the mannose receptor. *J Exp Med.* (2012) 209:1753–67. doi: 10.1084/jem.20111381

113. Meevissen MH, Wuhrer M, Doenhoff MJ, Schramm G, Haas H, Deelder AM, et al. Structural characterization of glycans on omega-1, a major *Schistosoma mansoni* egg glycoprotein that drives Th2 responses. *J Proteome Res.* (2010) 9:2630–42. doi: 10.1021/pr100081c

114. Bhargava P, Li C, Stanya KJ, Jacobi D, Dai L, Liu S, et al. Immunomodulatory glycan LNFPIII alleviates hepatosteatosis and insulin resistance through direct and indirect control of metabolic pathways. *Nat Med.* (2012) 18:1665–72. doi: 10.1038/nm.2962

115. Velupillai P, Harn DA. Oligosaccharide-specific induction of interleukin 10 production by B220$^+$ cells from schistosome-infected mice: a mechanism for regulation of CD4$^+$ T-cell subsets. *Proc Natl Acad Sci USA.* (1994) 91:18–22. doi: 10.1073/pnas.91.1.18

116. Kooij G, Braster R, Koning JJ, Laan LC, van Vliet SJ, Los T, et al. *Trichuris suis* induces human non-classical patrolling monocytes via the mannose receptor and PKC: implications for multiple sclerosis. *Acta Neuropathol Commun.* (2015) 3:45. doi: 10.1186/s40478-015-0223-1

117. Cvetkovic J, Ilic N, Sofronic-Milosavljevic L, Gruden-Movsesijan A. Glycans expressed on *Trichinella spiralis* excretory-secretory antigens are important for anti-inflamatory immune response polarization. *Comp Immunol Microbiol Infect Dis.* (2014) 37:355–67. doi: 10.1016/j.cimid.2014.10.004

118. van Die I, Cummings RD. The mannose receptor in regulation of helminth-mediated host immunity. *Front Immunol.* (2017) 8:1677. doi: 10.3389/fimmu.2017.01677

119. van Stijn CM, Meyer S, van den Broek M, Bruijns SC, van Kooyk Y, Geyer R, et al. *Schistosoma mansoni* worm glycolipids induce an inflammatory phenotype in human dendritic cells by cooperation of TLR4 and DC-SIGN. *Mol Immunol.* (2010) 47:1544–52. doi: 10.1016/j.molimm.2010.01.014

120. Meyer-Wentrup F, Cambi A, Joosten B, Looman MW, de Vries IJ, Figdor CG, et al. DCIR is endocytosed into human dendritic cells and inhibits TLR8-mediated cytokine production. *J Leukoc Biol.* (2009) 85:518–25. doi: 10.1189/jlb.0608352

121. Trinchieri G, Sher A. Cooperation of Toll-like receptor signals in innate immune defence. *Nat Rev Immunol.* (2007) 7:179–90. doi: 10.1038/nri2038

122. Geijtenbeek TB, Van Vliet SJ, Koppel EA, Sanchez-Hernandez M, Vandenbroucke-Grauls CM, Appelmelk B, et al. Mycobacteria target DC-SIGN to suppress dendritic cell function. *J Exp Med.* (2003) 197:7–17. doi: 10.1084/jem.20021229

123. Vanhoutte F, Breuilh L, Fontaine J, Zouain CS, Mallevaey T, Vasseur V, et al. Toll-like receptor (TLR)2 and TLR3 sensing is required for dendritic cell activation, but dispensable to control *Schistosoma mansoni* infection and pathology. *Microbes Infect.* (2007) 9:1606–13. doi: 10.1016/j.micinf.2007.09.013

124. Kane CM, Jung E, Pearce EJ. *Schistosoma mansoni* egg antigen-mediated modulation of Toll-like receptor (TLR)-induced activation occurs independently of TLR2, TLR4, and MyD88. *Infect Immun.* (2008) 76:5754–9. doi: 10.1128/IAI.00497-08

125. Breuilh L, Vanhoutte F, Fontaine J, van Stijn CM, Tillie-Leblond I, Capron M, et al. Galectin-3 modulates immune and inflammatory responses during helminthic infection: impact of galectin-3 deficiency on the functions of dendritic cells. *Infect Immun.* (2007) 75:5148–57. doi: 10.1128/IAI.02006-06

126. Van Liempt E, Imberty A, Bank CM, Van Vliet SJ, Van Kooyk Y, Geijtenbeek TB, et al. Molecular basis of the differences in binding properties of the highly related C-type lectins DC-SIGN and L-SIGN to Lewis X trisaccharide and *Schistosoma mansoni* egg antigens. *J Biol Chem.* (2004) 279:33161–7. doi: 10.1074/jbc.M404988200

127. Gringhuis SI, den Dunnen J, Litjens M, van Het Hof B, van Kooyk Y, Geijtenbeek TB. C-type lectin DC-SIGN modulates Toll-like receptor signaling via Raf-1 kinase-dependent acetylation of transcription factor NF-kappaB. *Immunity.* (2007) 26:605–16. doi: 10.1016/j.immuni.2007.03.012

128. Kuijk LM, van Die I. Worms to the rescue: can worm glycans protect from autoimmune diseases? *IUBMB Life* (2010) 62:303–12. doi: 10.1002/iub.304

129. Dillon S, Agrawal S, Banerjee K, Letterio J, Denning TL, Oswald-Richter K, et al. Yeast zymosan, a stimulus for TLR2 and dectin-1, induces regulatory antigen-presenting cells and immunological tolerance. *J Clin Invest.* (2006) 116:916–28. doi: 10.1172/JCI27203

130. Motran CC, Silvane L, Chiapello LS, Theumer MG, Ambrosio LF, Volpini X, et al. Helminth infections: recognition and modulation of the immune response by innate immune cells. *Front Immunol.* (2018) 9:664. doi: 10.3389/fimmu.2018.00664

131. Awad F, Assrawi E, Louvrier C, Jumeau C, Georgin-Lavialle S, Grateau G, et al. Inflammasome biology, molecular pathology and therapeutic implications. *Pharmacol Ther.* (2018) 187:133–49. doi: 10.1016/j.pharmthera.2018.02.011

132. Rzepecka J, Pineda MA, Al-Riyami L, Rodgers DT, Huggan JK, Lumb FE, et al. Prophylactic and therapeutic treatment with a synthetic analogue of a parasitic worm product prevents experimental arthritis and inhibits IL-1beta production via NRF2-mediated counter-regulation of the inflammasome. *J Autoimmun.* (2015) 60:59–73. doi: 10.1016/j.jaut.2015.04.005

133. Zaiss MM, Maslowski KM, Mosconi I, Guenat N, Marsland BJ, Harris NL. IL-1beta suppresses innate IL-25 and IL-33 production and maintains helminth chronicity. *PLoS Pathog.* (2013) 9:e1003531. doi: 10.1371/journal.ppat.1003531

134. Alhallaf R, Agha Z, Miller CM, Robertson AAB, Sotillo J, Croese J, et al. The NLRP3 inflammasome suppresses protective immunity to gastrointestinal helminth infection. *Cell Rep.* (2018) 23:1085–1098. doi: 10.1016/j.celrep.2018.03.097

135. Ferguson BJ, Newland SA, Gibbs SE, Tourlomousis P, Fernandes dos Santos P, Patel MN, et al. The *Schistosoma mansoni* T2 ribonuclease omega-1 modulates inflammasome-dependent IL-1beta secretion in macrophages. *Int J Parasitol.* (2015) 45:809–13. doi: 10.1016/j.ijpara.2015.08.005

136. Klotz C, Ziegler T, Danilowicz-Luebert E, Hartmann S. Cystatins of parasitic organisms. *Adv Exp Med Biol.* (2011) 712:208–21. doi: 10.1007/978-1-4419-8414-2_13

137. Manoury B, Gregory WF, Maizels RM, Watts C. Bm-CPI-2, a cystatin homolog secreted by the filarial parasite *Brugia malayi*, inhibits class II MHC-restricted antigen processing. *Curr Biol.* (2001) 11:447–51. doi: 10.1016/S0960-9822(01)00118-X

138. Hartmann S, Lucius R. Modulation of host immune responses by nematode cystatins. *Int J Parasitol.* (2003) 33:1291–302. doi: 10.1016/S0020-7519(03)00163-2

139. Lustigman S, Brotman B, Huima T, Prince AM, McKerrow JH. Molecular cloning and characterization of onchocystatin, a cysteine proteinase inhibitor of *Onchocerca volvulus*. *J Biol Chem.* (1992) 267:17339–46.

140. Hartmann S, Kyewski B, Sonnenburg B, Lucius R. A filarial cysteine protease inhibitor down-regulates T cell proliferation and enhances interleukin-10 production. *Eur J Immunol.* (1997) 27:2253–60. doi: 10.1002/eji.1830270920

141. Dainichi T, Maekawa Y, Ishii K, Zhang T, Nashed BF, Sakai T, et al. Nippocystatin, a cysteine protease inhibitor from Nippostrongylus brasiliensis, inhibits antigen processing and modulates antigen-specific immune response. *Infect Immun.* (2001) 69:7380–6. doi: 10.1128/IAI.69.12.7380-7386.2001

142. Pfaff AW, Schulz-Key H, Soboslay PT, Taylor DW, MacLennan K, Hoffmann WH. Litomosoides sigmodontis cystatin acts as an immunomodulator during experimental filariasis. *Int J Parasitol.* (2002) 32:171–8. doi: 10.1016/S0020-7519(01)00350-2

143. Schonemeyer A, Lucius R, Sonnenburg B, Brattig N, Sabat R, Schilling K, et al. Modulation of human T cell responses and macrophage functions by onchocystatin, a secreted protein of the filarial nematode *Onchocerca volvulus*. *J Immunol.* (2001) 167:3207–15. doi: 10.4049/jimmunol.167.6.3207

144. Schnoeller C, Rausch S, Pillai S, Avagyan A, Wittig BM, Loddenkemper C, et al. A helminth immunomodulator reduces allergic and inflammatory responses by induction of IL-10-producing macrophages. *J Immunol.* (2008) 180:4265–72. doi: 10.4049/jimmunol.180.6.4265

145. Rzepecka J, Rausch S, Klotz C, Schnoller C, Kornprobst T, Hagen J, et al. Calreticulin from the intestinal nematode *Heligmosomoides polygyrus* is a Th2-skewing protein and interacts with murine scavenger receptor-A. *Mol Immunol.* (2009) 46:1109–19. doi: 10.1016/j.molimm.2008.10.032

146. Everts B, Perona-Wright G, Smits HH, Hokke CH, van der Ham AJ, Fitzsimmons CM, et al. Omega-1, a glycoprotein secreted by Schistosoma mansoni eggs, drives Th2 responses. *J Exp Med.* (2009) 206:1673–80. doi: 10.1084/jem.20082460

147. Paul WE, Zhu J. How are T(H)2-type immune responses initiated and amplified? *Nat Rev Immunol.* (2010) 10:225–35. doi: 10.1038/nri2735

148. Pineda MA, Lumb F, Harnett MM, Harnett W. ES-62, a therapeutic anti-inflammatory agent evolved by the filarial nematode *Acanthocheilonema viteae*. *Mol Biochem Parasitol*. (2014) 194:1–8. doi: 10.1016/j.molbiopara.2014.03.003

149. Hosken NA, Shibuya K, Heath AW, Murphy KM, O'Garra A. The effect of antigen dose on CD4[+] T helper cell phenotype development in a T cell receptor-alpha beta-transgenic model. *J Exp Med*. (1995) 182:1579–84. doi: 10.1084/jem.182.5.1579

150. Appleby LJ, Nausch N, Heard F, Erskine L, Bourke CD, Midzi N, et al. Down regulation of the TCR Complex CD3zeta-Chain on CD3[+] T Cells: a potential mechanism for helminth-mediated immune modulation. *Front Immunol*. (2015) 6:51. doi: 10.3389/fimmu.2015.00051

151. Harnett W, Harnett MM. What causes lymphocyte hyporesponsiveness during filarial nematode infection? *Trends Parasitol*. (2006) 22:105–10. doi: 10.1016/j.pt.2006.01.010

152. Deehan MR, Harnett W, Harnett MM. A filarial nematode-secreted phosphorylcholine-containing glycoprotein uncouples the B cell antigen receptor from extracellular signal-regulated kinase-mitogen-activated protein kinase by promoting the surface Ig-mediated recruitment of Src homology 2 domain-containing tyrosine phosphatase-1 and Pac-1 mitogen-activated kinase-phosphatase. *J Immunol*. (2001) 166:7462–8. doi: 10.4049/jimmunol.166.12.7462

153. Harnett MM, Deehan MR, Williams DM, Harnett W. Induction of signalling anergy via the T-cell receptor in cultured Jurkat T cells by pre-exposure to a filarial nematode secreted product. *Parasite Immunol*. (1998) 20:551–63. doi: 10.1046/j.1365-3024.1998.00181.x

154. Pineda MA, McGrath MA, Smith PC, Al-Riyami L, Rzepecka J, Gracie JA, et al. The parasitic helminth product ES-62 suppresses pathogenesis in collagen-induced arthritis by targeting the interleukin-17-producing cellular network at multiple sites. *Arthritis Rheum*. (2012) 64:3168–78. doi: 10.1002/art.34581

155. Furuhashi Y, Imai S, Tezuka H, Fujita K. Recombinant dirofilaria immitis-derived antigen can suppress passive cutaneous anaphylaxis reactions. *Int Arch Allergy Immunol*. (2001) 125:144–51. doi: 10.1159/000053808

156. Jeong YI, Kim YJ, Ju JW, Hong SH, Lee MR, Cho SH, et al. Identification of anti-allergic effect of Clonorchis sinensis-derived protein venom allergen-like proteins (CsVAL). *Biochem Biophys Res Commun*. (2014) 445:549–55. doi: 10.1016/j.bbrc.2014.01.189

157. Imai S, Tezuka H, Fujita K. A factor of inducing IgE from a filarial parasite prevents insulin-dependent diabetes mellitus in nonobese diabetic mice. *Biochem Biophys Res Commun*. (2001) 286:1051–8. doi: 10.1006/bbrc.2001.5471

158. Griffith Q, Liang Y, Whitworth P, Rodriguez-Russo C, Gul A, Siddiqui AA, et al. Immuno-evasive tactics by schistosomes identify an effective allergy preventative. *Exp Parasitol*. (2015) 153:139–50. doi: 10.1016/j.exppara.2015.03.012

159. Johnston CJ, Smyth DJ, Dresser DW, Maizels RM. TGF-beta in tolerance, development and regulation of immunity. *Cell Immunol*. (2016) 299:14–22. doi: 10.1016/j.cellimm.2015.10.006

160. McSorley HJ, Grainger JR, Harcus Y, Murray J, Nisbet AJ, Knox DP, et al. daf-7-related TGF-beta homologues from Trichostrongyloid nematodes show contrasting life-cycle expression patterns. *Parasitology* (2010) 137:159–71. doi:10.1017/S0031182009990321

161. Johnston CJC, Smyth DJ, Kodali RB, White MPJ, Harcus Y, Filbey KJ, et al. A structurally distinct TGF-beta mimic from an intestinal helminth parasite potently induces regulatory T cells. *Nat Commun*. (2017) 8:1741. doi:10.1038/s41467-017-01886-6

162. Sulaiman AA, Zolnierczyk K, Japa O, Owen JP, Maddison BC, Emes RD, et al. A trematode parasite derived growth factor binds and exerts influences on host immune functions via host cytokine receptor complexes. *PLoS Pathog*. (2016) 12:e1005991. doi: 10.1371/journal.ppat.1005991

163. Fusco AC, Salafsky B, Kevin MB. *Schistosoma mansoni*: eicosanoid production by cercariae. *Exp Parasitol*. (1985) 59:44–50. doi: 10.1016/0014-4894(85)90055-4

164. Szkudlinski J. Occurrence of prostaglandins and other eicosanoids in parasites and their role in host-parasite interaction. *Wiad Parazytol*. (2000) 46:439–46.

165. Nakanishi M, Rosenberg DW. Multifaceted roles of PGE2 in inflammation and cancer. *Semin Immunopathol*. (2013) 35:123–37. doi: 10.1007/s00281-012-0342-8

166. Kalinski P. Regulation of immune responses by prostaglandin E2. *J Immunol*. (2012) 188:21–8. doi: 10.4049/jimmunol.1101029

167. Grencis RK, Entwistle GM. Production of an interferon-gamma homologue by an intestinal nematode: functionally significant or interesting artefact? *Parasitology* (1997) 115:S101–6.

168. Cliffe LJ, Grencis RK. The *Trichuris muris* system: a paradigm of resistance and susceptibility to intestinal nematode infection. *Adv Parasitol*. (2004) 57:255–307. doi: 10.1016/S0065-308X(04)57004-5

169. Smith P, Fallon RE, Mangan NE, Walsh CM, Saraiva M, Sayers JR, et al. *Schistosoma mansoni* secretes a chemokine binding protein with antiinflammatory activity. *J Exp Med*. (2005) 202:1319–25. doi: 10.1084/jem.20050955

170. Osbourn M, Soares DC, Vacca F, Cohen ES, Scott IC, Gregory WF, et al. HpARI protein secreted by a helminth parasite suppresses interleukin-33. *Immunity* (2017) 47:739–51. doi: 10.1016/j.immuni.2017.09.015

171. Chhabra S, Chang SC, Nguyen HM, Huq R, Tanner MR, Londono LM, et al. Kv1.3 channel-blocking immunomodulatory peptides from parasitic worms: implications for autoimmune diseases. *FASEB J*. (2014) 28:3952–64. doi: 10.1096/fj.14-251967

172. Chandy KG, DeCoursey TE, Cahalan MD, McLaughlin C, Gupta S. Voltage-gated potassium channels are required for human T lymphocyte activation. *J Exp Med*. (1984) 160:369–85. doi: 10.1084/jem.160.2.369

173. Wulff H, Calabresi PA, Allie R, Yun S, Pennington M, Beeton C, et al. The voltage-gated Kv1.3 K(+) channel in effector memory T cells as new target for MS. *J Clin Invest*. (2003) 111:1703–13. doi: 10.1172/JCI16921

174. Beeton C, Wulff H, Standifer NE, Azam P, Mullen KM, Pennington MW, et al. Kv1.3 channels are a therapeutic target for T cell-mediated autoimmune diseases. *Proc Natl Acad Sci USA*. (2006) 103:17414–9. doi: 10.1073/pnas.0605136103

175. Raposo G, Stoorvogel W. Extracellular vesicles: exosomes, microvesicles, and friends. *J Cell Biol*. (2013) 200:373–83. doi: 10.1083/jcb.201211138

176. Buzas EI, Gyorgy B, Nagy G, Falus A, Gay S. Emerging role of extracellular vesicles in inflammatory diseases. *Nat Rev Rheumatol*. (2014) 10:356–64. doi: 10.1038/nrrheum.2014.19

177. Kanada M, Bachmann MH, Contag CH. Signaling by extracellular vesicles advances cancer hallmarks. *Trends Cancer* (2016) 2:84–94. doi: 10.1016/j.trecan.2015.12.005

178. Robbins PD, Morelli AE. Regulation of immune responses by extracellular vesicles. *Nat Rev Immunol*. (2014) 14:195–208. doi: 10.1038/nri3622

179. Mulcahy LA, Pink RC, Carter DR. Routes and mechanisms of extracellular vesicle uptake. *J Extracell Vesicles* (2014) 3. doi: 10.3402/jev.v3.24641

180. Feng D, Zhao WL, Ye YY, Bai XC, Liu RQ, Chang LF, et al. Cellular internalization of exosomes occurs through phagocytosis. *Traffic* (2010) 11:675–87. doi: 10.1111/j.1600-0854.2010.01041.x

181. Kirchhausen T. Clathrin. *Annu Rev Biochem*. (2000) 69:699–727. doi: 10.1146/annurev.biochem.69.1.699

182. Doherty GJ, McMahon HT. Mechanisms of endocytosis. *Annu Rev Biochem*. (2009) 78:857–902. doi: 10.1146/annurev.biochem.78.081307.110540

183. Parolini I, Federici C, Raggi C, Lugini L, Palleschi S, De Milito A, et al. Sargiacomo and S. fais: microenvironmental pH is a key factor for exosome traffic in tumor cells. *J Biol Chem*. (2009) 284:34211–22. doi: 10.1074/jbc.M109.041152

184. Regev-Rudzki N, Wilson DW, Carvalho TG, Sisquella X, Coleman BM, Rug M, et al. Cell-cell communication between malaria-infected red blood cells via exosome-like vesicles. *Cell* (2013) 153:1120–33. doi: 10.1016/j.cell.2013.04.029

185. Marcilla A, Martin-Jaular L, Trelis M, de Menezes-Neto A, Osuna A, Bernal D, et al. Extracellular vesicles in parasitic diseases. *J Extracell Vesicles* (2014) 3:25040. doi: 10.3402/jev.v3.25040

186. Benchimol M. The release of secretory vesicle in encysting Giardia lamblia. *FEMS Microbiol Lett*. (2004) 235:81–7. doi: 10.1016/j.femsle.2004.04.014

187. Silverman JM, Clos J, de'Oliveira CC, Shirvani O, Fang Y, Wang C, et al. An exosome-based secretion pathway is responsible for protein export from Leishmania and communication with macrophages. *J Cell Sci*. (2010) 123:842–52. doi: 10.1242/jcs.056465

188. Twu O, de Miguel N, Lustig G, Stevens GC, Vashisht AA, Wohlschlegel JA, et al. *Trichomonas vaginalis* exosomes deliver cargo to host cells and mediate hostratioparasite interactions. *PLoS Pathog.* (2013) 9:e1003482. doi: 10.1371/journal.ppat.1003482

189. Szempruch AJ, Sykes SE, Kieft R, Dennison L, Becker AC, Gartrell A, et al. Extracellular vesicles from *Trypanosoma brucei* mediate virulence factor transfer and cause host anemia. *Cell* (2016) 164:246–57. doi: 10.1016/j.cell.2015.11.051

190. Garcia-Silva MR, Cabrera-Cabrera F, das Neves RF, Souto-Padron T, de Souza W, Cayota A. Gene expression changes induced by Trypanosoma cruzi shed microvesicles in mammalian host cells: relevance of tRNA-derived halves. *Biomed Res Int.* (2014) 305239 doi: 10.1155/2014/305239

191. Trelis M, Galiano A, Bolado A, Toledo R, Marcilla A, Bernal D. Subcutaneous injection of exosomes reduces symptom severity and mortality induced by Echinostoma caproni infection in BALB/c mice. *Int J Parasitol.* (2016) 46:799–808. doi: 10.1016/j.ijpara.2016.07.003

192. Samoil V, Dagenais M, Ganapathy V, Aldridge J, Glebov A, Jardim A, et al. Vesicle-based secretion in schistosomes: analysis of protein and microRNA (miRNA) content of exosome-like vesicles derived from *Schistosoma mansoni*. *Sci Rep.* (2018) 8:3286. doi: 10.1038/s41598-018-21587-4

193. Eichenberger RM, Talukder MH, Field MA, Wangchuk P, Giacomin P, Loukas A, et al. Characterization of *Trichuris muris* secreted proteins and extracellular vesicles provides new insights into host-parasite communication. *J Extracell Vesicles* (2018) 7:1428004. doi: 10.1080/20013078.2018.1428004

194. Kifle DW, Sotillo J, Pearson MS, Loukas A. Extracellular vesicles as a target for the development of anti-helminth vaccines. *Emerg Topics Life Sci.* (2017) 1:659–65. doi: 10.1042/ETLS20170095

195. Silverman JM, Clos J, Horakova E, Wang AY, Wiesgigl M, Kelly I, et al. Leishmania exosomes modulate innate and adaptive immune responses through effects on monocytes and dendritic cells. *J Immunol.* (2010) 185:5011–22. doi: 10.4049/jimmunol.1000541

196. Combes V, Coltel N, Alibert M, van Eck M, Raymond C, Juhan-Vague I, et al. ABCA1 gene deletion protects against cerebral malaria: potential pathogenic role of microparticles in neuropathology. *Am J Pathol.* (2005) 166:295–302. doi: 10.1016/S0002-9440(10)62253-5

197. Cwiklinski K, de la Torre-Escudero E, Trelis M, Bernal D, Dufresne PJ, Brennan GP, et al. Biogenesis pathways and cargo molecules involved in parasite pathogenesis. *Mol Cell Proteomics* (2015) 14:3258–73. doi: 10.1074/mcp.M115.053934

198. Simoes MC, Lee J, Djikeng A, Cerqueira GC, Zerlotini A, da Silva-Pereira RA, et al. Identification of *Schistosoma mansoni* microRNAs. *BMC Genomics* (2011) 12:47. doi: 10.1186/1471-2164-12-47

199. Roig J, Saiz ML, Galiano A, Trelis M, Cantalapiedra F, Monteagudo C, et al. Extracellular vesicles from the *Helminth Fasciola* hepatica prevent DSS-induced acute ulcerative colitis in a T-lymphocyte independent mode. *Front Microbiol.* (2018) 9:1036. doi: 10.3389/fmicb.2018.01036

200. Eichenberger RM, Ryan S, Jones L, Buitrago G, Polster R, Montes de Oca M, et al. Hookworm secreted extracellular vesicles interact with host cells and prevent inducible colitis in mice. *Front Immunol.* (2018) 9:850. doi: 10.3389/fimmu.2018.00850

201. Eichenberger RM, Sotillo J, Loukas A. Immunobiology of parasitic worm extracellular vesicles. *Immunol Cell Biol.* (2018) 96:704–13. doi: 10.1111/imcb.12171

202. Coakley G, McCaskill JL, Borger JG, Simbari F, Robertson E, Millar M, et al. Extracellular vesicles from a helminth parasite suppress macrophage activation and constitute an effective vaccine for protective immunity. *Cell Rep.* (2017) 19:1545–57. doi: 10.1016/j.celrep.2017.05.001

203. Schorey JS, Cheng Y, Singh PP, Smith VL. Smith: Exosomes and other extracellular vesicles in host-pathogen interactions. *EMBO Rep.* (2015) 16:24–43. doi: 10.15252/embr.201439363

204. Lustigman S, Grote A, Ghedin E. Ghedin: The role of 'omics' in the quest to eliminate human filariasis. *PLoS Negl Trop Dis.* (2017) 11:e005464. doi: 10.1371/journal.pntd.0005464

205. Zhu L, Liu J, Dao J, Lu K, Li H, Gu H, et al. Molecular characterization of *S. japonicum* exosome-like vesicles reveals their regulatory roles in parasite-host interactions. *Sci Rep.* (2016) 6:5885. doi: 10.1038/srep25885

206. Mekonnen GG, Pearson M, Loukas A, Sotillo J. Extracellular vesicles from parasitic helminths and their potential utility as vaccines. *Expert Rev Vaccines* (2018) 17:197–205. doi: 10.1080/14760584.2018.1431125

207. Weber JA, Baxter DH, Zhang S, Huang DY, Huang KH, Lee MJ, et al. The microRNA spectrum in 12 body fluids. *Clin Chem.* (2010) 56:1733–41. doi: 10.1373/clinchem.2010.147405

208. Berezikov E. Evolution of microRNA diversity and regulation in animals. *Nat Rev Genet.* (2011) 12:846–60. doi: 10.1038/nrg3079

209. Zheng Y, Cai X, Bradley JE. microRNAs in parasites and parasite infection. *RNA Biol.* (2013) 10:371–9. doi: 10.4161/rna.23716

210. Gutierrez-Loli R, Orrego MA, Sevillano-Quispe OG, Herrera-Arrasco L, Guerra-Giraldez C. MicroRNAs in *Taenia solium* neurocysticercosis: insights as promising agents in host-parasite interaction and their potential as biomarkers. *Front Microbiol.* (2017) 8:1905. doi: 10.3389/fmicb.2017.01905

211. Darnell DK, Kaur S, Stanislaw S, Konieczka JH, Yatskievych TA, Antin PB. MicroRNA expression during chick embryo development. *Dev Dyn.* (2006) 235:3156–65. doi: 10.1002/dvdy.20956

212. Aranha MM, Santos DM, Xavier JM, Low WC, Steer CJ, Sola S, et al. Apoptosis-associated microRNAs are modulated in mouse, rat and human neural differentiation. *BMC Genomics* (2010) 11:514. doi: 10.1186/1471-2164-11-514

213. Le MT, Xie H, Zhou B, Chia PH, Rizk P, Um M, et al. MicroRNA-125b promotes neuronal differentiation in human cells by repressing multiple targets. *Mol Cell Biol.* (2009) 29:5290–305. doi: 10.1128/MCB.01694-08

214. Nguyen HT, Dalmasso G, Yan Y, Laroui H, Dahan S, Mayer L, et al. MicroRNA-7 modulates CD98 expression during intestinal epithelial cell differentiation. *J Biol Chem.* (2010) 285:1479–89. doi: 10.1074/jbc.M109.057141

215. Tsitsiou E, Lindsay MA. microRNAs and the immune response. *Curr Opin Pharmacol.* (2009) 9:514–20. doi: 10.1016/j.coph.2009.05.003

216. O'Connell RM, Taganov KD, Boldin MP, Cheng G, Baltimore D. MicroRNA-155 is induced during the macrophage inflammatory response. *Proc Natl Acad Sci USA.* (2007) 104:1604–9. doi: 10.1073/pnas.0610731104

217. Turner ML, Schnorfeil FM, Brocker T. MicroRNAs regulate dendritic cell differentiation and function. *J Immunol.* (2011) 187:3911–7. doi: 10.4049/jimmunol.1101137

218. Johnnidis JB, Harris MH, Wheeler RT, Stehling-Sun S, Lam MH, Kirak O, et al. Regulation of progenitor cell proliferation and granulocyte function by microRNA-223. *Nature* (2008) 451:1125–9. doi: 10.1038/nature06607

219. Pobezinsky LA, Etzensperger R, Jeurling S, Alag A, Kadakia T, McCaughtry TM, et al. Let-7 microRNAs target the lineage-specific transcription factor PLZF to regulate terminal NKT cell differentiation and effector function. *Nat Immunol.* (2015) 16:517–24. doi: 10.1038/ni.3146

220. Lu J, Guo S, Ebert BL, Zhang H, Peng X, Bosco J, et al. MicroRNA-mediated control of cell fate in megakaryocyte-erythrocyte progenitors. *Dev Cell.* (2008) 14:843–53. doi: 10.1016/j.devcel.2008.03.012

221. Nutt SL, Kee BL. The transcriptional regulation of B cell lineage commitment. *Immunity* (2007) 26:715–25. doi: 10.1016/j.immuni.2007.05.010

222. Vigorito E, Perks KL, Abreu-Goodger C, Bunting S, Xiang Z, Kohlhaas S, et al. microRNA-155 regulates the generation of immunoglobulin class-switched plasma cells. *Immunity* (2007) 27:847–59. doi: 10.1016/j.immuni.2007.10.009

223. Cobb BS, Nesterova TB, Thompson E, Hertweck A, O'Connor E, Godwin J, et al. T cell lineage choice and differentiation in the absence of the RNase III enzyme dicer. *J Exp Med.* (2005) 201:1367–73. doi:10.1084/jem.20050572

224. Li QJ, Chau J, Ebert PJ, Sylvester G, Min H, Liu G, et al. miR-181a is an intrinsic modulator of T cell sensitivity and selection. *Cell* (2007) 129:147–61. doi: 10.1016/j.cell.2007.03.008

225. Hansen EP, Kringel H, Williams AR, Nejsum P. Secretion of RNA-containing extracellular vesicles by the porcine whipworm, *Trichuris suis*. *J Parasitol.* (2015) 101:336–40. doi: 10.1645/14-714.1

226. Wang L, Li Z, Shen J, Liu Z, Liang J, Wu X, et al. Exosome-like vesicles derived by *Schistosoma japonicum* adult worms mediates M1 type immune- activity of macrophage. *Parasitol Res.* (2015) 114:1865–73. doi: 10.1007/s00436-015-4373-7

227. Gu HY, Marks ND, Winter AD, Weir W, Tzelos T, McNeilly TN, et al. Conservation of a microRNA cluster in parasitic nematodes and

profiling of miRNAs in excretory-secretory products and microvesicles of *Haemonchus contortus*. *PLoS Negl Trop Dis.* (2017) 11:e0006056. doi: 10.1371/journal.pntd.0006056

228. Nowacki FC, Swain MT, Klychnikov OI, Niazi U, Ivens A, Quintana JF, et al. Protein and small non-coding RNA-enriched extracellular vesicles are released by the pathogenic blood fluke Schistosoma mansoni. *J Extracell Vesicles* (2015) 4:28665. doi:10.3402/jev.v4.28665

229. Coakley G, Maizels RM, Buck AH. Exosomes and other extracellular vesicles: the new communicators in parasite infections. *Trends Parasitol.* (2015) 31:477–89. doi: 10.1016/j.pt.2015.06.009

230. Subra C, Grand D, Laulagnier K, Stella A, Lambeau G, Paillasse M, et al. Exosomes account for vesicle-mediated transcellular transport of activatable phospholipases and prostaglandins. *J Lipid Res.* (2010) 51:2105–20. doi: 10.1194/jlr.M003657

231. Grainger JR, Smith KA, Hewitson JP, McSorley HJ, Harcus Y, Filbey KJ, et al.Helminth secretions induce *de novo* T cell Foxp3 expression and regulatory function through the TGF-beta pathway. *J Exp Med.* (2010) 207:2331–41. doi: 10.1084/jem.20101074

232. Moreno Y, Geary TG. Stage- and gender-specific proteomic analysis of *Brugia malayi* excretory-secretory products. *PLoS Negl Trop Dis.* (2008) 2:e326. doi: 10.1371/journal.pntd.0000326

233. Chehayeb JF, Robertson AP, Martin RJ, Geary TG. Proteomic analysis of adult *Ascaris suum* fluid compartments and secretory products. *PLoS Negl Trop Dis.* (2014) 8:e2939. doi: 10.1371/journal.pntd.0002939

234. de la Torre-Escudero E, Bennett APS, Clarke A, Brennan GP, Robinson MW. Extracellular vesicle biogenesis in helminths: more than one route to the surface? *Trends Parasitol.* (2016) 32:921–9. doi: 10.1016/j.pt.2016.09.001

235. Bernal D, Carpena I, Espert AM, De la Rubia JE, Esteban JG, Toledo R, et al. Identification of proteins in excretory/secretory extracts of Echinostoma friedi (Trematoda) from chronic and acute infections. *Proteomics* (2006) 6:2835–43. doi: 10.1002/pmic.200500571

236. Pratt AJ, MacRae IJ. The RNA-induced silencing complex: a versatile gene-silencing machine. *J Biol Chem.* (2009) 284:17897–901. doi: 10.1074/jbc.R900012200

237. Robinson MW, Hutchinson AT, Donnelly S, Dalton JP. Worm secretory molecules are causing alarm. *Trends Parasitol.* (2010) 26:371–2. doi: 10.1016/j.pt.2010.05.004

238. Robinson MW, Menon R, Donnelly SM, Dalton JP, Ranganathan S. An integrated transcriptomics and proteomics analysis of the secretome of the helminth pathogen *Fasciola hepatica*: proteins associated with invasion and infection of the mammalian host. *Mol Cell Proteomics* (2009) 8:1891–907. doi: 10.1074/mcp.M900045-MCP200

239. Geiger A, Hirtz C, Becue T, Bellard E, Centeno D, Gargani D, et al. Exocytosis and protein secretion in Trypanosoma. *BMC Microbiol.* (2010) 10:20. doi: 10.1186/1471-2180-10-20

240. Roma-Rodrigues C, Fernandes AR, Baptista PV. Exosome in tumour microenvironment: overview of the crosstalk between normal and cancer cells. *BioMed Res. Int.* (2014) 2014: 179486. doi: 10.1155/2014/179486

241. Xiang X, Poliakov A, Liu C, Liu Y, Deng ZB, Wang J, et al. Induction of myeloid-derived suppressor cells by tumor exosomes. *Int J Cancer* (2009) 124:2621–33. doi: 10.1002/ijc.24249

242. Yoon YJ, Kim OY, Gho YS. Extracellular vesicles as emerging intercellular communicasomes. *BMB Rep.* (2014) 47:531–9. doi: 10.5483/BMBRep.2014.47.10.164

243. Simbari F, McCaskill J, Coakley G, Millar M, Maizels RM, Fabrias G, et al. Plasmalogen enrichment in exosomes secreted by a nematode parasite versus those derived from its mouse host: implications for exosome stability and biology. *J Extracell Vesicles* (2016) 5:30741. doi: 10.3402/jev.v5.30741

244. Hotez PJ, Brindley PJ, Bethony JM, King CH, Pearce EJ, Jacobson J. Helminth infections: the great neglected tropical diseases. *J Clin Invest.* (2008) 118:1311–21. doi: 10.1172/JCI34261

245. Hewitson JP, Maizels RM. Vaccination against helminth parasite infections. *Expert Rev Vaccines* (2014) 13:473–87. doi: 10.1586/14760584.2014.893195

246. Shears RK, Bancroft AJ, Hughes GW, Grencis RK, Thornton DJ. Extracellular vesicles induce protective immunity against *Trichuris muris*. *Parasite Immunol.* (2018) 40:e12536. doi: 10.1111/pim.12536

247. Beauvillain C, Juste MO, Dion S, Pierre J, Dimier-Poisson I. Exosomes are an effective vaccine against congenital toxoplasmosis in mice. *Vaccine* (2009) 27:1750–7. doi: 10.1016/j.vaccine.2009.01.022

248. Schnitzer JK, Berzel S, Fajardo-Moser M, Remer KA, Moll H. Fragments of antigen-loaded dendritic cells (DC) and DC-derived exosomes induce protective immunity against *Leishmania* major. *Vaccine* (2010) 28:5785–93. doi: 10.1016/j.vaccine.2010.06.077

249. Sotillo J, Pearson M, Potriquet J, Becker L, Pickering D, Mulvenna J, et al. Extracellular vesicles secreted by *Schistosoma mansoni* contain protein vaccine candidates. *Int J Parasitol.* (2016) 46:1–5. doi: 10.1016/j.ijpara.2015.09.002

250. Carriere J, Barnich N, Nguyen HT. Exosomes: from functions in host-pathogen interactions and immunity to diagnostic and therapeutic opportunities. *Rev Physiol Biochem Pharmacol.* (2016) 172:39–75. doi: 10.1007/112_2016_7

251. Hu G, Drescher KM, Chen XM. Exosomal miRNAs: biological properties and therapeutic potential. *Front Genet.* (2012) 3:56. doi: 10.3389/fgene.2012.00056

252. Tokuhisa M, Ichikawa Y, Kosaka N, Ochiya T, Yashiro M, Hirakawa K, et al. Exosomal miRNAs from peritoneum lavage fluid as potential prognostic biomarkers of peritoneal metastasis in gastric cancer. *PLoS ONE* (2015) 10:e0130472. doi: 10.1371/journal.pone.0130472

253. Singh PP, Smith VL, Karakousis PC, Schorey JS. Exosomes isolated from mycobacteria-infected mice or cultured macrophages can recruit and activate immune cells *in vitro* and *in vivo*. *J Immunol.* (2012) 189:777–85. doi: 10.4049/jimmunol.1103638

254. Jorgensen M, Baek R, Pedersen S, Sondergaard EK, Kristensen SR, Varming K. Extracellular Vesicle (EV) array: microarray capturing of exosomes and other extracellular vesicles for multiplexed phenotyping. *J Extracell Vesicles* (2013) 2:1–9. doi: 10.3402/jev.v2i0.20920

255. Wang Y, Cheng Z, Lu X, Tang C. *Echinococcus multilocularis*: proteomic analysis of the protoscoleces by two-dimensional electrophoresis and mass spectrometry. *Exp Parasitol.* (2009) 123:162–7. doi: 10.1016/j.exppara.2009.06.014

256. Knudsen GM, Medzihradszky KF, Lim KC, Hansell E, McKerrow JH. Proteomic analysis of *Schistosoma mansoni* cercarial secretions. *Mol Cell Proteomics* (2005) 4:1862–75. doi: 10.1074/mcp.M500097-MCP200

257. Harnett W. Secretory products of helminth parasites as immunomodulators. *Mol Biochem Parasitol.* (2014) 195:130–6. doi: 10.1016/j.molbiopara.2014.03.007

258. Sripa J, Brindley PJ, Sripa B, Loukas A, Kaewkes S, Laha T. Evaluation of liver fluke recombinant cathepsin B-1 protease as a serodiagnostic antigen for human opisthorchiasis. *Parasitol Int.* (2012) 61:191–5. doi: 10.1016/j.parint.2011.05.009

259. Kojima M, Gimenes-Junior JA, Chan TW, Eliceiri BP, Baird A, Costantini TW, et al. Exosomes in postshock mesenteric lymph are key mediators of acute lung injury triggering the macrophage activation via Toll-like receptor 4. *FASEB J.* (2018) 32:97–110. doi: 10.1096/fj.201700488R

260. S ELA, Mager I, Breakefield XO, Wood MJ. Extracellular vesicles: biology and emerging therapeutic opportunities. *Nat Rev Drug Discov.* (2013) 12:347–57. doi: 10.1038/nrd3978

261. Aline F, Bout D, Amigorena S, Roingeard P, Dimier-Poisson I. *Toxoplasma gondii* antigen-pulsed-dendritic cell-derived exosomes induce a protective immune response against *T. gondii* infection. *Infect Immun.* (2004) 72:4127–37. doi: 10.1128/IAI.72.7.4127-4137.2004

10

Salivarian Trypanosomosis: A Review of Parasites Involved, their Global Distribution and their Interaction with the Innate and Adaptive Mammalian Host Immune System

Magdalena Radwanska[1], Nick Vereecke[1,2], Violette Deleeuw[2], Joar Pinto[2] and Stefan Magez[1,2]*

[1] Laboratory for Biomedical Research, Ghent University Global Campus, Incheon, South Korea, [2] Laboratory of Cellular and Molecular Immunology, Vrije Universiteit Brussel, Brussels, Belgium

*Correspondence:
Stefan Magez
stefan.magez@vub.be

Salivarian trypanosomes are single cell extracellular parasites that cause infections in a wide range of hosts. Most pathogenic infections worldwide are caused by one of four major species of trypanosomes including (i) *Trypanosoma brucei* and the human infective subspecies *T. b. gambiense* and *T. b. rhodesiense*, (ii) *Trypanosoma evansi* and *T. equiperdum*, (iii) *Trypanosoma congolense* and (iv) *Trypanosoma vivax*. Infections with these parasites are marked by excessive immune dysfunction and immunopathology, both related to prolonged inflammatory host immune responses. Here we review the classification and global distribution of these parasites, highlight the adaptation of human infective trypanosomes that allow them to survive innate defense molecules unique to man, gorilla, and baboon serum and refer to the discovery of sexual reproduction of trypanosomes in the tsetse vector. With respect to the immunology of mammalian host-parasite interactions, the review highlights recent findings with respect to the B cell destruction capacity of trypanosomes and the role of T cells in the governance of infection control. Understanding infection-associated dysfunction and regulation of both these immune compartments is crucial to explain the continued failures of anti-trypanosome vaccine developments as well as the lack of any field-applicable vaccine based anti-trypanosomosis intervention strategy. Finally, the link between infection-associated inflammation and trypanosomosis induced anemia is covered in the context of both livestock and human infections.

Keywords: trypanosomosis, immunology, pathology, anemia, transmission

INTRODUCTION

Human African Trypanosomosis and Animal African Trypanosomosis are two well-known diseases that affect sub-Saharan Africa and have historically prevented the development of vast lands of the African continent into highly productive agricultural areas. However, the first salivarian pathogenic trypanosome to be discovered was *T. evansi*, a parasite identified by Dr. Griffith Evans in 1880, in horses and camels suffering from a disease called Surra on the Indian subcontinent (1). Almost 140 years after this initial discovery, a wealth of world-wide epidemiological data on pathogenic trypanosomes shows they are present on four different continents. Molecular parasite mechanisms, that allow the escape from the hosts' immune and non-immune defense systems, have been discovered and various interactions in the context of vector biology have been described. However, in the end the data available today has still not given us a way to intervene in trypanosomosis transmission by means of an effective anti-parasite vaccination strategy. Hence, control still relies on a combination of active case diagnosis and treatment, as well as vector control (2, 3). In this review we cover the classification of trypanosomes, which has recently become under scrutiny (4), as well as new discoveries with respect to genetic exchange between trypanosomes that takes place in the insect vector (5, 6). In addition, the paper provides an update on recent discoveries with respect to the B cell destructive potential of trypanosomes (7, 8), T cell biology (9), and the impact of trypanosomosis on red blood cell (RBC) homeostasis and infection-associated anemia (10). Throughout the data review, both animal trypanosomosis (AT) and human trypanosomosis (HT) have been considered. However, as most recent data shows, this "artificial" distinction might be less useful than previously thought, as atypical human trypanosomosis (a-HT), which can be caused by various animal trypanosomes, is now gaining more and more attention in the field (11).

SETTING THE SCENE FOR SALIVARIAN TRYPANOSOMOSIS

Trypanosomes are unicellular protozoan organisms of the class Kinetoplastida that cause a wide range of infections in a broad range of hosts. The latter includes not just mammals but also fish (12), birds (13), and reptiles (14), while insect vectors actually should be considered not just as transmission "tools" but also as definite hosts. Indeed, it is only here that sexual reproduction stages have been reported, as comprehensively outlined in a recent review by Gibson W. (5). In mammals, both salivarian and stercorarian trypanosomes cause diseases that affect the health status of the infected host in multiple ways. While the stercorarian trypanosomes are an important group of parasites, the main focus of this review is directed toward the pathogenic salivarian trypanosomes that cause infections in human, livestock, and game animals. These infections are marked by the extracellular nature of the infecting agent, causing pathologies and health complications that are very different from the features that characterize intracellular pathogenic infections such as those caused by the stercorarian *T. cruzi* parasite. An additional complication that arises when describing trypanosomosis, is the use of the term *African Trypanosomosis*. This denomination is very often used in an incorrect way. Indeed, as will be described in this review, all major pathogenic salivarian trypanosome infections do occur on the African continent. However several of the pathogens responsible for these diseases have moved "out of Africa" and infections are progressing throughout the world. A last introductory remark for this paper is the fact that Human African Trypanosomosis or HAT has recently been brought under control in a very significant manner

by huge consorted international efforts of the last decennium (15). Hence, this might give the impression that trypanosomosis has become a disease of the past. This however could very well be a wrong assumption for three main reasons. First, there are no reports that suggest that AT is near to being controlled on a world-wide scale. Second, the most aggressive form of HAT caused by *T. b. rhodesiense* has a zoonotic origin, so as long as human infective trypanosomes are present in a wildlife reservoir, re-emergence of the disease remains a risk (16, 17). This holds true even if the majority of infections caused by *T. b gambiense* are being brought under control. Third, reports of a-HT in- and outside Africa show that "African" trypanosomosis is only part of the problem (11). Hence, for now trypanosome diseases still remain a threat to human health and to agriculture systems of emerging economies. In the absence of any vaccine strategy preventing the spread of these infections, continued research into host-parasite interactions is needed. This will provide a better understanding of trypanosome diseases itself, the mechanisms of disease resistance, modes of immune evasion, and ultimately the reasons for continued failure of vaccination attempts.

CLASSIFICATION OF THE MAIN PATHOGENIC SALIVARIAN TRYPANOSOMES

Trypanosomes belong to the sub-kingdom Protozoa, the order Kinetoplastida, the family Trypanosomatidae, and genus *Trypanosoma*. The large numbers of different species belonging to this genus have been classified in several subgenera according to their morphology. For the salivarian pathogenic trypanosomes the subgenera include *Trypanozoon, Duttonella, Nannomonas,* and *Pycnomonas*, of which the first three account for the vast majority of human and animal infections and are the subject of this review. Their combined geographic spread covers most of the developing world (**Figure 1**).

The first trypanosome subgenus, *Trypanozoon,* is composed of several *Trypanosoma* species, which are human and animal infective and includes the first pathogenic trypanosome ever to be discovered i.e. *Trypanosoma evansi*. Today, *T. evansi* is a parasite that is considered to have mainly a veterinary importance (1), causing the disease Surra in a wide range of economically important mammals such as horses, cattle, goats, buffalos, dogs, and camels. In addition, the parasite can be found in game animals such as deer, wild pigs, and capybaras, representing a reservoir that often might escape attention. Today, *T. evansi* is found across Central and South America, North Africa, the Russian territories, the Indian subcontinent, China, and Southeast Asia (23). Transmission mainly occurs mechanically through the bite of bloodsucking insects from the family Tabanidae (genus *Tabanus*) (24), Chrysops (25), Atylotus (26), and Muscidae (genus *Stomoxys* and *Haematobia*) (18). It is this mechanical transmission that has allowed the parasite to move beyond the tsetse fly region and out of Africa. Morphologically, *T. evansi* has long been considered as a monomorphic parasite with the main bloodstream form appearing as so called "long slender" forms. However, the appearance of short intermediate

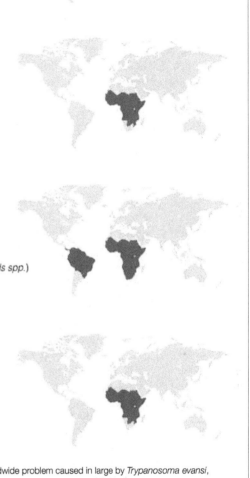

Scientific Name: *Trypanosoma evansi*
Subgenera: *Trypanozoon*
Main host: Equines; bovines and camelids
Main Vector: Tsetse flies (*Glossina spp.*);Stable-flies (*Stomoxys spp.*); Horse-flies (*Tabanids spp.*)
Transmission: Mechanical

Scientific Name: *Trypanosoma brucei*
Subgenera: *Trypanozoon*
Main host: Bovines and humans
Main Vector: Tsetse flies (*Glossina spp.*)
Transmission: Cyclical

Scientific Name: *Trypanosoma vivax*
Subgenera: *Duttonella*
Main host: Bovines ovines, caprines, equines
Main Vector: Tsetse flies (*Glossina spp.*);Stable-flies (*Stomoxys spp.*); Horse-flies (*Tabanids spp.*)
Transmission: Cyclical and mechanical

Scientific Name: *Trypanosoma congolense*
Subgenera: *Nannomonas*
Main host: Bovines
Main Vector: Tsetse flies (*Glossina spp.*)
Transmission: Cyclical

FIGURE 1 | Geographic distribution of salivarian trypanosomosis. Salivarian trypanosomosis is a worldwide problem caused in large by *Trypanosoma evansi*, *Trypanosoma brucei* (including the human infective subspecies *T. b. gambiense* and *T. b. rhodesiense*), *Trypanosoma vivax* and *Trypanosoma congolense*. *T. brucei*, and *T. congolense* infections are limited to the sub-Saharan tsetse belt. In contrast, as *T. vivax* and *T. evansi* can be mechanically transmitted, these parasites have migrate beyond the tsetse belt, out of Africa and into South America and Asia [adapted from (18–22)].

forms has also been reported, but only in blood smears of infected cat and monkey (27). Important is that the parasite has a peculiar kinetoplast, characterized by either a reduced (lack of maxi-circles and homogenous mini-circles) or a total absence of kinetoplast DNA (kDNA) (28). This deficiency is thought to lock *T. evansi* in the bloodstream form, as they are unable to transcribe the kDNA genes required to perform the oxidative phosphorylation required for the developmental processes in the midgut of the tsetse (29). For long, this altered kDNA characteristic has been used to differentiate *T. evansi* from African *T. brucei* subspecies. Recently however, genetic analysis of a large battery of both *T. evansi* and *T. brucei* parasites has

shown that the situation is more complex, and that many *T. evansi* parasites are closely related to *T. brucei*, even more closely than the relation between *T. evansi* parasites from different geographic locations (30–32). In addition, these data suggest that *T. evansi* arose multiple times from a different *T. brucei* ancestor. Hence, this has sparked a debate about the nomenclature of the *Trypanozoon* parasites. While it has been suggested by some to consider *T. evansi* as a *T. brucei* variant, a most recent revision has been proposed based on the proper application of the principles of biological nomenclature. This proposal suggests to rename all *T. brucei* subspecies as *T. evansi* subspecies, and even adopt the use of *T. evansi gambiense* and *T. evansi rhodesiense* for human infective African Trypanosomes (4). Important in the context of the parasite-host interplay of *T. evansi* is the notion that several human *T. evansi* infections have been reported in- and outside Africa (11). However, despite the wide geographic distribution of *T. evansi*, the reports on human non-African trypanosomosis are overall extremely rare. However, it cannot be excluded that one of the reasons for the scarce amount of data on a-HT is simply due to the lack of proper diagnostic practices that are able to correctly identify human trypanosomosis in *T. evansi* endemic areas.

The second *Trypanozoon* subspecies to be discovered was *T. brucei*, endemic to sub-Saharan Africa and transmitted by biting flies of the genus *Glossina*, commonly known as tsetse, with tsetse meaning "fly" in the Tswana language of Southern Africa. *T. brucei* parasites present a major health problem for humans, as the causative agent of the disease called HAT, or sleeping sickness. Domestic animals such as cattle, pigs, small ruminants, and game animals are also common hosts for *T. brucei*, in which the latter serve as a natural reservoir of the parasite. Three morphological indistinguishable subspecies of *T. brucei* are known (namely *T. b. gambiense*, *T. b. rhodesiense*, and *T. b. brucei.*) with *T. b. gambiense* and *T. b. rhodesiense* responsible for human trypanosome diseases in West/Central and East Africa, respectively. Uganda is one of the only countries where the two forms of HAT appear in adjacent regions. *T. b. brucei*, on the other hand, is unable to infect humans and is responsible for animal trypanosomosis only. The correct identification of the *T. brucei* subspecies is nearly impossible when solely based on their morphology or geographical origin. Indeed, all three subspecies appear as pleomorphic bloodstream parasites, having both long slender and short stumpy forms. However, molecular approaches have shown that this group is highly heterogeneous (33). The exclusive presence of the serum resistance associated (SRA) gene in *T. b. rhodesiense* has been used as a marker for the identification of this subspecies (34, 35). *T. b. gambiense* specific identification can be done through PCR amplification of the *T. b. gambiense*-specific glycoprotein (*TgsGP*) gene that encodes for a receptor-like glycoprotein, which is also involved in normal human serum resistance (36).

The third species within the subgenera of *Trypanozoon*, responsible for livestock infections, is *Trypanosoma equiperdum*. This parasite can be sexually transmitted amongst species from the family Equidae (horses and donkey), causing a venereal disease known as Dourine. Due to this transmission mode, the parasite has also acquired a wide geographic distribution. As for *T. evansi*, to which it is very closely related, also the classification of *T. equiperdum* as a separate species has been under scrutiny for many years (37), and several authors have suggested that there is no scientific argument to make a species level distinction between the two.

The second trypanosome subgenus responsible for salivarian trypanosomosis is *Dutonella*, which is mainly composed of two species, i.e., *T. vivax* and *T. uniforme*. Due to the global socio-economic impact caused by *T. vivax* infections in domestic animals, most of the studies of this subgenus have been carried out on this particular parasite species. This trypanosome is a pathogenic parasite species mainly found in Africa and South America (38). So far, only a single human infection has ever been

reported (11). In Africa, transmission occurs in large through the bite of tsetse flies, having the highest infection rate of any tsetse-transmitted trypanosome species (39, 40). This high infectivity could be attributed to the relatively simple cycle of development in the vector's mouthparts. The transmission beyond Africa is mainly carried out mechanically by hematophagous flies from the genus *Stomoxys* and *Tabanus*, which transmit the disease to domestic animals such as cattle and goats, as well as to endemic wild animals such as capybaras, deer, and bubaline antelopes. Despite its large economic impact, especially in South America, *T. vivax* remains one of the less studied animal-infective *Trypanosoma* species. The main issue with *T. vivax* in the context of experimental parasitology and immunology research is the fact that virtually no parasites of this species are capable to be grown in mice. Hence, virtually all laboratory infections in mouse models (incl. Tv700, STIB 719, STIB 731-A, ILRAD 560, IL 1392) are being executed with the derivatives of Y468 *T. vivax* clone that was originally isolated in Nigeria that happened to "grow well" in mice after extensive adaptation (41). Hence, it remains to be seen if the TvY486 *T. vivax* reference strain is a good representative parasite for the general population of parasites found both in Africa and South America regarding host-parasite interaction mechanisms.

The third subgenus of pathogenic salivarian trypanosomes is *Nannomonas*, encompassing three species of animal-infective trypanosomes, i.e., *Trypanosoma simiae*, *Trypanosoma godfreyi*, and *Trypanosoma congolense*. The two first species are mainly infective to mammals belonging to the Suidae family (domestic pigs, warthogs etc.) while *T. congolense* has a broader range of hosts including livestock and game animals, but is generally accepted to be non-infective to humans. It should however be mentioned that a mixed *T. b. gambiense*/*T. congolense* infection has been reported in a human (42) and that *in vitro* testing of human serum-induced trypanolysis has shown a resistance phenotype in several stocks (43). *T. congolense* is the major tsetse transmitted pathogenic salivarian livestock trypanosome present in sub-Saharan Africa and causes large economical losses in the countries where it is endemic. The disease caused by this parasite is referred to as Nagana, meaning *depressed spirit* in the Zulu language of Southern Africa. During transmission, *T. congolense* develops in the midgut and proboscis of the tsetse vector. Mechanical transmission can occur, involving mainly *Tabanus* and *Stomoxys* species (44). In general, *T. congolense* is considered to be a monomorphic parasite. The host-parasite interaction as well as immunopathology associated with *T. congolense* infections has been better studied than in the case of *T. evansi* and *T. vivax*. However, it is important to point out the fact that while the molecular parasite surface structure has been well-described and compared to *T. brucei* (45), the regulation and kinetics of surface coat variation, as well as the infection of the coat with the immune system have never been analyzed in detail. Hence, most statements about these interactions and regulations are based on the assumption that *T. congolense* should behave the same way as *T. brucei*. A second scientific issue that plagues the *T. congolense* research literature is the fact that it is often used as a "chronic" model in comparison to "acute" *T. brucei* infections. This artifact originates from the fact that a specific chronic *T. congolense* clone, i.e., Tc13, has been used in major immunological investigations for almost three decades (46). In contrast, the vast majority of experimental host-parasite research in *T. brucei brucei* and *T. brucei rhodesiense* models has been done with much more virulent *T. b.* AnTat 1 or LouTat 1 clones (47–49). While these studies by themselves all resulted in valid experimental data, it should be said that there are virulent *T. congolense* strains, resulting in infections in mice which display very similar survival times as the *T. brucei* clones mentioned above (50). Unfortunately, these more virulent *T. congolense* isolates have not been systematically used in comparative studies with *T. brucei*. Hence, reports that compare highly virulent *T. brucei* infections with low virulent *T. congolense* infections, and subsequently provide conclusion in which infection outcome is linked to the species-specific background of the parasite, should be taken with utmost caution. Of note is that the high genetic heterogeneity of *T. congolense* has led to the division of this parasite in three different subgroups i.e., Savannah, Kilifi, and Forest within the same species (51).

GENERAL LIFE CYCLE OF SALIVARIAN TRYPANOSOMES AND INTERACTION WITH BOTH INSECT AND MAMMALIAN HOSTS

The life cycle of cyclically transmitted salivarian trypanosomes inside their vector shows the plasticity of those parasites to adapt to new environments (**Figure 2**). Today, most of the knowledge on parasite transmission comes from the *T. brucei* model in which infection of tsetse flies occurs when the non-dividing short stumpy bloodstream form parasites are taken up during a fly's blood meal, reaching the fly's midgut and transforming into procyclic trypomastigotes (52). Once the parasite infection is established in the fly's midgut, the parasites migrate anteriorly to the proventriculus of the fly. Here, elongated trypomastigotes start to divide asymmetrically into both long and short epimastigotes of which the latter migrate toward the salivary glands and attach to the epithelial cells of the gland. Next, a final division occurs giving rise to the host-infective metacyclic forms. Once in the host's bloodstream, metacyclic parasites transform into long slender shaped bloodstream form parasites, which further divide by binary fission and represent the active dividing parasite form during the mammalian infection stage. It is at this stage that trypanosomes express the Variant Surface Glycoprotein (VSG) (55). This coat protein is encoded by a battery of over 1,000 different genes, mosaics and pseudogenes (56) and serves as an antibody decoy defense system (57). Indeed, VSGs are highly immunogenic and induce VSG-specific antibody responses. Hence, by regularly altering VSG variant expression, the parasite avoids efficient immune recognition and destruction (58). Genetic regulation of antigenic variation has been studied in detail and has been shown to involve various mechanisms of DNA recombination and transcription regulation of VSG genes (59, 60). With respect to mechanisms of genetic variation in trypanosomes, there is now ample evidence supporting the fact that *T. brucei* parasite mating or sexual reproduction does take place in the tsetse (5, 6). Hence, while the tsetse is conventionally referred as the insect vector for trypanosomosis, it should actually be considered as the definite host for the parasite. To put it in other words: mammals are merely the vessel that is used to ensure that trypanosomes are able to migrate from one tsetse to the next, and in addition provide long-term reservoirs that allow trypanosomes to survive seasonal periods in which fly populations are diminished. Sexual reproduction inside the insect vector offers the parasite in theory the chance of generating new hybrids, combining different parental characteristics. Important to note however is the fact that the effectiveness of trypanosome infection in the fly rapidly decreases with the age of the fly, hence also affecting the chance to generate hybrid descendants. Using both green and red fluorescent trypanosomes to study hybrid formation, it was shown that midgut and salivary gland infection rates were highest when flies were exposed to parasites in their first feed (53). Waiting $2^{1/2}$ weeks for a first parasite exposure reduced the infection success by half. Interestingly, exposing tsetse flies to two different trypanosome lines in a consecutive feeding experiment resulted most often in the establishment of the first infection only, as if the primary infection was able to push the vector to mount a protective immune response preventing secondary infection. Under natural circumstances, this would greatly reduce the chance of hybrids being formed, although the experimental conditions used above showed that in all combinations tested, hybrid formation did take place (53). As will be outlined later in this review, even the rarest hybrid formation events can have a significant impact on the transition from AAT to HAT, as it allows generation of a continuous pool of new human infective *T. rhodesiense* parasite strains (54). With respect to the vector immunity mentioned above, several studies published in the recent past have made contributions to the understanding of the mechanism underlying tsetse anti-trypanosome immunity. It is interesting to note that tsetse immunity development *per se* requires the presence of the obligate symbiont *Wigglesworthia* in the larval stage of the fly, transmitted through maternal milk gland secretion (61, 62). This finding complements the notion that the development of a fully functional innate immune system of the mature adult tsetse fly depends on the establishment of a bacterial microbiome population, and that the immaturity of the immune system is responsible for the high susceptibility to trypanosome infections during a first blood feeding (63). The fly immunity itself relies on multiple mechanisms. Indeed, the action of scavenger receptor peptidoglycan-recognition protein LB (PGRP-LP) is crucial for the colonization of the fly by its *Wigglesworthia* symbiont, and in addition has a direct trypanocidal activity on both procyclic and bloodstream form trypanosomes (64, 65). In addition, anti-trypanosome immunity relies on activation of the immune deficiency regulated pathway and antimicrobial peptides (66, 67), as well as reactive oxygen species (ROS) mediated defenses (68), which provides combined protective immunity at the level of the midgut and hemocoel. Interesting here is that for some time the peritrophic matrix, which is a chitinous protective layer lining the insect gut, has been considered as a physical barrier that could provide protection against invading infections. However, RNA interference-based reversed genetic approaches have shown that the matrix is a true immunological regulator. Its integrity is necessary to build a proper immune context in the defense against different microbes, including trypanosomes, through its role in the expression of the antimicrobial peptide attacin as well as dual oxidase and iNOS, both involved in the production of reactive oxygen intermediates (ROIs) (65). Finally, the tsetse fly's specific TsetseEP protein was shown to provide anti-trypanosome protection at the level of the midgut (69). Interestingly, starvation of flies reduces immune responsiveness and increases susceptibility toward trypanosome infections both in young and older flies (70–72).

Naturally, from a human and economic point of view, it is the mammalian infection stage that has attracted most attention in the past. It is only more recently that the parasite-vector interaction and biology has received more detailed attention and that also non-*T. brucei* infections have been studied in tsetse (73, 74). These reports show that in fact both *T. congolense* and *T. vivax* are much more effective in establishing tsetse infections than *T. brucei*. In particular, for *T. congolense* it has been shown that this parasite is particularly effective in reaching the proboscis of the fly, where the trypomastigote-epimastigote transformation takes place. In this case, migration from the foregut to the mouthparts appeared to occur with high efficiency. In contrast, *T. brucei* is much less efficient in colonizing the tsetse, as most parasites do not survive the migration from the foregut to the salivary glands. Investigating both *T. brucei* and *T. congolense* infections in parallel have suggested that *T. brucei* adopted to final survival in the salivary gland, as this niche would not be preoccupied by the much more efficiently growing *T. congolense* parasites. Hence, despite the fact that both parasites use the same transmission vector, and that also for *T. congolense* meiotic reproduction has been reported in the teste vector (75), there are remarkable differences in the way the two trypanosomes infect and occupy the body of the insect host. In recent years, specific attention has also been given to the immunological events that take place at the bite site of the tsetse, in order to explain how successful mammalian infections are initiated. Here, it has become clear that there is a crucial role for tsetse saliva components in preventing local blood clothing, vasodilation, and neutrophil influx, all leading to the successful establishment of a primary infection and allowing metacyclic saliva parasites to be transformed successfully into long slender bloodstream form parasites (76, 77).

Besides the biological vector transmission described above, mechanical transmission is a second way of ensuring parasites can move from one mammalian host to the next. This mode has been described for *T. congolense*, *T. evansi*, and *T. vivax*, but only the latter two have successfully used this way of transmission to migrate out of Africa, into other continents. The main vectors that have been reported today for both trypanosome species are the horsefly, stable fly, horn fly, and deerfly. In all cases, mechanical transmission occurs when a fly with blood-contaminated mouthparts, containing living bloodstream form parasites, rapidly changes feeding hosts allowing the parasites to be transmitted without any intermediate insect-specific forms. To date, virtually no information is available on possible immune interactions that could make this way of parasite transmission

more or less successful. Interestingly, also nothing is known about the immune events that aid in parasite transfer back to the fly. Indeed, it is remarkable that livestock parasitaemia levels are often extremely low, presenting blood parasite load levels that are hardly detectable by microscopy. Yet, even when circulating parasite numbers are extremely low, flies still manages to successfully pick up parasites while taking very small blood meal volumes. Whether this is due to the fact that parasitaemia in the skin microvasculature is uniquely high as compared to the general blood circulation, or whether fly saliva has unique and potent trypanosome chemoattractant, remains to be elucidated.

HUMAN TRYPANOSOMOSIS IN AFRICA IS ONLY PART OF THE PROBLEM

In 2009, the number of reported HAT cases dropped below 10.000 for the first time in 50 years, and the most recent figures available for 2015 indicate that the global incidence of HAT has dropped below 3.000. It is now estimated that by 2020 HAT will no longer be considered as a major human health problem in Africa and hence will also no longer be listed as a neglected disease (78). With HAT being caused by either *Trypanosoma brucei gambiense* (>97%) or *Trypanosoma brucei rhodesiense* (<3%) (79), these numbers and assumptions are mainly based on the current West/Central African situation. Considering however that *T. b. rhodesiense* is a zoonotic parasite with a cattle and wildlife reservoir, re-emergence of HAT is going to remain a crucial concern in Africa. Indeed, whether or not the reservoir of *T. b rhodesiense* has been brought under control is hard to verify due to the insufficient systemic reporting on *T. b. rhodesiense* game and cattle infections. In addition, beyond the borders of the African continent the existence of non-*T. brucei* human trypanosomosis could become a future problem as *T. evansi* infections spread around the globe. Despite the reports of *T. evansi* infections in humans (80–83), this parasite is still not widely considered as a human pathogen. The lack of interest in these infections, combined with the continued spread of these trypanosomes mainly in South America, the Indian subcontinent, and Asia, risks of exposing humans to a new type of "unconventional" disease that will require a whole new approach to trypanosomosis world-wide. In addition, the lack of experimental studies on *T. evansi* infections as compared to *T. brucei* infections makes it harder to link the discussion about the genetic classification of *T. evansi* as a *T. brucei* subspecies to data dealing with the cellular and molecular mechanisms that govern host-pathogen interactions, pathology development, and zoonotic behavior.

Taken the importance of the zoonotic aspect of most remaining human trypanosome infections, it is clear that (African) Animal Trypanosomosis (AAT) *per se* deserves particular attention. In fact, there is a wealth of information available with respect to geographic distribution of AAT, immune pathologies including anemia and vaccine efforts as well as failures. These reports outnumber the scientific data published on host-pathogen aspect of human trypanosomosis. However, this contrasts very much the situation with respect to the actual

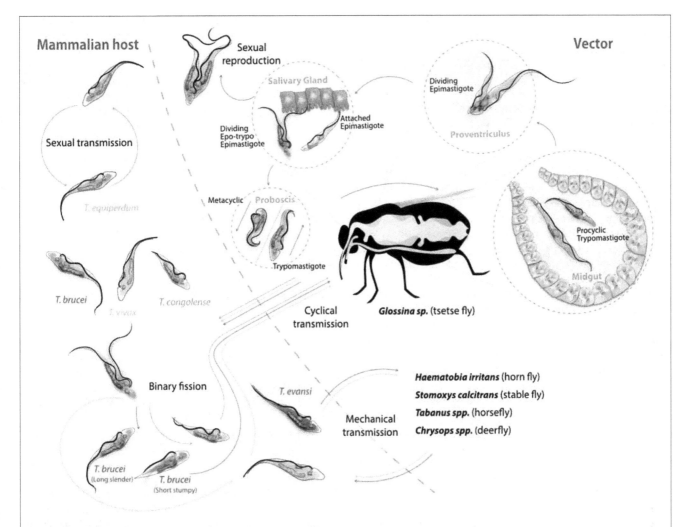

FIGURE 2 | Cyclic transmission of salivarian trypanosomes mediated by tsetse and other biting flies. Most lifecycle data of African Trypanosomes is based on the *T. brucei* cycle involving the tsetse (52). Here, short stumpy form parasite are taken up by the fly, progress through the body of the insect vector passing via the midgut, proventiculus and salivary gland, to be re-injected though the proboscis as infective metacyclic trypomastigotes into a new target. In the bloodstream, differentiation to long slender forms occurs followed by binary fission proliferation. Differentiation back to short stumpy forms will complete the cycle. While *T. congolense* and *T. vivax* can follow a similar cyclic transmission mode, the latter also is known to be spread through mechanical transmission (53, 54), as is the case for *T. evansi* (1). *T. equiperdum* spreads through sexual transmission only (37). Sexual reproduction of trypanosomes itself has been reported to take part in the teste, and has been reported for both *T. brucei* and *T. congolense* (5).

understanding of trypanosome diseases. Indeed, while many have focused on experimental models to understand human trypanosomosis in the past, much less effort has been made to understand the fundamentals of animal trypanosomosis. A fine example to illustrate this is the issue of antigenic variation. For more than four decades, scientists have been studying antigenic variation of the VSG coat used by trypanosomes to deliver a protective response against the host antibody defense system. All work that included genetic approaches as well as molecular biology approaches combined with computer modeling, has been done for *T. brucei*, largely ignoring the fact that the main cattle parasites i.e., *T. congolense* and *T. vivax* are very different trypanosomes that might use other systems of regulation and defense. For example, comparative studies of the VSG repertoire conducted in *T. congolense* and *T. vivax* indicated

that the scale of the VSG recombination differs between two species, being more frequent in *T. congolense* than in *T. vivax*. Moreover, *T. vivax* populations were shown to be consistent with clonal reproduction (84), while the *T. congolense* ability to undergo sexual reproduction generates opportunities for allelic recombination among VSG genes (85). Hence, to date we are left with molecular tools that are very suitable to study a wide range of host-parasite interactions in mice which could model human infections, but at the same time we have very little experimental models and tools to study AT. One striking example is *T. equiperdum, which* is hardly studied in comparison to other infections due to the fact that it causes a disease characterized by sexual transmission in horses, a feature so far not reported in mice. In fact, only a single report is available on experimental sexual transmission of trypanosomosis in mice, and this report is dealing with *T. b. gambiense* (86). However, whether sexual transmission of *T. brucei gambiense* is a real issue in human trypanosomosis, remains a matter of debate (87) and more species-specific research is needed to resolve these issues.

ADAPTATIONS OF ANIMAL INFECTIVE TRYPANOSOMES TO HUMAN HOST

Humans are considered naturally resistant to pathogenic animal trypanosomes such as *T. b. brucei, T. evansi, T. equiperdum, T. congolense,* and *T. vivax.* The mechanism of human resistance to those trypanosomes is based on the presence of cytolytic factors in the high density lipoprotein (HDL) fraction of normal human serum (NHS) (88) and is attributed to two fractions called trypanosome lytic factor 1 and 2 (TLF1 and TLF2), with the latter being the major active compound (89). The human infective *T. brucei* subspecies *T. b. gambiense* and *T. b. rhodesiense* are known to be resistant to TLF lysis through various mechanisms. A number of reports demonstrating *T. evansi* infections in humans has triggered a new wave of interest in molecular mechanisms underlying human infectivity in the context of the transition from an animal infective trypanosome to a zoonotic pathogen causing disease in humans. While TLF1 and TLF2 have slightly different compositions, they both contain the haptoglobin related protein (HPR) and Apolipoprotein L1 (ApoL1), of which the latter is considered the main active lytic compound. Furthermore, TLF2 is complexed with IgM molecules and has a much higher molecular mass than TLF1, but is lipid poor (90). With respect to the mechanisms of lysis and resistance to NHS, initial data was obtained in an experimental model for *T. b. rhodesiense.* Here, it was shown that resistant and susceptible sub-clones can be derived from a common ancestor by passaging trypanosomes in either the presence or absence of human serum. This work gave rise to the discovery of the *SRA* gene, encoding a truncated VSG and located within the VSG expression site (91). Transfer of the gene to *T. b. brucei* showed that the presence of this single gene indeed was enough to confer resistance to NHS (92). Subsequently, the identity of SRA allowed to characterize ApoL1 as the active serum compound (93) that acts through both lysosomal and mitochondrial membrane permeabilization (94). The inhibitory mechanism of SRA was shown to rely on its capacity to block the membrane pore-forming capacity of ApoL1 upon entering the acid compartments of the lysosomal system (95–98). Finally, the haptoglobin-hemoglobin receptor (HpHbR), localized in the flagellar pocket, was identified as the trypanosome receptor involved in TLF1 uptake (99), while the mechanism for TLF2 uptake has still not been elucidated (100). Indeed, HpHbR knock down *T. b. brucei* parasites remain sensitive to both NHS and TLF2 lysis (101). However, as both TLFs contain the same active ApoL1 compound, the SRA is capable of blocking all NHS activity. Interestingly, the *SRA* gene is only present in *T. b. rhodesiense* and hence has been used in a string of different diagnostic approaches for HAT, including PCR and LAMP, targeting not just human samples but also livestock and game reservoirs as well as the tsetse vector, in various regions in Eastern Africa. Of note is a report in which

a Ugandan HAT survey indicated that 20% of parasitologicaly confirmed *T. b. rhodesiense* cases resulted from infections that could not be detected by any of the *SRA* PCR methods described so far. Whether this indicates that *SRA*-negative human infective *T. b. rhodesiense* parasites exist, implying these parasites have alternative NHS resistance mechanisms, or whether the negative results were due to *SRA* gene polymorphism that prevented PCR primer annealing, remains a matter of debate (102). The existence of such *SRA* gene polymorphisms has been studied in the context of human disease severity (54). Most recently, using *SRA* as a genetic tracer, it has been shown that genetic recombination between *T. b rhodesiense* and the much larger pool of *T. b. brucei* animal trypanosomes allows for the continuous generation of new *SRA*-positive human infective parasites (103, 104). This once again indicates that in order to really bring HAT under control, AAT and particularly the animal *T. b. rhodesiense* reservoir has to be eliminated as well.

Interestingly, more than 97% of all human trypanosomosis infections are caused by *SRA*-negative *T. b. gambiense* (79), a parasite that is subdivided in Group 1 and Group 2 *T. b. gambiense* (105). While Group 1 parasites have an invariant phenotype toward NHS resistance, Group 2 parasites show a variable degree of resistance, modulated by the actual exposure to NHS. Neither Group 1, nor Group 2 parasites have the *SRA* gene (8), indicating that there are multiple ways to mount resistance to NHS. Literature of the last 5 years has mainly focused on the Group 1 *T. b. gambiense* resistance, showing that these parasites have acquired a combination of defense systems which allows them to resist the lytic action of NHS. This includes a specific point mutation in the HpHbR in combination with reduced receptor expression, reducing TLF1 uptake (106, 107). However, as this receptor is not a main player in TLF2 uptake, *T. b. gambiense* needs additional mechanisms to survive in human blood. These involve the alteration of lipid membrane fluidity by the *T. b. gambiense*-specific glycoprotein (TgsGP) (108, 109), as well as increased cysteine protease activity in the digestive vacuoles of the parasite. The latter is believed to directly affect ApoL1 activity (110). Today, it remains unclear how *T. b. gambiense* Group 2 parasites deal with the toxicity of NHS.

T. evansi parasites express neither SRA, nor TgsGP, but now have been reported in several instances as human pathogens causing a-HT (11, 18, 80, 82, 111). Similarly to *T. b. rhodesiense* and *T. b. gambiense* Group 2 parasites, a remarkable phenotypic plasticity of *T. evansi* has been described upon exposure to NHS, with resistance occurring after prolonged NHS exposure and being absent when NHS selective pressure is removed. Screenings of various *T. evansi* isolates indicated that some even display natural resistance to NHS, while others were found to be fully sensitive (112). In line with these observations in *T. evansi*, even *T. b. brucei* NHS resistance has now been reported. In the latter, a switch to a resistant phenotype was recorded to occur upon repetitive exposure to NHS or TLF1 in the absence of the *SRA* gene (113). However, a fragment homolog to *SRA*, named SRA basic copy (SRAbc), was found in the *T. brucei brucei* TREU927/4 strain, which exhibits low resistance to NHS (114). Similarly, one of the human infective *T. evansi* isolates was shown to contain the *SRAbc* homolog (115). Interestingly, the *T. b. brucei* parasites exhibiting increased NHS resistance had a significant reduction in TLF1 uptake, which coincided with downregulation of *T. b. brucei HpHbR* mRNA levels (100). Hence, it seems that the resistance mechanism in these parasites shows a mixed but attenuated phenotype of those found in either *T. b. gambiense* or *T. b. rhodesiense*, as if the latter could have been selected as "optimized" derivatives of *T. b. brucei* semi-resistant predecessors.

With respect to human *T. evansi,* it is important to highlight that at least one human infective case has been attributed to the lack of functional ApoL1 (81). Indeed, a frameshift mutation, found in both *ApoL1* alleles of the patient, resulted in the ability of trypanosomes to establish infection and to survive in the human bloodstream. This strongly suggests that human trypanosome resistance in large relies on a non-classical immune mechanism, i.e., lipid membrane disruption by TLF. However, a Vietnamese a-HT *T. evansi* victim was shown to have fully functional *ApoL1* alleles and a normal concentration of serum ApoL1 (116). Hence, this shows that there is an additional role for the immune system in the overall defense against trypanosomes, most likely involving a combination of the action of antibodies, cytokines, and complement factors. In at least two confirmed human *T. evansi* infections, the infected individuals were shown to have a compromised immune system. One case relates to a pregnant woman from Mumbai, India suffering from HIV/AIDS, anemia, and upper respiratory tract infection (117). The second case relates to the above mentioned Vietnamese woman who had just given birth (116), with pregnancy itself being known as a unique immune condition that is modulated by fetus development resulting in immune alterations that in some cases in facilitation of parasite growth. Important is that also in experimental *T. evansi* infections in mice, in particular IgM antibodies are crucial for parasitaemia control (118). This indicates that when "natural resistance" such as the resistance conferred by ApoL1 fails, the antibody-mediated immune response does provide a second defense barrier against the progressing of infection.

Finally, it should also be mentioned that several reports in the past have indicated the existence of a-HT caused by the stercorarian *T. lewisi* parasite (119). Here, resistance to NHS lysis was correlated with resistance to human ApoL1 as well. Hence, it seems that while multiple mechanisms have been acquired by various trypanosomes to block the lysosomal pore-forming catalytic activity of NHS, this activity itself is executed in large by a single factor, i.e., ApoL1. This finding itself has attracted scientific attention over the last years with respect to primate evolution (120), and has resulted in the findings that (i) ApoL1 is the common lytic factor in human, gorilla, and baboon primate sera (7, 8, 121), (ii) the chimpanzee, orangutan, and macaque, which are susceptible to all *T. brucei* subspecies, lack functional ApoL1 (121), and (iii) the baboon ApoL1 variant is capable of killing even *T. b. gambiense* and *T. b. rhodesiense*, as opposed to the human ApoL1 (122, 123). The latter finding has prompted an attempt to generate genetically modified TLF transgenic livestock that

would be able to resist all known pathogenic trypanosome species (122).

THE ROLE OF B CELLS AND ANTIBODIES IN SALIVARIAN TRYPANOSOMOSIS

As outlined above, VSG switching and antigenic variation, including the generation of VSG mosaic genes, have generally be considered as the major defense systems that parasites have developed against the host's adaptive immune system (56, 124, 125). However, in recent years it has become clear that trypanosomes have developed several precautionary adaptations that provide a rescue in case they do get recognized by antibodies. The reason for this is obvious: even if different VSG variants exhibit different hypervariable loops, and even if mosaic VSG present new epitopes to the immune system, there is no reason to assume that the overall pool of infection-induced antibodies is not at all capable of detecting new parasite variants. In fact, the existence of the cross-reactive nature of anti-VSG antibodies has been used since the beginning of trypanosome immunology research. Here, the VSG of the first arising variant or living cloned parasites, expressing a single VSG, have been used to monitor fluctuating anti-VSG titers throughout infection for weeks or months (57, 126). More interestingly maybe is the fact that reinfection models have shown that weeks into a primary infection, mice can be killed by a secondary infection with virulent trypanosomes expressing exactly the same VSG as the primary infection (127). In order to understand these results, three major host-parasite interactions mechanisms have to be considered. First, trypanosomes have developed a very efficient way of driving endocytosis. This system allows to continuously clear surface bound antibodies from the VSG coat, preventing antibody-mediated lysis (128). Secondly, while antibody/complement-mediated lysis has long been proposed to result in antibody-mediated trypanosome killing, it is important to note that AKR mice, which are natural C5 complement knockout mice, are able to clear peaks of parasitaemia in a similar way as other mice. This shows that the lack of complement-mediated lysis does not prevent the immune system of controlling peak stage parasite levels (129). Third, there is now ample evidence that trypanosomes cause a B cell depletion pathology, which is initiated by the very rapid disappearance of immature B cells in the bone marrow, as well as transitional and IgM$^+$ marginal zone B cells from the spleen, followed by a gradual depletion of Follicular B cells (FoB) (127, 130). This has now been reported for *T. b. gambiense* and *T. congolense* infections (50, 131). Mechanisms involved in the depletion process have been linked to IFNγ-mediated inflammation (132), NK-mediated B cell destruction (133), and direct cell-cell contact-mediated B cell apoptosis (111, 127). Once FoB cell depletion is accomplished by the parasite, it becomes impossible for the host to generate new efficient antibody responses against newly arising VSG variants (**Figure 3**). In addition, it hampers anti-VSG memory recall responses against previously encountered variants, hence making the host susceptible to secondary infections with old variants. This might also explain the accumulation of mosaic VSG variants during later stages of infection (56). Indeed, the question whether later variants are immunologically distinct (or not) from their ancestral variants, which has so far not been answered, might not be important at all. Possibly, these variants arise simply from the continuous gene rearrangements that are ongoing at the telomeric ends of the VSG expression sites and are tolerated, due to the lack of antibody-mediated elimination by the host, rather than being produced in order to evade the already existing antibodies.

B cell dysfunction, associated to trypanosomosis, also has a secondary detrimental effect on the mammalian host, i.e., the elimination of vaccine-induced memory recall responses. Indeed, in an experimental model for DTPa vaccination, it was shown that *T. b. brucei* is capable of destroying immunological memory rendering vaccinated mice susceptible to infections with *Bordetella pertussis* (130). This was not a result of an infection-associated immunosuppression, as it persisted after anti-trypanosome drug treatment and the elimination of active trypanosome infections. This detrimental effect of trypanosomes on non-related vaccine efficacy has also been reported in other models and natural infections. Although not thoroughly studied in human infections, one study has shown that antibody titers induced by the anti-measles vaccine are significantly downregulated in HAT patients, and that curative HAT treatment did not result in a restauration of antibody titers (**Figure 4**). For obvious ethical reasons, this study stopped short of assessing whether or not the remaining titers would still confer protection. In addition, the study did not address the question whether vaccine-induced memory recall responses were affected (138). With respect to AT, more data is available in particular with respect to *T. evansi* and *T. congolense* infections. Indeed, such infections in pigs were shown to abrogate protective immune responses generated against the classical swine fever vaccine (139). They were characterized by significantly reduced antibody responses, leukopenia, and high fever. Similarly, *T. evansi* infections in water buffalos, vaccinated against *Pasteurella multocida* (hemorrhagic septicemia), showed impaired capacity to mount a humoral and cell-mediated immune response upon challenge (140). When cattle, harboring *T. congolense* and *T. vivax*, were given a *Brucella abortus* vaccine or were vaccinated against contagious bovine pleuropneumonia, specific antibody responses to the vaccine were shown to be severely depressed (135, 141–143). Similarly, *T. congolense* infected goats vaccinated with *Bacillus anthracis* showed a profoundly diminished anti-anthrax antibody responses (144), while *T. congolense* infected cattle were shown to suffer from immunosuppression and failed recall responses in a foot-and-mouth vaccination setting (145). Taken together, these studies, conducted in natural hosts for animal trypanosomes such as cattle, water buffalos, goats, and pigs, confirmed studies in mice showing that trypanosome infection induces severe impairment of B cell responses and antibody production to a number of non-trypanosome related commercial veterinary vaccines.

THE ROLE OF T CELLS AND T CELL-DERIVED CYTOKINES IN SALIVARIAN TRYPANOSOMOSIS

Taken the extracellular nature of salivarian trypanosome infections, initial thoughts on the control of infection were naturally focused on the role of antibodies and B cells. However, already early in the 1980's it became obvious that while the virulence of experimental trypanosomosis was not linked to the expression of a specific VSG variant, or the use of a specific MHC-II type, CD4$^+$ T cells played an absolutely crucial role in infection control (146). Twenty-five years after this initial discovery, it was shown that major T cell responses against cryptic T cell epitopes play a major role in trypanosomosis control (147, 148). This observation caused a major paradigm shift in the way trypanosomosis control is thought to occur, as it shows that T cell help is not just needed to support effective B cell functioning and antibody production, but that it plays a crucial second B cell-independent role during the progression of infection. This role of T cell biology might initially have been underestimated, as a multitude of studies had shown that trypanosomosis, both in mice and cattle, results in the occurrence of T cell immunosuppression (49, 149). However, these reports mostly referred to suppression of T cell proliferation and not to cytokine secretion. To date, the active disease controlling role of T cells is mainly attributed to the cytokine production in which polarization toward a Th1-type response is crucial for initial parasitaemia control (137). Detailed analysis of both *T. brucei* and *T. congolense* infections has indeed shown that early IFNγ production is crucial for the control of the onset of infection (**Figure 3**). This hypothesis was initially driven by the description of the cytokine production profile of CD4$^+$T cells, and was later corroborated by the use of neutralizing anti-IFNγ antibodies as well as the use of IFNγ knockout mice (150, 151). The latter were shown to have an impaired control of the first peak of parasitaemia, followed by their inability to clear increasing parasite numbers, leading to the early death of the mice using the C57Bl/6 model (152). In experimental *T. congolense* infections, it was demonstrated that while hyper-susceptible BALB/c mice preferentially mount an infection associated Th2-type response against the Tc13 *T. congolense* parasite, Th1-biased C57Bl/6 mice were able to survive for up to 6 months when infected with the same clone (136). Also here it was shown that altering immune balances, by treatment with neutralizing anti-cytokine (or cytokine receptor) monoclonal antibodies, drastically alters the outcome of infection (153). Most recently, it was reported for *T. brucei* that the CD4$^+$ IFNγ response is preceded by the production of this cytokine by NK and NKT cells, followed by a marked upregulation of IFNγ production by CD8$^+$ T cells (154). This was observed in both the spleen and the liver of infected mice. However, by 10 days post infection it was clear that these cell populations were either drastically reduced in numbers or became totally depleted, leaving the CD4$^+$ T cells to execute the major task of cytokine production. A comprehensive report on the overall role of IFNγ in various trypanosome infection models was recently published by Wu *et al.* (155). Interestingly,

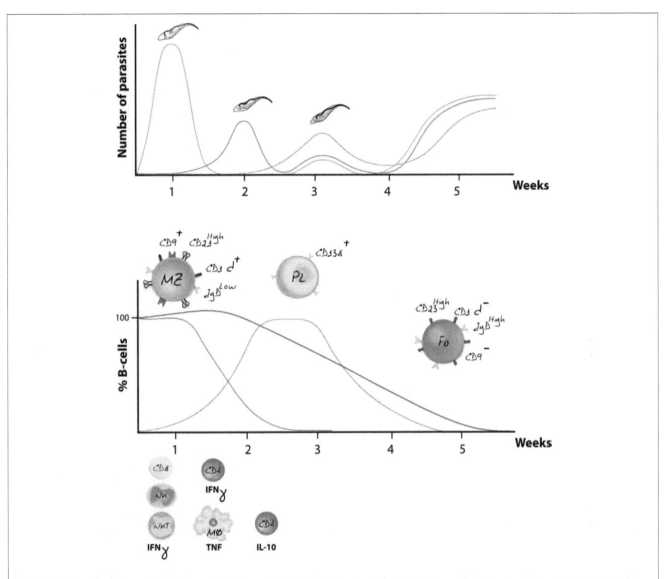

FIGURE 3 | Antigenic variation and host immune destruction are closely linked. Antigenic variation of the trypanosome VSG surface coat enables trypanosomes to escape specific antibody-mediated destruction, resulting in immunologicaly distinct parasites occurring at regular intervals (upper panel). To prevent total eradication, trypanosomes undermine the immune system by ablation of the B cell compartment. In mice, this results in abrogation of an efficient antibody mediated immune defense system, allowing different parasite variants to occur simultaneously (schematically represented as the week 3 situation). Despite to co-occurrence of several variants, later-stage parasitaemia peaks usually have a reduced magnitude in terms of actual parasite numbers as various non-B cell defense systems aid in parasiteamia control [upper panel, adapted from (134)]. The lower panel schematically represent the finding that onset of infection is followed by a rapid depletion of the MZ B cell compartment (purple), followed by a gradual destruction of the FoB cell compartment (red) (116, 119). While the initially host immune response generates effector Plasma B cells, later waves of newly arising parasite variants fail to be efficiently depleted due to the impaired capacity of the host to deliver a renewed Plasma B cell response (green). Overall immunopathology is initiated by excessive production of IFNγ during the first week of infection, involving mainly CD8$^+$ T cells, NK cells, and NKT cells. By 7 days post infection, IFNγ production is taken over by CD4$^+$ T cells, while activated macrophages now produce excessive amounts of TNF that contribute to pathology (135, 136). Later-on in infection, production of IL-10 has been documented to counteract the initial inflammation (137).

to date only one single trypanosome factor has been identified as being able to induce IFNγ production by T cells, CD8$^+$ T cells in particular. This molecule, named TLTF (trypanosome lymphocyte triggering factor) (10) has been characterized in *T. brucei* and *T. evansi* parasites (156), but a homolog has not been described for other trypanosomes. TLTF was shown to be capable of inducing IFNγ production by astrocytes, suggesting a direct role of the molecule in the pathology development of sleeping

sickness (157). This hypothesis has been further supported by the finding that IFNγ deficient mice show reduced CD4$^+$ and CD8$^+$ T cell influx into the brain parenchyma of *T. brucei* infected mice (158). Important is that when the role of T cells and IFNγ are considered within a trypanosomosis context, IL-10 was shown to be the main counter regulator of infection-associated inflammation in both *T. brucei* and *T. congolense* models. The source of the latter was proposed to be the regulatory

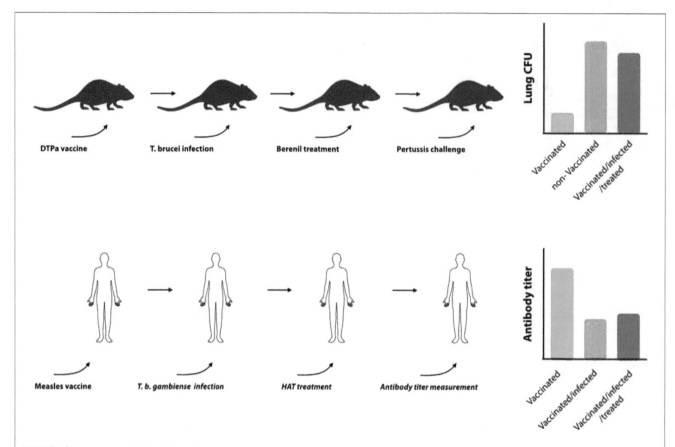

FIGURE 4 | Trypanosomosis-induced B cell destruction results in prolonged B cell dysfunction. Experimental infections in mice have shown that trypanosomes can destroy non-related DTPa induced vaccine responses (upper panel). Vaccinated mice that have been confronted with trypanosomes fail to clear diphtheria bacteria from their lungs, even when the bacterial challenge is performed after the trypanosome infection has been cleared by drug treatment [adapted from (119)]. Indeed is was shown that while the commercial vaccine Boostrix® provides significant protection against a *B. pertussis* challenge (green bar: vaccinated, blue bar: non-vaccinated), exposure to trypanosomes abrogated vaccine-induced protection (red bar). In humans (lower panel), trypanosome infections were shown to suppress vaccine induced anti-measles antibodies. Serum antibody titers in vaccinated *T. gambiense* HAT patients (blue bar) were shown to be significantly lower as compared to vaccinated control individuals (green bar), and specific antibody titers did not recover after curative anti-HAT treatment (red bar) (121).

T cells (9). However, a most recent effort to understand the full kinetics of IL-10 production during trypanosomosis, using the IL-10 reporter mouse system, has indicated that a whole range of cells is capable of producing IL-10 during infection and that most notably CD4$^+$ T cells, that do not have a defined regulatory phenotype, are the main producers of this cytokine (159).

As for the role of IFNγ in parasitaemia control, early reports characterized this cytokine as a trypanosome growth factor (160). In contrast, a number of follow-up reports have indicated that IFNγ is crucial for inhibition of trypanosome growth, as well as for trypanosomosis-associated NO production and TNF production that both limit trypanosome growth (152, 161, 162). Both these factors have subsequently been identified as direct players in the control of peak parasitaemia levels in *T. brucei* as well as *T. congolense* infections. Using TNF knockout mice, it was shown that parasitaemia control in relatively resistant C57Bl/6 mice depends on TNF production during the first peak of parasitaemia (163, 164). This confirmed initial reports in which neutralizing anti-TNF antibodies had a negative effect on *T. brucei* parasitaemia control (165). Subsequently, a comparative

infection model using BALB/c, C57Bl/6, C3H/HeN, and CBA/Ca mice showed that while TNF production *per se* was required for proper parasitaemia control, infected mice responded to TNF-associated inflammation with the shedding of TNF-R2 receptors. This, in turn resulted in limiting the TNF-mediated infection-associated immunopathology (166). Based on these results, and placing these observations in the wider context of trypanosome infections using various gene-deficient mouse models, it has been proposed that while soluble TNF could plays a pivotal role in parasitaemia control, it is the membrane-bound form of the cytokine that has a major impact on progressing inflammation and inducing pathology (167). When analyzing the possible direct effect of TNF on trypanosomes, results showed a differential outcome depending upon the model studied. First, it was reported for the *T. brucei brucei* AnTat 1.1 clone that TNF has a direct trypanolytic effect. The latter is mediated by a lectin binding domain of the TNF molecule that is located at the opposite site of the molecule as compared to the mammalian receptor binding site (168). Interestingly, the lectin specificity of TNF exhibits a high affinity for complex branched mannose sugars, such as those found on the trypanosome VSG molecule (169). Using a model for *T. brucei gambiense*, these findings were independently confirmed in an *in vitro* co-culture system (170). In contrast, experimental mouse studies with the human infective *T. brucei rhodesiense* LouTat 1 clone did not show a direct effect of TNF (171), suggesting that various trypanosome stocks can exhibit different levels of susceptibility to host cytokine-mediated growth regulation, as might be the case for IFNγ. Studies in trypanotolerant vs. trypanosusceptible cattle, using a *T. congolense* model, confirmed the possible role of TNF in parasitaemia control in natural infections (172), but here no link was made to a possible direct trypanolytic effect of the cytokine. Also, for the *T. congolense* infection mouse model, the direct action of TNF has not been reported but here TNF-R1 signaling has been associated to the combined release of soluble TNF and NO by activated macrophages. Those two combined were shown to play a crucial role in parasitaemia control, in conjunction with infection-induced anti-trypanosome antibodies (118). Interesting to note here is that in contrast to the limited knowledge on the molecular mechanisms of trypanosomosis-driven T cell IFNγ production, detailed research into the mechanisms of macrophage-derived TNF induction have been able to provide a more in-depth understanding of the host-parasite interplay. Indeed, first the VSG-GPI anchor was identified as the major trypanosome molecule responsible for TNF induction, with the trypanosome-specific galactose side-branch of the anchor playing a major role in macrophage activation (173, 174). Subsequently, it was shown that IFNγ could prime macrophages to become responsive to GPI-VSG and trypanosome stimulation (175). These results are in line with *in vivo* data showing that a rise in serum IFNγ values precedes the induction of infection-associated TNF (154). However, when macrophages are primed with VSG, prior to IFNγ, the cells are de-sensitize with respect to cytokine secretion (175). This may represent a way to prevent hyper-inflammation during the phase that corresponds to peak parasitaemia clearance, in which massive amounts of VSG are being released into the hosts' circulation. This information has been used to try and design an anti-disease vaccination approach for trypanosomosis (176). Although it was shown that repeated exposure to VSG-GPI prior to infection could indeed reduce the infection-associated pathology related to excessive macrophage activation, the results indicated that the vaccine approach did not result in the buildup of immunological memory involving antibodies or B cells. Instead, the reduction of inflammation, following the repeated GPI exposure related to an alteration of macrophage phenotypes, shifted the balance from infection-induced inflammatory type 1 cells to more anti-inflammatory type 2 cells or macrophages. This response was short-lived. Moreover, as the beneficial effect of the VSG-GPI treatment was observed to the same extent in both B cell deficient mice and in wild-type littermates, it became clear the approach could no longer be considered as a possible vaccine approach (177). In addition to the VSG-GPI, trypanosome DNA that contains high levels of unmethylated CpG sequences has been reported to be responsible for driving NF-κB an MAPK signaling pathways, resulting in the transcription of pro-inflammatory cytokine genes including *tnf*, in case of *T.*

brucei infection(178). As for infection with *T. evansi*, the information on the role of IFNγ is limited, but data has shown that in addition to anti-trypanosome antibodies, this cytokine is required for parasitaemia control (179). Most recently, a comparative cytokine analysis using different *T. evansi* infections confirmed the induction of IFNγ in all infections (180). For *T. vivax* infections, there is a general lack of published information on the role of T cells and their cytokines in the control of onset in infection, but it appears reasonable to assume that a similar cytokine environment is needed to obtain the best parasitaemia control possible. As for human (*T. b. rhodesiense*) and cattle (*T. congolense*) infection, the role of IFNγ in inducing inflammatory pathology has been confirmed in both (181, 182), and as already outlined above, IFNγ has been shown to play a major role in the actual cerebral complications that characterize human sleeping sickness (183).

ANEMIA IS A MAJOR PATHOLOGICAL FEATURE OF ANIMAL TRYPANOSOMOSIS

From the data reviewed above, it has become clear that the IFNγ/TNF driven immunopathology is a hallmark of trypanosomosis in both human and livestock. When focusing on the latter it has been amply documented that TNF-linked infection-associated anemia is the major pathological feature that marks both *T. congolense* and *T. vivax* trypanosomosis. In fact, the classification of so-called trypanotolerant and trypanosusceptible animals is based on the relative capacity to control anemia during infection which consequently is directly linked to whether or not animals remain productive while infected with trypanosomes (184). Mechanisms that underlie this tolerance are complex and to date still not clearly understood, but most likely include differences in erythropoeitic potential and hemodilution (185), factors involved in erythrolysis (186), eryhtrophagocytosis (187), the regulation of the erythropoietin homeostasis (188), the host's potential to raise neutralizing antibodies against secreted trypanosome virulence factors (189), and the general mechanism involved in inflammation control such as the regulation of the IFNγ/IL-10 balance as well as other cytokines (167). With respect to cytokine regulation during infection, it is worth mentioning that MIF (Macrophage migration Inhibitory Factor) was recently shown to be one of the key trypanosomosis-associated inflammation inducing cytokines involved in the promotion of so-called anemia of inflammation, in which classically activated macrophages also play a major role (190). Indeed, it was shown that MIF promotes the storage of iron in liver myeloid cells, subsequently depriving iron from the eythropoeitic system and preventing the maturation of RBCs. Important here is that the *T. congolense* C57Bl/6 mouse model has been proven useful over the years to unravel the molecular mechanisms that govern anemia pathology. Gene expression profiling studies in these mice have pinpointed infection-induced deregulation of erythropoiesis as well as the involvement of stress-induced acute phase responses linked to *T. congolense*-associated anemia (191). More recently, the C57Bl/6 model was also shown to be suitable for unraveling the pathology of *T.*

vivax infections (129, 192, 193). In addition, the use of various knockout mouse strains generated on the C56Bl/6 background, such as TNF$^{-/-}$ and Lymphytoxin$^{-/-}$ (194), TNFp75$^{-/-}$ (166), IFNγR$^{-/-}$ (152), IL-10$^{-/-}$ (195), and Gal3$^{-/-}$ (196) have all been used to study specific aspects of the inflammatory cascade that drive trypanosomosis-associated inflammation. One of the most recent finding here has shown that the reduced PCV, associated with experimental mouse trypanosomosis, is not just the result of reduced circulating RBC numbers, but also of increased plasma volume, leading to hemodilution. The reduction of platelet concentrations in *T. congolense*-infected mice has also been reported in *T. congolense*-infected cattle and sheep (197, 198) suggesting that hemodilution could be a major pathogenic characteristic of livestock trypanosomosis, as well.

To date, the characteristics of anemia are probably the most and best described features of AT. Whenever new surveillance efforts result in the discovery of new infection foci, anemia is usually the parameter that is used to describe disease severity. This is the case for *T. evansi, T. congolense,* and *T. vivax* independently of the geographic location of infection or host species. As described for *T. congolense, T. evansi*-induced anemia was linked to infection-associated deregulation of the iron metabolism as well (199), although the number of detailed mechanistic studies available for this infection are rare. Interestingly, trypanosomosis-associated anemia has even been observed in more rare infection cases of wildlife in the Australian little red flying fox infected with *T. minasense* and *T. rangeli* (200). Together, all these reports indicate that the general occurrence of trypanosomosis-associated anemia is most likely due to the multitude of inflammatory pathways, and linked to various aspects of impaired RBC development and clearance. Taken this into account, it is very intriguing that reports of severe infection-associated anemia are missing in the case of HAT. Indeed, most reports documenting HAT-associated anemia describe the induction of RBC lysis and acute anemia as the result of treatment rather than the infection itself. This is particularly the case for *T. b. gambiense* infections (201–204). For *T. b. rhodesiense* rare reports do exist on the occurrence of infection-associated anemia and hemolysis (205), and models have been developed using vervet monkeys to investigate this aspect of acute HAT pathology in details (206). However, at the same time other reports have shown the lack of any correlation between *T. b. rhodesiense* severity in humans and the presence or absence of anemia (207–209). Hence, it seems that the human immune system might have found unique ways of dealing with trypanosomosis both in terms of dealing with parasite killing through the TLF1/2 ApoL1 mechanisms, as well as the control of infection-associated anemia.

CONCLUSION

Over the past years, international joint efforts to control Human African Trypanosomosis have resulted in a drastic reduction

in the number of confirmed disease cases. In addition, it might be feasible that by 2020 the incidence of this neglected tropic disease will be reduced to levels where it is no longer considered as a public health threat. However, at the same time the incidence of animal trypanosomosis is on the rise, affecting animal productivity through the detrimental health effects caused by excessive host-parasite immune interactions. This has now become a world-wide issue that affects agricultural infrastructures in emerging economy countries, not just in Africa but also in Asia and South America. In addition, AT even threatens the livestock industry of developed countries when sudden outbreaks occur due to importation of the disease either through infected vectors or host animals. To date, not a single vaccine strategy is available to control AT. Detrimental infection-associated mechanisms undermine both T cell and B cell compartments, making it virtually impossible to develop methods that allow the generation of long-term sustainable immunological memory. It appears that in the evolutionary battle between the trypanosome and the host immune system, the parasite has not only been able to find ways to evade innate trypanosome killing mechanisms, but has also acquired tools to undermine the crucial immunological defense and memory systems of the host. Only recently, it has become obvious that one of the major strengths of the African Trypanosomes' defense system is the capacity of genetic exchanges between individual parasites, while residing in the insect vector. Through this mechanism, new human-infective parasites can be generated and this by combining resistant genes from existing *T. b. rhodesiense* parasites with the vast repertoire of the *T. b. brucei* animal parasite reservoir. In addition, it has become clear that mechanisms of genetic plasticity also have allowed *T. b. brucei* to transform into *T. equiperdum* and *T. evansi*, parasites that have now successfully conquered large areas of the developing world, as they no longer need the tsetse vector for transmission. In particular, the latter risks to become a future health problem, as human infective cases of *T. evansi* have already been reported in India, Vietnam, Egypt, and Algeria. Together, these results show that while classic *T. gambiense* trypanosomosis is becoming rare, AT and new atypical human trypanosomosis remain a serious risk for the human population. Future research into the host-parasite interactions and trypanosomosis- associated inflammation of these new atypical infections should allow to obtain a better understanding of problems, including vaccine failure, and hopefully lead us to a long-term solution that can deal with both human and livestock infections, as well as the ever surviving wildlife trypanosome reservoir.

AUTHOR CONTRIBUTIONS

All authors contributed to the writing of the paper. In addition all artwork was prepared by JP.

REFERENCES

1. Desquesnes M, Holzmuller P, Lai D, Dargantes A, Lun Z, Jittaplapong S. *Trypanosoma evansi* and surra: a review and perspectives on origin, history, distribution, taxonomy, morphology, hosts, and pathogenic effects. *Biomed Res Int.* (2013) 2013:194176. doi: 10.1155/2013/194176

2. Büscher P, Cecchi G, Jamonneau V, Priotto G. Human African trypanosomiasis. *Lancet* (2017) 390:2397–409. doi: 10.1016/S0140-6736(17)31510-6

3. Diall O, Cecchi G, Wanda G, Argilés-Herrero R, Vreysen MJB, Cattoli G, et al. Developing a progressive control pathway for African animal trypanosomosis. *Trends Parasitol.* (2017) 33:499–509. doi: 10.1016/j.pt.2017.02.005

4. Molinari J, Moreno SA. *Trypanosoma brucei* Plimmer & Bradford, 1899 is a synonym of T. evansi (Steel, 1885) according to current knowledge and by application of nomenclature rules. *Syst Parasitol.* (2018) 95:249–56. doi: 10.1007/s11230-018-9779-z

5. Gibson W. Liaisons dangereuses: sexual recombination among pathogenic trypanosomes. *Res Microbiol.* (2015) 166:459–66. doi: 10.1016/j.resmic.2015.05.005

6. Peacock L, Ferris V, Sharma R, Sunter J, Bailey M, Carrington M, et al. Identification of the meiotic life cycle stage of *Trypanosoma brucei* in the tsetse fly. *Proc Natl Acad Sci USA.* (2011) 108:3671–6. doi: 10.1073/pnas.1019423108

7. Lugli EB, Pouliot M, Portela MDPM, Loomis MR, Raper J. Characterization of primate trypanosome lytic factors. *Mol Biochem Parasitol.* (2004) 138:9–20. doi: 10.1016/j.molbiopara.2004.07.004

8. Capewell P, Cooper A, Clucas C, Weir W, MacLeod A. A co-evolutionary arms race: trypanosomes shaping the human genome, humans shaping the trypanosome genome. *Parasitology* (2015) 142:S108–19. doi: 10.1017/S0031182014000602

9. Guilliams M, Bosschaerts T, Hérin M, Hünig T, Loi P, Flamand V, et al. Experimental expansion of the regulatory T cell population increases resistance to African trypanosomiasis. *J Infect Dis.* (2008) 198:781–91. doi: 10.1086/590439

10. Bakhiet M, Mix E, Kristensson K, Wigzell H, Olsson T. T cell activation by a*Trypanosoma brucei* brucei-deriyed lymphocyte triggering factor is dependent on tyrosine protein kinases but not on protein kinase C and A. *Eur J Immunol.* (1993) 23:1535–1539. doi: 10.1002/eji.1830230721

11. Truc P, Büscher P, Cuny G, Gonzatti MI, Jannin J, Joshi P, et al. A typical human infections by animal trypanosomes. *PLoS Negl Trop Dis.* (2013) 7:e2256. doi: 10.1371/journal.pntd.0002256

12. Overath P, Haag J, Mameza MG, Lischke A. Freshwater fish trypanosomes: definition of two types, host control by antibodies and lack of antigenic variation. *Parasitology* (1999) 119(Pt 6):591–601. doi: 10.1017/S0031182099005089

13. Zídková L, Cepicka I, Szabová J, Svobodová M. Biodiversity of avian trypanosomes. *Infect Genet Evol.* (2012) 12:102–12. doi: 10.1016/j.meegid.2011.10.022

14. Haag J, O'hUigin C, Overath P. The molecular phylogeny of trypanosomes: evidence for an early divergence of the Salivaria. *Mol Biochem Parasitol.* (1998) 91:37–49. doi: 10.1016/S0166-6851(97)00185-0

15. Pandey A, Galvani A. Strategies for *Trypanosoma brucei gambiense* elimination. *Lancet Glob Health* (2017) 5:e10–1. doi: 10.1016/S2214-109X(16)30284-4

16. Holmes P. On the road to elimination of rhodesiense human African trypanosomiasis: first WHO meeting of stakeholders. *PLoS Negl Trop Dis.* (2015) 9:10–12. doi: 10.1371/journal.pntd.0003571

17. Informal Expert Group on Gambiense HAT Reservoirs, Büscher P, Bart J-M, Boelaert M, Bucheton B, Cecchi G, et al. Do cryptic reservoirs threaten gambiense-sleeping sickness elimination? *Trends Parasitol.* (2018) 34:197–207. doi: 10.1016/j.pt.2017.11.008

18. Desquesnes M, Dargantes A, Lai D-H, Lun Z-R, Holzmuller P, Jittapalong S. *Trypanosoma evansi* and Surra: a review and perspectives on transmission, epidemiology and control, impact, and zoonotic aspects. *Biomed Res Int.* (2013) 1–20. doi: 10.1155/2013/321237

19. Morrison LJ, Vezza L, Rowan T, Hope JC. Animal African trypanosomiasis: time to increase focus on clinically relevant parasite and host species. *Trends Parasitol.* (2016) 32:599–607. doi: 10.1016/j.pt.2016.04.012

20. Auty H, Torr SJ, Michoel T, Jayaraman S, Morrison LJ. Cattle trypanosomosis: the diversity of trypanosomes and implications for disease epidemiology and control. *Rev Sci Tech.* (2015) 34:587–98.

21. Giordani F, Morrison LJ, Rowan TG, DE Koning HP, Barrett MP. The animal trypanosomiases and their chemotherapy: a review. *Parasitology* (2016) 143:1862–89. doi: 10.1017/S0031182016001268

22. P. Finelle. African animal trypanosomiasis transmission of trypanosomes. *World Anim Rev.* (1973) 7:1–6.

23. Lun ZR, Lai DH, Li FJ, Lukeš J, Ayala FJ. *Trypanosoma brucei*: two steps to spread out from Africa. *Trends Parasitol.* (2010) 26:424–7. doi: 10.1016/j.pt.2010.05.007

24. Baldacchino F, Desquesnes M, Mihok S, Foil LD, Duvallet G, Jittapalpong S. Tabanids: neglected subjects of research, but important vectors of disease agents! *Infect Genet Evol.* (2014) 28:596–615. doi: 10.1016/j.meegid.2014.03.029

25. Banerjee D, Kumar V, Maity A, Ghosh B, Tyagi K, Singha D, et al. Identification through DNA barcoding of Tabanidae (Diptera) vectors of surra disease in India. *Acta Trop.* (2015) 150:52–8. doi: 10.1016/j.actatropica.2015.06.023

26. Taioe MO, Motloang MY, Namangala B, Chota A, Molefe NI, Musinguzi SP, et al. Characterization of tabanid flies (Diptera: Tabanidae) in South Africa and Zambia and detection of protozoan parasites they are harboring. *Parasitology* (2017) 144:1162–78. doi: 10.1017/S0031182017000440

27. Misra KK, Roy S, Choudhury A. Biology of *Trypanosoma* (Trypanozoon) evansi in experimental heterologous mammalian hosts. *J Parasit Dis.* (2016) 40:1047–61. doi: 10.1007/s12639-014-0633-1

28. Borst P, Fase-Fowler F, Gibson WC. Kinetoplast DNA of *Trypanosoma evansi*. *Mol Biochem Parasitol.* (1987) 23:31–8.

29. Paris Z, Hashimi H, Lun S, Alfonzo JD, Lukeš J. Futile import of tRNAs and proteins into the mitochondrion of *Trypanosoma brucei evansi*. *Mol Biochem Parasitol.* (2011) 176:116–20. doi: 10.1016/j.molbiopara.2010.12.010

30. Carnes J, Anupama A, Balmer O, Jackson A, Lewis M, Brown R, et al. Genome and phylogenetic analyzes of *Trypanosoma evansi* reveal extensive similarity to T. brucei and multiple independent origins for dyskinetoplasty. *PLoS Negl Trop Dis.* (2015) 9:e3404. doi: 10.1371/journal.pntd.0003404

31. Cuypers B, Van den Broeck F, Van Reet N, Meehan CJ, Cauchard J, Wilkes JM, et al. Genome-Wide SNP analysis reveals distinct origins of *Trypanosoma evansi* and *Trypanosoma equiperdum*. *Genome Biol Evol.* (2017) 9:1990–7. doi: 10.1093/gbe/evx102

32. Richardson JB, Lee K-Y, Mireji P, Enyaru J, Sistrom M, Aksoy S, et al. Genomic analyses of African Trypanozoon strains to assess evolutionary relationships and identify markers for strain identification. *PLoS Negl Trop Dis.* (2017) 11:e0005949. doi: 10.1371/journal.pntd.0005949

33. Gibson W. Molecular characterization of field isolates of human pathogenic trypanosomes. *Trop Med Int Health* (2001) 6:401–6. doi: 10.1046/j.1365-3156.2001.00711.x

34. Radwanska M, Chamekh M, Vanhamme L, Claes F, Magez S, Magnus E, et al. The serum resistance-associated gene as a diagnostic tool for the detection of *Trypanosoma brucei rhodesiense*. *Am J Trop Med Hyg.* (2002) 67:684–90. doi: 10.4269/ajtmh.2002.67.684

35. Welburn SC, Picozzi K, Fèvre EM, Coleman PG, Odiit M, Carrington M, et al. Identification of human-infective trypanosomes in animal reservoir of sleeping sickness in Uganda by means of serum-resistance-associated (SRA) gene. *Lancet* (2001) 358:2017–9. doi: 10.1016/S0140-6736(01)07096-9

36. Radwanska M, Claes F, Magez S, Magnus E, Perez-Morga D, Pays E, et al. Novel primer sequences for polymerase chain reaction-based detection of *Trypanosoma brucei gambiense*. *Am J Trop Med Hyg.* (2002) 67:289–95. doi: 10.4269/ajtmh.2002.67.289

37. Claes F, Büscher P, Touratier L, Goddeeris BM. *Trypanosoma equiperdum*: master of disguise or historical mistake? *Trends Parasitol.* (2005) 21:316–21. doi: 10.1016/j.pt.2005.05.010

38. Jones TW, Dávila AMR. *Trypanosoma vivax*–out of Africa. *Trends Parasitol.* (2001) 17:99–101. doi: 10.1016/S1471-4922(00)01777-3

39. Moloo SK, Sabwa CL, Kabata JM. Vector competence of Glossina pallidipes and G. morsitans centralis for *Trypanosoma vivax*, *T. congolense* and *T. b. brucei*. *Acta Trop.* (1992) 51:271–80. doi: 10.1016/0001-706X(92)90045-Y

40. Croft SL, Kuzoe FA, Ryan L, Molyneux DH. Trypanosome infection rates of *Glossina* spp. (Diptera: Glossinidae) in transitional forest-savanna near Bouaflé, Ivory Coast. *Tropenmed Parasitol.* (1984) 35:247–50.

41. Gibson W. The origins of the trypanosome genome strains *Trypanosoma brucei brucei* TREU 927, *T. b. gambiense* DAL 972, *T. vivax* Y486 and *T. congolense* IL3000. *Parasit Vectors* (2012) 5:71. doi: 10.1186/1756-3305-5-71

42. Truc P, Jamonneau V, N'Guessan P, N'Dri L, Diallo PB, Cuny G. *Trypanosoma brucei* ssp. and *T congolense*: mixed human infection in Côte d'Ivoire. *Trans R Soc Trop Med Hyg.* (1996) 92:537–8.

43. Van Xong H, De Baetselier P, Pays E, Magez S. Selective pressure can influence the resistance of *Trypanosoma congolense* to normal human serum. *Exp Parasitol.* (2002) 102:61–5. doi: 10.1016/S0014-4894(03)00032-8

44. Wiesenhütter E. Research into the relative importance of tabanidae (Diptera) in mechanical disease transmission I. the seasonal occurrence and relative abundance of tabanidae in a dar es salaam dairy farm. *J Nat Hist.* (1975) 9:377–84. doi: 10.1080/00222937500770271

45. Gerold P, Striepen B, Reitter B, Geyer H, Geyer R, Reinwald E, et al. Glycosyl-phosphatidylinositols of *Trypanosoma congolense*: two common precursors but a new protein-anchor. *J Mol Biol.* (1996) 261:181–94. doi: 10.1006/jmbi.1996.0451

46. Okwor I, Onyilagha C, Kuriakose S, Mou Z, Jia P, Uzonna JE. Regulatory T cells enhance susceptibility to experimental *Trypanosoma Congolense* infection independent of mouse genetic background. *PLoS Negl Trop Dis.* (2012) 6:e1761. doi: 10.1371/journal.pntd.0001761

47. Inverso JA, De Gee AL, Mansfield JM. Genetics of resistance to the African trypanosomes. VII. Trypanosome virulence is not linked to variable surface glycoprotein expression. *J Immunol.* (1988) 140:289–93.

48. Magez S, Stijlemans B, Radwanska M, Pays E, Ferguson MA, De Baetselier P. The glycosyl-inositol-phosphate and dimyristoylglycerol moieties of the glycosylphosphatidylinositol anchor of the trypanosome variant-specific surface glycoprotein are distinct macrophage-activating factors. *J Immunol.* (1998) 160:1949–56. doi: 10.4049/jimmunol.164.4.2070

49. Sileghem M, Flynn JN. Suppression of interleukin 2 secretion and interleukin 2 receptor expression during tsetse-transmitted trypanosomiasis in cattle. *Eur J Immunol.* (1992) 22:767–73. doi: 10.1002/eji.1830220321

50. Obishakin E, de Trez C, Magez S. Chronic *Trypanosoma congolense* infections in mice cause a sustained disruption of the B-cell homeostasis in the bone marrow and spleen. *Parasite Immunol.* (2014) 36:187–98. doi: 10.1111/pim.12099

51. Garside LH, Gibson WC. Molecular characterization of trypanosome species and subgroups within subgenus Nannomonas. *Parasitology* (1995) 111(Pt 3):301–12. doi: 10.1017/S0031182000081853

52. Vickerman K. Developmental cycles and biology of pathogenic trypanosomes. *Br Med Bull.* (1985) 41:105–14. doi: 10.1093/oxfordjournals.bmb.a072036

53. Peacock L, Bailey M, Gibson W. Dynamics of gamete production and mating in the parasitic protist *Trypanosoma brucei*. *Parasit Vectors* (2016) 9:404. doi: 10.1186/s13071-016-1689-9

54. Maclean L, Chisi JE, Odiit M, Gibson WC, Ferris V, Picozzi K, et al. Severity of human African trypanosomiasis in East Africa is associated with geographic location, parasite genotype, and host in ammatory cytokine response pro le. *Infect Immun.* (2004) 72:7040–4. doi: 10.1128/IAI.72.12.7040

55. Murphy WJ, Brentano ST, Rice-Ficht AC, Dorfman DM, Donelson JE. DNA rearrangements of the variable surface antigen genes of the trypanosomes1. *J Protozool* (1984) 31:65–73. doi: 10.1111/j.1550-7408.1984.tb04291.x

56. Hall JPJ, Wang H, David Barry J. Mosaic VSGs and the scale of *Trypanosoma brucei* antigenic variation. *PLoS Pathog.* (2013) 9:e1003502. doi: 10.1371/journal.ppat.1003502

57. Levine RF, Mansfield JM. Genetics of resistance to the African trypanosomes. III. Variant-specific antibody responses of H-2-compatible resistant and susceptible mice. *J Immunol.* (1984) 133:1564–9.

58. Mugnier MR, Stebbins CE, Papavasiliou FN. Masters of disguise: antigenic variation and the VSG coat in *Trypanosoma brucei*. *PLoS Pathog.* (2016) 12:e1005784. doi: 10.1371/journal.ppat.1005784

59. Pays E. Regulation of antigen gene expression in *Trypanosoma brucei*. *Trends Parasitol.* (2005) 21:517–20. doi: 10.1016/j.pt.2005.08.016

60. Horn D. Antigenic variation in African trypanosomes. *Mol Biochem Parasito* (2014) 195:123–9. doi: 10.1016/j.molbiopara.2014.05.001

61. Weiss BL, Wang J, Aksoy S. Tsetse immune system maturation requires the presence of obligate symbionts in larvae. *PLoS Biol.* (2011) 9:e1000619. doi: 10.1371/journal.pbio.1000619

62. Weiss BL, Maltz M, Aksoy S. Obligate symbionts activate immune system development in the tsetse fly. *J Immunol.* (2012) 188:3395–403. doi: 10.4049/jimmunol.1103691

63. Weiss BL, Wang J, Maltz MA, Wu Y, Aksoy S. Trypanosome infection establishment in the tsetse fly gut is influenced by microbiome-regulated host immune barriers. *PLoS Pathog.* (2013) 9:e1003318. doi: 10.1371/journal.ppat.1003318

64. Wang J, Wu Y, Yang G, Aksoy S. Interactions between mutualist Wigglesworthia and tsetse peptidoglycan recognition protein (PGRP-LB) influence trypanosome transmission. *Proc Natl Acad Sci USA.* (2009) 106:12133–8. doi: 10.1073/pnas.0901226106

65. Weiss BL, Savage AF, Griffith BC, Wu Y, Aksoy S. The peritrophic matrix mediates differential infection outcomes in the tsetse fly gut following challenge with commensal, pathogenic, and parasitic microbes. *J Immunol.* (2014) 193:773–82. doi: 10.4049/jimmunol.1400163

66. Hao Z, Kasumba I, Lehane MJ, Gibson WC, Kwon J, Aksoy S. Tsetse immune responses and trypanosome transmission: implications for the development of tsetse-based strategies to reduce trypanosomiasis. *Proc Natl Acad Sci USA.* (2001) 98:12648–53. doi: 10.1073/pnas.221363798

67. Hu C, Aksoy S. Innate immune responses regulate trypanosome parasite infection of the tsetse fly glossina morsitans morsitans. *Mol Microbiol.* (2006) 60:1194–204. doi: 10.1111/j.1365-2958.2006.05180.x

68. Hao Z, Kasumba I, Aksoy S. Proventriculus (cardia) plays a crucial role in immunity in tsetse fly (Diptera: Glossinidiae). *Insect Biochem Mol Biol.* (2003) 33:1155–64. doi: 10.1016/j.ibmb.2003.07.001

69. Haines LR, Lehane SM, Pearson TW, Lehane MJ. Tsetse EP protein protects the fly midgut from trypanosome establishment. *PLoS Pathog.* (2010) 6:e1000793. doi: 10.1371/journal.ppat.1000793

70. Akoda K, Van Den Abbeele J, Marcotty T, De Deken R, Sidibe I, Van den Bossche P. Nutritional stress of adult female tsetse flies (Diptera: Glossinidae) affects the susceptibility of their offspring to trypanosomal infections. *Acta Trop.* (2009) 111:263–7. doi: 10.1016/j.actatropica.2009.05.005

71. Akoda K, Van den Bossche P, Marcotty T, Kubi C, Coosemans M, De Deken R, et al. Nutritional stress affects the tsetse fly's immune gene expression. *Med Vet Entomol.* (2009) 23:195–201. doi: 10.1111/j.1365-2915.2009.00799.x

72. Akoda K, Van den Bossche P, Lyaruu E A, De Deken R, Marcotty T, Coosemans M, et al. Maturation of a *Trypanosoma Brucei* infection to the infectious metacyclic stage is enhanced in nutritionally stressed tsetse flies : table 1. *J Med Entomol.* (2009) 46:1446–9. doi: 10.1603/033.046.0629

73. Peacock L, Cook S, Ferris V, Bailey M, Gibson W. The life cycle of Trypanosoma (Nannomonas) congolense in the tsetse fly. *Parasit Vectors* (2012) 5:109. doi: 10.1186/1756-3305-5-109

74. Gibson W, Peacock L, Hutchinson R. Microarchitecture of the tsetse fly proboscis. *Parasit Vectors* (2017) 10:430. doi: 10.1186/s13071-017-2367-2

75. Morrison LJ, Tweedie A, Black A, Pinchbeck GL, Christley RM, Schoenefeld A, et al. Discovery of mating in the major African livestock pathogen trypanosoma congolense. *PLoS ONE* (2009) 4:e5564. doi: 10.1371/journal.pone.0005564

76. Caljon G, Van Den Abbeele J, Stijlemans B, Coosemans M, De Baetselier P, Magez S. Tsetse fly saliva accelerates the onset of *Trypanosoma brucei* infection in a mouse model associated with a reduced host inflammatory response. *Infect Immun.* (2006) 74:6324–30. doi: 10.1128/IAI.01046-06

77. Caljon G, De Ridder K, De Baetselier P, Coosemans M, Van Den Abbeele J. Identification of a tsetse fly salivary protein with dual inhibitory action on human platelet aggregation. *PLoS ONE* (2010) 5:e9671. doi: 10.1371/journal.pone.0009671

78. Sutherland CS, Stone CM, Steinmann P, Tanner M, Tediosi F. Seeing beyond 2020: an economic evaluation of contemporary and emerging strategies for elimination of *Trypanosoma brucei gambiense*. *Lancet Glob Health* (2017) 5:e69–79. doi: 10.1016/S2214-109X(16)30237-6

79. Simarro PP, Diarra A, Postigo JAR, Franco JR, Jannin JG. The human african trypanosomiasis control and surveillance program of the World Health Organization 2000-2009: the way forward. *PLoS Negl Trop Dis.* (2011) 5:e1007. doi: 10.1371/journal.pntd.0001007

80. Joshi PP, Shegokar VR, Powar RM, Herder S, Katti R, Salkar HR, et al. Human trypanosomiasis caused by *Trypanosoma evansi* in India: the first case report. *Am J Trop Med Hyg.* (2005) 73:491-5. doi: 10.4269/ajtmh.2005.73.491

81. Vanhollebeke B, Truc P, Poelvoorde P, Pays A, Joshi PP, Katti R, et al. Human *Trypanosoma evansi* infection linked to a lack of apolipoprotein L-I. *N Engl J Med.* (2006) 355:2752-6. doi: 10.1056/NEJMoa063265

82. Truc P, Gibson W, Herder S. Genetic characterization of *Trypanosoma evansi* isolated from a patient in India. *Infect Genet Evol.* (2007) 7:305-7. doi: 10.1016/j.meegid.2006.07.004

83. Haridy FM, El-Metwally MT, Khalil HHM, Morsy TA. *Trypanosoma evansi* in dromedary camel: with a case report of zoonosis in greater Cairo, Egypt. *J Egypt Soc Parasitol.* (2011) 41:65-76.

84. Duffy CW, Morrison LJ, Black A, Pinchbeck GL, Christley RM, Schoenefeld A, et al. *Trypanosoma vivax* displays a clonal population structure. *Int J Parasitol.* (2009) 39:1475-83. doi: 10.1016/j.ijpara.2009.05.012

85. Jackson AP, Berry A, Aslett M, Allison HC, Burton P, Vavrova-Anderson J, et al. Antigenic diversity is generated by distinct evolutionary mechanisms in African trypanosome species. *Proc Natl Acad Sci USA.* (2012) 109:3416-21. doi: 10.1073/pnas.1117313109

86. Biteau N, Asencio C, Izotte J, Rousseau B, Fèvre M, Pillay D, et al. *Trypanosoma brucei* gambiense infections in mice lead to tropism to the reproductive organs, and horizontal and vertical transmission. *PLoS Negl Trop Dis.* (2016) 10:1-15. doi: 10.1371/journal.pntd.0004350

87. Rocha G, Martins A, Gama G, Brandão F, Atouguia J. Possible cases of sexual and congenital transmission of sleeping sickness [5]. *Lancet* (2004) 363:247. doi: 10.1016/S0140-6736(03)15345-7

88. Seed JR, Sechelski JB, Ortiz JC, Chapman JF. Relationship between human serum trypanocidal activity and host resistance to the African trypanosomes. *J Parasitol.* (1993) 79:226-32. doi: 10.1016/j.molbiopara.2015.03.007

89. Raper J, Fung R, Ghiso J, Nussenzweig V, Tomlinson S. Characterization of a novel trypanosome lytic factor from human serum. *Infect Immun.* (1999) 67:1910-6.

90. Raper J, Portela MP, Lugli E, Frevert U, Tomlinson S. Trypanosome lytic factors: novel mediators of human innate immunity. *Curr Opin Microbiol.* (2001) 4:402-8. doi: 10.1016/S1369-5274(00)00226-5

91. De Greef C, Hamers R. The serum resistance-associated (SRA) gene of *Trypanosoma brucei* rhodesiense encodes a variant surface glycoprotein-like protein. *Mol Biochem Parasitol.* (1994) 68:277-84. doi: 10.1016/0166-6851(94)90172-4

92. Xong H V, Vanhamme L, Chamekh M, Chimfwembe CE, Van Den Abbeele J, Pays A, et al. A VSG expression site-associated gene confers resistance to human serum in *Trypanosoma rhodesiense*. *Cell* (1998) 95:839-46.

93. Vanhamme L, Paturiaux-Hanocq F, Poelvoorde P, Nolan DP, Lins L, Abbeele J Van Den, et al. Apolipoprotein L-1 is the trypanosome lytic factor of human serum. *Nature* (2003) 422:83-7. doi: 10.1038/nature01457.1.

94. Vanwalleghem G, Fontaine F, Lecordier L, Tebabi P, Klewe K, Nolan DP, et al. Coupling of lysosomal and mitochondrial membrane permeabilization in trypanolysis by APOL1. *Nat Commun .*(2015) 6:8078. doi: 10.1038/ncomms9078

95. Pérez-Morga D, Vanhollebeke B, Paturiaux-Hanocq F, Nolan DP, Lins L, Homblé F, et al. Apolipoprotein L-I promotes trypanosome lysis by forming pores in lysosomal membranes. *Science* (2005) 309:469-72. doi: 10.1126/science.1114566

96. Vanhollebeke B, Lecordier L, Perez-Morga D, Amiguet-Vercher A, Pays E. Human serum lyses *Trypanosoma brucei* by triggering uncontrolled swelling of the parasite lysosome. *J Eukaryot Microbiol.* (2007) 54:448-51. doi: 10.1111/j.1550-7408.2007.00285.x

97. Oli MW, Cotlin LF, Shiflett AM, Hajduk SL. Serum resistance-associated protein blocks lysosomal targeting of trypanosome lytic factor in *Trypanosoma brucei*. *Eukaryot Cell* (2006) 5:132-9. doi: 10.1128/EC.5.1.132-139.2006

98. Greene AS, Hajduk SL. Trypanosome lytic factor-1 initiates oxidation-stimulated osmotic lysis of *Trypanosoma brucei brucei*. *J Biol Chem.* (2016) 291:3063-75. doi: 10.1074/jbc.M115.680371

99. DeJesus E, Kieft R, Albright B, Stephens NA, Hajduk SL. A single amino acid substitution in the group 1 *Trypanosoma brucei* gambiense haptoglobin-hemoglobin receptor abolishes TLF-1 binding. *PLoS Pathog.* (2013) 9:1-10. doi: 10.1371/journal.ppat.1003317

100. Bullard W, Kieft R, Capewell P, Veitch NJ, Macleod A, Hajduk SL. Haptoglobin-hemoglobin receptor independent killing of African trypanosomes by human serum and trypanosome lytic factors. *Virulence* (2012) 3:72-6. doi: 10.4161/viru.3.1.18295

101. Vanhollebeke B, De Muylder G, Nielsen MJ, Pays A, Tebabi P, Dieu M, et al. A haptoglobin-hemoglobin receptor conveys innate immunity to *Trypanosoma brucei* in humans. *Science* (2008) 320:677-81. doi: 10.1126/science.1156296

102. Enyaru JCK, Matovu E, Nerima B, Akol M, Sebikali C. Detection of *T.b. rhodesiense* trypanosomes in humans and domestic animals in South East Uganda by amplification of serum resistance-associated gene. *Ann N Y Acad Sci.* (2006) 1081:311-9. doi: 10.1196/annals.1373.041

103. Gibson W, Peacock L, Ferris V, Fischer K, Livingstone J, Thomas J, et al. Genetic recombination between human and animal parasites creates novel strains of human pathogen. *PLoS Negl Trop Dis.* (2015) 9:1-16. doi: 10.1371/journal.pntd.0003665

104. Echodu R, Sistrom M, Bateta R, Murilla G, Okedi L, Aksoy S, et al. Genetic diversity and population structure of <italic>Trypanosoma brucei</italic> in uganda: implications for the epidemiology of sleeping sickness and nagana. *PLoS Negl Trop Dis.* (2015) 9:e0003353. doi: 10.5061/dryad.m7q4c

105. Capewell P, Veitch NJ, Turner CMR, Raper J, Berriman M, Hajduk SL, et al. Differences between *Trypanosoma brucei* gambiense groups 1 and 2 in their resistance to killing by trypanolytic factor 1. *PLoS Negl Trop Dis.* (2011) 5:e1287. doi: 10.1371/journal.pntd.0001287

106. Higgins MK, Tkachenko O, Brown A, Reed J, Raper J, Carrington M. Structure of the trypanosome haptoglobin-hemoglobin receptor and implications for nutrient uptake and innate immunity. *Proc Natl Acad Sci USA.* (2013) 110:1905-10. doi: 10.1073/pnas.1214943110

107. Kieft R, Capewell P, Turner CMR, Veitch NJ, MacLeod A, Hajduk S. Mechanism of *Trypanosoma brucei* gambiense (group 1) resistance to human trypanosome lytic factor. *Proc Natl Acad Sci USA.* (2010) 107:16137-41. doi: 10.1073/pnas.1007074107

108. Berberof M, Pérez-Morga D, Pays E. A receptor-like flagellar pocket glycoprotein specific to *Trypanosoma brucei* gambiense. *Mol Biochem Parasitol.* (2001) 113:127-38. doi: 10.1016/S0166-6851(01)00208-0

109. Capewell P, Clucas C, DeJesus E, Kieft R, Hajduk S, Veitch N, et al. The TgsGP gene is essential for resistance to human serum in *Trypanosoma brucei* gambiense. *PLoS Pathog.* (2013) 9:2-7. doi: 10.1371/journal.ppat.1003686

110. Uzureau P, Uzureau S, Lecordier L, Fontaine F, Tebabi P, Homblé F, et al. Mechanism of *Trypanosoma brucei* gambiense resistance to human serum. *Nature* (2013) 501:430-4. doi: 10.1038/nature12516

111. Radwanska M, Bockstal V, Brombacher F, Magez S. Parasite-induced B-cell apoptosis results in loss of specific protective anti-trypanosome antibody responses, and abolishment of vaccine induced protective memory. In: *XII INTERNATIONAL CONGRESS OF PARASITOLOGY (ICOPA)* (Melbourne, VIC). (2010). p. 31–38.

112. Lai D-H, Wang Q-P, Li Z, Luckins AG, Reid SA, Lun Z-R. Investigations into human serum sensitivity expressed by stocks of *Trypanosoma brucei evansi*. *Int J Parasitol.* (2010) 40:705-10. doi: 10.1016/j.ijpara.2009.11.009

113. Faulkner SD, Oli MW, Kieft R, Cotlin L, Widener J, Shiflett A, et al. *In vitro* generation of human high-density-lipoprotein-resistant *Trypanosoma brucei*. *Eukaryot Cell* (2006) 5:1276-86. doi: 10.1128/EC.00116-06

114. Vanhamme L, Renauld H, Lecordier L, Poelvoorde P, Van Den Abbeele J, Pays E. The *Trypanosoma brucei* reference strain TREU927/4 contains T. brucei rhodesiense-specific SRA sequences, but displays a distinct phenotype of relative resistance to human serum. *Mol Biochem Parasitol.* (2004) 135:39-47. doi: 10.1016/j.molbiopara.2004.01.004

115. Lai D, Wang Q, Li Z, Julius L, Lun Z. Evolution of the serum resistance-associated SRA gene in African trypanosomes. *Sci Bull.* (2009) 54:1275-8. doi: 10.1007/s11434-009-0137-z

116. Van Vinh Chau N, Buu Chau L, Desquesnes M, Herder S, Phu Huong Lan N, Campbell JI, et al. A clinical and epidemiological investigation of the first reported human infection with the zoonotic parasite *Trypanosoma evansi* in Southeast Asia. *Clin Infect Dis.* (2016) 62:1002–8. doi: 10.1093/cid/ciw052

117. Wabale V, Nalage P, Joshi A, Bharadwaj R, Deshpande K, Chowdhary A. Human Asian Trypanosomiasis due to *Trypanosoma evansi*: a rare case. *J Adv Parasitol.* (2015) 3:65–8. doi: 10.14737/journal.jap/2015/2.3.65.68

118. Baral TN, De Baetselier P, Brombacher F, Magez S. Control of *Trypanosoma evansi* infection is IgM mediated and does not require a type I inflammatory response. *J Infect Dis.* (2007) 195:1513–20. doi: 10.1086/515577

119. Desquesnes M, Yangtara S, Kunphukhieo P, Chalermwong P, Jittapalapong S, Herder S. Zoonotic trypanosomes in South East Asia: attempts to control *Trypanosoma lewisi* using veterinary drugs. *Exp Parasitol.* (2016) 165:35–42. doi: 10.1016/j.exppara.2016.03.009

120. Thomson R, Genovese G, Canon C, Kovacsics D, Higgins MK, Carrington M, et al. Evolution of the primate trypanolytic factor APOL1. *Proc Natl Acad Sci USA.* (2014) 111:E2130–9. doi: 10.1073/pnas.1400699111

121. Smith EE, Malik HS. The apolipoprotein L family of programmed cell death and immunity genes rapidly evolved in primates at discrete sites of host-pathogen interactions. *Genome Res.* (2009) 19:850–8. doi: 10.1101/gr.085647.108

122. Thomson R, Molina-Portela P, Mott H, Carrington M, Raper J. Hydrodynamic gene delivery of baboon trypanosome lytic factor eliminates both animal and human-infective African trypanosomes. *Proc Natl Acad Sci USA.* (2009) 106:19509–14. doi: 10.1073/pnas.0905669106

123. Cooper A, Capewell P, Clucas C, Veitch N, Weir W, Thomson R, et al. A primate APOL1 variant that kills *Trypanosoma brucei gambiense*. *PLoS Negl Trop Dis.* (2016) 10:e0004903. doi: 10.1371/journal.pntd.0004903

124. Borst P. Antigenic variation and allelic exclusion. *Cell* (2002) 109:5–8. doi: 10.1016/S0092-8674(02)00711-0

125. Pays E, Vanhamme L, Pérez-Morga D. Antigenic variation in *Trypanosoma brucei*: facts, challenges and mysteries. *Curr Opin Microbiol.* (2004) 7:369–74. doi: 10.1016/j.mib.2004.05.001

126. Radwanska M, Magez S, Michel A, Stijlemans B, Geuskens M, Pays E. Comparative analysis of antibody responses against HSP60, invariant surface glycoprotein 70, and variant surface glycoprotein reveals a complex antigen-specific pattern of immunoglobulin isotype switching during infection by *Trypanosoma brucei*. *Infect Immun.* (2000) 68:848–60. doi: 10.1128/IAI.68.2.848-860.2000

127. Bockstal V, Guirnalda P, Caljon G, Goenka R, Telfer JC, Frenkel D, et al. *T. brucei* infection reduces B lymphopoiesis in bone marrow and truncates compensatory splenic lymphopoiesis through transitional B-cell apoptosis. *PLoS Pathog.* (2011) 7:e1002089. doi: 10.1371/journal.ppat.1002089

128. Engstler M, Pfohl T, Herminghaus S, Boshart M, Wiegertjes G, Heddergott N, et al. Hydrodynamic flow-mediated protein sorting on the cell surface of trypanosomes. *Cell* (2007) 131:505–15. doi: 10.1016/j.cell.2007.08.046

129. La Greca F, Haynes C, Stijlemans B, De Trez C, Magez S. Antibody-mediated control of *Trypanosoma vivax* infection fails in the absence of tumor necrosis factor. *Parasite Immunol.* (2014) 36:271–6. doi: 10.1111/pim.12106

130. Radwanska M, Guirnalda P, De Trez C, Ryffel B, Black S, Magez S. Trypanosomiasis-induced B cell apoptosis results in loss of protective anti-parasite antibody responses and abolishment of vaccine-induced memory responses. *PLoS Pathog.* (2008) 4:e1000078. doi: 10.1371/journal.ppat.1000078

131. Cnops J, Kauffmann F, De Trez C, Baltz T, Keirsse J, Radwanska M, et al. Maintenance of B cells during chronic murine *Trypanosoma brucei gambiense* infection. *Parasite Immunol.* (2016) 38:642–7. doi: 10.1111/pim.12344

132. Cnops J, De Trez C, Bulte D, Radwanska M, Ryffel B, Magez S. IFN-γ mediates early B-cell loss in experimental African trypanosomosis. *Parasite Immunol.* (2015) 37:479–84. doi: 10.1111/pim.12208

133. Frenkel D, Zhang F, Guirnalda P, Haynes C, Bockstal V, Radwanska M, et al. *Trypanosoma brucei* Co-opts NK cells to kill splenic B2 B cells. *PLoS Pathog.* (2016) 12:e1005733. doi: 10.1371/journal.ppat.1005733

134. Cnops J, Magez S, De Trez C. Escape mechanisms of African trypanosomes: why trypanosomosis is keeping us awake. *Parasitology* (2015) 142:417–27. doi: 10.1017/S0031182014001838

135. Tizard IR, Mittal KR, Nielsen K. Depressed immunoconglutinin responses in calves experimentally infected with *Trypanosoma congolense*. *Res Vet Sci.* (1980) 28:203–6.

136. Uzonna JE, Kaushik RS, Gordon JR, Tabel H. Cytokines and antibody responses during *Trypanosoma congolense* infections in two inbred mouse strains that differ in resistance. *Parasite Immunol.* (1999) 21:57–71. doi: 10.1046/j.1365-3024.1999.00202.x

137. Schopf LR, Filutowicz H, Bi XJ, Mansfield JM. Interleukin-4-dependent immunoglobulin G1 isotype switch in the presence of a polarized antigen-specific Th1-cell response to the trypanosome variant surface glycoprotein. *Infect Immun.* (1998) 66:451–61.

138. Lejon V, Mumba Ngoyi D, Kestens L, Boel L, Barbé B, Kande Betu V, et al. Gambiense human african trypanosomiasis and immunological memory: effect on phenotypic lymphocyte profiles and humoral immunity. *PLoS Pathog.* (2014) 10:e1003947. doi: 10.1371/journal.ppat.1003947

139. Holland WG, Do TT, Huong NT, Dung NT, Thanh NG, Vercruysse J, et al. The effect of *Trypanosoma evansi* infection on pig performance and vaccination against classical swine fever. *Vet Parasitol.* (2003) 111:115–23. doi: 10.1016/S0304-4017(02)00363-1

140. Holland WG, My LN, Dung TV, Thanh NG, Tam PT, Vercruysse J, et al. The influence of T. evansi infection on the immuno-responsiveness of experimentally infected water buffaloes. *Vet Parasitol.* (2001) 102:225–34. doi: 10.1016/S0304-4017(01)00534-9

141. Rurangirwa FR, Musoke AJ, Nantulya VM, Tabel H. Immune depression in bovine trypanosomiasis: effects of acute and chronic *Trypanosoma congolense* and chronic *Trypanosoma vivax* infections on antibody response to *Brucella abortus* vaccine. *Parasite Immunol.* (1983) 5:267–76. doi: 10.1111/j.1365-3024.1983.tb00743.x

142. Rurangirwa FR, Tabel H, Losos GJ, Tizard IR. Suppression of antibody response to Leptospira biflexa and Brucella abortus and recovery from immunosuppression after Berenil treatment. *Infect Immun.* (1979) 26:822–6.

143. Ilemobade AA, Adegboye DS, Onoviran O, Chima JC. Immunodepressive effects of trypanosomal infection in cattle immunized against contagious bovine pleuropneumonia. *Parasite Immunol.* (1982) 4:273–82. doi: 10.1111/j.1365-3024.1982.tb00438.x

144. Mwangi DM, Munyua WK, Nyaga PN. Immunosuppression in caprine trypanosomiasis: effects of acute *Trypanosoma congolense* infection on antibody response to anthrax spore vaccine. *Trop Anim Health Prod.* (1990) 22:95–100. doi: 10.1007/BF02239832

145. Sharpe RT, Langley AM, Mowat GN, Macaskill JA, Holmes PH. Immunosuppression in bovine trypanosomiasis: response of cattle infected with *Trypanosoma congolense* to foot-and-mouth disease vaccination and subsequent live virus challenge. *Res Vet Sci.* (1982) 32:289–293.

146. De Gee L, Levine RF, Mansfield JM. Genetics of resistance to the African trypanosomes. VI. Heredity of resistance and variable surface glycoprotein-specific immune responses. *J Immunol.* (1988) 140:283–8.

147. Dagenais TR, Demick KP, Bangs JD, Forest KT, Paulnock DM, Mansfield JM. T-cell responses to the trypanosome variant surface glycoprotein are not limited to hypervariable subregions. *Infect Immun.* (2009) 77:141–51. doi: 10.1128/IAI.00729-08

148. Dagenais TR, Freeman BE, Demick KP, Paulnock DM, Mansfield JM. Processing and presentation of variant surface glycoprotein molecules to T cells in African trypanosomiasis. *J Immunol.* (2009) 183:3344–55. doi: 10.4049/jimmunol.0802005

149. Schleifer KW, Mansfield JM. Suppressor macrophages in African trypanosomiasis inhibit T cell proliferative responses by nitric oxide and prostaglandins. *J Immunol.* (1993) 151:5492–503.

150. Hertz CJ, Filutowicz H, Mansfield JM. Resistance to the African trypanosomes is IFN-gamma dependent. *J Immunol.* (1998) 161:6775–83.

151. Hertz CJ, Mansfield JM. IFN-gamma-dependent nitric oxide production is not linked to resistance in experimental African trypanosomiasis. *Cell Immunol.* (1999) 192:24–32. doi: 10.1006/cimm.1998.1429

152. Magez S, Radwanska M, Drennan M, Fick L, Baral TN, Brombacher F, et al. Interferon-gamma and nitric oxide in combination with antibodies are key protective host immune factors during *trypanosoma congolense* Tc13 infections. *J Infect Dis.* (2006) 193:1575–83. doi: 10.1086/503808

153. Uzonna JE, Kaushik RS, Gordon JR, Tabel H. Experimental murine *Trypanosoma congolense* infections. I. Administration of anti-IFN-gamma antibodies alters trypanosome-susceptible mice to a resistant-like phenotype. *J Immunol.* (1998) 161:5507–15.

154. Cnops J, De Trez C, Stijlemans B, Keirsse J, Kauffmann F, Barkhuizen M, et al. NK-, NKT- and CD8-Derived IFNγ drives myeloid cell activation and erythrophagocytosis, resulting in trypanosomosis-associated acute anemia. *PLoS Pathog.* (2015) 11:e1004964. doi: 10.1371/journal.ppat.1004964

155. Wu H, Liu G, Shi M. Interferon gamma in African Trypanosome infections: friends or foes? *Front Immunol.* (2017) 8:1105. doi: 10.3389/fimmu.2017.01105

156. Bakhiet M, Büscher P, Harris RA, Kristensson K, Wigzell H, Olsson T. Different trypanozoan species possess CD8 dependent lymphocyte triggering factor-like activity. *Immunol Lett.* (1996) 50:71–80. doi: 10.1016/0165-2478(96)02521-7

157. Bakhiet M, Hamadien M, Tjernlund A, Mousal A, Seiger A. African trypanosomes activate human fetal brain cells to proliferation and IFN-gamma production. *Neuroreport* (2002) 13:53–6. doi: 10.1097/00001756-200201210-00015

158. Masocha W, Robertson B, Rottenberg ME, Mhlanga J, Sorokin L, Kristensson K. Cerebral vessel laminins and IFN-gamma define *Trypanosoma brucei* brucei penetration of the blood-brain barrier. *J Clin Invest.* (2004) 114:689–94. doi: 10.1172/JCI22104

159. Liu G, Sun D, Wu H, Zhang M, Huan H, Xu J, et al. Distinct contributions of CD4+ and CD8+ T cells to pathogenesis of *Trypanosoma brucei* infection in the context of gamma interferon and interleukin-10. *Infect Immun.* (2015) 83:2785–95. doi: 10.1128/IAI.00357-15

160. Olsson T, Bakhiet M, Edlund C, Höjeberg B, Van der Meide PH, Kristensson K. Bidirectional activating signals between *Trypanosoma brucei* and CD8+ T cells: a trypanosome-released factor triggers interferon-gamma production that stimulates parasite growth. *Eur J Immunol.* (1991) 21:2447–54. doi: 10.1002/eji.1830211022

161. Sternberg JM, Mabbott NA. Nitric oxide-mediated suppression of T cell responses during*Trypanosoma brucei* infection: soluble trypanosome products and interferon-γ are synergistic inducers of nitric oxide synthase. *Eur J Immunol.* (1996) 26:539–43. doi: 10.1002/eji.1830260306

162. Lopez R, Demick KP, Mansfield JM, Paulnock DM. Type I IFNs play a role in early resistance, but subsequent susceptibility, to the African trypanosomes. *J Immunol.* (2008) 181:4908–17. doi: 10.4049/jimmunol.181.7.4908

163. Magez S, Radwanska M, Beschin A, Sekikawa K, De Baetselier P. Tumor necrosis factor alpha is a key mediator in the regulation of experimental *Trypanosoma brucei* infections. *Infect Immun.* (1999) 67:3128–32.

164. Iraqi F, Sekikawa K, Rowlands J, Teale A. Susceptibility of tumor necrosis factor-alpha genetically deficient mice to *Trypanosoma congolense* infection. *Parasite Immunol.* (2001) 23:445–51. doi: 10.1046/j.1365-3024.2001.00401.x

165. Magez S, Lucas R, Darji A, Songa EB, Hamers R, De Baetselier P. Murine tumor necrosis factor plays a protective role during the initial phase of the experimental infection with *Trypanosoma brucei* brucei. *Parasite Immunol.* (1993) 15:635–41. doi: 10.1111/j.1365-3024.1993.tb00577.x

166. Magez S, Truyens C, Merimi M, Radwanska M, Stijlemans B, Brouckaert P, et al. P75 tumor necrosis factor-receptor shedding occurs as a protective host response during African trypanosomiasis. *J Infect Dis.* (2004) 189:527–39. doi: 10.1086/381151

167. Stijlemans B, De Baetselier P, Magez S, Van Ginderachter JA, De Trez C. African trypanosomiasis-associated anemia: the contribution of the interplay between parasites and the mononuclear phagocyte system. *Front Immunol.* (2018) 9:218. doi: 10.3389/fimmu.2018.00218

168. Lucas R, Magez S, De Leys R, Fransen L, Scheerlinck JP, Rampelberg M, et al. Mapping the lectin-like activity of tumor necrosis factor. *Science* (1994) 263:814–7. doi: 10.1126/science.8303299

169. Magez S, Radwanska M, Stijlemans B, Xong H V, Pays E, De Baetselier P. A conserved flagellar pocket exposed high mannose moiety is used by African trypanosomes as a host cytokine binding molecule. *J Biol Chem.* (2001) 276:33458–64. doi: 10.1074/jbc.M103412200

170. Daulouède S, Bouteille B, Moynet D, De Baetselier P, Courtois P, Lemesre JL, et al. Human macrophage tumor necrosis factor (TNF)-alpha production induced by *Trypanosoma brucei* gambiense and the role of TNF-alpha in parasite control. *J Infect Dis.* (2001) 183:988–91. doi: 10.1086/319257

171. Paulnock DM, Freeman BE, Mansfield JM. Modulation of innate immunity by African trypanosomes. *Parasitology* (2010) 137:2051–63. doi: 10.1017/S0031182010001460

172. O'Gorman GM, Park SDE, Hill EW, Meade KG, Mitchell LC, Agaba M, et al. Cytokine mRNA profiling of peripheral blood mononuclear cells from trypanotolerant and trypanosusceptible cattle infected with *Trypanosoma congolense*. *Physiol Genomics* (2006) 28:53–61. doi: 10.1152/physiolgenomics.00100.2006

173. Magez S, Stijlemans B, Baral T, De Baetselier P. VSG-GPI anchors of African trypanosomes: their role in macrophage activation and induction of infection-associated immunopathology. *Microbes Infect.* (2002) 4:999–1006. doi: 10.1016/S1286-4579(02)01617-9

174. Leppert BJ, Mansfield JM, Paulnock DM. The soluble variant surface glycoprotein of African trypanosomes is recognized by a macrophage scavenger receptor and induces I kappa B alpha degradation independently of TRAF6-mediated TLR signaling. *J Immunol.* (2007) 179:548–56. doi: 10.4049/jimmunol.179.1.548

175. Coller SP, Mansfield JM, Paulnock DM. Glycosylinositolphosphate soluble variant surface glycoprotein inhibits IFN- -induced nitric oxide production via reduction in STAT1 phosphorylation in African Trypanosomiasis. *J Immunol.* (2003) 171:1466–72. doi: 10.4049/jimmunol.171.3.1466

176. Stijlemans B, Baral TN, Guilliams M, Brys L, Korf J, Drennan M, et al. A glycosylphosphatidylinositol-based treatment alleviates trypanosomiasis-associated immunopathology. *J Immunol.* (2007) 179:4003–14. doi: 10.4049/jimmunol.179.6.4003

177. Stijlemans B, Vankrunkelsven A, Brys L, Raes G, Magez S, De Baetselier P. Scrutinizing the mechanisms underlying the induction of anemia of inflammation through GPI-mediated modulation of macrophage activation in a model of African trypanosomiasis. *Microbes Infect.* (2010) 12:389–99. doi: 10.1016/j.micinf.2010.02.006

178. Harris TH, Cooney NM, Mansfield JM, Paulnock DM. Signal transduction, gene transcription, and cytokine production triggered in macrophages by exposure to trypanosome DNA. *Infect Immun.* ₐ(2006) 74:4530–7. doi: 10.1128/IAI.01938-05

179. Barkhuizen M, Magez S, Ryffel B, Brombacher F. Interleukin-12p70 deficiency increases survival and diminishes pathology in *Trypanosoma congolense* infection. *J Infect Dis.* (2008) 198:1284–91. doi: 10.1086/592048

180. Krishnamoorthy P, Sengupta PP, Das S, Ligi M, Shome BR, Rahman H. Cytokine gene expression and pathology in mice experimentally infected with different isolates of *Trypanosoma evansi*. *Exp Parasitol.* (2016) 170:168–76. doi: 10.1016/j.exppara.2016.09.019

181. Flynn JN, Sileghem M. The role of the macrophage in induction of immunosuppression in *Trypanosoma congolense*-infected cattle. *Immunology* (1991) 74:310–6.

182. Maclean L, Odiit M, Macleod A, Morrison L, Sweeney L, Cooper A, et al. Spatially and genetically distinct African Trypanosome virulence variants defined by host interferon-gamma response. *J Infect Dis.* (2007) 196:1620–8. doi: 10.1086/522011

183. Kennedy PGE. Cytokines in central nervous system trypanosomiasis: cause, effect or both? *Trans R Soc Trop Med Hyg.* (2009) 103:213–4. doi: 10.1016/j.trstmh.2008.08.013

184. Murray M, Morrison WI, Whitelaw DD. Host susceptibility to African trypanosomiasis: trypanotolerance. *Adv Parasitol.* (1982) 21:1–68. doi: 10.1016/S0065-308X(08)60274-2

185. Naessens J. Bovine trypanotolerance: a natural ability to prevent severe anemia and haemophagocytic syndrome? *Int J Parasitol.* (2006) 36:521–8. doi: 10.1016/j.ijpara.2006.02.012

186. Rifkin MR, Landsberger FR. Trypanosome variant surface glycoprotein transfer to target membranes: a model for the pathogenesis of trypanosomiasis. *Proc Natl Acad Sci USA.* (1990) 87:801–5. doi: 10.1073/pnas.87.2.801

187. Guegan F, Plazolles N, Baltz T, Coustou V. Erythrophagocytosis of desialylated red blood cells is responsible for anemia during *Trypanosoma vivax* infection. *Cell Microbiol.* (2013) 15:1285–303. doi: 10.1111/cmi.12123

188. Suzuki T, Ueta YY, Inoue N, Xuan X, Saitoh H, Suzuki H. Beneficial effect of erythropoietin administration on murine infection with *Trypanosoma congolense. Am J Trop Med Hyg.* (2006) 74:1020–5. doi: 10.4269/ajtmh.2006.74.1020

189. Authié E, Boulangé A, Muteti D, Lalmanach G, Gauthier F, Musoke AJ. Immunisation of cattle with cysteine proteinases of *Trypanosoma congolense*: targetting the disease rather than the parasite. *Int J Parasitol.* (2001) 31:1429–33. doi: 10.1016/S0020-7519(01)00266-1

190. Stijlemans B, Brys L, Korf H, Bieniasz-Krzywiec P, Sparkes A, Vansintjan L, et al. MIF-mediated hemodilution promotes pathogenic anemia in experimental African trypanosomosis. *PLOS Pathog.* (2016) 12:e1005862. doi: 10.1371/journal.ppat.1005862

191. Thompson PD, Tipney H, Brass A, Noyes H, Kemp S, Naessens J, et al. Claudin 13, a member of the claudin family regulated in mouse stress induced erythropoiesis. *PLoS ONE* (2010) 5:e12667. doi: 10.1371/journal.pone.0012667

192. Blom-Potar MC, Chamond N, Cosson A, Jouvion G, Droin-Bergère S, Huerre M, et al. *Trypanosoma vivax* infections: pushing ahead with mouse models for the study of Nagana. II. Immunobiological dysfunctions. *PLoS Negl Trop Dis.* (2010) 4:e793. doi: 10.1371/journal.pntd.0000793

193. Chamond N, Cosson A, Blom-Potar MC, Jouvion G, D'Archivio S, Medina M, et al. *Trypanosoma vivax* infections: pushing ahead with mouse models for the study of Nagana. I. Parasitological, hematological and pathological parameters. *PLoS Negl Trop Dis.* (2010) 4:e792. doi: 10.1371/journal.pntd.0000792

194. Magez S, Stijlemans B, Caljon G, Eugster H-P, De Baetselier P. Control of experimental *Trypanosoma brucei* infections occurs independently of lymphotoxin-alpha induction. *Infect Immun.* (2002) 70:1342–51. doi: 10.1128/IAI.70.3.1342

195. Bosschaerts T, Guilliams M, Noel W, Hérin M, Burk RF, Hill KE, et al. Alternatively activated myeloid cells limit pathogenicity associated with African trypanosomiasis through the IL-10 inducible gene selenoprotein P. *J Immunol.* (2008) 180:6168–75. doi: 10.1186/1756-3305-4-74

196. Vankrunkelsven A, De Ceulaer K, Hsu D, Liu F-T, De Baetselier P, Stijlemans B. Lack of galectin-3 alleviates trypanosomiasis-associated anemia of inflammation. *Immunobiology* (2016) 215:833–41. doi: 10.1016/j.imbio.2010.05.028

197. Katunguka-Rwakishaya E, Murray M, Holmes PH. Pathophysiology of *Trypanosoma congolense* infection in two breeds of sheep, Scottish blackface and Finn dorset. *Vet Parasitol.* (1997) 68:215–25. doi: 10.1016/S0304-4017(96)01075-8

198. Katunguka-Rwakishaya E, Murray M, Holmes PH. Pathophysiology of ovine trypanosomiasis: ferrokinetics and erythrocyte survival studies. *Res Vet Sci.* (1992) 53:80–6. doi: 10.1016/0034-5288(92)90089-K

199. da Silva CB, Wolkmer P, Paim FC, Da Silva AS, Siqueira LC, de Souza CL, et al. Iron metabolism and its relationship to anemia and immune system in *Trypanosoma evansi* infected rats. *Exp Parasitol.* (2013) 133:357–64. doi: 10.1016/j.exppara.2012.12.010

200. Mackie JT, Stenner R, Gillett AK, Barbosa A, Ryan U, Irwin PJ. Trypanosomiasis in an Australian little red flying fox (*Pteropus scapulatus*). *Aust Vet J.* (2017) 95:259–61. doi: 10.1111/avj.12597

201. Doua F, Yapo FB. Human trypanosomiasis in the Ivory Coast: therapy and problems. *Acta Trop.* (1993) 54:163–8. doi: 10.1016/0001-706X(93)90090-X

202. Doua F, Boa FY, Schechter PJ, Miézan TW, Diai D, Sanon SR, et al. Treatment of human late stage gambiense trypanosomiasis with alpha-difluoromethylornithine (eflornithine): efficacy and tolerance in 14 cases in Côte d'Ivoire. *Am J Trop Med Hyg.* (1987) 37:525–33.

203. Burri C, Brun R. Eflornithine for the treatment of human African trypanosomiasis. *Parasitol Res.* (2003) 90(Supp 1):S49–52. doi: 10.1007/s00436-002-0766-5

204. Milord F, Pépin J, Loko L, Ethier L, Mpia B. Efficacy and toxicity of eflornithine for treatment of *Trypanosoma brucei* gambiense sleeping sickness. *Lancet* (1992) 340:652–5. doi: 10.1016/0140-6736(92)92180-N

205. Paul M, Stefaniak J, Smuszkiewicz P, Van Esbroeck M, Geysen D, Clerinx J. Outcome of acute East African trypanosomiasis in a polish traveler treated with pentamidine. *BMC Infect Dis.* (2014) 14:111. doi: 10.1186/1471-2334-14-111

206. Ngotho M, Kagira JM, Kariuki C, Maina N, Thuita JK, Mwangangi DM, et al. Influence of trypanocidal therapy on the hematology of vervet monkeys experimentally infected with *Trypanosoma brucei* rhodesiense. *Acta Trop.* (2011) 119:14–8. doi: 10.1016/j.actatropica.2011.02.013

207. Chisi JE, Misiri H, Zverev Y, Nkhoma A, Sternberg JM. Anaemia in human African trypanosomiasis caused by *Trypanosoma brucei* rhodesiense. *East Afr Med J.* (2004) 81:505–8. doi: 10.4314/eamj.v81i10.9232

208. MacLean L, Chisi JE, Odiit M, Gibson WC, Ferris V, Picozzi K, et al. Severity of human African trypanosomiasis in east Africa is associated with geographic location, parasite genotype, and host inflammatory cytokine response profile. *Infect Immun.* (2004) 72:7040–4. doi: 10.1128/IAI.72.12.7040-7044.2004

209. Songa EB, Hamers R, Rickman R, Nantulya VM, Mulla AF, Magnus E. Evidence for widespread asymptomatic *Trypanosoma rhodesiense* human infection in the Luangwa Valley (Zambia). *Trop Med Parasitol.* (1991) 42:389–93.

11

Indole Treatment Alleviates Intestinal Tissue Damage Induced by Chicken Coccidiosis Through Activation of the Aryl Hydrocarbon Receptor

Woo H. Kim[1], Hyun S. Lillehoj[1]* and Wongi Min[2]

[1] Animal Biosciences and Biotechnology Laboratory, U. S. Department of Agriculture, Beltsville Agricultural Research Center, ARS, Beltsville, MD, United States, [2] College of Veterinary Medicine and Institute of Animal Medicine, Gyeongsang National University, Jinju, South Korea

*Correspondence:
Hyun S. Lillehoj
hyun.lillehoj@ars.usda.gov

Indoles, as the ligands of aryl hydrocarbon receptor (AhR), have been shown to possess immune-modulating property in terms of the balancing between regulatory T cells (Treg) and T helper 17 cells (Th17) activities. In the present study, we examined the effects of dietary indoles, 3,3′-diindolylmethane (DIM) and indole-3-carbinol (I3C), on CD4$^+$T cell population and functions in chickens. Furthermore, the effects of dietary DIM treatment on chicken coccidiosis caused by an apicomplexan parasite were investigated. Dietary treatment of healthy chickens with DIM and I3C induced increased CD4$^+$CD25$^+$ (Treg) cells and the mRNA expression of IL-10, while decreasing number of CD4$^+$IL-17A$^+$ (Th17) cells and Th17-related cytokines transcripts expression in the intestine. In addition, we explored the role of AhR in indole-treated splenic lymphocytes by using AhR antagonist and our results suggested that DIM is a ligand for chicken AhR. In chicken coccidiosis, treatment of DIM increased the ratio of Treg/Th17 cells and significantly reduced intestinal lesion although no significant changes in body weight and fecal oocyst production were noted compared to non-treated control group. These results indicate that DIM is likely to affect the ratios of Treg/Th17 reducing the level of local inflammatory response induced by *Eimeria* or facilitate repairing process of inflamed gut following *Eimeria* infection. The results described herein are thus consistent with the concept that AhR ligand modulates the T cell immunity through the alteration of Treg/Th17 cells with Treg dominance. To our knowledge, present study is the first scientific report showing the effects of dietary indole on T cell immunity in poultry species.

Keywords: indole, CD4$^+$ T cells, Treg cells, Th17 cells, chicken, coccidiosis

INTRODUCTION

Coccidiosis which is caused by apicomplexan protozoan parasites of *Eimeria* spp. is one of the most economically important diseases affecting poultry production (1). After chickens ingest sporulated oocysts, sporozoites are released in the intestinal tract, invading intestinal epithelial cells for intracellular development. Invasion and egress of sporozoites and merozoites, which are, two major invasive form of *Eimeria* lead to the destruction of the intestinal mucosa, thus resulting in local inflammation in the intestine (2). In *E. tenella*-infected chickens, the number of CD4$^+$ lymphocytes in the intestine significantly increases (3). Early studies have shown that T lymphocytes and their cytokines are essential for immunity against *Eimeria* infection in chickens

(4, 5). *Eimeria* infection elicits strong IFN-γ-driven immune responses by T cells, and it plays a crucial role in control of coccidiosis (6). However, a growing body of literature implicates Th17- and Treg-related cytokines in host defense by the intestinal lymphocytes during *Eimeria* infection in chickens (7–10).

Indoles are phytochemicals that are very common in the body and diet and are abundant in Brassica (cruciferous) vegetables, including broccoli, Brussels sprouts, cabbage, and cauliflower (11). After ingestion, indole compounds such as 3,3'-diindolymethane (DIM) and indole-3-carbinol (I3C) are converted from glucosinolates, which are abundant in cruciferous vegetables (11). Both DIM and I3C are ligands for the aryl hydrocarbon receptor (AhR) and have been found to exhibit anti-inflammatory and anticancer properties through AhR activation (12, 13). AhR is a ligand-activated transcription factor recognizing a consensus xenobiotic responsive element binding site located in the upstream regulatory regions of target genes including cytochrome P450 family 1 members such as CYP1A1 and CYP1A2 (14–16). Recently, several studies have focused on activation of AhR by indoles in $CD4^+$ T cell immunity; interestingly, the findings have indicated different effects on the differentiation of T cell subsets, particularly regulatory T (Treg) and T helper 17 (Th17) cells, depending on the type of indole, although the underlying mechanism is not fully established (17–21). For example, 6-formylindolo[3,2-b]carbazole (FICZ), the tryptophan photoproduct containing two indole rings, specifically induces the differentiation of Th17 cells (21–23), whereas DIM and I3C promote the generation of Treg cells and the suppression of Th17 cells (17, 18). Treg and Th17 cells are relatively newly described lineages of $CD4^+$ T helper cells. Although Treg and Th17 cells share a common precursor cell (the naïve CD4 T cell) and require a common tumor growth factor (TGF)-β signal for initial differentiation, Treg cells play a role in the maintenance of T cell homeostasis and regulation of self-tolerance, whereas Th17 cells are involved in the inflammatory response by producing proinflammatory cytokines such as interleukin (IL)-17. The interplay or balance between Treg and Th17 cells is a major factor in inflammation (24).

The effects of indole compounds in chickens and the roles of Treg and Th17 cells in chicken coccidiosis have not been extensively studied. Given the ability of indoles to regulate the T cell immune response and the importance of T cell immunity in coccidiosis, in the present study, we investigated whether dietary indoles might regulate $CD4^+$ T cell immunity in chicken coccidiosis. We hypothesized that DIM and I3C administered orally would activate AhR in chicken and lead to Treg-dominance, thereby decreasing the intestinal inflammatory response and preventing tissue damage.

MATERIALS AND METHODS

Reagents and Antibodies

DIM (D9568, CAS no. 1968-05-04) and I3C (I7256, CAS no. 700-06-1) were purchased from Sigma (St. Louis, MO). Both DIM and I3C were suspended in DMSO (D2650, Sigma) for *in vitro* studies and diluted with corn oil purchased from a local market

for *in vivo* studies. Concanavalin A (Con A, C5275), phorbol-12-myristate-13-acetate (PMA, P8139) ionomycin (I9657), and CH223191 (C8124) were purchased from Sigma. Antibodies (Abs) with the following specificities were used for flow cytometry: CD4-PE (CT-4), CD8-Alexa Fluor 700 (CT-8), CD3-Pacific blue (CT-3), and CD45-APC (LT40) (Southern Biotech, Birmingham, AL). The following antibodies were purified and conjugated in-house: CD25-FITC (#32) and IL-17A-FITC (1G8) (25, 26).

Chickens

Newly hatched broiler chickens (Ross/Ross) were purchased from Longnecker's Hatchery (Elizabethtown, PA) and housed in electrically heated battery starter cages (Petersime, Gettysburg, OH). All chickens were raised in starter cages until 14 days of age and transferred to finisher cages, where they were kept until they are sacrificed. Feed and water were provided *ad libitum* under coccidian-free conditions. We used 150 birds for *in vivo* *E. tenella* infection study and another 12 healthy birds were used for preparation of lymphocytes from spleen and cecal tonsil. Animal husbandry followed the guidelines for the care and use of animals in agricultural research. All experiments were approved and followed by the United States Department of Agriculture (USDA)-Agricultural Research Service Beltsville Institutional Animal Care and Use Committee (protocol number: 18-019).

Cell Culture

Chicken primary lymphocytes from cecal tonsils or spleen were isolated as previously described with modifications (8). Briefly, spleen and cecal tonsils were collected aseptically from healthy chicken and homogenized using gentleMACS Dissociator (Miltenyi Biotec, Gaithersburg, USA). The lymphocytes were purified by a Histopaque-1077(Sigma) density gradient method. Freshly purified primary lymphocytes from cecal tonsils or spleen were cultured in complete RPMI-1640 (GE Healthcare, Pittsburgh, PA) supplemented with 10% FBS (GE Healthcare), penicillin/streptomycin (10,000 unit/ml, Invitrogen, Carlsbad, CA), 50 μg/ml gentamycin (Sigma), 25 mM HEPES (Gibco, Gaithersburg, MD), and 55 μM 2-Mercaptoethanol (Gibco). For sporozoite viability test, chicken epithelial cell line (MM-CHiC clone, 8E11) was purchased and cultured in DMEM/F-12 (1:1, Sigma) supplemented with 2 mM L-glutamine (Sigma), 10 % FBS, and 10,000 unit/ml penicillin/streptomycin.

Parasite Propagation and Preparation of Sporozoite Antigen

To obtain sporulated *E. tenella* oocysts (ARS strain) for *in vivo* study, unsporulated were purified from the feces of infected chickens, and sporulation was conducted with incubation in 2.5% potassium dichromate solution for 48 h. Sporozoites of *E. tenella* were obtained by excystation of sporulated oocysts (27). Briefly, freshly sporulated oocysts were disrupted with 0.5-mm glass beads for 5–7 s by using a Mini-beadbeater (BioSpec Products, Bartlesville, OK). The released sporocysts were purified by isopycnic centrifugation in a Percoll gradient and washed in ice-cold Hank's balanced salt solution (HBSS, Sigma), and the excystation of sporozoites was induced by treatment with 0.25%

trypsin and 0.014 M taurocholic acid (Sigma) at 41°C for 90 min. The excysted sporozoites were collected, washed three times with HBSS at 3,000 × g for 10 min at 4°C and resuspended to 1.0 × 10^7/ml in HBSS. *E. tenella* sporozoite antigen (EtSzAg) was obtained through a series of sonication and freeze and thaw cycles followed by filtration with a 0.22 μm filter. The concentration was measured with a Pierce BCA Protein Assay kit (Thermo Fisher Scientific, Frederick, MD), and samples were stored at −80°C until use.

Intracellular Staining and Flow Cytometry

For the intracellular staining of IL-17A, lymphocytes were stimulated with PMA (10 ng/ml) and ionomycin (500 μg/ml) in complete RPMI-1640 for 4 h in the presence of golgiplug (1 μl/1 × 10^6 cells, BD, Franklin Lakes, NJ). Cells were analyzed with a Cytoflex flow cytometer (Beckman Coulter, Brea, CA). Lymphocytes from single-cell suspensions were identified according to their light scattering properties and the CD45+ population. Potential doublet cells were discriminated by FSC-H/FSC-W, and dead cells were excluded by using Fixable Viability Stain 780 (BD). Treg cells and Th17 cells were designated as CD45+CD3+CD4+CD25+ and CD45+CD3+CD4+IL-17A+ cells, respectively. Unfortunately, foxp3, a signature transcription factor for Treg, has not been cloned in chickens; thus, we had to consider the CD4+CD25+ phenotype as being indicative of Treg cells (28, 29).

Quantitative Real-Time PCR

RNA was isolated from primary lymphocytes from the cecal tonsils or spleen by using an RNeasy Isolation Kit (Qiagen, Germantown, MD), per the manufacturer's instructions, then treated with RNase-free DNase (Qiagen) and eluted in RNase-free water (Qiagen). The concentration and purity of the RNA were measured using a NanoDrop spectrophotometer (Thermo Fisher Scientific). cDNA was synthesized using random hexamer primers and a QuantiTect Reverse Transcription Kit (Qiagen). Real-time RT-PCR was performed using a Stratagene Mx3000P thermocycler (Agilent Technologies, USA) with a QuantiTect SYBR Green PCR Kit (Qiagen) and the various chicken chemokine and cytokine primers listed in **Table 1**. A melting curve was obtained at the end of each run to verify the presence of a single amplification product without primer dimers. Standard curves were generated using serial five-fold dilutions of cDNA to validate the amplification efficiency. The fold changes in each transcript were normalized to β-actin and are reported relative to the transcript expression in the vehicle control group or non-infected group (normalized to 1), on the basis of the comparative ΔΔCt method, as previously described (27).

Eimeria tenella Infection Model

For *in vivo* study, One-hundred-fifty 1-day-old birds were randomly distributed into five groups (n = 30): non-infected control (NI), non-infected, DIM treated (NIDIM), *E. tenella*-infected (ET), *E. tenella*-infected, vehicle treated (ETVH), and *E. tenella*-infected, DIM treated (ETDIM). The schematic outline of *in vivo* study is shown in **Figure 4A**. The chickens in ET, ETVH and ETDIM groups were orally infected with *E. tenella*

TABLE 1 | List of quantitative real-time RT-PCR primers used in this study.

Target	Primer and sequence	References
IL-10	(For) 5′-ACATCCAACTGCTCAGCTCT-3′	(30)
	(Rev) 5′-ATGCTCTGCTGATGACTGGT-3′	
IL-17A	(For) 5′-GAGAAGAGTGGTGGGAAAG-3′	(31)
	(Rev) 5′-TCTACAAACTTGTTTATCAGCAT-3′	
IL-17F	(For) 5′-TGAAGACTGCCTGAACCA-3-3′	(31)
	(Rev) 5′-AGAGACCGATTCCTGATGT-3′	
IL-21	(For) 5′-CAACTTCACCAAAAGCAATGAAAT-3′	(32)
	(Rev) 5′-ATCCATCCCCAGGGTTTTCT-3′	
IL-22	(For) 5′-TGTTGTTGCTGTTTCCCTCTTC-3′	(33)
	(Rev) 5′-CACCCCTGTCCCTTTTGGA-3′	
CYP1A4	(For) 5′-CCGTGACAACCGCCCTGTCC-3′	(34)
	(Rev) 5′-GAGTTCGGTGCCGGCTGCAT-3′	
CYP1A5	(For) 5′-GGACCGTTGCGTGTTTAT-3′	(35)
	(Rev) 5′-CTCCCACTTGCCTATGTTTT-3′	
IL-1β	(For) 5′-TGGGCATCAAGGGCTACA-3′	(31)
	(Rev) 5′-CGGCCCACGTAGTAAATGAT-3′	
IL-6	(For) 5′-CAAGGTGACGGAGGAGGAC-3′	(31)
	(Rev) 5′-TGGCGAGGAGGGGATTTCT-3′	
CXCLi2	(For) 5′-GGCTTGCTAGGGGAAATGA-3′	(31)
	(Rev) 5′-AGCTGACTCTGACTAGGAAACTGT-3′	
TL1A	(For) 5′-CCTGAGTTATTCCAGCAACGCA-3′	(36)
	(Rev) 5′-ATCCACCAGCTTGATGTCACTAAC-3′	
JAM2	(For) 5′-AGCCTCAAATGGGATTGGATT-3′	(37)
	(Rev) 5′-CATCAACTTGCATTCGCTTCA-3′	
ZO1	(For) 5′-CCGCAGTCGTTCACGATCT-3′	(37)
	(Rev) 5′-GGAGAATGTCTGGAATGGTCTGA-3′	
β-actin	(For) 5′-CACAGATCATGTTTGAGACCTT-3′	(38)
	(Rev) 5′-CATCACAATACCAGTGGTACG-3′	

sporulated oocysts (1 × 10^4/bird) at 7 days old and the other groups were given HBSS as a control. The chickens in the NIDIM and ETDIM groups were treated every other day (starting at 5 days old) with DIM (200 mg/kg) and the other groups were given corn oil as a vehicle control by oral gavage until the end of experimental period (20 days old). Body weight gain (BWG) was measured at 0 and 13 days post infection (DPI) (n = 15). Cecal tissues were collected from four chickens of each group at 1, 4, 7, 10, and 13 days post infection (DPI) to extract RNA, and the expression of Treg- and Th17-related mRNAs was analyzed (n = 4). Five chickens from each group were randomly selected for gut lesion scoring in the cecum at 7 DPI (n = 5). Lesion scores were evaluated by three independent observers based on scoring techniques previously described (39). Each chicken received a numerical value from 0 to 4. Same cecal samples were used for histological examination (n = 5). Briefly, the tissues were fixed in 4% paraformaldehyde (Sigma), and paraffin blocks were prepared, microtome sections were made, and sections were stained using hematoxylin and eosin. The sections were examined for intestinal structure, parasites and infiltration of inflammatory cells using an Eclipse 80i microscope (Nikon, Japan). To count fecal *Eimeria* oocyst shedding, collection of feces from three cages of each group was started at 5 DPI until

9 DPI ($n = 3$), and the number of *E. tenella* oocyst in the feces was calculated, as previously described, by using a McMaster counting chamber (Marienfeld-Superior, Germany) (40). The total number of oocysts was calculated according to the following formula: total oocysts = oocysts counted × dilution factor × fecal sample volume/counting chamber volume. The values were converted as oocyst per gram of feces.

Sporozoite Viability Test

To assess the viability of sporozoites, purified sporozoites were incubated with DIM (0–500 μM) for 24 h, the viability was measured using CyQuant direct cell proliferation assay (41). To infect sporozoites into chicken epithelial cell line (8E11), purified sporozoites were stained with carboxyfluorescein succinimidyl ester (CFSE, Thermo Fisher Scientific) according to manufacturer's instructions. 8E11 was cultured in DMEM/F12 supplemented with 10% FBS, penicillin/streptomycin, and 25 mM HEPES and the sporozoites was infected at a multiplicity of infection of 1.0 (sporozoite/cell ratio of 1:1). Free sporozoites were washed after 3 h incubation and new media was replaced. After further incubation for 21 h, the number of sporozoites was measured at 485/528 nm.

Statistical Analysis

The data were analyzed using Prism Version 5.01 (GraphPad Software, La Jolla, CA). The normality of each data was tested by Kolmogorov–Smirnov test. Parametric tests were used to compare between groups with one-way ANOVA and Dunnett's multiple comparison test and non-parametric tests were conducted with Kruskal–Wallis test and Dunn's multiple comparison test. The data are expressed as the mean ± standard error for parametric analysis and median with interquartile range for non-parametric analysis and the differences were considered significant at $p < 0.05$ or $p < 0.01$.

RESULTS

Increased Treg Cells and Th17/Treg Ratio in Indole-Treated Chickens

To determine the dietary effects of indole treatment on CD4[+] T cells in healthy chickens, we firstly investigated the frequencies of CD4[+]CD25[+] (Treg) and CD4[+]IL-17A[+] (Th17) cells from the spleen and intestine after oral treatment of either DIM or I3C. In the indole-treated groups compared with the vehicle control group, Treg cells were significantly higher, whereas the treatment with indoles induced a decrease in Th17 cells in both the spleen and cecal tonsils (**Figures 1A,B**). The ratio of Th17/Treg cells decreased in both indole-treated groups (**Figure 1C**). There was no significant difference in the frequencies of Treg or Th17 cells between the treatments with DIM and I3C. Furthermore, the real-time qPCR results showed that indoles increased the mRNA expression of the Treg-related cytokine IL-10 and decreased Th17-related cytokines such as IL-17F, IL-21, and IL-22 in cecal tonsils (**Figure 1D**).

The *in vitro* Effects of Indoles on Treg Cells and Aryl Hydrocarbon Receptor

To validate *in vivo* findings on the role of indoles on CD4+ T cell subsets, we performed *in vitro* experiments to investigate the effects of indole treatment on Treg cells in chicken lymphocytes. Chicken splenic lymphocytes were purified and stimulated with Con A or EtSzAg in the presence or absence of both indoles for 72 h. The data indicated that cell proliferation induced by Con A was inhibited by both DIM or I3C, as compared with the results for Con A-stimulated cells. Interestingly, indole treatment also inhibited the proliferation induced by EtSzAg, thus suggesting a role in coccidiosis in chickens (**Figure 2A**). We further investigated the mRNA expression of Treg-related (IL-10) or Th17-related (IL-17A) cytokine mRNAs in those cells. Both indole treatments significantly up-regulated expression of IL-10 while down-regulating IL-17A (**Figures 2B,C**). In agreement with data from *in vivo* experiments, the proportion of Treg cells in *in vitro* assays was increased in splenic lymphocytes incubated with DIM or I3C (**Figure 2D**). To test the hypothesis that indoles are ligands for AhR and can cause AhR activation in chickens as in mammals (42), we determined the mRNA expression levels of the chicken cytochrome P-450 enzymes CYP1A4 and CYP1A5, which are orthologous to mammalian CYP1A1 and CYP1A2, in indole-treated cecal tonsil lymphocytes. Both are AhR-regulated genes and markers of AhR activation (43). As shown in **Figure 3A**, the expression of CYP1A4 and CYP1A5 increased after treatment with DIM or I3C, and normal expression was restored in the presence of the AhR-specific antagonist CH223191 (**Figure 3A**). Furthermore, the frequency of Treg cells was higher in DIM-treated cecal tonsil lymphocytes than in non-treated cells in the presence of CH223191 (**Figure 3B**).

Effects of DIM on Treg and Th17 Cells in *E. tenella* Infection

Because our findings indicated that indoles induced Treg cells while suppressing Th17 cells in chickens, and Th17 is known to play a pathological role in coccidiosis (7, 44), we designed the *in vivo* experiment to determine the effect of DIM on the regulation of CD4[+] T cells in *E. tenella* infection in chickens (**Figure 4A**). Treatment of chickens with DIM, compared with vehicle control, induced a significant increase in intestinal Treg cells while decreasing Th17 cells. Compared with the ET group, the ETDIM group showed an increase in Treg cells at from 4 DPI, and Treg cells remained elevated until the end of experiment, whereas the decrease in Th17 cells was seen only early in infection, such as at 4 DPI (**Figures 4B,C**). The ratio of Th17/Treg cells exhibited significant decrease at 1, 4, and 7 DPI (**Figure 4D**). We also found that DIM inhibited the proliferation of lymphocytes. As shown in **Figure 4E**, the ETDIM group showed lower proliferation than the other groups during the re-activation of the lymphocytes with DIM *in vitro*. Notably, the NIDIM group did not show any significant inhibition of proliferation, thus suggesting that the inhibitory effect of DIM is much stronger when the lymphocytes are pre-activated with *Eimeria* antigen.

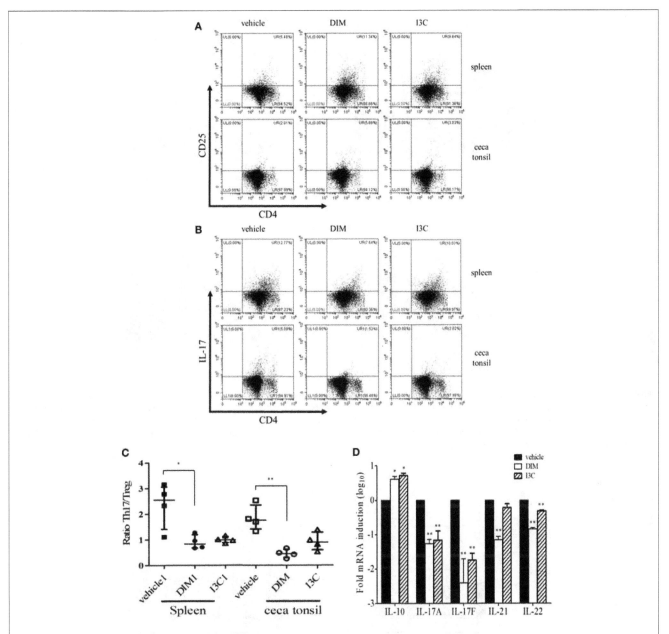

FIGURE 1 | Effects of indoles to induce Treg cells in indole-treated chickens. Two-weeks-old chickens were given orally corn oil as a vehicle control, DIM (200 mg/kg), or I3C (200 mg/kg) for 14 days on a daily basis. Lymphocytes were isolated from the spleen and cecal tonsils, and stained with CD3, CD45, CD4, and CD25, or CD3, CD45, CD4, and IL-17A for analyzing Treg **(A)** and Th17 **(B)** populations, respectively, and gated CD4+ T cells. Cells were stimulated with PMA and ionomycin for the determination of Th17 cells. Data show the representative staining from two independent experiments. **(C)** The ratio of Th17/Treg cells in the spleen and cecal tonsils. The data represent median with interquartile range after Kruskal-Wallis test with Dunn's multiple comparison test. **(D)** RNA was isolated from cecal tonsils and used for real-time qPCR to measure Treg- (IL-10) and Th17-related (IL-17A, IL-17F, IL-21, and IL-22) mRNA expression. The data represent the mean ± SE from two independent experiments. *$p < 0.05$ and **$p < 0.01$ were considered statistically significant compared to the vehicle control in each sample or target.

mRNA Expression of Treg- and Th17-Related Genes in DIM-Treated Chickens

To determine the cytokines involved in T cell regulation by DIM, we carried out real-time qPCR to measure the mRNA expression of Treg- and Th17-related genes in T cells. In agreement with our *in vitro* findings, the expression of IL-10 increased after treatment of DIM. Following *E. tenella* infection, IL-10 expression increased in the ET group and the increased IL-10 expression in the ET groups persisted until the end of the experiment. Compared with DIM, ETDIM induced greater IL-10 expression after 1 DPI, thus suggesting that DIM induces more Treg cells in coccidiosis (**Figure 5A**). However, the expression of Th17-related cytokines was generally down-regulated in the DIM and ETDIM

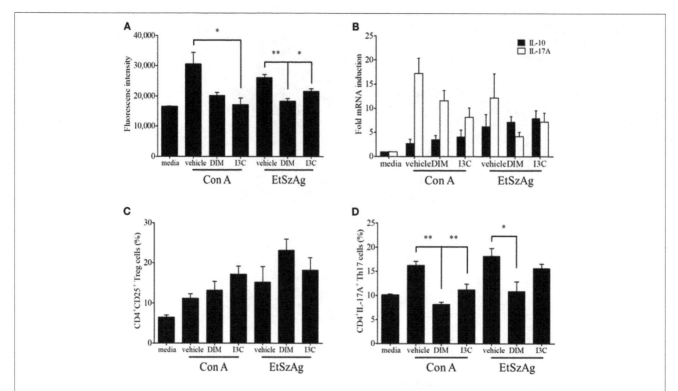

FIGURE 2 | Effects of indoles to induce Treg cells *in vitro*. **(A)** Lymphocytes from spleen of healthy chickens were isolated and stimulated with DMSO as a vehicle control, DIM (100 μM), or I3C (100 μM) in the presence of Con A (10 μg/ml) or EtSzAg for 24 h and the proliferation was measured by CyQuant direct cell proliferation assay. **(B)** The mRNA expressions of Treg- and Th17-related cytokine were measured after 24 h by real-time qPCR. The frequency of Treg **(C)** and Th17 cells **(D)** were analyzed by flow cytometry. The data represent the mean ± SE from two independent experiments. *p < 0.05 and **p < 0.01 were considered statistically significant compared to the vehicle control of each treatment.

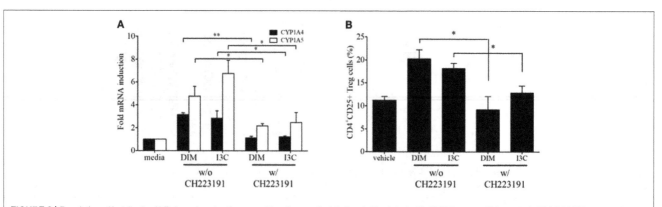

FIGURE 3 | Regulation of indoles by AhR. Lymphocytes from cecal tonsils were isolated and stimulated with DMSO as a vehicle control, DIM (100 M/ml), or I3C (100 M/ml) in the absence of presence of specific AhR antagonist, CH223191 for 24 h. **(A)** The mRNA expressions of CYP1A4 and CYP1A5 were measure by real-time qPCR. **(B)** The frequency of Treg cells were analyzed by flow cytometry. The data represent the mean ± SE from two independent experiments. *p < 0.05 and **p < 0.01 were considered statistically significant compared to the samples.

groups (**Figure 5B**). Interestingly, we found high expression of IL-17A in the ET group between 7 and 13 DPI, but the increases in expression of these cytokines were diminished in the ETDIM group (**Figure 5B**). These results suggest that *E. tenella* infection induces Th17 cells at a later stage of infection, and the suppression of Th17 cells by DIM seems to depend on the level of Th17 cytokine.

Effects of DIM on Growth Performance, Oocyst Production, and Intestinal Lesions

Next, we examined the effects of dietary DIM on BWG, oocyst production, and intestinal lesions in *E. tenella*-infected chickens. The NIDIM group showed no difference in BWG compared with the NI group, thus indicating that DIM has no effect on growth performance. Furthermore, the ETDIM and ET groups

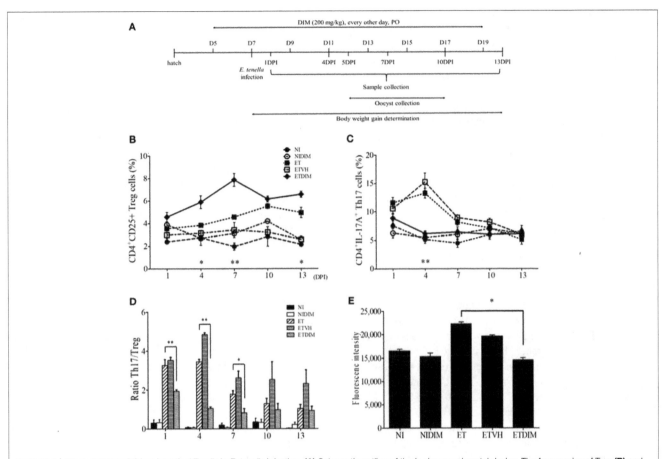

FIGURE 4 | Effect of dietary DIM on intestinal T cells in *E. tenella* infection. **(A)** Schematic outline of the *in vivo* experimental design. The frequencies of Treg **(B)** and Th17 cells **(C)** of cecal tonsil lymphocytes were analyzed at indicated DPIs by flow cytometry. *$p < 0.05$ and **$p < 0.01$ were considered statistically significant compared between the ET and ETDIM groups at each time point. **(D)** The ratio of Th17/Treg cells in and cecal tonsils. **(E)** Lymphocytes were stimulated with Con A (10 μg/ml) and the proliferation of cecal tonsil lymphocytes was measured by CyQuant direct cell proliferation assay in EtSzAg-activated cells. *$p < 0.05$ and **$p < 0.01$ were considered statistically significant compared to the samples.

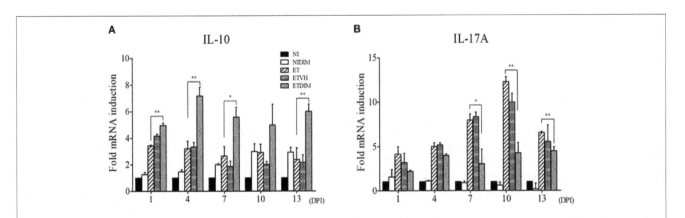

FIGURE 5 | Effect of dietary DIM on mRNA expressions of Treg- and Th17-related genes in *E. tenella* infection. The mRNA expressions of IL-10 **(A)** and IL-17A **(B)** were measure in cecal tonsils by real-time qPCR. The data represent the mean ± SE from two independent experiments. *$p < 0.05$ and **$p < 0.01$ were considered statistically significant compared to the samples.

showed comparable BWG (**Figure 6A**). In agreement with the BWG data, the ETDIM group, compared with the ET group, did not exhibit significantly less oocyst shedding from feces (**Figure 6B**). Interestingly, however, the severity of intestinal lesions was significantly lower in the ETDIM group than the ET group (**Figure 6C**). In H&E staining, the NI and NIDIM groups displayed a normal structure and no visible changes. In all ET groups, there was structural disorder, epithelial loss, and inflammatory cell infiltration; however, the ETDIM group showed less severity in terms of abnormality of villi structure and inflammatory cell number (**Figure 6D**). These has been validated by our histological finding that showed the gross morphological changes in the cecum of ETDIM group showed less hemorrhage in the mucosa and less watery ingesta mixed with mucus than did the ET group (data not shown).

mRNA Expression of Proinflammatory Genes in DIM-Treated Chickens

From the findings from our *in vivo* experiments, we hypothesized that DIM treatment decreases inflammation in the intestine through the regulation of Treg and Th17 cells. To this end, we determined the mRNA expression profiles of proinflammatory genes in intestinal tissues by using real-time qPCR. As expected, *E. tenella* infection induced robust expression of proinflammatory genes such as IL-1β, IL-6, and CXCLi2 (a homolog of mammalian CXCL8) but not TNFSF15 (TL1A, a functional homolog of mammalian TNF-α) (36). Compared with the ET group, the ETDIM group showed lower expression of those genes (**Figure 7A**). Next, we measured the expression of tight junction proteins such as JAM2, and ZO1 to determine whether DIM treatment is involved in intestinal barrier function. Following *E. tenella* infection, mRNA expression of JAM2, and ZO1 significantly decreased, but their expression was restored to a much greater extent in the ETDIM group than the ET or ETVEH groups (**Figure 7B**). Together, these results suggest that treatment of DIM in coccidiosis may be beneficial to reduce intestinal inflammation and to help to restore the damage from coccidiosis.

Direct Effect of DIM on *E. tenella*

Finally, we determined whether DIM has any direct activity against *Eimeria* sporozoites, an invasive form of parasites. First, we incubated *E. tenella* sporozoites with various concentrations of DIM. **Figure 8A** shows that DIM had no effect on sporozoites viability. Second, we infected sporozoites to the chicken epithelial cell line 8E11, then treated DIM to the cells harboring sporozoites. DIM treatment did not alter the viability of sporozoites inside of cells (**Figure 8B**). It suggests that the beneficial effects of DIM on *E. tenella* infection are not associated with its activity against parasite itself.

DISCUSSION

I3C is derived from cruciferous vegetables, which contain abundant indoles. When digested, it produces several biologically active I3C oligomers such as DIM. Earlier studies of dietary indole derivatives have focused on their anti-cancer effect, given that they have been shown to reduce the risk of cancer (45–47). Indoles have been shown to induce antioxidant activity and apoptosis of cancer cells, and to regulate hormone metabolism (48–51). Recently, several studies have reported that indoles also have immunoregulatory properties, especially on T cells. For example, Singh et al. (17) have reported that dietary indoles suppress the delayed-type hypersensitivity (DTH) response through the regulation of Treg and Th17 cells in mice. Dietary supplementation of indoles also has been shown to suppress neuroinflammation by induction of reciprocal differentiation of Treg and Th17 cells in experimental autoimmune encephalomyelitis (EAE) mice (18). These abilities of indoles to modulate the immune response are related to AhR signaling (21). AhR was first discovered as a transcription factor mediating the toxicity of chemicals such as 2,3,7,8-tetrachlorodibenzo-*p*-dioxin (TCDD) (52). Recent studies have suggested that AhR activation plays diverse roles in cellular function including the regulation of the immune system (53, 54). Interestingly, there are two types of AhR found in chickens, AhR1 and AhR2, and AhR1 is the dominant form in cormorants (*Phalacrocorax carbo*) (55). In the chicken intestine, both mRNA were expressed; however further studies will be required to elucidate their role in T cell regulation (56). Moreover, there is a distinct set of cytochrome P450 family members in chickens: CYP1A4 and CYP1A5. On the basis of their amino acid sequences, they can be classified in the CYP1A family, but both are more like CYP1A1 than CYP1A2 (57). Because they are induced by AhR activation in chickens (34, 58), we identified their expression levels after DIM treatment in cecal tonsil lymphocytes. Inhibition assays using AhR-specific inhibitor confirmed that DIM and its precursor I3C induce AhR activation in chickens. Unfortunately, we did not find any evidence of an effect of chicken CYP1As on T cell regulation, thus suggesting that the mechanism of AhR activation in modulating Treg and Th17 cells may differ from the one that mediating the toxicity of environmental toxins. Quintana et al. (21) have identified an evolutionarily conserved binding site for AhR in the foxp3 gene and three non-evolutionarily conserved AhR-binding sites in the promoter regions of foxp3 genes in zebrafish, mice, and humans. Their subsequence studies proved that AhR controls foxp3 expression, which induces the generation of Treg cells. Another report has explained the possible AhR activation mechanism. Singh et al. (17) have investigated microRNA profiles in DTH mice treated with several AhR ligands and found that several microRNAs targeting foxp3 and IL-17 mRNA are important in regulating Treg and Th17 cells. The activation of AhR to regulate T cells is dependent on the type of AhR ligands. For example, TCDD induces Treg cells in EAE mice to reduce the EAE score, whereas FICZ increases Th17 cell differentiation and the severity of EAE (21, 59). DIM, an AhR ligand that we used in this study, has therapeutic effects in oxazolone-induced colitis and mBSA-induced DTH in mice through Treg cell induction and suppression of Th2 or Th17 cells (17, 60). In chickens, compared to mammals, very little is known about the effect of dietary indoles as AhR ligands on the immune response. In this study, we provide the first demonstration in chickens of

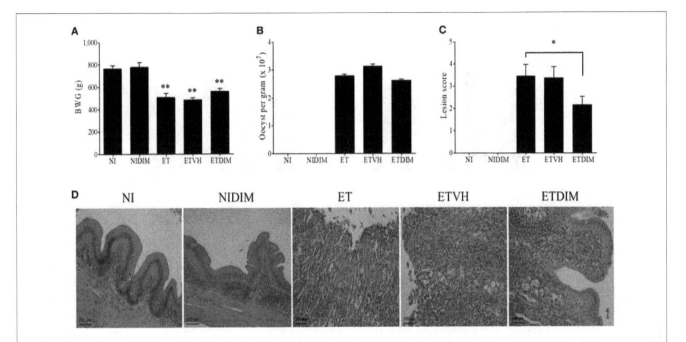

FIGURE 6 | Effect of dietary DIM on growth performance, oocyst production and intestinal lesions in *E. tenella* infection. **(A)** Body weight gain was measured from 0 to 13 DPI ($n = 15$). **(B)** Fecal oocysts were collected and pooled from 5 to 9 DPI and counted using McMaster counting chamber ($n = 15$). *$p < 0.05$ and **$p < 0.01$ were considered statistically significant compared to the samples. **(C)** Lesion score was determined from cecum at 7 DPI ($n = 5$). **(D)** Histological sections prepared from the cecum (X400).

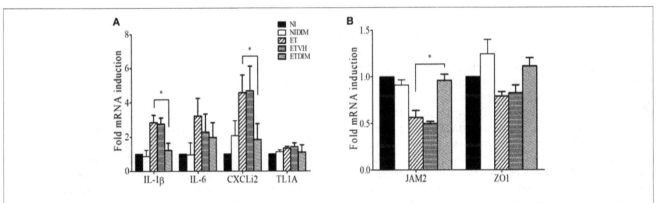

FIGURE 7 | Effect of dietary DIM on mRNA expressions of proinflammatory and tight junction protein genes in *E. tenella* infection. The mRNA expressions of proinflammatory genes; IL-1β, IL-6, CXCLi2, and TL1A **(A)** and tight junction protein gene; JAM2 and ZO1 **(B)** were measure in cecum by real-time qPCR. *$p < 0.05$ and was considered statistically significant compared to the samples.

how AhR ligand modulates T cells in terms of Treg and Th17 cells. As we expected, DIM and I3C increased the number of CD4$^+$CD25$^+$ cells in chicken lymphocytes *in vivo* as well as *in vitro*, thus suggesting that they have comparable effects to those in mammals. Regarding the Th17 cells, the data showed a decrease in CD4$^+$IL-17A$^+$ cells, but to a lesser extent than the increase in intestinal Treg cells. Moreover, the expression of each lineage of Th cell-related cytokines was consistent with data obtained from flow cytometry. The anti-inflammatory cytokine IL-10 showed increased expression in DIM-treated groups, whereas the expression of the IL-17A, IL-17F, IL-21, and IL-22 was downregulated in the DIM-treated groups. These data

suggest that the cytokine profile for each Th lineage is likely to overlap in chickens and mammals.

We further investigated the effects of indole in regulating Treg and Th17 cells in coccidiosis. Coccidiosis caused by *Eimeria* spp. induces an inflammatory response in parasitized intestinal tissues (61). Profiling of cytokines in coccidiosis revealed that most T cell cytokines are increased along with the inflammation in the intestine (62, 63). Moreover, our previous studies have indicated that Th17-related cytokines such as IL-17A and IL-17F, and IL-17 receptor signaling are involved in inflammation induced by coccidiosis, although the predominant protective response in coccidiosis is considered to be an IFN-γ-related

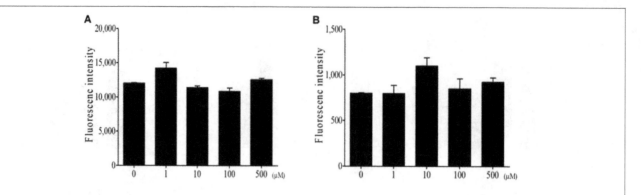

FIGURE 8 | Direct effect of DIM on *E. tenella* parasite. **(A)** DIM was incubated with *E. tenella* sporozoites for 24 h and measured viability using CyQuant direct cell proliferation assay. **(B)** *E. tenella* sporozoites were stained with CFSE and infected to intestinal epithelial cells (8E11). Following infection, DIM was treated and fluorescence was measured. The data represent the mean ± SE from two independent experiments.

Th1 response (6, 8, 31, 64). We investigated the changes in Th1 cells as CD4$^+$IFN-γ^+ cells in *E. tenella* infection. Initially, we expected that DIM would also affect the Th1 response, because several studies have shown that AhR agonists can also modulate the differentiation of Th1 cells (65, 66). As shown in **Figure S1**, Th1 cells were highly induced at 1 and 4 DPI following *E. tenella* infection although they did not change as much as Treg and Th17 cells in the DIM-treated groups. Therefore, Th1 response may play a role during the early phase of coccidiosis by initiating local inflammatory response started by the host cell invasion of sporozoites of *Eimeria* with subsequent intracellular development in early to intermediate phase. Compared to the NI group, Treg and Th17 cells in the ET groups were induced in a later phase, thus suggesting that they might be involved in tissue recovery from the damage induced by Th17 responses or have an important function in gut homeostasis. Several studies have reported that chicken IL-17A plays a pathogenic role in *Eimeria* infection (7, 44). Likewise, in the ETDIM group, which showed a lower degree of intestinal lesions, Th17 cells were downregulated compared with their levels in the NI or DIM group, and it is likely Th17 cells are involved in pathogenicity or inhibiting recovery from inflammation. At the same time points, Treg cells showed increased populations in the ETDIM group, thus indicating that DIM increased the Treg populations and decreased the inflammation in the parasitized intestine. IL-10 has been considered to play an important role to evade host immune response in coccidiosis. One possible mechanism is that coccidial parasites have evolved to stimulate Treg cells to express IL-10 and it helps parasites to facilitate invasion and survival in chickens through the suppression of protective response mediating IFN-γ-expressing Th1 cells. Using two inbred lines of chicken differing in their resistance or susceptibility to *Eimeria* infection, it is revealed that the expression of IL-10 was the major difference between those two lines. The expression of IL-10 was highly induced in susceptible line of chickens among the genes related to different helper T cell lineages such as IFN-γ for Th1, IL-4 for Th2, and IL-10 and TGF-β for Treg cells while it is suppressed in age-matched resistant line (10). The administration of IL-10 antibody in *Eimeria*-infected chicken showed improved

growth rate compared to control antibody group but it did not influence fecal oocyst production (67, 68). These results are indicating that the regulation of protective immune response to *Eimeria* spp. by Treg cells is critical and IL-10 contributes to pathogenesis in coccidiosis. In the current study, on the other aspect of Treg cells, we found another role of Treg cells that involves in anti-inflammatory response through suppress inflammatory Th17 cells. It is thought that the anti-inflammatory Treg cells could be participate in the self-limiting mechanism of *Eimeria* spp. that prevents the collateral intestinal damage caused by exaggerated inflammation. Other evidences of reduced intestinal inflammation we found in this study was the expression of proinflammatory genes and tight junction protein. Chicken IL-17A and IL-17F have known to induce proinflammatory cytokines such as IL-1β, IL-6, and CXCLi2 as in mammals (31) thus decrease of Th17 cytokines might involve the anti-inflammatory process in the intestine. As a marker of intestinal integrity, tight junction protein play an important role in the regulation of intestinal permeability by sealing the paracellular space between intestinal epithelial cells (69). The recovery of tight junction protein expressions was induced by dietary treatment of DIM and it might be associated with that mammalian IL-17A and IL-17F reported to disrupt the distribution of tight junction protein (70).

As the main source of indoles in cruciferous vegetables, Glucosinolates (GLS) have been used to measure the biologically active constituent. McNaughton and Mark reported GLS content of various cruciferous vegetables (71). It varies depending on the species (e.g., cress for the highest GLS content as 389 mg/100 g while the lowest content for Pe-tsai chinese cabbage; 20 mg/100 g) and there is large variation in the values reported for the same vegetable by different studies (71, 72). Since the US Food and Drug Administration permitted the use of claims acknowledging the relationship between increased vegetable consumption and decreased cancer risk in 1993, there has been a growing literature reporting human health benefits of cruciferous vegetables, more specifically, indoles (73, 74). In poultry research, however, there is a lack of information of the effects of any forms of indole supplementation. In addition, the production of indoles, especially food-grade indole naturally derived is very highly priced, due to an expensive chemical conversion process which makes commercial chicken supplementation unfeasible at this phase. Nonetheless, the present study could support the scientific evidences for beneficial effects of indole supplementation in human as well as animal. From the present study, DIM treatment exhibited significantly upregulated Treg cells and IL-10 expression in *Eimeria*-infected chicken while DIM-treated chickens with no *Eimeria* infection did not increase as much as the group infected indicating that DIM likely displays of better effectiveness in *Eimeira*-infected gut rather than those of healthy ones. In the approach to such a drug to prevent/treat chicken gut inflamed by coccidiosis, indoles might have potentials since coccidiosis is considered one of most problematic disease in the poultry industry.

In summary, this is the first evidence to show the effect of dietary indole in reducing intestinal damage induced by coccidiosis in chickens occurs through the regulation of Treg and Th17 cells in the intestine. Because of the lack of immune reagents to detect chicken cytokines related to the T cell response, the study of T cell immunology in chickens has been lagging far behind that in mammals. In this study, we validated that monoclonal antibodies which we previously developed (6, 26) for flow cytometry application could be easily applied to study T cell immune response by determining specific cytokine-expressing T cell phenotypes and in our knowledge, this is the first report to stain chicken lymphocytes with four different fluorescent dyes.

AUTHOR CONTRIBUTIONS

WK designed the project, performed the experiments, analyzed the data, and wrote the manuscript. HL supervised the research. WM and HL revised the manuscript.

REFERENCES

1. Shirley MW, Lillehoj HS. The long view: a selective review of 40 years of coccidiosis research. *Avian Pathol.* (2012) 41:111–21. doi: 10.1080/03079457.2012.666338
2. Dong X, Abdelnabi GH, Lee SH, Li G, Jin H, Lillehoj HS, et al. Enhanced Egress of Intracellular *Eimeria tenella* Sporozoites by splenic lymphocytes from coccidian-infected chickens. *Infect Immun.* (2011) 79:3465–70. doi: 10.1128/IAI.01334-10
3. Vervelde L, Vermeulen AN, Jeurissen SH. *In situ* characterization of leucocyte subpopulations after infection with *Eimeria tenella* in chickens. *Parasite Immunol.* (1996) 18:247–56.
4. Wakelin D, Rose ME, Hesketh P, Else KJ, Grencis RK. Immunity to coccidiosis: genetic influences on lymphocyte and cytokine responses to infection with *Eimeria vermiformis* in inbred mice. *Parasite Immunol.* (1993) 15:11–9.
5. Lillehoj HS, Trout JM. CD8+ T cell-coccidia interactions. *Parasitol Today.* (1994) 10:10–4.
6. Yun CH, Lillehoj HS, Choi KD. *Eimeria tenella* infection induces local gamma interferon production and intestinal lymphocyte subpopulation changes. *Infect Immun.* (2000) 68:1282–8. doi: 10.1128/IAI.68.3.1282-1288.2000
7. Zhang L, Liu R, Song M, Hu Y, Pan B, Cai J, Wang M. *Eimeria tenella*: interleukin 17 contributes to host immunopathology in the gut during experimental infection. *Exp Parasitol.* (2013) 133:121–30. doi: 10.1016/j.exppara.2012.11.009
8. Kim WH, Jeong J, Park AR, Yim D, Kim S, Chang HH, et al. Downregulation of chicken interleukin-17 receptor A during *Eimeria* infection. *Infect Immun.* (2014) 82:3845–54. doi: 10.1128/IAI.02141-14
9. Min W, Kim WH, Lillehoj EP, Lillehoj HS. Recent progress in host immunity to avian coccidiosis: IL-17 family cytokines as sentinels of the intestinal mucosa. *Dev Comp Immunol.* (2013) 41:418–428. doi: 10.1016/j.dci.2013.04.003
10. Rothwell L, Young JR, Zoorob R, Whittaker CA, Hesketh P, Archer A, et al. Cloning and characterization of chicken IL-10 and its role in the immune response to *Eimeria maxima*. *J Immunol.* (2004) 173:2675–82. doi: 10.4049/jimmunol.173.4.2675
11. Verhoeven DT, Verhagen H, Goldbohm RA, van den Brandt PA, van Poppel G. A review of mechanisms underlying anticarcinogenicity by brassica vegetables. *Chem Biol Interact.* (1997) 103:79–129.
12. Ribaux P, Irion O, Cohen M. An active product of cruciferous vegetables, 3,3′-diindolylmethane, inhibits invasive properties of extravillous cytotrophoblastic cells. *Neuro Endocrinol Lett.* (2012) 33:133–7. Available online at: http://www.nel.edu/an-active-product-of-cruciferous-vegetables-3-3-diindolylmethane-inhibits-invasive-properties-of-extravillous-cytotrophoblastic-cells-752/
13. Taylor-Harding B, Agadjanian H, Nassanian H, Kwon S, Guo X, Miller C, et al. Indole-3-carbinol synergistically sensitises ovarian cancer cells to bortezomib treatment. *Br J Cancer.* (2012) 106:333–43. doi: 10.1038/bjc.2011.546
14. Schmidt J V, Su GH, Reddy JK, Simon MC, Bradfield CA. Characterization of a murine Ahr null allele: involvement of the Ah receptor in hepatic growth and development. *Proc Natl Acad Sci USA.* (1996) 93:6731–6.
15. Hankinson O. The aryl hydrocarbon receptor complex. *Annu Rev Pharmacol Toxicol.* (1995) 35:307–40. doi: 10.1146/annurev.pa.35.040195.001515
16. Whitlock JP. Induction of cytochrome P4501A1. *Annu Rev Pharmacol Toxicol.* (1999) 39:103–25. doi: 10.1146/annurev.pharmtox.39.1.103
17. Singh NP, Singh UP, Rouse M, Zhang J, Chatterjee S, Nagarkatti PS, et al. Dietary indoles suppress delayed-type hypersensitivity by inducing a switch from proinflammatory Th17 cells to anti-inflammatory regulatory T cells through regulation of MicroRNA. *J Immunol.* (2016) 196:1108–22. doi: 10.4049/jimmunol.1501727
18. Rouse M, Singh NP, Nagarkatti PS, Nagarkatti M. Indoles mitigate the development of experimental autoimmune encephalomyelitis by induction of reciprocal differentiation of regulatory T cells and Th17 cells. *Br J Pharmacol.* (2013) 169:1305–21. doi: 10.1111/bph.12205
19. Funatake CJ, Marshall NB, Steppan LB, Mourich DV, Kerkvliet NI. Cutting edge: activation of the aryl hydrocarbon receptor by 2,3,7,8-tetrachlorodibenzo-p-dioxin generates a population of CD4+ CD25+ cells with characteristics of regulatory T cells. *J Immunol.* (2005) 175:4184–8. doi: 10.4049/jimmunol.175.7.4184
20. Esser C, Rannug A, Stockinger B. The aryl hydrocarbon receptor in immunity. *Trends Immunol.* (2009) 30:447–54. doi: 10.1016/j.it.2009.06.005
21. Quintana FJ, Basso AS, Iglesias AH, Korn T, Farez MF, Bettelli E, et al. Control of Treg and TH17 cell differentiation by the aryl hydrocarbon receptor. *Nature.* (2008) 453:65–71. doi: 10.1038/nature06880
22. Veldhoen M, Hirota K, Christensen J, O'Garra A, Stockinger B. Natural agonists for aryl hydrocarbon receptor in culture medium are essential for optimal differentiation of Th17 T cells. *J Exp Med.* (2009) 206:43–49. doi: 10.1084/jem.20081438
23. Kimura A, Naka T, Nohara K, Fujii-Kuriyama Y, Kishimoto T. Aryl hydrocarbon receptor regulates Stat1 activation and participates in the development of Th17 cells. *Proc Natl Acad Sci USA.* (2008) 105:9721–6. doi: 10.1073/pnas.0804231105
24. Diller ML, Kudchadkar RR, Delman KA, Lawson DH, Ford ML. Balancing inflammation: the link between Th17 and regulatory T cells. *Mediators Inflamm.* (2016) 2016:1–8. doi: 10.1155/2016/6309219
25. Lee SH, Lillehoj HS, Jang SI, Baldwin C, Tompkins D, Wagner B, et al. Development and characterization of mouse monoclonal antibodies reactive

with chicken interleukin-2 receptor alpha chain (CD25). *Vet Immunol Immunopathol.* (2011) 144:396–404. doi: 10.1016/j.vetimm.2011.08.001

26. Yoo J, Chang HH, Bae YH, Seong C-N, Choe N-H, Lillehoj HS, et al. Monoclonal antibodies reactive with chicken interleukin-17. *Vet Immunol Immunopathol.* (2008) 121:359–63. doi: 10.1016/j.vetimm.2007.10.004

27. Kim WH, Lillehoj HS, Min W. Evaluation of the immunomodulatory activity of the chicken NK-lysin-derived peptide cNK-2. *Sci Rep.* (2017) 7:45099. doi: 10.1038/srep45099

28. Shanmugasundaram R, Selvaraj RK. Regulatory T cell properties of chicken CD4⁺CD25⁺ Cells. *J Immunol.* (2011) 186:1997–2002. doi: 10.4049/jimmunol.1002040

29. Denyer MP, Pinheiro DY, Garden OA, Shepherd AJ. Missed, not missing: phylogenomic evidence for the existence of Avian FoxP3. *PLoS ONE.* (2016) 11:e0150988. doi: 10.1371/journal.pone.0150988

30. John DA, Williams LK, Kanamarlapudi V, Humphrey TJ, Wilkinson TS. The bacterial species *Campylobacter jejuni* induce diverse innate immune responses in human and avian intestinal epithelial cells. *Front Microbiol.* (2017) 8:1840. doi: 10.3389/fmicb.2017.01840

31. Kim WH, Jeong J, Park AR, Yim D, Kim Y-H, Kim KD, et al. Chicken IL-17F: Identification and comparative expression analysis in *Eimeria*-infected chickens. *Dev Comp Immunol.* (2012) 38:401–9. doi: 10.1016/j.dci.2012.08.002

32. Shaughnessy RG, Meade KG, McGivney BA, Allan B, O'Farrelly C. Global gene expression analysis of chicken caecal response to *Campylobacter jejuni*. *Vet Immunol Immunopathol.* (2011) 142:64–71. doi: 10.1016/j.vetimm.2011.04.010

33. Kim S, Faris L, Cox CM, Sumners LH, Jenkins MC, Fetterer RH, et al. Molecular characterization and immunological roles of avian IL-22 and its soluble receptor IL-22 binding protein. *Cytokine.* (2012) 60:815–27. doi: 10.1016/j.cyto.2012.08.005

34. Bussmann UA, Pérez Sáez JM, Bussmann LE, Barañao JL. Aryl hydrocarbon receptor activation leads to impairment of estrogen-driven chicken vitellogenin promoter activity in LMH cells. *Comp Biochem Physiol Part C Toxicol Pharmacol.* (2013) 157:111–18. doi: 10.1016/j.cbpc.2012.10.006

35. Shang S, Jiang J, Deng Y. Chicken cytochrome P450 1A5 is the key enzyme for metabolizing T-2 toxin to 3′OH-T-2. *Int J Mol Sci.* (2013) 14:10809–18. doi: 10.3390/ijms140610809

36. Takimoto T, Sato K, Akiba Y, Takahashi K. Role of chicken TL1A on inflammatory responses and partial characterization of its receptor. *J Immunol.* (2008) 180:8327–32. doi: 10.4049/jimmunol.180.12.8327

37. Gadde UD, Oh S, Lee Y, Davis E, Zimmerman N, Rehberger T, et al. Dietary Bacillus subtilis- based direct-fed microbials alleviate LPS-induced intestinal immunological stress and improve intestinal barrier gene expression in commercial broiler chickens. *Res Vet Sci.* (2017) 114:236–43. doi: 10.1016/j.rvsc.2017.05.004

38. De Boever S, Vangestel C, De Backer P, Croubels S, Sys SU. Identification and validation of housekeeping genes as internal control for gene expression in an intravenous LPS inflammation model in chickens. *Vet Immunol Immunopathol.* (2008) 122:312–7. doi: 10.1016/J.VETIMM.2007.12.002

39. Johnson J, Reid WM. Anticoccidial drugs: lesion scoring techniques in battery and floor-pen experiments with chickens. *Exp Parasitol.* (1970) 28:30–6.

40. Lee SH, Lillehoj HS, Jang SI, Lillehoj EP, Min W, Bravo DM. Dietary supplementation of young broiler chickens with Capsicum and turmeric oleoresins increases resistance to necrotic enteritis. *Br J Nutr.* (2013) 110:840–7. doi: 10.1017/S0007114512006083

41. Jones LJ, Gray M, Yue ST, Haugland RP, Singer VL. Sensitive determination of cell number using the CyQUANT cell proliferation assay. *J Immunol Methods.* (2001) 254:85–98. doi: 10.1016/S0022-1759(01)00404-5

42. Hu J, Chang H, Wang L, Wu S, Shao B, Zhou J, et al. Detection, occurrence and fate of indirubin in municipal sewage treatment plants. *Environ Sci Technol.* (2008) 42:8339–44. doi: 10.1021/es801038y

43. Hu W, Sorrentino C, Denison MS, Kolaja K, Fielden MR. Induction of Cyp1a1 is a nonspecific biomarker of aryl hydrocarbon receptor activation: results of large scale screening of pharmaceuticals and toxicants *in vivo* and *in vitro*. *Mol Pharmacol.* (2007) 71:1475–86. doi: 10.1124/mol.106.032748

44. Del Cacho E, Gallego M, Lillehoj HS, Quílez J, Lillehoj EP, Ramo A, et al. IL-17A regulates *Eimeria tenella* schizont maturation and migration in avian coccidiosis. *Vet Res.* (2014) 45:25. doi: 10.1186/1297-9716-45-25

45. Traka MH. Health benefits of glucosinolates. *Adv Bot Res.* (2016) 80:247–79. doi: 10.1016/BS.ABR.2016.06.004

46. Higdon J, Delage B, Williams D, Dashwood R. Cruciferous vegetables and human cancer risk: epidemiologic evidence and mechanistic basis. *Pharmacol Res.* (2007) 55:224–36. doi: 10.1016/j.phrs.2007.01.009

47. Tang L, Zirpoli GR, Guru K, Moysich KB, Zhang Y, Ambrosone CB, et al. xConsumption of raw cruciferous vegetables is inversely associated with bladder. *Cancer Epidemiol Biomarkers Prev.* (2008) 17:938–44. doi: 10.1158/1055-9965.EPI-07-2502

48. Aggarwal BB, Ichikawa H. Molecular targets and anticancer potential of indole-3-carbinol and its derivatives. *Cell Cycle.* (2005) 4:1201–15. doi: 10.4161/cc.4.9.1993

49. Weng J-R, Bai L-Y, Chiu C-F, Wang Y-C, Tsai M-H. The dietary phytochemical 3,3′-diindolylmethane induces G2/M arrest and apoptosis in oral squamous cell carcinoma by modulating Akt-NF-κB, MAPK, and p53 signaling. *Chem Biol Interact.* (2012) 195:224–30. doi: 10.1016/j.cbi.2012.01.0031

50. Khwaja FS, Wynne S, Posey I, Djakiew D. 3,3′-Diindolylmethane Induction of p75NTR-dependent cell death via the p38 mitogen-activated protein kinase pathway in prostate cancer cells. *Cancer Prev Res.* (2009) 2:566–71. doi: 10.1158/1940-6207.CAPR-08-0202

51. Nachshon-Kedmi M, Yannai S, Haj A, Fares FA. Indole-3-carbinol and 3,3′-diindolylmethane induce apoptosis in human prostate cancer cells. *Food Chem Toxicol.* (2003) 41:745–52. doi: 10.1016/S0278-6915(03)00004-8

52. Fernandez-Salguero P, Pineau T, Hilbert DM, McPhail T, Lee SS, Kimura S, et al. Immune system impairment and hepatic fibrosis in mice lacking the dioxin-binding Ah receptor. *Science.* (1995) 268:722–6.

53. Singh NP, Hegde VL, Hofseth LJ, Nagarkatti M, Nagarkatti P. Resveratrol (trans-3,5,4′-trihydroxystilbene) ameliorates experimental allergic encephalomyelitis, primarily via induction of apoptosis in T cells involving activation of aryl hydrocarbon receptor and estrogen receptor. *Mol Pharmacol.* (2007) 72:1508–21. doi: 10.1124/mol.107.038984

54. Singh NP, Nagarkatti M, Nagarkatti P. Primary peripheral T cells become susceptible to 2,3,7,8-tetrachlorodibenzo-p-dioxin-mediated apoptosis *in vitro* upon activation and in the presence of dendritic cells. *Mol Pharmacol.* (2008) 73:1722–35. doi: 10.1124/mol.107.043406

55. Yasui T, Kim E-Y, Iwata H, Franks DG, Karchner SI, Hahn ME, et al. Functional characterization and evolutionary history of two aryl hydrocarbon receptor isoforms (AhR1 and AhR2) from avian species. *Toxicol Sci.* (2007) 99:101–17. doi: 10.1093/toxsci/kfm139

56. Lee J-S, Iwabuchi K, Nomaru K, Nagahama N, Kim E-Y, Iwata H. Molecular and functional characterization of a novel aryl hydrocarbon receptor isoform, AHR1β, in the Chicken (Gallus gallus). *Toxicol Sci.* (2013) 136:450–466. doi: 10.1093/toxsci/kft192

57. Gilday D, Gannon M, Yutzey K, Bader D, Rifkind AB. Molecular cloning and expression of two novel avian cytochrome P450 1A enzymes induced by 2,3,7,8-tetrachlorodibenzo-p-dioxin. *J Biol Chem.* (1996) 271:33054–9.

58. Sinclair PR, Gorman N, Walton HS, Sinclair JF, Lee CA, Rifkind AB. Identification of CYP1A5 as the CYP1A enzyme mainly responsible for uroporphyrinogen oxidation induced by AH receptor ligands in chicken liver and kidney. *Drug Metab Dispos.* (1997) 25:779–83.

59. Veldhoen M, Hirota K, Westendorf AM, Buer J, Dumoutier L, Renauld J-C, et al. The aryl hydrocarbon receptor links TH17-cell-mediated autoimmunity to environmental toxins. *Nature.* (2008) 453:106–9. doi: 10.1038/nature06881

60. Huang Z, Jiang Y, Yang Y, Shao J, Sun X, Chen J, et al. 3,3′-Diindolylmethane alleviates oxazolone-induced colitis through Th2/Th17 suppression and Treg induction. *Mol Immunol.* (2013) 53:335–44. doi: 10.1016/j.molimm.2012.09.007

61. Lillehoj HS, Trout JM. Coccidia: a review of recent advances on immunity and vaccine development. *Avian Pathol.* (1993) 22:3–31. doi: 10.1080/03079459308418897

62. Hong YH, Lillehoj HS, Lee SH, Dalloul RA, Lillehoj EP. Analysis of chicken cytokine and chemokine gene expression following *Eimeria acervulina* and *Eimeria tenella* infections. *Vet Immunol Immunopathol.* (2006) 114:209–23. doi: 10.1016/j.vetimm.2006.07.007

63. Hong YH, Lillehoj HS, Lillehoj EP, Lee SH. Changes in immune-related gene expression and intestinal lymphocyte subpopulations following *Eimeria*

maxima infection of chickens. *Vet Immunol Immunopathol.* (2006) 114:259–72. doi: 10.1016/j.vetimm.2006.08.006

64. Min W, Lillehoj HS. Isolation and Characterization of Chicken Interleukin-17 cDNA. *J Interf Cytokine Res.* (2002) 22:1123–8. doi: 10.1089/10799900260442548

65. Negishi T, Kato Y, Ooneda O, Mimura J, Takada T, Mochizuki H, et al. Effects of aryl hydrocarbon receptor signaling on the modulation of TH1/TH2 balance. *J Immunol.* (2005) 175:7348–56. doi: 10.4049/jimmunol.175.11.7348

66. Beamer CA, Shepherd DM. Role of the aryl hydrocarbon receptor (AhR) in lung inflammation. *Semin Immunopathol.* (2013) 35:693–704. doi: 10.1007/s00281-013-0391-7

67. Sand JM, Arendt MK, Repasy A, Deniz G, Cook ME. Oral antibody to interleukin-10 reduces growth rate depression due to *Eimeria* spp. infection in broiler chickens. *Poult Sci.* (2016) 95:439–46. doi: 10.3382/ps/pev352

68. Arendt MK, Sand JM, Marcone TM, Cook ME. Interleukin-10 neutralizing antibody for detection of intestinal luminal levels and as a dietary additive in *Eimeria* challenged broiler chicks. *Poult Sci.* (2016) 95:430–438. doi: 10.3382/ps/pev365

69. Anderson JM. Molecular structure of tight junctions and their role in epithelial transport. *News Physiol Sci.* (2001) 16:126–30. doi: 10.1152/physiologyonline.2001.16.3.126

70. Chen Y, Yang P, Li F, Kijlstra A. The effects of Th17 cytokines on the inflammatory mediator production and barrier function of ARPE-19 cells. *PLoS ONE.* (2011) 6:e18139. doi: 10.1371/journal.pone.0018139

71. McNaughton SA, Marks GC. Development of a food composition database for the estimation of dietary intakes of glucosinolates, the biologically active constituents of cruciferous vegetables. *Br J Nut.* (2003) 90:687–97. doi: 10.1079/BJN2003917

72. Ciska E, Martyniak-Przybyszewska B, Kozlowska H. Content of glucosinolates in cruciferous vegetables grown at the same site for two years under different climatic conditions. *J Agric Food Chem.* (2000) 48:2862–7. doi: 10.1021/jf981373a

73. *FDA Specific Requirements for Health Claims*, 21 C.F.R § 101.78 (1993).

74. Minich DM, Bland JS. A review of the clinical efficacy and safety of cruciferous vegetable phytochemicals. *Nutr Rev.* (2007) 65:259–67. doi: 10.1111/j.1753-4887.2007.tb00303.x

12

The Influence of Parasite Infections on Host Immunity to Co-Infection with Other Pathogens

Neil A. Mabbott*

The Roslin Institute & Royal (Dick) School of Veterinary Studies, University of Edinburgh, Edinburgh, United Kingdom

*Correspondence:
Neil A. Mabbott
neil.mabbott@roslin.ed.ac.uk

Parasites have evolved a wide range of mechanisms that they use to evade or manipulate the host's immune response and establish infection. The majority of the *in vivo* studies that have investigated these host-parasite interactions have been undertaken in experimental animals, especially rodents, which were housed and maintained to a high microbiological status. However, in the field situation it is increasingly apparent that pathogen co-infections within the same host are a common occurrence. For example, chronic infection with pathogens including malarial parasites, soil-transmitted helminths, *Mycobacterium tuberculosis* and viruses such as HIV may affect a third of the human population of some developing countries. Increasing evidence shows that co-infection with these pathogens may alter susceptibility to other important pathogens, and/or influence vaccine efficacy through their effects on host immune responsiveness. Co-infection with certain pathogens may also hinder accurate disease diagnosis. This review summarizes our current understanding of how the host's immune response to infection with different types of parasites can influence susceptibility to infection with other pathogenic microorganisms. A greater understanding of how infectious disease susceptibility and pathogenesis can be influenced by parasite co-infections will enhance disease diagnosis and the design of novel vaccines or therapeutics to more effectively control the spread of infectious diseases.

Keywords: parasite, helminth, co-infection, pathogenesis, susceptibility, immunity

INTRODUCTION

The important host-parasite interactions that influence the progression and control of infection to individual pathogenic microorganisms have been studied in much detail, especially in laboratory mice. However, since many pathogens are acquired through similar routes of exposure (e.g., orally following ingestion of contaminated water, food, or pasture) infection of natural host species in field situations and humans with multiple pathogens is common, especially in regions with poor sanitation and/or limited access to clean drinking water. In order to sustain chronic infections, the parasitic microorgansisms have evolved a diverse range of mechanisms to enable them to evade or manipulate the host's immune response. As a consequence, by-stander effects due to infection with certain parasite species can significantly alter susceptibility to other important pathogens, and/or influence the development of pathology. Discussed throughout this review are examples of the many studies that have investigated the effects of parasitic helminth infections on host susceptibility to co-infection with a diverse range other pathogenic microorganisms.

Helminths are large, multicellular parasitic microorganisms. Estimates suggest that approximately a third of the global human population may be infected with helminth parasites, causing important public health concerns, especially in regions with poor sanitation or limited access to clean drinking water. Helminths are commonly referred to as parasitic worms and can include the following groupings: roundworms (nematodes), such as *Ascaris lumbricoides*; whipworms, such as *Trichuris trichiura* in humans and *T. muris* in mice; hookworms, such as *Necator americanus*; flukes (trematodes), such as *Facsiola hepatica* and *Schistosoma mansoni*; and cestodes (tapeworms). Many of these helminth parasites are soil-transmitted and cause gastrointestinal infections following ingestion of pasture or water contaminated with their eggs. The schistosomes, in contrast, can establish chronic infection within the host's bloodstream. Infections with helminth parasites often cause significant pathology, for example as they migrate through host tissues following infection via the skin (e.g., schistosomes), or feed on the gut epithelium (e.g., *Trichuris* spp.) (1). These chronic infections are often associated with the development of systemic and mucosal CD4$^+$ T helper cell type 2 (Th2) polarized immune responses. These are typically characterized by increased expression of cytokines such as interleukin-4 (IL-4), IL-13, eosinophilia, production of immunoglobulin E (IgE), and stimulation of alternatively activated (M2) macrophages and type 2 innate lymphoid cells (ILC2) (2, 3). The alternatively activated macrophages are considered to play an important role in repairing the tissue damage caused by the helminth infection.

However, the characteristics of the immune response to infection with other types of parasites can differ substantially. Trypanosomes and malaria parasites are important vector-borne unicellular protozoan parasites, and are the causative agents of trypanosomiasis and malaria, respectively, in humans and animals. Each of these parasite species can establish chronic infections in the host's bloodstream: the trypanosomes living extracellularly, whereas the malaria parasites establish cyclical rounds of intracellular infection within erythrocytes. Host immune responses to infection with these protozoan parasites are usually fundamentally distinct from the predominantly Th2-polarized responses induced by helminth infections. Malaria infections, for example, are associated with elevated levels of pro-inflammatory cytokines such as interferon-γ (IFNγ), IL-12, increased levels of CD4$^+$ Th1 cells, CD8$^+$ T cells, and NK cells and the stimulation of pro-inflammatory classically activated (M1) macrophages (4, 5).

An increasing body of data indicates that alterations to these responses due to co-infection with other pathogens can dramatically influence disease susceptibility. Many of the examples presented below suggest links between parasite-induced disturbances to the Th1/Th2 balance and/or macrophage phenotype (alternatively activated vs. classically activated) and altered susceptibility or pathogenesis following subsequent co-infection with other pathogens. The effects of the parasite infection on the host's immune response may also have serious implications for the accurate diagnosis of other infections within the same individual. Bovine tuberculosis is an important infectious disease of cattle caused by the pathogenic

bacterium *Mycobacterium bovis*. Current measures to control this disease include the regular testing of cattle and removal of infected stock from herds. A widely used diagnostic test for this disease is based on the detection of *M. bovis*-specific IFNγ production by peripheral blood lymphocytes. However, as helminth infections can modulate host IFNγ responses, co-infections with these parasites could have serious consequences for the reliable detection of other important pathogens (see section *Mycobacterium tuberculosis*).

This review therefore discusses how the induction of an immune response to infection with distinct types of parasites may modulate the development of effective immunity and/or disease pathogenesis to co-infections with other important pathogenic microorganisms. Many of the data obtained in the studies described below was derived from experimental mouse models, but studies from humans and natural host species are included where data were available.

MALARIA

Malaria, caused by infection with unicellular protozoan *Plasmodium* parasites, is an important infectious disease of humans and animals that inflicts significant morbidity and mortality in tropical and sub-tropical regions throughout the world. Infections are transmitted through the deposition of sporozoite parasite stages into the skin via the bite of infected mosquito vectors. These then travel via the bloodstream to the liver, where they infect hepatocytes and undergo morphological change and replication before subsequently infecting erythrocytes. The parasites then undergo extensive cycles of replication and infection in erythrocytes leading to anemia. During the erythrocytic stage of malaria infection, IFNγ production from CD4$^+$ Th1-cells and CD4$^+$ T-cell help for the B-cell response are each required for effective control and elimination of the parasitaemia. The actions of CD4$^+$ T cells are also important for controlling the pre-erythrocytic stages of infection through the activation of parasite-specific CD8$^+$ T cells [for in-depth review see (5)]. However, excessive inflammatory responses in response to malaria infection can also lead to significant immunopathology.

Effects of Malaria on Helminth Co-infection
Malaria patients in endemic regions are often co-infected with soil-transmitted helminths. Following infection of the mammalian host the larval stages of certain parasitic helminth species migrate to the lungs of the host where they cause pathology. The larvae typically induce strong pulmonary Th2 immune responses and are accompanied by the induction of alternatively activated macrophages. The combined actions of these immune responses are considered to help mediate parasite clearance and the repair of host tissues. In BALB/c mice infected with hookworms parasites such as *Nippostrongylus brasiliensis*, the development of a Th2-polarized immune response to the hookworm infection was impaired in those co-infected with *P. chabaudi chabaudi* malaria parasites. This effect also coincided with the reduced expression of alternatively activated macrophage-derived factors in the lung such as chitinase and

resistin family members (6). Similarly, in a separate study the incidence of lung granulomas induced by infection with *Litomosoides sigmodontis* microfilariae was reduced in mice co-infected with either *P. chabaudi* or *P. yoelii* malaria parasites (7). These experimental mouse studies suggest that malaria infection can negatively impact on the ability of the host to induce a Th2-polarized specific immune response to co-infection with helminths. How malaria infection mediates these effects is not known. Further experiments are clearly necessary to determine whether they are a consequence of direct effects of the malaria parasites themselves or are an indirect consequence of the induction of a strong Th1-polarized immune response/cytokine milieu in response to the malaria infection.

Effects of Helminth Co-infection on Malaria

Co-infections with parasites such as helminths may also have a significant impact on malaria pathogenesis and susceptibility (8). In mice infected with *N. brasiliensis* 2 weeks before subsequent infection with *P. berghei* malaria parasites, the induction of a malaria-driven Th1 cytokine response was impeded, affecting the activation phenotype of the macrophages in the lung (8). Helminth infections can promote the secretion of IL-10 by regulatory T cells (9, 10), and this can downregulate the expression of pro-inflammatory cytokines such as IL-12p70 and IFNγ. Since IFNγ plays an important role in protective immunity to *P. falciparum* infection, it is plausible that expression of an anti-inflammatory cytokine milieu during helminth infection might exacerbate malaria pathogenesis and susceptibility. In support of this hypothesis, co-infection of mice with the hookworm parasite *N. brasiliensis* was reported to impede the induction of a pro-inflammatory classically activated macrophage phenotype in the lungs of mice subsequently infected with malaria parasites (8). The induction of an effective Th1 response to *P. berghei* infection was similarly reduced in mice co-infected with schistosomes (*S. mansoni*). As a consequence, the co-infected mice were less able to control the malaria infection, displaying increased parasitemias during the early phase of *P. berghei* infection and increased fatality (11). Mice chronically infected with the gastrointestinal helminth pathogen *Heligmosomoides polygyrus* before a subsequent *P. chabaudi* AS infection likewise displayed reduced immunity to the bloodstream stage of malaria infection, including decreased production of IFNγ and malaria-specific Th1-associated IgG2a antibody production (12).

Parasite co-infections may also affect the magnitude of the pathology that develops in host tissues. For example, an exacerbation of immunopathology during *P. chabaudi* infection was observed in mice co-infected with *L. sigmodontis* microfilariae (13). The incidence of pathology in the co-infected mice was found to be associated with the absence of microfilaraemia. This implies that the presence of the microfilariae stimulates an immunomodulatory response in the host that can partially protect against severe malaria (13). However, helminth co-infections may differentially regulate murine malarial infections in a malaria strain-dependent way. For example, co-infection of mice with *L. sigmodontis* impaired

the development of lesions in the kidneys caused by infection with either *P. chabaudi* or *P. yoelii*. However, the peak of malaria parasitaemia was decreased in mice co-infected *P. yoelii*, but not in those co-infected with *P. chabaudi* (7). Conversely, the growth of *P. yoelii* in the liver was inhibited in mice co-infected with *S. mansoni*, and malaria parasite gametocyte infectivity was much reduced (14).

Whether co-infections with helminths such as schistosomes can modulate susceptibility to malaria in humans is uncertain, but an experimental study in baboons (*Papio anubis*) suggests that this also plausible. This study showed that the baboons that were chronically infected with *S. mansoni* had significantly lower *P. knowlesi* malaria parasite burdens and were protected from anemia (15). A study of Senegalese children similarly showed that those with light *S. haematobium* infection had lower burdens of *P. falciparum* when compared to those that weren't co-infected with schistosomes (16). The mechanisms responsible for mediating these effects are not known. It is possible that the reduced levels of regulatory T cells or a Th2-polarized cytokine milieu in *S. haematobium* infected children may provide protection against falciparum malaria by modulating systemic expression of Th1 cytokines (17).

Effects of Parasite Co-infection on Experimental Cerebral Malaria

Severe forms of malaria are leading causes of mortality in infected children and pregnant mothers, presenting as cerebral malaria, severe anemia, or acidosis (18). The sequestration of malaria parasites across the blood-brain barrier leads to the influx of immune lymphocytes and leukocytes into the brain, particularly parasite-specific CD8$^+$ T cells, which ultimately leads to the development of neuropathology. Studies using a murine experimental cerebral malaria (ECM) model show that co-infection with Chikungunya virus can impede the sequestration of malaria parasites into the brain and provide some protection against ECM (19). In this model co-infection system, the malaria parasite-specific pathogenic CD8$^+$ T cells appeared to be retained in the spleens of mice co-infected with Chikungunya virus due to their reduced expression of the CXCR3 chemokine receptor (19). This implied that the reduced early migration of pathogenic CD8$^+$ T cells into the brains of the virus co-infected mice may have impeded the development of ECM and brain pathology.

Systemic co-infection of mice with the schistosomes (*S. mansoni*) seven weeks before infection with *P. berghei* malaria parasites was similarly shown to reduce the severity of ECM (11, 20). In this study, protection from ECM was dependent on the relative doses of the parasites used in the co-infections. Here, infection with a high dose of schistosome cercariae resulted in higher protection against ECM when co-infected with a low dose of *P. berghei* malaria paratites. Conversely, when the mice were co-infected with *S. mansoni* and a higher dose of *P. berghei*, the development of ECM was unaffected when compared to mice infected with malaria parasites alone (21). Development of ECM in mice is considered to be Th1-associated. The switch toward a Th2-polarized cytokine profile in the *S. mansoni* co-infected mice suggests a mechanism by which the effects on ECM pathogenesis may have been mediated. Clearly further experiments are required to specifically confirm the identify of the cellular and molecular factors responsible for these effects. A predominantly Th1-polarized cytokine profile is observed in mice by 4 weeks after *S. mansoni* infection (before significant egg production occurs). When mice were co-infected with malaria parasites 4 weeks after *S. mansoni* infection (prior to the onset of the Th1/Th2 switch), no improvements to ECM pathogenesis were observed (20), supporting the hypothesis that a Th2-polarized cytokine response may have a protective role.

Co-infections with the helminth parasites *A. lumbricoides* and *T. trichiura* have also been associated with reductions in risk of cerebral malaria in humans (22). However, it is interesting to note that the beneficial effects of *T. trichiura* were reduced when the individuals were also co-infected with hookworms (22). This study reveals an additional layer of complexity in naturally affected host-species where the outcome on the host of interactions between two parasite species can be modified by the presence of a third. These data emphasize how the relationships between multiple parasite communities in an individual host can significantly affect disease outcomes.

TREMATODES (FLUKES)

Liver Fluke

The liver fluke *Fasciola hepatica* is highly prevalent in ruminant livestock species, but can also establish infection in a wide range of other mammalian species including humans. Infection of livestock with *F. hepatica* occurs through the ingestion of pasture contaminated with encysted cercariae. The parasites then migrate through the gut wall and peritoneal cavity to the liver and bile ducts, where they mature and produce large numbers of eggs that are excreted into the environment. In common with many helminth infections, the migrating juvenile parasite stages induce a strong Th2-polarized immune response in the mammalian host. Infection of mice with *F. hepatica* can down-regulate Th1-responses *in vivo*, even in IL-4-deficient mice (23) suggesting this is not simply due to the actions of Th2 cells or cytokines. Indeed, the parasites produce a large range of excretory/secretory (ES) molecules that help them to mediate tissue invasion, feeding and immunomodulation (24) including the suppression of IFNγ responses (25).

Bovine tuberculosis (BTB), caused by infection with the bacterium *M. bovis* is an important pathogen of cattle worldwide and has zoonotic potential. Although some countries have reduced or eliminated BTB, wildlife *M. bovis* reservoirs and the limitations of diagnostic tests have hindered successful eradication in other regions. The single intradermal comparative cervical tuberculin test (SICCT) and the *in vitro* IFNγ assay are commonly used to identify *M. bovis* infected cattle. However, certain parasite co-infections can reduce the sensitivity of these assays. A large-scale epidemiological study in England and Wales showed that in dairy herds with a high incidence of

F. hepatica fewer animals were detected as positive reactors against BTB (26). Experiments in cattle confirmed that infection with *F. hepatica* reduces the sensitivity of the standard BTB tests (SICCT test and IFNγ test) through reduced *M. bovis*-specific Th1 immune responses (27). However, *F. hepatica* co-infection did not influence the detection of visible lesions in BTB infected cows (28). These data clearly show how the immunomodulatory effects of *F. hepatica* on the bovine host can reduce the sensitivity of current pre-mortem BTB tests. This may significantly influence the ability of practical measures to eliminate BTB infections in regions with high prevalence of *F. hepatica*.

Despite the reduced *M. bovis*-specific Th1 immunity in cows co-infected with *F. hepatica*, mycobacterial burdens were shown to be reduced (29). The mechanisms responsible for this are uncertain, but the authors proposed that the actions of alternatively-activated macrophages induced in response to *F. hepatica* infection may act to limit the proliferation of *M. bovis*.

In sheep, infections with the liver flukes *Dicrocoelium dentriticum* or *F. hepatica* can predispose the ewes to mastitis in the immediate *post-partum* period (30). Abnormal metabolism of carbohydrates during the later stages of pregnancy in ewes can cause pregnancy toxemia. This disease is associated with hyperketonaeimia, and blood concentrations of the ketone body β-hydroxybutyrate can help detect ewes at risk of developing pregnancy toxemia. Higher concentrations of β-hydroxybutyrate were recorded in trematode-infected ewes (30). Since β-hydroxybutyrate may have immunomodulatory effects, the authors hypothesized that its increased levels in infected ewes may suppress immunity in the udder enhancing the risk of infection at this site (30). This has raised the hypothesis that the use of anthelmintic drugs may also help reduce the incidence of mastitis in trematode-affected flocks.

Finally, infection with the human liver fluke *Opisthorchis viverrini* is endemic in the Greater Mekong sub-region. This fluke is classified as a group 1 carcinogen by the International Agency for Research on Cancer because chronic infections with *O. viverrini* can lead to the development of cholangiocarcinoma, a malignant cancer of the bile ducts. In areas of Thailand where flukes are endemic, the Gram-negative bacterium *Helicobacter pylori* was found in 66.7% of the patients studied that had cholangiocarcinoma (31). This raised the hypothesis that co-infections with *H. pylori* and with *O. viverrini* synergistically increases the severity of hepatobiliary abnormalities. Indeed, in an experimental hamster model the severity of the hepatobiliary abnormalities was increased in those that were co-infected with *O. viverrini* (32).

Effects on Schistosome (Blood Fluke) Infections

Infections with schistosomes cause chronic inflammatory disease in humans and animals. The diseases they cause can lead to the development of severe pathology, significant morbidity, and economic loss. Schistosomes are transmitted through the skin via contact with infected water sources inhabited by the snail vector. The parasites establish chronic infections in the mammalian host's bloodstream where they mature, mate, and produce substantial quantities of eggs. The eggs enter the intestines and bladder where they are excreted via feces and urine. Deposition of the eggs in host tissues can cause chronic inflammation, tissue damage and fibrosis. Schistosomes typically induce a Th2-polarized immune response in the mammalian host that enables them to establish chronic infections where they can persist for years (33).

Experiments in mice have shown that a gastrointestinal nematode infection can influence the pathogenesis of a subsequent schistosome infection. A chronic *Trichuris muris* infection within the large intestine enhanced the survival and migration of *S. mansoni* schistosomula to the portal system. Consequently, schistosome worm and egg burdens and associated pathology were enhanced when compared to mice infected with *S. mansoni* alone (34). This suggests that the immunomodulatory effects elicited in the mucosa of the large intestine to enable the gastrointestinal helminth to establish chronic infection can extend to other host tissues. This may exacerbate host susceptibility to subsequent co-infection with other helminth parasites. A similar effect has been reported to occur in a naturally-affected livestock species. A longitudinal study of free-ranging African buffalo reported that animals infected with *Cooperia fuelleborni* had greater burdens of schistosomes (*Schistosoma mattheei*) than those where this nematode species was not detected (35). The mechanisms that mediate these effects in the co-infected animals remain to be determined. This could simply represent host variation in susceptibility to gastrointestinal nematodes. However, since infection of cattle with the related gastrointestinal nematode species *C. oncophora* enhanced their susceptibility to lungworm (*Dictyocaulus viviparus*) infection (36), it is plausible that nematode-mediated effects on the buffalo immune response may similarly impede the establishment of immunity to schistosomes.

However, it is important to note that data from mouse studies show that differences in the species of the co-infecting parasite may have contrasting effects on schistosome infections (34, 37). The gastrointestinal helminth *H. polygyrus* establishes infection specifically within the murine duodenum. In mice infected with *H. polygyrus* a marked reduction in schistosome egg-induced hepatic pathology was observed. This effect appeared to correlate with significant decreases in the expression of pro-inflammatory cytokines responsible for the induction of the egg-induced immunopathology (37). Thus, although co-infection with gastrointestinal helminths may significantly impact on schistosomiasis, the currently available data do not help us to reliably predict whether they are likely to exacerbate or reduce the disease pathogenesis.

TRYPANOSOMES

African Trypanosomes

African trypanosomes are single-cell extracellular hemoflagellate protozoan parasites and are transmitted between mammalian hosts via blood-feeding tsetse flies of the genus *Glossina*. The *Trypanosoma brucei rhodesiense* and *T. b. gambiense* subspecies cause human African trypanosomiasis in endemic regions within the tsetse fly belt across sub-Saharan Africa. Animal African trypanosomiasis is caused by *T. congolense*, *T. vivax*, and *T. brucei* and inflicts substantial economic strains on the African livestock industry. The parasitic life cycle within the mammalian host is initiated by the intradermal injection of metacyclic trypomastigotes by the tsetse fly vector. The extracellular parasites then reach the draining lymph nodes, presumably via invasion of the afferent lymphatics and then disseminate systemically (38, 39). During this process the metacyclic trypanosome forms differentiate into long slender bloodstream forms that are adapted for survival within the mammalian host. When C57BL/6 mice are infected with *T. brucei* the initial parasitaemic wave coincides with the expression of high levels of IFNγ by the host in an attempt to control the infection. However, the trypanosomes also cause significant immunosuppression enabling them to establish chronic infections in the hostile environment of the host's bloodstream.

A study has shown that the severity of malaria and trypanosomiasis was exacerbated in mice co-infected with *P. berghei* and *T. brucei* (40). In the co-infected mice survival rates were reduced and the parasitaemias were greater, with more severe anemia and hypoglycaemia. Each of these infections induces a strong pro-inflammatory response with high levels of IFNγ. Further studies are necessary to determine whether additive/synergistic effects of each infection on IFNγ expression are responsible for the increased disease severity observed in the co-infected mice.

Trypanosome infections may also modulate host susceptibility to infection with some pathogenic bacteria. For example, in mice chronically-infected with either *Brucella melitensis*, *B. abortus*, or *B. suis*, the burden of bacteria in the spleen was reduced if the mice were also co-infected with *T. brucei* (41). The effects of *T. brucei* infection on *Brucella* burdens in co-infected mice were impeded in the absence of functional IL-12p35/IFNγ signaling. This suggests that the strong pro-inflammatory IFNγ-mediated immune response induced by the *T. brucei* infection aided the clearance of *Brucella*. Thus, although infections with *T. brucei* can induce significant levels of immunosuppression and immunopathology, this study shows that under some circumstances the host's response to *T. brucei* infection may provide protection against co-infection with other pathogens (41). However, this not true for all pathogenic bacteria. Although Th1 responses are essential for protection against *Mycobacterium tuberculosis*, *T. brucei* infection did not ameliorate the susceptibility of mice to co-infection with this pathogenic bacterium (41).

T. cruzi

Infection with the obligate intracellular parasite *T. cruzi* causes Chagas' disease and is an important cause of morbidity and mortality in humans in Central and South America (42). Concurrent infection of mice with *S. mansoni* can significantly affect disease pathogenesis and susceptibility following infection with *T. cruzi* (43). The co-infected mice were shown to be unable to effectively control the *T. cruzi* infection, and the increased parasitic load was accompanied by substantial inflammation in their livers. Infections with *T. cruzi* are associated with the establishment of a Th1-polarized immune response, and the production of macrophage-derived NO from arginine by inducible NO synthetase (iNOS) is important for parasite clearance. However, during the chronic phase of schistosomiasis high levels of arginase-1 are instead expressed by alternatively activated macrophages. In the *S. mansoni* co-infected mice, the reduced protection against *T. cruzi* coincided with the reduced production of IFN-γ and NO (43). This study illustrates how macrophage polarity and the relative expression levels of iNOS and arginase-1 in response to infection with one parasite could influence the host's ability to co-infection with other parasites.

APICOMPLEXAN PARASITES

Toxoplasma gondii

T. gondii is an orally-acquired obligate intracellular protozoan parasite affecting ∼30% of the human population. Following oral infection, the parasites typically disseminate systemically and convert into dormant stages in muscle tissues and the brain. Infection with *T. gondii* elicits a strong Th1-polarized immune response characterized by production of IFNγ, IL-12, and parasite specific IgG2a antibodies. Studies in mice suggest these responses are important for host protection. Infections are typically asymptomatic in immunocompetent humans, but can reactivate in immunocompromised individuals and result in the development of a life-threatening encephalitis.

Although a study has shown that gastrointestinal helminth (*H. polygyrus*) co-infection did not affect the induction of a protective Th1 response to *T. gondii* infection (44), the Th2-response to the *H. polygyrus* infection was impeded. Co-infection with *T. gondii* in these mice was instead accompanied by a shift toward a non-protective helminth-specific Th1 response (44). Conversely, separate studies have shown that *H. polygyrus* co-infection can negatively impact upon CD8$^+$ T cell differentiation and cytokine production in response to *T. gondii* infection (45, 46). Conventional dendritic cells from the *H. polygyrus* co-infected mice also had reduced expression of IL-12 (46). The reasons for the contrasting outcomes in these two studies are not immediately apparent, but are perhaps explained by important differences in their experiment design. In the first study (44), the mice were first infected with *T. gondii* and 14 days later orally co-infected with *H. polygyrus*. However, in the other studies (45, 46), the mice were first infected with *H. polygyrus* and subsequently co-infected with *T. gondii* parasites.

Although further experiments are necessary to confirm the cellular and molecular mechanisms that underpin these effects, these studies suggest that differences in the order and timing of the infections with two distinct oral pathogens, can significantly influence the host's response to the second. In particular these data imply that the presence of a strong Th1-polarized immune response to an ongoing *T. gondii* infection can impede the development of Th2-polarized immune responses to a subsequent helminth co-infection (44). However, the induction of CD8+ T-cell responses against *T. gondii* co-infection is impeded in the presence of an existing Th2-polarized immune response to a gastrointestinal helminth infection.

Eimeria

Eimeria tenella is a major pathogen of chickens causing intestinal coccidiosis. Infection with *E. tenella* is restricted to the caecum and causes significant morbidity and mortality, including diarrhea, mucosal lesions and weight loss. The prevalence of *E. tenella* and *T. gondii* is widespread, suggesting co-infections with these two pathogens may be common. The effect of co-infection of chickens with *Eimeria* and *T. gondii* has been addressed in an experimental study (47). However, the pathology and immune response following co-infection with these parasites did not differ significantly from that observed in chickens infected with *Eimeria* alone. Co-infection with *Eimeria* also did not affect the abundance of *T. gondii*-positive tissue samples or the clinical course of *T. gondii* infection. Distinct *T. gondii* strain types have been characterized in Europe and North America (type I, II, and III) and these can significantly influence the virulence and severity of the disease in different host species (48). For example, chickens are generally considered refractory to infection with type I or II oocysts (49, 50), but they may cause severe disease in other host species such as mice (51). Whereas, co-infection of chickens with two common apicomplexan parasites did not reveal any significant mutual effects on disease pathogenesis (47), a study of wild rabbits in Scotland suggested a link between *T. gondii* infection and higher burdens of *E. stiedae* (52). Whether differences in the virulence of *T. gondii* infection in different host species could have a significant impact on their susceptibility to co-infection with other pathogens remains to be determined. Of course, the possibility also cannot be excluded that the rabbits with high *Eimeria* burdens had high susceptibility to orally-acquired parasite infections.

Giardia

Infection with *Giardia duodenalis* (syn. *G. intestinalis*, or *G. lamblia*) is a leading cause of waterborne diarrhoeal disease. The characteristic signs of Giardiasis include diarrhea, abdominal pain, nausea, vomiting, and anorexia, with some individuals also developing extra-intestinal and post-infectious complications. Little is currently known of the effects of parasite co-infections on susceptibility to giardiasis. A study of 3 year old children in the Quininde district of Ecuador has shown that those co-infected with the gastrointestinal helminth *A. lumbricoides* had plasma cytokine profiles indicative of an increased Th2/Th1 cytokine bias, and significantly lower plasma levels of IL-2 and TNF-α when compared to those infected with *G. lamblia* alone (53). Studies from mouse models have shown that expression of TNF-α is essential for resistance to *G. lamblia* infection (54). Little is known of the mechanisms that are essential for protection of humans against *Giardia* infections. However, it is plausible that the effects of *Ascaris* infection on TNF-α expression may have negatively affected the ability of the children to eradicate *Giardia*.

EFFECTS ON BACTERIAL INFECTIONS

Effects on Salmonella Pathogenesis

Oral infections with the Gram negative bacterium *Salmonella*, through consumption of contaminated food such as meat, eggs, or milk are amongst the most common causes of diarrhea.

Co-infections with distinct parasites, helminths, and malaria parasites, have each been shown to exacerbate susceptibility to, or the pathogenesis of, salmonellosis.

Many of the examples discussed above have suggested a link between the induction of a Th2-polarized immune response to helminth infection and the reduced development of Th1-polarized immunity to co-infection with other pathogens. However, co-infection of mice with the gastrointestinal helminth *H. polygyrus* has also been shown to enhance the pathogenesis of infection with *Salmonella enterica* serovar Typhimurium independently of the actions of Th2 cells and regulatory T cells (55). Here, co-infection with *H. polygyrus* has been reported to disrupt the metabolic profile within the small intestine, and by doing so, directly affect the invasive capacity of *S. typhimurium*. This helminth infection was shown to mediate this effect through the enhancement of bacterial expression of *Salmonella* pathogenicity island 1 (SPI-1) genes (55). This study reveals a novel immune system-independent mechanism by which a helminth-modified metabolome in the host's intestine can promote susceptibility to bacterial co-infection.

Invasive nontyphoid *Salmonella* (NTS) bacteraemia is a common cause of community-acquired bacteraemia in the human populations of several regions of sub-Saharan Africa (56). Associations between NTS co-infection and high malaria mortality have been reported (57), and a study of hospitalized children in north-eastern Tanzania showed that a decline in malaria cases was associated with a similar decline in the incidence of NTS and other forms of bacteraemia (58).

Since malaria parasites establish infection within erythrocytes, the daily rounds of parasite replication within these cells can cause high levels of erythrocyte lysis and haemolysis, resulting in anemia. The association of NTS infection with haemolysis is well-established in humans with malaria, especially in patients with severe malarial anemia (59). This haemolysis releases large quantities of cell-free haeme which is toxic to the host. To counter this cytotoxicity, haeme oxygenase 1 (HO-1) expression is induced to degrade the haeme and provide tolerance toward some of the pathological consequences of malaria infection. The actions of HO-1 also provide an additional cytoprotective role by limiting the production of reactive oxygen species (60). However, data from mice (61) and from the analysis of neutrophils from malaria-infected children (62) show that the actions of HO-1 in granulocytes in response to haemolysis during malaria infection impedes their oxidative burst activity and production of reactive oxygen species. This leads to dysfunctional granulocyte mobilization and long-term neutrophil dysfunction. As a consequence, *Salmonella* are able to survive and proliferate within neutrophils during malaria infection due to their decreased oxidative burst activity, leading to increased NTS susceptibility (61, 62). These data clearly show how a host-induced cytoprotective response to one of the pathological consequences of malaria infection (haemolysis) can significantly impair neutrophil-mediated resistance to co-infection with another pathogen.

Mycobacterium tuberculosis

Infection with the obligate intracellular bacterium *M. tuberculosis* causes tuberculosis (TB), a chronic disease affecting ∼2 billion people worldwide. This infection typically affects the lungs, and the majority of individuals infected with *M. tuberculosis* have latent infections and are asymptomatic. However, data from various clinical studies in humans have raised the hypothesis that helminth co-infections may affect TB susceptibility and the risk of developing latent *M. tuberculosis* infection, as co-infected patients often displayed more advanced disease (63, 64). Gastrointestinal helminth infections may also modulate susceptibility and/or disease pathogenesis to co-infection with other pathogenic *Mycobacteria* spp. Infection with *M. leprae* or *M. lepromatis* causes leprosy, a chronic granulomatous infectious disease. A study of Indonesian patients infected with *M. lepromatis* reported that those with gastrointestinal helminth infections (e.g., *T. trichiura*, *Stongyloides sterocalis*) similarly presented with more severe types of leprosy (65).

Studies from animal models, especially mice, indicate that protection against TB infection is dependent upon the induction of a strong pro-inflammatory Th1-polarized immune response and production of IFNγ, IL-12, and TNF-α, as well as contribution from Th17 cells and IL-17 and IL-23 (66, 67). The immune response induced by co-infection with gastrointestinal helminths may affect immunity to *M. tuberculosis* through a range of distinct mechanisms, including the induction of regulatory T cell responses (68), modulation of Th1 and Th17 responses to the bacterial infection and reduced expression of effector cytokines (69–71). The increased expression of Th2 cytokines, especially IL-4, in mice co-infected with helminths also promotes the induction of alternatively activated macrophages. These cells have been shown to be less effective than pro-inflammatory IFNγ-stimulated macrophages in controlling *M. tuberculosis* (72, 73). Indeed, antigens from helminths such as *T. muris* and *Hymenolepis diminuta* (tapeworms) can induce an alternatively activated phenotype in human macrophages, reducing their ability to control *M. tuberculosis* infection *in vitro* (74). However, mouse studies show that under some circumstances the acute host response to helminth infection might enhance the early control of *M. tuberculosis* infection by alveolar macrophages (75).

Although the induction of T cell responses is considered essential for protective immunity against TB infection, B cells, and the production of mycobacterial-specific antibodies have also been proposed to play an important role (76). However, helminth infections can also influence B cell responses to *M. tuberculosis* infection. Co-infection of humans with *Strongyloides stercoralis* has been shown to affect B cell responses during latent tuberculosis infection, significantly reducing B cell numbers, the induction of mycobacterial-specific IgM and IgG resopnses and expression levels of the B-cell growth factors APRIL and BAFF (77). These helminth-associated impairments to mycobacteria-specific B cell responses could have significant implications for the efficacy of vaccine-induced immune responses to TB in affected regions. However, a clinical trial study in healthy, previously BCG vaccinated adolescents reported that helminth co-infection (*S. mansoni* did not impact on the efficacy of a candidate viral vector-based TB vaccine (78).

Pneumonia

A study of goats in Nigeria revealed that the incidence of pneumonia corresponded with the presence of gastrointestinal parasitism in the same animals (79). Furthermore, a strong association was observed between the occurrence of helminth infections and granulomatous pneumonia. In this study the affected goats were often hydrated, implying that the gastrointestinal helminth infections may have caused pulmonary oedema due to increased fluid accumulation in the lung. The authors suggested that may this have reduced the efficacy of immunity in the lung, enabling other pathogenic microorganisms (bacteria and/or viruses) to establish infection and the subsequent development of pneumonia (79).

Pathogenic *Escherichia coli*

The zoonotic bacterium *E. coli* O157 is a worldwide problem for public health causing haemorrhagic diarrhea in infected humans. Cattle are considered the major reservoir for human infection, and infection in these animals is usually asymptomatic. A study of 14 British farms suggested that co-infection with the liver fluke *F. hepatica* may increase the risk of *E. coli* O157 shedding (80). This implies that strategies aimed at controlling *F. hepatica* infection may have additional benefit by reducing the shedding of *E. coli* O157.

Giardia lamblia and enteroaggregative *E. coli* are two of the most commonly isolated pathogens in malnourished children. Mice fed on a protein-deficient diet were used to model the pathogenesis of co-infection with these pathogens in malnourished individuals (81). The malnourished mice fed a protein-deficient diet exhibited significantly greater weight loss following co-infection with *G. lamblia* and enteroaggregative *E. coli* when compared to co-infected mice that received a normal diet. This study reveals how the combined effects of the composition of the host's diet and pathogen infection can affect disease pathogenicity. Studies using a laboratory biofilm system to mimic the human gut microbiota have revealed that *G. duodenalis* can cause significant dysbiosis. These effects were mediated in part through the actions of secretory-excretory *Giardia* cysteine proteases, and these could promote gut epithelial cell apoptosis, tight junction disruption, and bacterial translocation across the gut epithelium (82).

Despite the ability of *Giardia* infection to cause intestinal dysbiosis, in countries with poor standards of sanitation *Giardia* infection has been associated with decreased incidence of diarrhoeal disease. This raised the hypothesis that infection with *Giardia* spp. might modulate host responses to co-infection with attaching and effacing enteropathogens. Weight loss, pathological signs of colitis and bacterial colonization and translocation were significantly attenuated in mice co-infected with *G. muris* and the attaching and effacing enteropathogen *Citrobacter rodentium* (83). These effects coincided with enhanced secretion of the antimicrobial factors β-defensin 2 and trefoil factor 3 by gut epithelial cells during co-infection (83). This suggests that components of the host response to

infection with *Giardia* spp. (e.g., production of antimicrobial factors) may reduce susceptibility to gastrointestinal co-infection with certain pathogenic bacteria. These studies also highlight how differences in the anatomical niches that the parasites inhabit may also have a significant influence on the disease pathogenesis of a bacterial co-infection. When pathogens infect the same niche such as the gastrointestinal tract, infection with *Giardia* spp. may provide protection against bacterial co-infection (83). Conversely, infection with *F. hepatica* in the liver was associated with the enhanced pathogenesis of a bacterial co-infection in the intestine (80).

EFFECTS ON VIRAL INFECTIONS

Several studies have revealed how parasite co-infections, especially helminths, can reduce immunity to important viral pathogens. In many of these instances the induction of a Th2-polarized immune response to the parasite infection appears to impede the development of effective antiviral immunity. For example, mice co-infected with the gastrointestinal helminths *Trichinella spiralis* or *H. polygyrus* and mouse norovirus (MNV) had increased viral loads and reduced levels of virus-specific CD4+ T cells expressing IFNγ and TNF-α when compared to mice infected with norovirus alone (84). The production of Th2 cytokines during helminth infection is associated with the expression of the transcription factor signal transducer and activator of transcription 6 (STAT6) by alternatively activated macrophages. In mice deficient in STAT6, viral loads were reduced when compared to wild-type controls indicating that the induction of STAT6-dependent alternatively activated macrophages during helminth infection can impede the induction of antiviral innate and adaptive immunity (85). As well as impeding the efficacy of anti-viral immunity, the expression of IL-4 and activation of the transcription factor STAT6 during helminth infection in mice can also promote the reactivation of a latent γ-herpesvirus infection (85). The sections below describe how parasite co-infections may impede immunity to certain viral pathogens, but examples are also provided where potential host-protective effects have been proposed.

Impeding Viral Immunity
Hepatitis C Virus (HCV)

Infections with HCV can cause liver fibrosis and cirrhosis and are major causes of chronic liver disease throughout the world. A study of Egyptian HCV patients co-infected with *S. mansoni* showed that these individuals had significantly higher concentrations of HCV proteins in distinct stages of the virus-mediated hepatic fibrosis (86). Co-infected individuals may also have an increased rate of progressing through the different pathological stages of HCV-mediated hepatic fibrosis than those infected with HCV alone. The authors suggested that the immune response induced in response to *S. mansoni* infection may have led to enhanced HCV propagation and increased concentration of HCV proteins. This implies that that components of the immune response to the schistosome infection may have suppressed the HCV-induced Th1 cytokine production, reducing antiviral immunity. Treatment of co-infected patients with anti-schistosome therapy may therefore help to decrease the progression rate of the HCV-induced hepatic fibrosis.

Human Immunodeficiency Virus (HIV)

African adults infected with HIV are often co-infected with gastrointestinal parasites. A study of HIV-infected Ugandans showed a high prevalence of parasitic infections (especially *Necator americanus*), and co-infection with hookworms correlated with much lower peripheral blood CD4$^+$ T cell levels than those infected with HIV alone (87). This raises the suggestion that individuals co-infected with hookworms and HIV are at a distinct immunologic disadvantage when compared to those infected with HIV alone. This hypothesis has been experimentally tested in mice using a helminth/retrovirus co-infection model (88). Although the ability of the mice to control the *L. sigmodontis* infection was not affected in the co-infected mice, helminth infection did interfere with the host's ability to the control of the viral infection. Levels of virus-specific CD8$^+$ T cells, FoxP3$^+$ regulatory T cells, and cytokines were similar in co-infected mice and those infected with Friend virus alone. The increased viral loads in co-infected mice were instead associated with reduced titres of neutralizing virus-specific IgG2b and IgG2c antibodies. However, earlier studies in humans have reported no beneficial effect of antihelminthic treatment on HIV viral loads [plasma HIV-1 RNA concentrations; (89)], and other studies have suggested that helminth co-infections do not exacerbate HIV infection (90). On face value, the prospective studies undertaken in humans suggest that antihelmitic treatments or helminth-specific vaccines are unlikely to have any beneficial effects in regions with high incidence of helminth and HIV infections. However, further studies are necessary to determine whether additional factors such as host age, the intensity of the helminth infection or magnitude of the viral load affect the efficacy of such approaches.

Human T-Cell Lymphotropic Virus-1 (HTLV-1)

Strongyloides stercoralis is a soil-transmitted intestinal helminth parasite of humans. Infection occurs following penetration of the skin by filiform larvae. The majority of *S. stercoralis* infections are asymptomatic to mild, but a life-threatening hyper-infection syndrome can develop in immunosuppressed hosts. This is accompanied by the massive dissemination of the filariform larvae from the colon to the lungs, liver, central nervous system, or kidneys. Co-infection with HTLV-1 can impede the induction of Th2-polarized immunity (91, 92), and patients infected with HTLV-1 have more frequent and more severe forms of strongyloidiasis. Patients co-infected with HTLV-1 and *S. stercoralis* were shown to have higher parasite burdens than those with strongyloidiasis alone (93). Mouse models have shown that IL-5-mediated eosinophil production and activation is important for protection against infection with *S. stercoralis* (94). In patients co-infected with HTLV-1 and *S. stercoralis* both parasite antigen-specific IL-5 responses and eosinophil levels were significantly decreased, suggesting an additional means by which the virus

infection may impede immunity to helminths. However, rare incidences of acute respiratory distress syndrome have been encountered in HTLV-1-infected patients following treatment with antihelminthics (95). The mechanisms responsible for the development of this pathology are unknown, but it is plausible that acute immune reactions to the intrapulmonary destruction of the large parasite burden following antihelminthic treatment may play a role in triggering this response (95).

Vaccinia Virus

A study in BALB/c mice has shown that co-infection with *Ascaris* in *Vaccinia* virus-infected hosts enhances the virus-associated pathology due to impaired *Vaccinia* virus-specific immunity (96). The levels of splenic CD8+ T cells in the co-infected mice were significantly reduced, as was the frequency of IFN-γ-producing virus-specific CD4$^+$ and CD8$^+$ T cells. Similar effects have also been reported in mice co-infected with *S. mansoni* (97). In this study *Vaccinia* virus-specific CD8$^+$ cytotoxic T-cell responses were reduced in the mice co-infected with *S. mansoni*, suggesting a mechanistic link between the increased viral loads and reduced viral clearance. Since many chronic helminth infections induce a strong Th2-polarized immune response, the above examples suggest that the presence of this cytokine milieu at the time of virus co-infection may play an important role in impeding the induction of the IFNγ-mediated control of virus replication.

Respiratory Syncytial Virus (RSV)

In contrast to the above reports, it is plausible that in some circumstances that co-infection with helminths may enhance protection against viruses. Respiratory syncytial virus (RSV) is a major respiratory pathogen, and nearly all infants are infected with this virus by the age of 2 years old. However, because the virus does not induce lasting immunity recurrent RSV infections can occur throughout life. A study has shown how a gastrointestinal helminth infection can promote protective antiviral effects in the lung (98). Mice infected with *H. polygyrus* had reduced viral loads after co-infection with RSV and developed significantly less disease and pulmonary inflammation. These effects were not a considered to be a consequence of the induction of a Th2-polarized immune response to the worm infection. Instead, *H. polygyrus* infection coincided with the upregulated expression of type I IFN in the gut and the lung in a microbiota-dependent manner. Furthermore, the protective effects of helminth infection on RSV co-infection were impeded in mice lacking type I IFN receptor signaling (*Ifnar1*-deficient mice).

Virus Infection in Amphibians

All the above studies have described parasite virus co-infections in mammals or birds, but similar interactions have been reported in experimental amphibians. Prior infection of the larval stages (tadpole) of four distinct amphibian species with trematode parasites (*Echinoparyphium* spp.) significantly reduced viral loads following co-infection with ranavirus (99). Furthermore, *Echinoparyphium* co-infection coincided with reduced ranavirus transmission within a community of larval wood frogs (*Lithobates sylvaticus*). The cellular and molecular mechanisms by which helminth co-infection mediated these effects on ranavirus pathogenesis remain to be determined.

INFECTIONS WITH PRIONS (TRANSMISSIBLE SPONGIFORM ENCEPHALOPATHIES)

Prions are a unique group of pathogens that can cause infectious, chronic, neurodegenerative diseases in humans and some domesticated and free-ranging animal species. The precise nature of the infectious prion is uncertain, but an abnormal, relatively proteinase-resistant isoform (PrP^{Sc}) of the host cellular prion protein (PrP^C), co-purifies with prion infectivity in diseased tissues (100). Many natural prion diseases are acquired by oral consumption of contaminated food or pasture. The gut-associated lymphoid tissues (GALT) within the lining of the intestine such as the tonsils, Peyer's patches, appendix, colonic, and caecal patches, together with the mesenteric lymph nodes, help to provide protection against intestinal pathogens. However, the early replication of prions within the Peyer's patches in the small intestine is essential for their efficient spread of from the gut to the brain (a process termed *neuroinvasion*) (101–104).

Natural prion disease susceptible hosts such as sheep, deer, and cattle are regularly exposed to helminths but it is uncertain whether co-infections with these pathogens can influence oral prion disease pathogenesis, for example by causing damage to the gut epithelium and enhancing the uptake of prions into the GALT. In one study, lambs with high genetic susceptibility to natural sheep scrapie were experimentally co-infected with *Teladorsagia circumcincta* at monthly intervals from 6 to 11 months old and effects on prion disease determined (105). Although no mechanistic insights were reported, the authors suggested that the onset of prion disease was shortened in the co-infected lambs. However, the significance of data reported in this study is unclear as the animals were co-infected with *T. circumcincta* long after prion neuroinvasion from the intestine had occurred (106, 107). Conversely, when mice were co-infected with the large intestine-restricted helminth pathogen *T. muris* around the time of oral prion exposure, no effects on prion disease duration were observed (104). This is most likely because the large intestinal GALT are not important early sites of prion accumulation and neuroinvasion (104). Clearly additional studies are required to determine whether the pathology specifically in small intestine caused by a helminth infection may influence the prion neuroinvasion from the gut to the brain.

CONCLUDING REMARKS

Infectious diseases are commonly studied in experimental animals exposed to individual pathogenic microorganisms. However, this review described many examples of how infection with certain parasites can have a dramatic influence on host susceptibility or disease pathogenesis to co-infection with other pathogens. Many of these studies have reported correlations between alterations to specific immune parameters (T cell polarity etc.) and pathogen susceptibility, raising the hypothesis that many of the effects of co-infection are immune mediated. For example, alterations to the polarity of the T-cell response or macrophage phenotype induced by the parasite infection could affect the induction of protective immunity to co-infection with another pathogen. Further scrutiny of these studies shows that in many instances definitive demonstrations that the effects are indeed immune-mediated are lacking. Addressing these issues in natural host species is technically challenging. However, a large array of murine *in vivo* tractable systems are now available that enable the contributions of specific cellular and molecular immune components to be determined.

Laboratory mice housed to high microbiological status in specific-pathogen free conditions have proved to be highly tractable model systems in which to study the pathogenesis of many infectious diseases. How representative these mice are to natural host species in field conditions is questionable, since wild mice are typically infected with numerous micro- and macro-parasite species. The immune status of laboratory mice and wild mice differs significantly (108). Wild mice are markedly more antigen-experienced than laboratory mice, displaying on-going immune activation and the presence of an inflammatory myeloid cell subset that has not been detected in laboratory mice. Wild mice also express cytokine responses to microbial ligands that are similar or lower when compared to laboratory mice, and have highly heterogeneous gut microbiomes (108, 109). This suggests that the high level of pathogen exposure is a major driver of the enhanced immune activation in wild mice.

Many of the above examples suggest links between alterations to Th2/Th1 polarity or the nature of the innate immune response and susceptibility to pathogen co-infection. However, the underlying rules that dictate whether these interactions are likely to confer increased susceptibility or protection are not always apparent and are likely influenced by multiple factors. For example, susceptibility to these co-infections may be dependent on the individual niches that each pathogen inhabits in the host e.g., the same niche, or mucosal (gastrointestinal) vs. systemic. In other situations, the induction of a strong pro-inflammatory response to a parasite infection may exacerbate susceptibility and/or pathology following co-infection with another pathogen that induces a similar pro-inflammatory response. Chronic helminth infection in mice also promoted the reactivation of a latent virus infection. But not all the effects on co-infection appear to be directly immune mediated, as disruptions to the metabolic profile within the gastrointestinal tract following helminth infection promoted susceptibility to co-infection with certain pathogenic bacteria. As well as influencing host susceptibility to pathogen co-infection, the immune response to certain parasite infections may have other important health issues by negatively affecting the induction of antigen-specific immunity to vaccine antigens, reducing vaccine efficacy.

A greater understanding of how infectious disease susceptibility and pathogenesis are influenced by concurrent parasite infections will help the design of more effective treatments to control the spread of infectious diseases. For example, some helminth-derived ES products possess potent immunoregulatory properties, and these could be sufficient to suppress allograft rejection (110). Whether similar parasite-derived molecules can suppress host-responses to other pathogens, or conversely can be used therapeutically to enhance their clearance, remains to be determined.

AUTHOR CONTRIBUTIONS

The author confirms being the sole contributor of this work and has approved it for publication.

REFERENCES

1. Inclan-Rico JM, Siracusa MC. First responders: innate immunity to helminths. *Trends Parasitol.* (2018) 34:861–80. doi: 10.1016/j.pt.2018.08.007
2. Allen JE, Maizels RM. Diversity and dialogue in immunity to helminths. *Nat Rev Immunol.* (2011) 11:375–88. doi: 10.1038/nri2992
3. Gerbe F, Sidot E, Smyth DJ, Ohmoto M, Matsumoto I, Dardalhon V, et al. Intestinal epithelial tuft cells initiate type 2 mucosal immunity to helminth parasites. *Nature* (2016) 529:226–30. doi: 10.1038/nature16527
4. Langhorne J, Ndungu FM, Sponaas AM, Marsh K. Immunity to malaria: more questions than answers. *Nat Immunol.* (2008) 9:725–32. doi: 10.1038/ni.f.205
5. Perez-Mazliah D, Langhorne J. CD4 T-cell subsets in malaria: TH1/TH2 revisited. *Front Immunol.* (2015) 5:671. doi: 10.3389/fimmu.2014.00671
6. Hoeve MA, Mylonas KJ, Fairlie-Clarke KJ, Mahajan SM, Allen JE, Graham AL. *Plasmodium chabaudi* limits early *Nippostrongylus brasiliensis*-induced pulmonary immune activation and Th2 polarization in co-infected mice. *BMC Immunol.* (2009) 10:60. doi: 10.1186/1471-2172-10-60
7. Karadjian G, Berrebi D, Dogna N, Vallarino-Lhermitte N, Bain O, Landau I, et al. Co-infection restrains *Litomosoides sigmodontis* filarial load and plasmodial *P. yoelii* but not *P. chabaudi parasitaemia* in mice. *Parasite* (2014) 21:16. doi: 10.1051/parasite/2014017
8. Craig JM, Scott AL. Antecedent *Nippostrongylus* infection alters the lung immune response to *Plasmodium berghei*. *Parasite Immunol.* (2016) 39:e12441. doi: 10.1111/pim.12441
9. Hartmann W, Haben I, Fleischer B, Breloer M. Pathogenic nematodes suppress humoral responses to third-party antigens *in vivo* by IL-10-mediated interference with Th cell function. *J Immunol.* (2011) 187:4088–99. doi: 10.4049/jimmunol.1004136
10. Metenou S, Dembele B, Konate S, Dolo H, Coulibaly YI, Diallo AA, et al. Filarial infection suppresses malaria-specific multifunctional Th1 and Th17 responses in malaria and filarial coinfections. *J Immunol.* (2011) 186:4725–33. doi: 10.4049/jimmunol.1003778
11. Bucher K, Dietz K, Lackner P, Pasche B, Fendel R, Mordmüller B, et al. Schistosoma co-infection protects against brain pathology but does not prevent severe disease and death in a murine model of cerebral malaria. *Int J Parasitol.* (2011) 41:21–31. doi: 10.1016/j.ijpara.2010.06.008
12. Su Z, Segura M, Morgan K, Loredo-Osti JC, Stevenson MM. Impairment of protective immunity to blood-stage malaria by concurrent nematode infection. *Infect Immun.* (2005) 73:3531–9. doi: 10.1128/IAI.73.6.3531-3539.2005
13. Graham AL, Lamb TJ, Read AF, Allen JE. Malaria-filaria coninfection in mice makes malarial disease more severe unless filarial infection achieves patency. *J Infect Dis.* (2005) 191:410–21. doi: 10.1086/426871
14. Moriyasu T, Nakamura R, Deloer S, Senba M, Kubo M, Inoue M, et al. *Schistosoma mansoni* infection suprresses the growth of *Plasmodium yoelli* parasites in the liver and reduces gametocyte infectivity in mosquitoes. *PLoS Neglect Trop Dis.* (2018) 12:e0006197. doi: 10.1371/journal.pntd.0006197
15. Nyakundi RK, Nyamongo O, Maamun J, Akinyi M, Mulei I, Farah IO, et al. Protective effect of chronic schistosomiasis in baboons coinfected with *Schistosoma mansoni* and *Plasmondium knowlesi*. *Infect Immun.* (2016) 84:1320–30. doi: 10.1128/IAI.00490-15
16. Lemaitre M, Watier L, Briand V, Garcia A, Le Hesran JY, Cot M. Coinfection with *Plasmodium falciparum* and *Schistosoma haematobium*: additional evidence of the protective effect of schistosomiasis on malaria in Senegalese children. *Am J Trop Med Hyg.* (2014) 90:329–34. doi: 10.4269/ajtmh.12-0431
17. Lyke KE, Dabo A, Arama C, Daou M, Diarra I, Wang A, et al. Reduced T regulatory cell response during acute *Plasmodium falciparum* infection in Malian children co-infected with *Schistosoma haematobium*. *PLoS ONE* (2012) 7:e31647. doi: 10.1371/journal.pone.0031647
18. Cunnington AJ, Walther M, Riley EM. Piecing together the puzzle of malaria. *Sci Trans Med.* (2013) 5:211–8. doi: 10.1126/scitranslmed.3007432
19. Teo T-H, Howland SW, Claser C, Gun SY, Poh CM, Lee WW, et al. Conversely, co-infection with Chikungunya virus alters the trafficking of pathogenic CD8$^+$ T cells into the brain and prevents *Plasmodium*-induced neuropathology. *EMBO Mol Med.* (2018) 10:121–38. doi: 10.15252/emmm.201707885
20. Waknine-Grinberg JH, Gold D, Ohayon A, Flescher E, Heyfets A, Doenhoff MJ, et al. *Schistosoma mansoni* infection reduces the incidence of murine cerebral malaria. *Malaria J.* (2010) 9:5. doi: 10.1186/1475-2875-9-5
21. Wang ML, Feng YH, Pang W, Qi ZM, Zhang Y, Guo YJ, et al. Parasite densities modulate susceptibility of mice to cerebral malaria during co-infection with *Schistosoma japonicum* and *Plasmodium berghei*. *Malaria J.* (2014) 13:116. doi: 10.1186/1475-2875-13-116
22. Abbate JL, Ezenwa VO, Guégan JF, Choisy M, Nacher M, Roche B. Disentangling complex parasite interactions: protection against cerebral malaria by one helminth species is jeopardized by co-infection with another. *PLoS Neglect Trop Dis.* (2018) 12:e0006483. doi: 10.1371/journal.pntd.0006483
23. O'Neill SM, Brady MT, Callanan JJ, Mulcahy G, Joyce P, Mills KH, et al. *Fasciola hepatica* infection downregulates Th1 responses in mice. *Parasite Immunol.* (2000) 22:147–55. doi: 10.1046/j.1365-3024.2000.00290.x
24. Lucena AN, Cuatero LG, Mulcahy G, Zintl A. The immunomodulatory effects of co-infection with *Fasciola hepatica*: from bovine tuberculosis to Johne's disease. *Vet J.* (2017) 222:9–16. doi: 10.1016/j.tvjl.2017.02.007
25. O'Neill SM, Mills KH, Dalton JP. *Fasciola hepatica* cathepsin L cysteine proteinase suppresses *Bordatella pertussis*-specific interferon-gamma production *in vivo*. *Parasite Immunol.* (2001) 23:541–7. doi: 10.1046/j.1365-3024.2001.00411.x
26. Claridge J, Diggle P, McCann CM, Mulcahy G, Flynn R, McNair J, et al. *Fasciola hepatica* is associated with the failure to detect bovine tuberculosis in dairy cattle. *Nat Commun.* (2012) 3:853. doi: 10.1038/ncomms1840
27. Flynn RJ, Mannion C, Golden O, Hacariz O, Mulcahy G. Experimental *Fasciola hepatica* infection alters responses to tests used for diagnosis of bovine tuberculosis. *Infect Immun.* (2007) 75:1373–81. doi: 10.1128/IAI.01445-06
28. Byrne AW, Graham J, Brown C, Donaghy A, Guelbenzu-Gonzalo M, McNair J, et al. Bovine tuberculosis visible lesions in cattle culled during herd breakdowns: the effects of individual characteristics trade movement and co-infecion. *BMC Vet Res.* (2017) 13:400. doi: 10.1186/s12917-017-1321-z
29. Garza-Cuartero L, O'Sullivan J, Blanco A, McNair J, Welsh M, Flynn RJ, et al. *Fasciola hepatica* infection reduces *Mycobacterium bovis* burden and mycobacterial uptake and suppresses the pro-inflammatory response. *Parasite Immunol.* (2016) 38:387–402. doi: 10.1111/pim.12326
30. Mavrogianni VS, Papadopoulos E, Spanos SA, Mitsoura A, Ptochos S, Gougoulis DA, et al. Trematode infections in pregnant ewes can predispose to mastitis during the subsequent lactation period. *Res Vet Sci.* (2014) 96:171–9. doi: 10.1016/j.rvsc.2013.11.009
31. Boonyanugomol W, Chomvarin C, Sripa B, Bhudhisawasdi V, Khuntikeo N, Hahnvajanawong C, et al. *Helicobacter pylori* in Thai patients with cholangiocarcinoma and its association with biliary inflammation and proliferation. *HPB* (2012) 14:177–84. doi: 10.1111/j.1477-2574.2011.00423.x

32. Dangtakot R, Pinlaor S, Itthitaetrakool U, Chaidee A, Chomvarin C, Sangka A, et al. Coinfection with *Helicobacter pylori* and *Opisthorchis viverrini* enhances the severity of hepatobiliary abnormalities in hamsters. *Infect Immun.* (2017) 85:e00009–19. doi: 10.1128/IAI.00009-17

33. Pearce EJ, MacDonald AS. The immunobiology of schistosomiasis. *Nat Rev Immunol.* (2002) 2:499–511. doi: 10.1038/nri843

34. Bickle QD, Solum J, Helmby H. Chronic intestinal nematode infection exacerbates experimental *Schistosoma mansoni* infection. *Infect Immun.* (2008) 76:5802–9. doi: 10.1128/IAI.00827-08

35. Beechler BR, Jolles AE, Budischak SA, Corstjens PLAM, Ezenwa VO, Smith M, et al. Host immunity, nutrition and coinfection alter longitudinal infection patterns of schistosomes in a free ranging African buffalo population. *PLoS Neglect Trop Dis.* (2017) 11:e0006122. doi: 10.1371/journal.pntd.0006122

36. Kloosterman A, Frankena K, Ploeger HW. Increased establishment of lungworms (*Dictyocaulus viviparus*) in calves after previous infections with gastrointestinal nematodes (*Ostertagia ostertagi* and *Cooperia oncophora*). *Vet Parasitol.* (1989) 33:155–63. doi: 10.1016/0304-4017(89)90063-0

37. Bazzone LE, Smith PM, Rutitzky LI, Shainheit MG, Urban JF, Setiawan T, et al. Coinfection with the intestinal nematode *Heligmosomoides polygyrus* markedly reduces hepatic egg-induced immunopathology and proinflammatory cytokines in mouse models of severe schistosomiasis. *Infect Immun.* (2008) 76:5164–72. doi: 10.1128/IAI.00673-08

38. Tabel H, Wei G, Bull HJ. Immunosuppression: cause for failures of vaccines against African trypanosomiases. *PLoS Neglect Trop Dis.* (2013) 7:e2090. doi: 10.1371/journal.pntd.0002090

39. Caljon G, Van Reet N, De Trez C, Vermeersch M, Pérez-Morga D, Van Den Abbeele J. The dermis as a delivery site of *Trypanosoma brucei* for tsetse flies. *PLoS Pathog.* (2016) 12:e1005744. doi: 10.1371/journal.ppat.1005744

40. Ademola IO, Odeniran PO. Co-infection with *Plasmodium berghei* and *Trypanosoma brucei* increases severity of malaria and trypanosomiasis in mice. *Acta Trop.* (2016) 159:29–35. doi: 10.1016/j.actatropica.2016.03.030

41. Machelart A, Van Vyve M, Potemberg G, Demars A, De Trez C, Tima HG, et al. *Trypanosoma* infection favors *Brucella* elimination via IL-12/IFNγ-dependent pathways. *Front Immunol.* (2017) 8:903. doi: 10.3389/fimmu.2017.00903

42. Teixeira AR, Hecht MM, Guimaro MC, Sousa AO, Nitz N. Pathogenesis of Chagas' disease: parasite persistence and autoimmunity. *Clin Microbiol Rev.* (2011) 24:592–630. doi: 10.1128/CMR.00063-10

43. Rodriguez JPF, Caldas IS, Goncalves V, Almeida LA, Souza RLM, Novaes R. *S. mansoni-T. cruzi* co-infection modulates arginase-1/iNOS expression, liver and heart disease in mice. *Nitric Oxide* (2017) 66:43–52. doi: 10.1016/j.niox.2017.02.013

44. Ahmed N, French T, Rausch S, Kühl A, Hemminger K, Dunay IR, et al. Toxoplasma co-infection prevents Th2 differentiation and leads to a helminth-specific Th1 response. *Front Cell Infect Microbiol.* (2017) 7:341. doi: 10.3389/fcimb.2017.00341

45. Khan IA, Hakak R, Eberle K, Sayles P, Weiss LM, Urban JF. Coninfection with *Heligmosomoides polygyrus* fails to establish CD8+ T-cell immunity against *Toxoplasma gondii*. *Infect Immun.* (2008) 76:1305–13. doi: 10.1128/IAI.01236-07

46. Marple A, Wu W, Shah S, Zhao Y, Du P, Gause WC, et al. Cutting edge: helminth coinfection blocks effector differentiation of CD8 T cells through alternatate host Th2- and IL-10-mediated responses. *J Immunol.* (2016) 198:634–9. doi: 10.4049/jimmunol.1601741

47. Hiob L, Koethe M, Schares G, Goroll T, Daugschies A, Bangoura B. Experimental *Toxoplasma gondii* and *Eimeria tenella* co-infection in chickens. *Parasitol Res.* (2017) 116:3189–203. doi: 10.1007/s00436-017-5636-2

48. Xiao J, Yolken RH. Strain hypothesis of *Toxoplasma gondii* infection on the outcome of human disease. *Acta Physiol.* (2015) 213:828–45. doi: 10.1111/apha.12458

49. Dubey JP, Ruff MD, Camargo ME, Shen SK, Wilkins GL, Kwok OC, et al. Serologic and parasitologic responses of domestic chickens after oral inoculation with *Toxoplasma gondii* oocysts. *Am J Vet Res.* (1993) 54:1668–72.

50. Kaneto CN, Costa AJ, Paulillo AC, Moraes FR, Murakami TO, Meireles MV. Experimental toxoplasmosis in broiler chicks. *Vet Parasitol.* (1997) 69:203–10. doi: 10.1016/S0304-4017(96)01126-0

51. Saeij JP, Boyle JP, Boothroyd JC. Differences among the three major strains of *Toxoplasma gondii* and their specific interactions with the infected host. *Trends Parasitol.* (2005) 21:476–81. doi: 10.1016/j.pt.2005.08.001

52. Mason S, Dubey JP, Smith JE, Boag B. *Toxoplasma gondii* coinfection with diseases and parasites in wild rabbits in Scotland. *Parasitology* (2015) 142:1415–21. doi: 10.1017/S003118201500075X

53. Weatherhead J, Cortes AA, Sandoval C, Vaca M, Chico M, Loor S, et al. Comparison of cytokine responses in Ecuadorian children infected with *Giardia*, *Ascaris*, or both parasites. *Am J Trop Med Hyg.* (2017) 96:1394–9. doi: 10.4269/ajtmh.16-0580

54. Zhou P, Li E, Shea-Donohue T, Singer SM. Tumour necrosis factor α contributes to protection against *Giardia lamblia* infection in mice. *Parasite Immunol.* (2007) 29:367–74. doi: 10.1111/j.1365-3024.2007.00953.x

55. Reynolds LA, Redpath SA, Yurist-Doutsch S, Gill N, Brown EM, van der Heijden J, et al. Enteric helminths promote *Salmonella* coninfection by altering the intestinal microbiome. *J Infect Dis.* (2017) 215:1245–54. doi: 10.1093/infdis/jix141

56. Morpeth SC, Ramadhani HO, Crump JA. Invasive non-Typhi *Salmonella* disease in Africa. *Clin Infect Dis.* (2009) 49:606–11. doi: 10.1086/603553

57. Berkley JA, Bejon P, Mwangi T, Gwer S, Maitland K, Williams TN, et al. HIV infection, malnutrition, and invasive bacterial infection among children with severe malaria. *Clin Infect Dis.* (2009) 49:336–43. doi: 10.1086/600299

58. Mtove G, Amos B, Nadjm B, Hendriksen IC, Dondorp AM, Mwambuli A, et al. Decreasing incidence of severe malaria and community-acquired bacteraemia among hospitalized children in Muhesa, north-eastern Tanzania, 2006–2010. *Malaria J.* (2011) 10:320. doi: 10.1186/1475-2875-10-320

59. Mabey DC, Brown A, Greenwood BM. *Plasmodium falciparum* malaria and *Salmonella* infections in Gambian children. *J Infect Dis.* (1987) 155:1319–21. doi: 10.1093/infdis/155.6.1319

60. Gozzelino R, Jeney V, Soares MP. Mechanisms of cell protection by heme oxygenase-1. *Ann Rev Pharmacol Toxicol.* (2010) 50:323–54. doi: 10.1146/annurev.pharmtox.010909.105600

61. Cunnington AJ, de Souza JB, Walther M, Riley EM. Malaria impairs resistance to *Salmonella* through heme- and heme oxygenase-dependent dysfunctional granulocyte mobilization. *Nat Med.* (2012) 18:120–7. doi: 10.1038/nm.2601

62. Cunnington AJ, Njie M, Correa S, Takem EN, Riley EM, Walther M. Prolonged neutrophil dysfunction after *Plasmodium falciparum* malaria is related to hemolysis and heme oxygenase-1 induction. *J Immunol.* (2012) 189:5336–46. doi: 10.4049/jimmunol.1201028

63. Resende Co T, Hirsch CS, Toossi Z, Dietze R, Ribeiro-Rodrigues R. Intestinal helminth co-infection has a negative impact on both anti-*Mycobacterium tuberculosis* immunity and clinical response to tuberculosis therapy. *Clin Exp Immunol.* (2007) 147:45–52. doi: 10.1111/j.1365-2249.2006.03247.x

64. Verhagen LM, Hermans PW, Warris A, de Groot R, Maes M, Villalba JA, et al. Helminths and skewed cytokine profiles increase tuberculin skin test positivity in Warao Amerindians. *Tuberculosis* (2012) 92:505–12. doi: 10.1016/j.tube.2012.07.004

65. Oktaria S, Effendi EH, Indriatmi W, van Hees CLM, Thio HB, Sjamsoe-Daili ES, et al. Soil-transmitted helminth infections and leprosy: a cross-sectional study of the association between two major neglected tropical diseases in Indonesia. *BMC Infect Dis.* (2016) 16:258. doi: 10.1186/s12879-016-1593-0

66. Flynn JL. Lessons from experimental *Mycobacterium tuberculosis* infections. *Microbes Infect.* (2006) 8:1179–88. doi: 10.1016/j.micinf.2005.10.033

67. Khader SA, Cooper AM. IL-23 and IL-17 in tuberculosis. *Cytokine* (2008) 41:79–83. doi: 10.1016/j.cyto.2007.11.022

68. Toulza F, Tsang L, Ottenhoff TH, Brown M, Dockrell HM. *Mycobacterium tuberculosis*-specific CD4+ T-cell response is increased, and Treg cells decreased, in anthelmintic-treated patients with latent TB. *Eur J Immunol.* (2016) 46:752–61. doi: 10.1002/eji.201545843

69. Babu S, Bhat SQ, Kumar NP, Jayantasri S, Rukmani S, Kumaran P, et al. Human type 1 and 17 responses in latent tuberculosis are modulated by coincident filarial infection through cytotoxic T lymphocyte antigen-4 and programmed death-1. *J Infect Dis.* (2009) 200:288–98. doi: 10.1086/599797

70. George PJ, Anuradha R, Kumaran PP, Chandrasekaran V, Nutman TB, Babu S. Modulation of mycobacterial-specific Th1 and Th17 cells in latent tuberculosis by coincident hookworm infection. *J Immunol.* (2013) 190:5161–8. doi: 10.4049/jimmunol.1203311

71. George PJ, Anuradha R, Kumar NP, Sridhar R, Banurekha VV, Nutman TB, et al. Helminth infections coincident with active pulmonary tuberculosis inhibit mono- and multifunctional CD4$^+$ and CD8$^+$ T cell responses in a process dependent on IL-10. *PLoS Pathog.* (2014) 10:e1004375. doi: 10.1371/journal.ppat.1004375

72. Kahnert A, Seiler P, Stein M, Bandermann S, Hahnke K, Mollenkopf H, et al. Alternative activation deprives macrophages of a coordinated defense program to *Mycobacterium tuberculosis. Eur J Immunol.* (2006) 36:631–47. doi: 10.1002/eji.200535496

73. Potian JA, Rafi W, Bhatt K, McBride A, Gause WC, Salgame P. Preexisting helminth infection induces inhibition of innate pulmonary anti-tuberculosis defense by engaging the IL-4 receptor pathway. *J Exp Med.* (2011) 208:1863–74. doi: 10.1084/jem.20091473

74. Aira N, Andersson AM, Singh SK, McKay DM, Blomgran R. Species dependent impact of helminthderived antigens on human macrophages infected with *Mycobacterium tuberculosis*: direct effect on the innate anti-mycobacterial response. *PLoS Neglect Trop Dis.* (2017) 11:e0005390. doi: 10.1371/journal.pntd.0005390

75. du Plessis N, Kleynhans L, Thiart L, van Helden PD, Brombacher F, Horsnell WG, et al. Acute helminth infection enhances early macrophage mediated control of mycobacterial infection. *Mucosal Immunol.* (2013) 6:931–41. doi: 10.1038/mi.2012.131

76. Achkar JM, Chan J, Casadevall A. B cells and antibodies in the defense against *Mycobacterium tuberculosis* infection. *Immunol Rev.* (2015) 264:167–81. doi: 10.1111/imr.12276

77. Anuradha R, Munisankar S, Bhootra Y, Dolla C, Kumaran P, Nutman TB, et al. Modulation of *Mycobacterium tuberculosis*-specific humoral immune responses is associated with *Strongyloides stercoralis* coinfection. *PLoS Neglect Trop Dis.* (2017) 11:e0005569. doi: 10.1371/journal.pntd.0005569

78. Wajja A, Kizito D, Nassanga B, Nalwoga A, Kabagenyi J, Kimuda S, et al. The effect of current *Schistosoma mansoni* infection on the immunogenicity of a candidate TB vaccine, MVA85A, in BCGvaccinated adolescents: an open-label trial. *PLoS Neglect Trop Dis.* (2017) 11:e0005440. doi: 10.1371/journal.pntd.0005440

79. Adeyemi MT, Morenikeji OA, Emikpe BO, Jarikre TA. Interactions between gastrointestinal parasitism and pneumonia in Nigerian goats. *J Parasit Dis.* (2017) 41:726–33. doi: 10.1007/s12639-017-0878-6

80. Howell AK, Tongue SC, Currie C, Evans J, Williams DJL, McNeilly TN. Co-infection with *Fasciola hepatica* may increase the risk of *Escherichia coli* O157 shedding in British cattle destined for the food chain. *Prevent Vet Med.* (2018) 150:70–6. doi: 10.1016/j.prevetmed.2017.12.007

81. Bartelt LA, Bolick DT, Mayneris-Perxachs J, Kolling GL, Medlock GL, Zaenker EI, et al. Cross-modulation of pathogen-specific pathways enhances malnutrition during enteric co-infection with *Giardia lamblia* and enteroaggregative *Escherichia coli. PLoS Pathog.* (2017) 13:e1006471. doi: 10.1371/journal.ppat.1006471

82. Beatty JK, Akierman SV, Motta JP, Muise S, Workentine ML, Harrison JJ, et al. *Giardia duodenalis* induces pathogenic dysbiosis of human intestinal microbiota biofilms. *Int J Parasitol.* (2017) 47:311–26. doi: 10.1016/j.ijpara.2016.11.010

83. Manko A, Motta JP, Cotton JA, Feener T, Oyeyemi A, Vallance BA, et al. *Giardia* co-infection promotes the secretion of antimicrobial peptides beta-defensin 2 and trefoil factor 3 and attenuates attaching and effacing bacteria-induced intestinal disease. *PLoS ONE* (2017) 12:e0178647. doi: 10.1371/journal.pone.0178647

84. Osborne LC, Monticelli LA, Nice TJ, Sutherland TE, Siracusa MC, Hepworth MR, et al. Virus-helminth coninfection reveals a microbiota-independent mechanism of immunomodulation. *Science* (2014) 345:579–82. doi: 10.1126/science.1256942

85. Reese TA, Wakeman BS, Choi HS, Hufford MM, Huang SC, Zhang X, et al. Helminth infection reactivates latent γ-herpesvirus via cytokine competition at a viral promoter. *Science* (2014) 345:573–7. doi: 10.1126/science.1254517

86. Attallah AM, Abdallah SO, Albannan MS, Omran MM, Attallah AA, Farid K. Impact of hepatitis C virus/*Schistosoma mansoni* coinfection on the circulating levels of HCV-NS4 protein and extracellular-matrix deposition in patients with different hepatic fibrosis stages. *Am J Trop Med Hyg.* (2016) 95:1044–50. doi: 10.4269/ajtmh.16-0129

87. Morawski BM, Yunus M, Kerukadho E, Turyasingura G, Barbra L, Ojok AM, et al. Hookworm infection is associated with decreased CD4$^+$ T cell counts in HIV-infected adult Ugandans. *PLoS Neglect Trop Dis.* (2017) 11:e0005634. doi: 10.1371/journal.pntd.0005634

88. Dietze KK, Dittmer U, Koudaimi DK, Schimmer S, Reitz M, Breloer M, et al. Filariae-retrovirus co-infection in mice is associated with suppressed virus-specific IgG immune responses and higher viral loads. *PLoS Neglect Trop Dis.* (2016) 10:e0005170. doi: 10.1371/journal.pntd.0005170

89. Modjarrad K, Zulu I, Redden DT, Njobvu L, Lane HC, Bentwich Z, et al. Treatment of intestinal helminths does not reduce plasma concentrations of HIV-1 RNA in coinfected Zambian adults. *J Infect Dis.* (2005) 192:1277–83. doi: 10.1086/444543

90. Elliott AM, Mawa PA, Joseph S, Namujju PB, Kizza M, Nakiyingi JS, et al. Association between helminth infection and CD4$^+$ T cell count, viral load and cytokine responses in HIV-1-infected Ugandan adults. *Trans R Soc Trop Med Hyg.* (2003) 97:103–8. doi: 10.1016/S0035-9203(03)90040-X

91. Carvalho EM, Da Fonseca Porto A. Epidemiological and clinical interaction between HTLV-1 and *Strongyloides stercoralis. Parasite Immunol.* (2004) 26:487–97. doi: 10.1111/j.0141-9838.2004.00726.x

92. Vadlamudi RS, Chi DS, Krishnaswamy G. Intestinal strongyloidiasis and hyperinfection syndrome. *Clin Mol Allergy* (2006) 4:8. doi: 10.1186/1476-7961-4-8

93. Montes M, Sanchez C, Verdonck K, Lake JE, Gonzalez E, Lopez G, et al. Regulatory T Cell expansion in HTLV-1 and strongyloidiasis co-infection is associated with reduced IL-5 responses to *Strongyloides stercoralis* antigen. *PLoS Neglect Trop Dis.* (2009) 3:e456. doi: 10.1371/journal.pntd.0000456

94. Herbert DR, Lee JJ, Lee NA, Nolan TJ, Schad GA, Abraham D. Role of IL-5 in Innate and adaptive immunity to larval *Strongyloides stercoralis* in mice. *J Immunol.* (2000) 165:4544–51. doi: 10.4049/jimmunol.165.8.4544

95. Choksi TT, Madison G, Dar T, Asif M, Fleming K, Clarke L, et al. Case report: multiorgan dysfunction syndrome from *Strongyloides stercoralis* hyperinfection in a patient with human T-cell lymphotrophic virus-1 coinfection after initiation of Ivermectin treatment. *Am J Trop Med Hyg.* (2016) 95:864–7. doi: 10.4269/ajtmh.16-0259

96. Gazzinelli-Guimarães PH, de Freitas LF, Gazzinelli-Guimarães AC, Coelho F, Barbosa FS, Nogueira D, et al. Concomitant helminth infection downmodulates the *Vaccinia* virus-specific immune response and potentiates virus-associated pathology. *Int J Parasitol.* (2017) 47:1–19. doi: 10.1016/j.ijpara.2016.08.007

97. Actor JK, Shirai M, Kullberg MC, Buller RM, Sher A, Berzofsky JA. Helminth infection results in decreased virus-specific CD8$^+$ cytotoxic T-cell and Th1 cytokine responses as well as delayed virus clearance. *Proc Nat Acad Sci USA.* (1993) 90:948–52. doi: 10.1073/pnas.90.3.948

98. McFarlane AJ, McSorley HJ, Davidson DJ, Fitch PM, Errington C, Mackenzie KJ, et al. Enteric helminth-induced type I interferon signaling protects against pulmonary virus infection through interaction with the microbiota. *J Allergy Clin Immunol.* (2017) 140:1068–78. doi: 10.1016/j.jaci.2017.01.016

99. Wuerthner VP, Hua J, Hoverman JT. The benefits of coinfection: trematodes alter disease outcomes associated with virus infection. *J Anim Ecol.* (2017) 86:921–31. doi: 10.1111/1365-2656.12665

100. Legname G, Baskakov IV, Nguyen HO, Riesner D, Cohen FE, DeArmond SJ, et al. Synthetic mammalian prions. *Science* (2004) 305:673–6. doi: 10.1126/science.1100195

101. Mabbott NA, Young J, McConnell I, Bruce ME. Follicular dendritic cell dedifferentiation by treatment with an inhibitor of the lymphotoxin pathway dramatically reduces scrapie susceptibility. *J Virol.* (2003) 77:6845–54. doi: 10.1128/JVI.77.12.6845-6854.2003

102. Glaysher BR, Mabbott NA. Role of the GALT in scrapie agent neuroinvasion from the intestine. *J Immunol.* (2007) 178:3757–66. doi: 10.4049/jimmunol.178.6.3757

103. McCulloch L, Brown KL, Bradford BM, Hopkins J, Bailey M, Rajewsky K, et al. Follicular dendritic cell-specific prion protein (PrPC) expression alone is sufficient to sustain prion infection in the spleen. *PLoS Pathog.* (2011) 7:e1002402. doi: 10.1371/journal.ppat.1002402

104. Donaldson DS, Else KJ, Mabbott NA. The gut-associated lymphoid tissues in the small intestine, not the large intestine, play a major role in oral prion disease pathogenesis. *J Virol.* (2015) 15:9532–47. doi: 10.1128/JVI. 01544-15

105. Gruner L, Elsen JM, Vu Tien Khang J, Eychenne F, Caritez JC, Jacquiet P, et al. Nematode parasites and scrapie: experiments in sheep and mice. *Parasitol Res.* (2004) 93:493–8. doi: 10.1007/s00436-004-1131-7

106. van Keulen LJ, Schreuder BE, Vromans ME, Langeveld JP, Smits MA. Pathogenesis of natural scrapie in sheep. *Arch Virol Suppl.* (2000) 16:57–71. doi: 10.1007/978-3-7091-6308-5_5

107. van Keulen LJ, Vromans ME, van Zijderveld FG. Ealry and late pathogenesis of natural scrapie infection in sheep. *APMIS* (2002) 110:23–32. doi: 10.1034/j.1600-0463.2002.100104.x

108. Abolins S, King EC, Lazarou L, Weldon L, Hughes L, Drescher P, et al. The comparative immunology of wild and laboratory mice, *Mus musculus domesticus. Nat Commun.* (2017) 8:14811. doi: 10.1038/ncomms14811

109. Weldon L, Abolins S, Lenzi L, Bourne C, Riley EM, Viney M. The gut microbiota of wild mice. *PLoS ONE* (2015) 10:e0134643. doi: 10.1371/journal.pone.0134643

110. Johnston C, McSorley H, Smyth D, Anderton S, Wigmore S, Maizels R. A role for helminth parasites in achieving immunological tolerance in transplantation. *Lancet* (2015) 385:S50. doi: 10.1016/S0140-6736(15)60365-8

13

Involvement of T Cell Immunity in Avian Coccidiosis

Woo H. Kim†, Atul A. Chaudhari† and Hyun S. Lillehoj*

Animal Biosciences and Biotechnology Laboratory, U.S. Department of Agriculture, Beltsville Agricultural Research Center, ARS, Beltsville, MD, United States

Correspondence:
Hyun S. Lillehoj
Hyun.Lillehoj@ars.usda.gov

†These authors have contributed equally to this work

Avian coccidiosis is caused by *Eimeria*, which is an intracellular apicomplexan parasite that invades through the intestinal tract to cause devastating disease. Upon invasion through the intestinal epithelial cells, a strong inflammatory response is induced that results in complete villous destruction, diarrhea, hemorrhage, and in severe cases, death. Since the life cycle of *Eimeria* parasites is complex and comprises several intra- and extracellular developmental stages, the host immune responses are diverse and complex. Interferon-γ-mediated T helper (Th)1 response was originally considered to be the predominant immune response in avian coccidiosis. However, recent studies on other avian T cell lineages such as Th17 and T regulatory cells have implicated their significant involvement in maintaining gut homeostasis in normal and disease states including coccidiosis. Therefore, there is a need to understand better their role in coccidiosis. This review focuses on research findings concerning the host immune response induced by avian coccidiosis in the context of T cell immunity, including expression of T-cell-related cytokines and surface molecules that determine the phenotype of T lymphocytes.

Keywords: chicken, coccidiosis, T cells, avian immunology, host immunity

INTRODUCTION

Avian coccidiosis is caused by intracellular protozoan parasites that belong to several different species of *Eimeria* (1, 2). This apicomplexan parasite invades intestinal epithelial tissues and causes severe damage in birds, resulting in enormous economic losses in the poultry industry. The major challenge in coccidiosis control is the diversity among several *Eimeria* species that target different specific regions of the intestine.

The coccidia exhibit a complex life cycle comprising both intracellular and extracellular stages as well as asexual and sexual reproduction (3, 4). The life cycle mainly consists of an exogenous stage, characterized by excretion of unsporulated oocysts, and endogenous stage of schizogony (asexual reproduction) and gametogony (sexual differentiation) (5, 6). During the exogenous stage, the unsporulated oocysts become sporulated (with four sporocysts, each containing two sporozoites) under the influence of external environmental factors such as moisture, oxygen, and warmth. The endogenous stage occurs inside the host, which involves several stages of asexual reproduction followed by sexual reproduction, fertilization, and shedding of the unsporulated oocysts. In general, two to four generations of asexual reproduction are followed by the sexual phase, in which zygote formation takes place that eventually matures into oocysts that are released in the intestinal mucosa and finally shed into feces (7). The coccidia life cycle is usually short (4–6 days depending on several different species) and production of sporulating oocysts can easily increase the infectivity of the parasites in a large population of chickens. After ingesting the sporulated oocysts, excystation of oocysts occurs in the gizzard and the sporozoites are released, invade the intestinal cells, and cause severe damage as the reproductive cycle of the parasite begins. As a result, symptoms such as bloody diarrhea and reduced body weight and feed intake are observed in the birds.

Upon exposure to developing schizonts, anti-*Eimeria* immunity develops and is subsequently boosted by multiple re-exposures to oocysts (7). The immunity to avian coccidiosis can be categorized as innate and adaptive (8). As a first line of defense, the innate immune response is activated in response to the conserved antigens. Innate immune responses include recognition of conserved pathogen-associated molecular patterns (PAMPs) by pattern recognition receptors (PRRs) such as Toll-like receptors (TLRs) (5, 9, 10). A major TLR ligand, profilin, is expressed in all the developmental stages of the life cycle of several *Eimeria* parasites and is conserved (11). Such ligands induce a robust innate response such as immune cell proliferation and cytokine production. The cells involved in innate immune responses to *Eimeria* parasites at different phases are natural killer (NK) cells, dendritic cells, epithelial cells, heterophils, and macrophages. In particular, macrophage migration inhibitory factor plays a crucial role in mediating innate immunity in coccidiosis (12).

On the other hand, adaptive immunity is specific and regulates the antigen-specific immune responses to prevent colonization and growth of the pathogen inside the host. Like mammals, two major lymphocyte types, B cells (producing surface immunoglobulins) and T cells (T cell receptors), are the major components of adaptive immune responses in birds (13). Anticoccidial antibodies in serum and mucosal secretions have been reported in avian coccidiosis (13). Although B cell depletion studies (14) have revealed that antibodies do not play a specific role in anticoccidial protective immunity, other studies have emphasized the importance of passively transferred humoral immunity in *Eimeria* infection in chickens (15–18). Cell-mediated immunity in avian coccidiosis is characterized by antigen-specific or non-specific activation of several immune cells such as T cells, NK cells, and macrophages. The CD4$^+$ T helper (Th) cells and CD8$^+$ cytotoxic T lymphocytes (CTLs) are the two major T-cell subsets that are involved in anticoccidial immunity (19–22). Although the role of several T-cell subpopulations in avian coccidiosis remains to be elucidated, T cells are the most important for protection against *Eimeria* infections in birds.

In this article, we reviewed the historical progress of immunological studies on the host immune response to avian coccidiosis, with an emphasis on recent findings in the understanding of the complexity of T-cell immune responses in avian coccidiosis, especially those mediated by Th17 and T regulatory (Treg) cells.

DEVELOPMENT OF IMMUNOLOGY IN AVIAN COCCIDIOSIS

Since the first report of chicken coccidiosis in the cecum in the late eighteenth century (1), immunity to several *Eimeria* parasites has been investigated thoroughly. An important contribution from Rose and colleagues (23) defined the basic principles of avian immunity to coccidial parasites in terms of specificity, wherein one species of *Eimeria* offers little protection against heterologous challenge with other species. Over the past few decades, studies focusing on investigating the role of avian immunity in response to various coccidial parasites has shown promising developments toward better understanding of avian immunity to coccidiosis (20, 24, 25). From all these studies, it was apparent that out of the two types of immunity, cellular immunity was more important than humoral immunity in coccidiosis, as the later offered little protection against the infection. Early investigations in both mammalian and avian species have revealed that the cellular immune responses through T cells and their associated cytokines play an important role in anticoccidial immunity (2, 26, 27). Acquired immunity to murine coccidiosis is attributed more to T cells than B cells (26). Several immune cell types including NK cells, dendritic cells, and macrophages are involved in innate immune responses to avian coccidiosis (8, 27). B-cell-deficient chickens have shown increased oocyst production after primary infection with *Eimeria* species. However, secondary infection does not yield clinical coccidiosis in the bursectomized chickens due to the protective immunity acquired by the primary infection (8). This indicates that the anticoccidial immunity acquired after primary infection is B cell independent. It is also apparent that chicken coccidiosis can be prevented by adaptive transfer of peripheral blood lymphocytes and splenocytes from *Eimeria*-infected chickens in the syngeneic recipients (28). Subsequently, the T-cell immunosuppressant cyclosporin A abolished the protective immunity offered by *Eimeria* re-infection, thus further emphasizing the integral role of cellular immune mechanisms in chicken coccidiosis (14).

The early findings indicated that T cells serve as a key factor to mediate anticoccidial immunity in chickens (8, 14). Greater numbers of CTLs expressing CD8 cell surface antigen were predominantly observed in chickens after primary infection (29–31). Furthermore, the differential role of CD4$^+$ and CD8$^+$ T lymphocytes in offering resistance to primary and secondary coccidial infection was also reported (32, 33). Increased populations of T cells are linked to elevated production of proinflammatory cytokine interferon (IFN)-γ, which has an immunoregulatory effect (34), as well as inhibiting intracellular development of the parasite (35, 36). The role of T cells in mediating host immunity to coccidiosis became more evident when flow cytometric analysis of intestinal epithelial lymphocytes (IELs), using lymphocyte-specific immune reagents, revealed their significance in innate immunity in naïve chickens and adaptive immunity in previously infected chickens (19, 37, 38). More studies showed that different IEL subtypes are involved in anti-*Eimeria* defense in the gut (39, 40). Research over the past several years has shown that, as a part of protective immunity against avian coccidiosis, T cells produce numerous secretions besides IFN-γ, such as cytokines interleukin (IL)-1, IL-2, IL-4–6, IL-8, IL-10, IL-12, IL-13, and IL-15–18, tumor necrosis factor (TNF)-α, lipopolysaccharide-induced TNF-α factor (LITAF), TNF-α superfamily 15 (TNFSF15), transforming growth factor

(TGF)-β1–4, and granulocyte–macrophage colony-stimulatory factor (GM-CSF). All these findings are based on research oriented toward investigating the immunoregulatory responses of these molecules after primary and/or secondary coccidiosis (40–60). More recent work has indicated the involvement of TLR4 and TLR15 as a part of the innate immune response to *Eimeria* infection (61). IL-17 also contributes to host immunopathology in response to experimental infection (62). The immunoproteomics analysis of three *Eimeria* species has identified several immunodominant antigens from these three species that could provide a useful breakthrough in exploring anticoccidial immunity, as some of these molecules cause profuse inflammatory and cellular immune response that contribute to pathogenesis and severity of infection (3, 63). Additionally, research on anticoccidial vaccines and natural alternatives has explored the immunobiology of coccidiosis in poultry (7). All these findings show the immunoregulatory effect of vaccines or several naturally occurring anti-inflammatory products such as curcumin and *Allium hookeri*. These findings also provide a useful insight into immunoregulation in avian coccidiosis, however, this is outside the scope of this review and has been reviewed previously (7). Much of this work has focused on immunomodulation by dietary ingredients in experimental *Eimeria* infections (64, 65).

Besides the above information, immunological variation among the different strains of the same *Eimeria* species has also been reported in chickens (66, 67). These findings show the characteristic intraspecific variations attributed to the biological features of *Eimeria*, such as morphology of oocysts, pathogenicity, and sensitivity to drugs (68). This inter- and intraspecies variation has been recently defined with the help of more advanced molecular approaches such as random amplification of polymorphic DNA–PCR, and restricted or amplified fragment length polymorphism (69). Analysis of these variations has led to the identification of several strain-specific immunoprotective antigens (70, 71). Similarly, more recent findings have also highlighted the variation in immune responses to *Eimeria tenella* infection in genetically distinct chicken lineages (72).

ROLE OF IFN-γ-MEDIATED IMMUNITY IN AVIAN COCCIDIOSIS

Among all the cytokines mentioned above, IFN-γ is a major cytokine that has anticoccidial effects (73). In mammals, parasitic infections are often characterized by increased levels of IFN-γ. Similarly, the functional role of this cytokine in *Eimeria* infections has been studied thoroughly (34, 74, 75). Until the cDNA cloning of chicken IFNs revealed the independent existence of type I (76) (IFN-α) and type II (77) (IFN-γ) IFNs, most of the findings on the role of IFN-like activity in *Eimeria* infections were believed to be associated with IFN-γ. All these IFN-dependent activities inhibit the invasion or development of *Eimeria* in cultured cells *in vitro* (73, 78). *In vivo* studies have also revealed the anticoccidial IFN-like activity in *Eimeria*-infected

birds (79, 80). The specific involvement of IFN-γ in anti-*Eimeria* immunity was later described by Breed et al. who showed that IFN-γ was produced specifically after stimulation of peripheral blood lymphocytes from *Eimeria*-infected birds (31). It was then discovered that mitogen- or antigen-stimulated specific T cells circulating in the blood of *Eimeria*-infected chickens specifically produced IFN-γ (81). Based on these findings, it was proposed that T-cell priming might occur at the site of infection, resulting in production of IFN-γ at the infection site, thus regulating anticoccidial immunity (81). It was also hypothesized that CD8+ cells produce IFN-γ, which is involved in immunoregulation in primary coccidiosis (81). These findings were extended by Rothwell et al. who showed that IFN-γ-producing cells were present in blood and the spleen and may migrate from the spleen after secondary infection (82). *In situ* hybridization has shown that, following *Eimeria* challenge, IFN-γ is produced by the cells (predominantly T cells) at the site of infection (cecum) and by splenocytes (82). Several studies have shown the potential application of IFN-γ in protecting against *Eimeria* infections (36, 83, 84). Birds immunized with recombinant IFN-γ show increased body weight gain during infection with *Eimeria acevirulina* (36, 83). Also, the development of *E. tenella* is inhibited by IFN-γ *in vitro* (36, 84). When chicken cells are treated with recombinant IFN-γ, intracellular development of *E. tenella* is inhibited, with no significant effect on sporozoite invasion of the cells (36). Similarly, *in vivo* administration of recombinant IFN-γ protects against *E. acevirulina* characterized by reduced oocyst production and increased body weight gain (36, 83).

Besides its immunoregulatory or immunoprotective effect against chicken coccidiosis, IFN-γ has also been shown to have an adjuvant effect on coccidial vaccine in *Eimeria*-infected chickens (85). The adjuvant effect of IFN-γ is characterized by enhanced immune response to the vaccine antigen that induces a microbicidal effect to resolve the parasitic infection, thus increasing vaccine efficacy (85). Some DNA vaccines administered with IFN-γ increased the immunity at intestinal level and protected against avian coccidiosis (36, 86, 87). Recent studies have also indicated the beneficial effect of IFN-γ on anticoccidial DNA vaccine (88, 89). A chimeric vaccine constructed by fusion of genes encoding the *E. tenella* surface antigen, and IFN-γ alleviated the cecal lesions and improved the anticoccidial index in experimentally infected chickens, further suggesting the adjuvant effect of IFN-γ (89). Thus, all these efforts indicate the anticoccidial role of IFN-γ, direct, or as an adjuvant, and underline the significance of IFN-γ in anticoccidial immunity.

Th17 CELLS AND THEIR CYTOKINES IN AVIAN COCCIDIOSIS

Besides the response elicited by IFN-γ-mediated Th1 cells against avian coccidiosis, the other CD4 T-cell subsets have also been studied since the discovery of their homologs in mammals (42). A lineage of IL-17-producing CD4+ T helper (Th)17 cells that are distinct from the previously well-characterized Th1/Th2 paradigm, has emerged and is involved in proinflammatory responses in various autoimmune diseases and infections (90). The biological activities of IL-17 as a signature cytokine of Th17 cells include recruitment of neutrophils, stimulation of antimicrobial peptide production, such as β-defensins and mucins, as well as induction of cytokines and chemokines, in particular IL-6, CXCL8 and GM-CSF (91). Chicken IL-17 isolated from *Eimeria*-infected IELs exerts a proinflammatory role in coccidiosis (8). The exact role of Th17 cells in chicken is poorly understood due to the lack of immunological reagents. This section describes studies that focused on the role of IL-17 as a signature cytokine in Th17 cells in chicken coccidiosis. Following infection by *E. acervulina* or *E. maxima*, IL-17 mRNA levels were increased in IELs compared to uninfected controls (40). In *E. tenella* infection, IL-17 expression in IELs was downregulated, except in the latter stage of infection (39). Similarly, Kim et al. reported that chicken IL-17 expression was downregulated in inflamed intestinal tissue following *E. tenella* infection, and treatment with IL-17 or IL-17F induced expression of proinflammatory cytokines in chicken fibroblasts (92). These results suggest that chicken coccidiosis induces IL-17 expression in the gut and is dependent on the species of *Eimeria*. Th17 response can play both protective and pathological roles in protozoan infections. The cloning of IL-17 receptor A (IL-17RA), which binds IL-17A and IL-17F in chickens, has revealed that *Eimeria* infection downregulates expression of IL-17RA, and modulation of this receptor facilitates the host to reduce intestinal pathogenesis amplified by IL-17/IL-17RA signaling. Several authors have proposed that Th17 cells or IL-17 promote pathogenesis in leishmaniasis, toxoplasmosis, and *Eimeria falciformis* infection (93–95), whereas others have demonstrated that they are involved in protective immunity against trypanosomiasis, toxoplasmosis and *Pneumocystis carinii* infection (96, 97). Recent evidence seems to support a role for Th17 cytokines in host immunopathology in coccidiosis in chickens. Treatment with IL-17 neutralizing antibody in *E. tenella* infection induces lower heterophil recruitment, inflammatory cytokine expression, and parasite burden in the intestinal tract, resulting in enhanced body weight gain, reduced oocyst production in feces, and intestinal lesions (62). IL-17 is also involved in the initiation and migratory response of epithelial cells during intracellular development, and maturation of parasites, contributing to pathogenesis in the intestinal tract. Following *E. tenella* infection, chickens treated with IL-17 neutralizing antibody have a reduced number of second-generation schizonts and cecal lesions (98).

ANTI-INFLAMMATORY IL-10 AND Treg CELLS IN AVIAN COCCIDIOSIS

Treg cells are a subset of T cells involved in immunosuppression. Mammalian Treg cells have the phenotype $CD4^+CD25^+FoxP3^+$ (99). In chickens, the ortholog of mammalian FoxP3 has yet

to be identified, although there is a report of an avian *foxp3* gene (100, 101). Thus, $CD4^+CD25^+$ T cells in chickens have been characterized as Treg cells showing suppression of activated immune cells (102). These cells produce high amounts of IL-10, TGF-β, CTLA-4, and LAG-3, as in mammals (103). IL-10 showed 29-fold higher expression in $CD4^+CD25^+$ cells compared to $CD4^+CD25^-$ cells and its immunosuppression in chickens has been extensively studied (102). In coccidiosis, IL-10 is considered to play an important role in evasion of the host immune response. One possible mechanism to explain its role in coccidiosis is that coccidial parasites have evolved to stimulate Treg cells to express IL-10, and it helps parasites to facilitate invasion and survival in chickens through suppression of the IFN-γ-related Th1 response that is critical for protective immunity against coccidial parasites. Two inbred lines of chickens that differ in their resistance or susceptibility to *Eimeria* infection have revealed that expression of IL-10 is the major difference between the two lines. Expression of IL-10 is highly induced in susceptible chickens among the genes related to different Th lineages, such as IFN-γ for Th1, IL-4 for Th2, and IL-10 and TGF-β for Treg cells, while IL-10 is suppressed in the age-matched resistant line (46). *Eimeria*-infected chickens treated with IL-10 neutralizing antibody show improved growth rate compared to those with control antibody but it has no effect on fecal oocyst production (104, 105). Morris et al. reported that supplementation of vitamin D induced IL-10 expression as well as Treg cells and showed decreased production losses associated with coccidial infection (106). These results indicate that regulation of the protective immune response to *Eimeria* infection by Treg cells is critical, and IL-10 plays a role in pathogenesis in chicken coccidiosis. We recently identified that Treg cells could help to reduce pathology in *Eimeria*-infected intestine by suppression of Th17 cells that induce tissue inflammation. Increased expression of $CD4^+CD25^+$ Treg cells has been found in *E. tenella*-infected chickens with increased IL-10 expression. After treatment with aryl hydrocarbon receptor such as 3,3'-diindolylmethane, Treg cells are increased in the intestine, whereas $CD4^+IL-17^+$ Th17 cells are suppressed. We have also found that generation of Th17 cells is suppressed by Treg cells, which leads to reduced pathogenicity in chicken coccidiosis (107).

CONCLUDING REMARKS

It is the consensus that the Th1 response is the most efficient host response in avian coccidiosis. However, studies on other aspects like Th17 and Treg responses are also important because the immune responses are not independent, but rather they are connected and work together in an integrated immune system. It is becoming clear that the outcome of an inflammatory process caused by infection depends on the balance of responses by several components of the immune system of particular relevance is the interplay between Treg and Th17 cells during immunoinflammatory events (108). Compared to mammalian immunology, little is known about the role of T cells in chickens, although the number of reports on coccidiosis is steadily growing. To understand better immunity against chicken coccidiosis, it is necessary to know how T cells are modulated and how they interplay since this intracellular pathogen predominantly induces a T-cell-associated immune response that involves several types of T cells. In regard to controlling coccidiosis, the best way might be development of alternatives to antibiotics because most effective anticoccidial drugs that produce resistance or residues will be banned from

the market in the future. Understanding the mechanism of how chickens respond to *Eimeria* will lead to new approaches to control coccidiosis.

AUTHOR CONTRIBUTIONS

All authors listed have made a substantial, direct and intellectual contribution to the work, and approved it for publication.

REFERENCES

1. Railliet ALA. Developpement experimental des coccidies de l'epithelium intestinal du lapin et de la poule. *C R Soc Biol Paris.* (1891) 36:820–3.
2. Rose ME, Hesketh P. Immunity to coccidiosis : t-lymphocyte- deficient animals B-lymphocyte-. *Immunology.* (1979) 26:630–7.
3. Lal K, Bromley E, Oakes R, Prieto JH, Sanderson SJ, Kurian D, et al. Proteomic comparison of four *Eimeria tenella* life-cycle stages: Unsporulated oocyst, sporulated oocyst, sporozoite and second-generation merozoite. *Proteomics.* (2009) 9:4566–76. doi: 10.1002/pmic.200900305
4. Norton CC, Chard MJ. The oocyst sporulation time of *Eimeria* species from the fowl. *Parasitology.* (1983) 86:193–8. doi: 10.1017/S00311820000 50368
5. Dalloul RA, Lillehoj HS. Recent advances in immunomodulation and vaccination strategies against coccidiosis. *Avian Dis.* (2005) 49:1–8. doi: 10.1637/7306-11150R
6. Gilbert ER, Cox CM, Williams PM, McElroy AP, Dalloul RA, Keith Ray W, et al. *Eimeria* species and genetic background influence the serum protein profile of broilers with coccidiosis. *PLoS ONE.* (2011) 6:e14636. doi: 10.1371/journal.pone.0014636
7. Quiroz-Castañeda RE, Dantán-González E. Control of avian coccidiosis: future and present natural alternatives. *BioMed Res Int.* (2015) 2015:430610. doi: 10.1155/2015/430610
8. Min W, Kim WH, Lillehoj EP, Lillehoj HS. Recent progress in host immunity to avian coccidiosis: IL-17 family cytokines as sentinels of the intestinal mucosa. *Dev Compar Immunol.* (2013) 41:418–28. doi: 10.1016/j.dci.2013.04.003
9. Kumar H, Kawai T, Akira S. Pathogen recognition by the innate immune system. *Int Rev Immunol.* (2011) 30:16–34. doi: 10.3109/08830185.2010.529976
10. Brownlie R, Allan B. Avian toll-like receptors. *Cell Tissue Res.* (2011) 343:121–30. doi: 10.1007/s00441-010-1026-0
11. Fetterer RH, Miska KB, Jenkins MC, Barfield RC. A conserved 19-kDa *Eimeria tenella* antigen is a profilin-like protein. *J Parasitol.* (2004) 90:1321–8. doi: 10.1645/GE-307R
12. Sun H-W, Bernhagentt J, Bucalat R, Lolis E. Crystal structure at 2.6-A resolution of human macrophage migration inhibitory factor. *Proc Natl Acad Sci USA.* (1996) 93:5191–6. doi: 10.1073/pnas.93.11.5191
13. Girard F, Fort G, Yvore P, Quere P. Kinetics of specific immunoglobulin A, M and G production in the duodenal and caecal mucosa of chickens infected with *Eimeria acervulina* or *Eimeria tenella. Int J Parasitol.* (1997) 27:803–9. doi: 10.1016/S0020-7519(97)00044-1
14. Lillehoj HS. Effects of immunosuppression on avian coccidiosis: cyclosporin A but not hormonal bursectomy abrogates host protective immunity. *Infect Immun.* (1987) 55:1616–21.
15. Wallach M, Halabi A, Pillemer G, Sar-Shalom O, Mencher D, Gilad M, et al. Maternal immunization with gametocyte antigens as a means of providing protective immunity against *Eimeria maxima* in chickens. *Infect Immun.* (1992) 60:2036–9.
16. Wallach M. Role of antibody in immunity and control of chicken coccidiosis. *Trends Parasitol.* (2010) 26:382–7. doi: 10.1016/j.pt.2010.04.004
17. Lee SH, Lillehoj HS, Park DW, Jang SI, Morales A, García D, et al. Induction of passive immunity in broiler chickens against *Eimeria acervulina*

by hyperimmune egg yolk immunoglobulin Y. *Poultry Science.* (2009) 88:562–6. doi: 10.3382/ps.2008-00340
18. Lee SH, Lillehoj HS, Park DW, Jang SI, Morales A, García D, et al. Protective effect of hyperimmune egg yolk IgY antibodies against *Eimeria tenella* and *Eimeria maxima* infections. *Vet Parasitol.* (2009) 163:123–6. doi: 10.1016/j.vetpar.2009.04.020
19. Lillehoj HS. Role of T lymphocytes and cytokines in coccidiosis. *Int J Parasitol.* (1998) 28:1071–81. doi: 10.1016/S0020-7519(98) 00075-7
20. Lillehoj HS, Lillehoj EP. Avian coccidiosis. A review of acquired intestinal immunity and vaccination strategies. *Avian Dis.* (2000) 44:408–25. doi: 10.2307/1592556
21. Trout JM, Lillehoj HS. T lymphocyte roles during *Eimeria acervulina* and *Eimeria tenella* infections. *Vet Immunol Immunopathol.* (1996) 53:163–72. doi: 10.1016/0165-2427(95)05544-4
22. Yun CH, Lillehoj HS, Lillehoj EP. Intestinal immune responses to coccidiosis. *Dev Compar Immunol.* (2000) 24:303–24. doi: 10.1016/S0145-305X(99)00080-4
23. Rose ME, Long PL. Immunity to four species of *Eimeria* in fowls. *Immunology.* (1962) 5:79–92.
24. Allen PC, Fetterer RH. Recent advances in biology and immunobiology of *Eimeria* species and in diagnosis and control of infection with these coccidian parasites of poultry. *Clin Microbiol Rev.* (2002) 15:58–65. doi: 10.1128/CMR.15.1.58-65.2002
25. Shirley MW, Lillehoj HS. The long view: a selective review of 40 years of coccidiosis research. *Avian Pathol.* (2012) 41:111–21. doi: 10.1080/03079457.2012.666338
26. Rose ME, Ogilvie BM, Hesketh P, Festing MFW. Failure of nude. (athymic) rats to become resistant to reinfection with the intestinal coccidian parasite *Eimeria nieschulzi* or the nematode *Nippostrongylus brasiliensis. Parasite Immunol.* (1979) 1:125–32. doi: 10.1111/j.1365-3024.1979. tb00700.x
27. Wakelin D, Rose ME, Hesketh P, Else KJ, Grencis RK. Immunity to coccidiosis: genetic influences on lymphocyte and cytokine responses to infection with *Eimeria vermiformis* in inbred mice. *Parasite Immunol.* (1993) 15:11–9. doi: 10.1111/j.1365-3024.1993.tb00567.x
28. Rose ME, Hesketh P, Ogilvie BM. Peripheral blood leucocyte response to coccidial infection: a comparison of the response in rats and chickens and its correlation with resistance to reinfection. *Immunology.* (1979) 36:71–9.
29. Lillehoj HS, Bacon LD. Increase of intestinal intraepithelial lymphocytes expressing CD8 antigen following challenge infection with *Eimeria acervulina. Avian Dis.* (1991) 35:294–301. doi: 10.2307/15 91179
30. Breed DGJ, Dorrestein J, Vermeulen AN. Immunity to *Eimeria tenella* in chickens: phenotypical and functional changes in peripheral blood T-cell subsets. *Avian Dis.* (1996) 40:37–48. doi: 10.2307/1592369
31. Breed DGJ, Dorrestein J, Schetters TPM, Waart LVD, Rijke E, Vermeulen AN. Peripheral blood lymphocytes from *Eimeria tenella* infected chickens produce gamma-interferon after stimulation *in vitro. Parasite Immunol.* (1997) 19:127–35. doi: 10.1046/j.1365-3024.1997.d01-191.x
32. Rose ME, Hesketh P, Wakelin D. Immune control of murine coccidiosis: CD4+ and CD8+ T lymphocytes contribute differentially in resistance

to primary and secondary infections. *Parasitology*. (1992) 105:349–354. doi: 10.1017/S0031182000074515

33. Rothwell L, Gramzinski RA, Rose ME, Kaiser P. Avian coccidiosis: changes in intestinal lymphocyte populations associated with the development of immunity to *Eimeria maxima*. *Parasite Immunol*. (1995) 17:525–33. doi: 10.1111/j.1365-3024.1995.tb00883.x

34. Rose ME, Wakelin D, Hesketh P. Interferon-gamma-mediated effects upon immunity to coccidial infections in the mouse. *Parasite Immunol*. (1991) 13:63–74. doi: 10.1111/j.1365-3024.1991.tb00263.x

35. Choi KD, Lillehoj HS, Song KD, Han JY. Molecular and functional characterization of chicken IL-15. *Dev Compar Immunol*. (1999) 23:165–77. doi: 10.1016/S0145-305X(98)00046-9

36. Lillehoj HS, Choi KD. Recombinant chicken interferon-gamma-mediated inhibition of Eimeria tenella development *in vitro* and reduction of oocyst production and body weight loss following *Eimeria acervulina* challenge infection. *Avian Dis*. (1998) 42:307–14. doi: 10.2307/1592481

37. Lillehoj HS. Lymphocytes involved in cell-mediated immune responses and methods to assess cell-mediated immunity. *Poultry Sci*. (1991) 70:1154–64. doi: 10.3382/ps.0701154

38. Lillehoj HS. Analysis of *Eimeria acervulina*-induced changes in the intestinal T lymphocyte subpopulations in two chicken strains showing different levels of susceptibility to coccidiosis. *Res Vet Sci*. (1994) 56:1–7. doi: 10.1016/0034-5288(94)90188-0

39. Hong YH, Lillehoj HS, Lillehoj EP, Lee SH. Changes in immune-related gene expression and intestinal lymphocyte subpopulations following *Eimeria maxima* infection of chickens. *Vet Immunol Immunopathol*. (2006) 114:259–72. doi: 10.1016/j.vetimm.2006.08.006

40. Hong YH, Lillehoj HS, Lee SH, Dalloul RA, Lillehoj EP. Analysis of chicken cytokine and chemokine gene expression following *Eimeria acervulina* and *Eimeria tenella* infections. *Vet Immunol Immunopathol*. (2006) 114:209–23. doi: 10.1016/j.vetimm.2006.07.007

41. Avery S, Rothwell L, Degen WDJ, Schijns VEJC, Young J, Kaufman J, et al. Characterization of the first nonmammalian T2 cytokine gene cluster: the cluster contains functional single-copy genes for IL-3, IL-4, IL-13, and GM-CSF, a gene for IL-5 that appears to be a pseudogene, and a gene encoding another cytokinelike transcript. *J Interf Cytokine Res*. (2004) 24:600–10. doi: 10.1089/jir.2004.24.600

42. Min W, Lillehoj HS. Isolation and characterization of chicken interleukin-17 cDNA. *J Interf Cytokine Res*. (2002) 22:1123–8. doi: 10.1089/10799900260442548

43. Min W, Lillehoj HS. Identification and characterization of chicken interleukin-16 cDNA. *Dev Compar Immunol*. (2004) 28:153–62. doi: 10.1016/S0145-305X(03)00133-2

44. Min W, Lillehoj HS, Fetterer RH. Identification of an alternatively spliced isoform of the common cytokine receptor γ chain in chickens. *Biochem Biophys Res Commun*. (2002) 299:321–7. doi: 10.1016/S0006-291X(02)02636-0

45. Pan H, Halper J. Cloning, expression, and characterization of chicken transforming growth factor β4. *Biochem Biophys Res Commun*. (2003) 303:24–30. doi: 10.1016/S0006-291X(03)00300-0

46. Rothwell L, Young JR, Zoorob R, Whittaker CA, Hesketh P, Archer A, et al. Cloning and characterization of chicken IL-10 and its role in the immune response to *Eimeria maxima*. *J Immunol*. (2004) 173:2675–82. doi: 10.4049/jimmunol.173.4.2675

47. Schneider K, Puehler F, Baeuerle D, Elvers S, Staeheli P, Kaspers B, et al. cDNA cloning of biologically active chicken interleukin-18. *J Interf Cytokine Res*. (2000) 20:879–83. doi: 10.1089/10799900050163244

48. Schneider K, Klaas R, Kaspers B, Staeheli P. Chicken interleukin-6: cDNA structure and biological properties. *Eur J Biochem*. (2001) 268:4200–6. doi: 10.1046/j.1432-1327.2001.02334.x

49. Song KD, Lillehoj HS, Choi KD, Zarlenga D, Han JY. Expression and functional characterization of recombinant chicken interferon-gamma. *Vet Immunol Immunopathol*. (1997) 58:321–33. doi: 10.1016/S0165-2427(97)00034-2

50. Yoo J, Jang SI, Kim S, Cho JH, Lee HJ, Rhee MH, et al. Molecular characterization of duck interleukin-17. *Vet Immunol Immunopathol*. (2009) 132:318–22. doi: 10.1016/j.vetimm.2009.06.003

51. Zhang S, Lillehoj HS, Ruff MD. Chicken tumor necrosis-like factor. I. *In vitro* production by macrophages stimulated with *Eimeria tenella* or bacterial lipopolysaccharide. *Poultry Sci*. (1995) 74:1304–10. doi: 10.3382/ps.0741304

52. Degen WGJ, van Daal N, van Zuilekom HI, Burnside J, Schijns VEJC. Identification and molecular cloning of functional chicken IL-12. *J Immunol*. (2004) 172:4371–80. doi: 10.4049/jimmunol.172.7.4371

53. Hong YH, Lillehoj HS, Hyen Lee S, Woon Park D, Lillehoj EP. Molecular cloning and characterization of chicken lipopolysaccharide-induced TNF-A factor. (LITAF). *Dev Compar Immunol*. (2006) 30:919–29. doi: 10.1016/j.dci.2005.12.007

54. Jakowlew SB, Dillard PJ, Winokur TS, Flanders KC, Sporn MB, Roberts AB. Expression of transforming growth factor-βs 1-4 in chicken embryo chondrocytes and myocytes. *Dev Biol*. (1991) 143:135–48. doi: 10.1016/0012-1606(91)90061-7

55. Jeong J, Lee C, Yoo J, Koh PO, Kim YH, Chang HH, et al. Molecular identification of duck and quail common cytokine receptor γ chain genes. *Vet Immunol Immunopathol*. (2011) 140:159–65. doi: 10.1016/j.vetimm.2010.11.023

56. Jeong J, Kim WH, Yoo J, Lee C, Kim S, Cho J-H, et al. Identification and comparative expression analysis of interleukin 2/15 receptor β chain in chickens infected with *E. tenella*. *PLoS ONE*. (2012) 7:e37704. doi: 10.1371/journal.pone.0037704

57. Koskela K, Kohonen P, Salminen H, Uchida T, Buerstedde JM, Lassila O. Identification of a novel cytokine-like transcript differentially expressed in avian γδ T cells. *Immunogenetics*. (2004) 55:845–54. doi: 10.1007/s00251-004-0643-8

58. Kaiser P, Poh TY, Rothwell L, Avery S, Balu S, Pathania US, et al. A genomic analysis of chicken cytokines and chemokines. *J Interf Cytokine Res*. (2005) 25:467–84. doi: 10.1089/jir.2005.25.467

59. Lillehoj HS, Min W, Dalloul RA. Recent progress on the cytokine regulation of intestinal immune responses to *Eimeria*. *Poultry Sci*. (2004) 83:611–23. doi: 10.1093/ps/83.4.611

60. Gadde U, Rathinam T, Erf GF, Chapman HD. Acquisition of immunity to the protozoan parasite *Eimeria adenoeides* in turkey poults and cellular responses to infection. *Poultry Sci*. (2013) 92:3149–57. doi: 10.3382/ps.2013-03406

61. Zhou Z, Wang Z, Cao L, Hu S, Zhang Z, Qin B, et al. Upregulation of chicken TLR4, TLR15 and MyD88 in heterophils and monocyte-derived macrophages stimulated with *Eimeria tenella in vitro*. *Exp Parasitol*. (2013) 133:417–33. doi: 10.1016/j.exppara.2013.01.002

62. Zhang L, Liu R, Song M, Hu Y, Pan B, Cai J, et al. *Eimeria tenella*: interleukin 17 contributes to host immunopathology in the gut during experimental infection. *Exp Parasitol*. (2013) 133:121–30. doi: 10.1016/j.exppara.2012.11.009

63. Liu L, Huang X, Liu J, Li W, Ji Y, Tian D, et al. Identification of common immunodominant antigens of *Eimeria tenella*, *Eimeria acervulina* and *Eimeria maxima* by immunoproteomic analysis. *Oncotarget*. (2017) 8:34935–45. doi: 10.18632/oncotarget.16824

64. Allen PC. Dietary supplementation with *Echinacea* and development of immunity to challenge infection with coccidia. *Parasitol Res*. (2003) 91:74–8. doi: 10.1007/s00436-003-0938-y

65. Lee SH, Lillehoj HS, Jang SI, Lee KW, Bravo D, Lillehoj EP. Effects of dietary supplementation with phytonutrients on vaccine-stimulated immunity against infection with *Eimeria tenella*. *Vet Parasitol*. (2011) 181:97–105. doi: 10.1016/j.vetpar.2011.05.003

66. Joyner LP. Immunological variation between two strains of *Eimeria acervulina*. *Parasitology*. (1969) 59L725–732. doi: 10.1017/S0031182000031243

67. Norton CC, Hein EH. *Eimeria maxima*: a comparison of two laboratory strains with a fresh isolate. *Parasitology*. (1976) 72:345–54. doi: 10.1017/S0031182000049544

68. Jeffers TK. Genetic transfer of anticoccidial drug resistance in *Eimeria tenella*. *J Parasitol*. (1974) 60:900–4. doi: 10.2307/3278505

69. Chapman HD, Barta JR, Blake D, Gruber A, Jenkins M, Smith NC, et al. A selective review of advances in coccidiosis research. *Adv Parasitol*. (2013) 83:93–171. doi: 10.1016/B978-0-12-407705-8.00002-1

70. Blake DP, Oakes R, Smith AL. A genetic linkage map for the apicomplexan protozoan parasite *Eimeria maxima* and comparison with *Eimeria tenella. Int J Parasitol.* (2011) 41:263–70. doi: 10.1016/j.ijpara.2010. 09.004

71. Blake DP, Billington KJ, Copestake SL, Oakes RD, Quail MA, Wan KL, et al. Genetic mapping identifies novel highly protective antigens for an apicomplexan parasite. *PLoS Pathog.* (2011) 7:e1001279. doi: 10.1371/journal.ppat.1001279

72. Lee SH, Dong X, Lillehoj HS, Lamont SJ, Suo X, Kim DK, et al. Comparing the immune responses of two genetically B-complex disparate Fayoumi chicken lines to *Eimeria tenella. British Poultry Sci.* (2016) 57:165–71. doi: 10.1080/00071668.2016.1141172

73. Kogut M, Lange C. Interferon-g-mediated inhibition of the development of *Eimeria tenella* in cultured cells. *J Parasitol.* (1989) 75:313–7. doi: 10.2307/3282782

74. Rose ME, Wakelin D, Hesketh P. Gamma imerferon controls *Eimeria vermiformis* primary infection in BALB/c mice. *Infect Immun.* (1989) 57:1599–603.

75. Smith AL, Hayday AC. Genetic analysis of the essential components of the immunoprotective response to infection with *Eimeria vermiformis. Int J Parasitol.* (1998) 28:1061–9. doi: 10.1016/S0020-7519(98)00 081-2

76. Sekellick MJ, Ferrandino AF, Hopkins DA, Marcus PI. Chicken interferon gene: cloning, expression, and analysis. *J Interf Res.* (1994) 14:71–9. doi: 10.1089/jir.1994.14.71

77. Digby M, Lowenthal J. Cloning and expression of the chicken interferon-gamma gene. *J Interf Cytokine Res.* (1995) 15:939–45. doi: 10.1089/jir.1995.15.939

78. Kogut MH, Lange C. Recombinant interferon-γ inhibits cell invasion by *Eimeria tenella. J Interf Res.* (1989) 9:67–77. doi: 10.1089/jir. 1989.9.67

79. Prowse SJ, Pallister J. Interferon release as a measure of the T-cell response to coccidial antigens in chickens. *Avian Pathol.* (1989) 18:619–30. doi: 10.1080/03079458908418637

80. Byrnes S, Emerson K, Kogut M. Dynamics of cytokine production during coccidial infections in chickens: colony-stimulating factors and interferon. *FEMS Immunol Med Microbiol.* (1993) 6:45–52. doi: 10.1111/j.1574-695X.1993.tb00302.x

81. Breed DGJ, Schetters TPM, Verhoeven NAP, Vermeulen AN. Characterization of phenotype related responsiveness of peripheral blood lymphocytes from *Eimeria tenella* infected chickens. *Parasite Immunol.* (1997) 19:536–69. doi: 10.1046/j.1365-3024.1997. d01-174.x

82. Rothwell L, Muir W, Kaiser P. Interferon-γ is expressed in both gut and spleen during *Eimeria tenella* infection. *Avian Pathol.* (2000) 29:333–42. doi: 10.1080/03079450050118467

83. Lowenthal JW, York JJ, O'Neil TE, Rhodes S. Prowse SJ, Strom DG, et al. *In vivo* effects of chicken interferon-γ during infection with *Eimeria. J Interf Cytokine Res.* (1997) 17:551–8. doi: 10.1089/jir.1997.17.551

84. Dimier IH, Quéré P, Naciri M, Bout DT. Inhibition of *Eimeria tenella* development *in vitro* mediated by chicken macrophages and fibroblasts treated with chicken cell supernatants with IFN-gamma activity. *Avian Dis.* (1998) 42:239–47. doi: 10.2307/1592473

85. Takehara K, Kobayashi K, Ruttanapumma R, Kamikawa M, Nagata T, Yokomizo Y, et al. Adjuvant effect of chicken interferon-gamma for inactivated *Salmonella Enteritidis* antigen. *J Vet Med Sci.* (2003) 65:1337–41. doi: 10.1292/jvms.65.1337

86. Lillehoj HS, Ding X, Quiroz MA, Bevensee E, Lillehoj EP. Resistance to intestinal coccidiosis following DNA immunization with the cloned 3-1E *Eimeria* gene plus IL-2, IL-15, and IFN-gamma. *Avian Dis.* (2005) 49:112–7. doi: 10.1637/7249-073004R

87. Min W, Lillehoj HS, Burnside J, Weining KC, Staeheli P, Zhu JJ. Adjuvant effects of IL-1β, IL-2, IL-8, IL-15, IFN-α, IFN-γ TGF-β4 and lymphotactin on DNA vaccination against *Eimeria acervulina. Vaccine.* (2001) 20:267–74. doi: 10.1016/S0264-410X(01)00270-5

88. Shah MAA, Song X, Xu L, Yan R, Song H, Ruirui Z, et al. The DNA-induced protective immunity with chicken interferon gamma against poultry coccidiosis. *Parasitol Res.* (2010) 107:747–50. doi: 10.1007/s00436-010-1940-9

89. Song X, Huang X, Yan R, Xu L, Li X. Efficacy of chimeric DNA vaccines encoding Eimeria tenella 5401 and chicken IFN-γ or IL-2 against coccidiosis in chickens. *Exp Parasitol.* (2015) 156:19–25. doi: 10.1016/j.exppara.2015.05.003

90. Martinez GJ, Nurieva RI, Yang XO, Dong C. Regulation and function of proinflammatory TH17 cells. *Annals N Y Acad Sci.* (2008) 1143:188–211. doi: 10.1196/annals.1443.021

91. Pappu R, Rutz S, Ouyang W. Regulation of epithelial immunity by IL-17 family cytokines. *Trends Immunol.* (2012) 33:343–9. doi: 10.1016/j.it.2012.02.008

92. Kim WH, Jeong J, Park AR, Yim D, Kim Y-H, Kim KD, et al. Chicken IL-17F: Identification and comparative expression analysis in *Eimeria*-infected chickens. *Dev Compar Immunol.* (2012) 38:401–9. doi: 10.1016/j.dci.2012.08.002

93. Bacellar O, Faria D, Nascimento M, Cardoso TM, Gollob KJ, Dutra WO, et al. Interleukin 17 production among patients with american cutaneous leishmaniasis. *J Infect Dis.* (2009) 200:75–8. doi: 10.1086/59 9380

94. Guiton R, Vasseur V, Charron S, Arias MT, Van Langendonck N, Buzoni-Gatel D, et al. Interleukin 17 receptor signaling is deleterious during *Toxoplasma gondii* infection in susceptible BL6 mice. *J Infect Dis.* (2010) 202:427–35. doi: 10.1086/653738

95. Stange J, Hepworth MR, Rausch S, Zajic L, Kühl AA, Uyttenhove C, et al. IL-22 mediates host defense against an intestinal intracellular parasite in the absence of IFN-γ at the cost of Th17-driven immunopathology. *J Immunol.* (2012) 188:2410–8. doi: 10.4049/jimmunol. 1102062

96. Miyazaki Y, Hamano S, Wang S, Shimanoe Y, Iwakura Y, Yoshida H. IL-17 is necessary for host protection against acute-phase *Trypanosoma cruzi* infection. *J Immunol.* (2010) 185:1150–7. doi: 10.4049/jimmunol. 0900047

97. Kelly MN, Kolls JK, Happel K, Schwartzman JD, Schwarzenberger P, Combe C, et al. Interleukin-17/interleukin-17 receptor-mediated signaling is important for generation of an optimal polymorphonuclear response against *Toxoplasma gondii* infection. *Infect Immun.* (2005) 73:617–21. doi: 10.1128/IAI.73.1.617-621.2005

98. Del Cacho E, Gallego M, Lillehoj HS, Quílez J, Lillehoj EP, Ramo A, et al. IL-17A regulates *Eimeria tenella* schizont maturation and migration in avian coccidiosis. *Vet Res.* (2014) 45:1–9. doi: 10.1186/1297-9716-45-25

99. Tiemessen MM, Jagger AL, Evans HG, van Herwijnen MJC, John S, Taams LS. CD4$^+$CD25$^+$Foxp3$^+$ regulatory T cells induce alternative activation of human monocytes/macrophages. *Proc Natl Acad Sci USA.* (2007) 104:19446–51. doi: 10.1073/pnas.0706924104

100. Shack LA, Buza JJ, Burgess SC. The neoplastically transformed. (CD30hi) Marek's disease lymphoma cell phenotype most closely resembles T-regulatory cells. *Cancer Immunol Immunother.* (2008) 57:1253–62. doi: 10.1007/s00262-008-0460-2

101. Denyer MP, Pinheiro DY, Garden OA, Shepherd AJ. Missed, not missing: phylogenomic evidence for the existence of avian foxP3. *PLoS ONE.* (2016) 11:e0150988. doi: 10.1371/journal.pone.0150988

102. Shanmugasundaram R, Selvaraj RK. Regulatory T cell properties of chicken CD4$^+$CD25$^+$ cells. *J Immunol.* (2011) 186:1997–2002. doi: 10.4049/jimmunol.1002040

103. Selvaraj RK. Avian CD4$^+$CD25$^+$ regulatory T cells: properties and therapeutic applications. *Dev Compar Immunol.* (2013) 41:397–402. doi: 10.1016/j.dci.2013.04.018

104. Sand JM, Arendt MK, Repasy A, Deniz G, Cook ME. Oral antibody to interleukin-10 reduces growth rate depression due to *Eimeria* spp. infection in broiler chickens. *Poultry Sci.* (2016) 95:439–46. doi: 10.3382/ps/pev352

105. Arendt MK, Sand JM, Marcone TM, Cook ME. Interleukin-10 neutralizing antibody for detection of intestinal luminal levels and as a dietary additive in *Eimeria* challenged broiler chicks. *Poultry Sci.* (2016) 95:430–8. doi: 10.3382/ps/pev365

106. Morris A, Shanmugasundaram R, McDonald J, Selvaraj RK. Effect of *in vitro* and *in vivo* 25-hydroxyvitamin D treatment on macrophages, T cells, and layer chickens during a coccidia challenge. *J Anim Sci.* (2015) 93:2894–903. doi: 10.2527/jas.2014-8866

107. Kim WH, Lillehoj HS, Min W. Indole treatment alleviates intestinal tissue damage induced by chicken coccidiosis through activation of the aryl hydrocarbon receptor. *Front Immunol.* (2019) 10:560. doi: 10.3389/fimmu.2019.00560

108. Sehrawat S, Rouse BT. Interplay of regulatory T cell and Th17 cells during infectious diseases in humans and animals. *Front Immunol.* (2017) 8:341. doi: 10.3389/fimmu.2017.00341

14

Acute *Toxoplasma Gondii* Infection in Cats Induced Tissue-Specific Transcriptional Response Dominated by Immune Signatures

Wei Cong [1,2†], Tania Dottorini [3,4†], Faraz Khan [4], Richard D. Emes [3,4], Fu-Kai Zhang [1], Chun-Xue Zhou [1], Jun-Jun He [1], Xiao-Xuan Zhang [1], Hany M. Elsheikha [3*] and Xing-Quan Zhu [1*]

[1] State Key Laboratory of Veterinary Etiological Biology, Key Laboratory of Veterinary Parasitology of Gansu Province, Lanzhou Veterinary Research Institute, Chinese Academy of Agricultural Sciences, Lanzhou, China, [2] Department of Marine Engineering, Marine College, Shandong University, Weihai, China, [3] Faculty of Medicine and Health Sciences, School of Veterinary Medicine and Science, University of Nottingham, Loughborough, United Kingdom, [4] Advanced Data Analysis Centre, University of Nottingham, Loughborough, United Kingdom

Correspondence:
Xing-Quan Zhu
xingquanzhu1@hotmail.com
Hany M. Elsheikha
hany.elsheikha@nottingham.ac.uk

†These authors have contributed equally to this work

RNA-sequencing was used to detect transcriptional changes in six tissues of cats, seven days after *T. gondii* infection. A total of 737 genes were differentially expressed (DEGs), of which 410 were up-regulated and 327 were down-regulated. The liver exhibited 151 DEGs, lung (149 DEGs), small intestine (130 DEGs), heart (123 DEGs), brain (104 DEGs), and spleen (80 DEGs)-suggesting tissue-specific transcriptional patterns. Gene ontology and KEGG analyses identified DEGs enriched in immune pathways, such as cytokine-cytokine receptor interaction, Jak-STAT signaling pathway, NOD-like receptor signaling pathway, NF-kappa B signaling pathway, MAPK signaling pathway, T cell receptor signaling pathway, and the cytosolic DNA sensing pathway. C-X-C motif chemokine 10 (CXCL10) was involved in most of the immune-related pathways. PI3K/Akt expression was down-regulated in all tissues, except the spleen. The genes for phosphatase, indoleamine 2,3-dioxygenase, Hes Family BHLH Transcription Factor 1, and guanylate-binding protein 5, playing various roles in immune defense, were co-expressed across various feline tissues. Multivariate K-means clustering analysis produced seven gene clusters featuring similar gene expression patterns specific to individual tissues, with lung tissue cluster having the largest number of DEGs. These findings suggest the presence of a broad immune defense mechanism across various tissues in cats against acute *T. gondii* infection.

Keywords: *Toxoplasma gondii*, host-parasite interaction, transcriptome, differential gene expression, biomarkers

INTRODUCTION

The intracellular protozoan *Toxoplasma gondii* infects almost all warm-blooded animals and approximately one-third of the world's human population, causing toxoplasmosis, a serious illness with fatal consequences in immune-compromised individuals and the unborn fetus (1–3). The emergence of drug-resistant parasite strains (4) together with the adverse effects of the currently-available drug therapies (5), and the inability to clear chronic infection highlight the need for improved treatment strategies to combat toxoplasmosis in humans and animals.

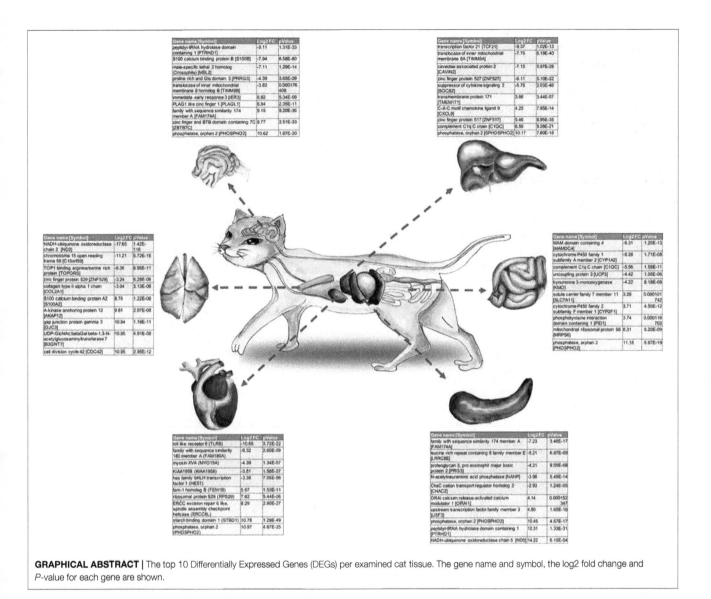

GRAPHICAL ABSTRACT | The top 10 Differentially Expressed Genes (DEGs) per examined cat tissue. The gene name and symbol, the log2 fold change and *P*-value for each gene are shown.

T. gondii has a complex lifecycle, wherein the parasite undergoes asexual reproduction in the intermediate host and sexual reproduction in the definitive host (members of the Felidae family). Cats acquire infection by ingesting prey tissue containing parasite cysts or, more rarely, oocysts. Prenatal infection may also occur in cats and humans (2, 6). Infected cats discharge oocysts (the product of parasite sexual reproduction in the cat's intestine) in their feces. The ability to accommodate both sexual and asexual reproduction of *T. gondii*, makes cats a significant source of infection to humans and animals (1, 7). *T. gondii* is a food-borne pathogen acquired via oral infection; however, it has a dispersive nature and can disseminate throughout the cat's body to infect multiple tissues (8–14).

Recognizing early transcriptional signatures of infection, while knowing the factors that determine tissue susceptibility to *T. gondii* infection in cats, would assist in planning preventative measures against environmental contamination with oocysts. Previous investigations have provided insights into the transcriptome of many intermediate host species

during *T. gondii* infection (15–21). However, knowledge of the mechanisms that underpin the feline host transcriptional response to *T. gondii* remains poorly understood; and no genome-wide expression profiling of multiple tissues from cat, has been reported. Single-tissue gene expression can provide information on how a specific tissue responds to infection; however, understanding the patterns of gene expression across various tissues may advance our understanding of *T. gondii* molecular-pathogenesis events occurring during acute infection in cats and reveal the mechanisms by which the definitive host counters a complex infection such as *T. gondii*. RNA sequencing (RNA-Seq) of the whole transcriptome has proved a powerful and versatile tool for global gene expression analysis (22–24), enabling a comparison of transcriptomes between the merozoite and tachyzoite stages of *T. gondii* infecting the cat's intestine (25).

Here, we hypothesized that tissues of *T. gondii*-infected cats exhibit characteristic transcriptional signatures which are dominated by a number of genes, and may be exclusive to a particular tissue with variance across tissues from the same individual. Differential gene expression and gene clustering analyses were performed on six tissues, individually or combined, in cats infected with *T. gondii*. Our studies provided novel information about the transcriptomic landscape of the major tissue types in cats during acute *T. gondii* infection and revealed tissue responsive signatures during acute *T. gondii* infection.

MATERIALS AND METHODS

Ethics Approval

All efforts were made to minimize suffering and to reduce the number of animals in the experiment. All work with live *T. gondii* was performed at biosafety level 2 and the animal experimental protocols were approved by The Animal Administration and Ethics Committee of Lanzhou Veterinary Research Institute, Chinese Academy of Agricultural Sciences (Protocol Permit Number: LVRIAEC-2014-001).

Animal Husbandry

Twelve domestic cats (*Felis catus;* 2 to 3-months-old; Chinese Li Hua breed) were purchased from a local breeder and housed individually in a controlled environment. Six cats each from two litters– were randomly allocated into four groups (2x infected and 2x control) with three cats per group. All of the cats were tested negative for feline immunodeficiency virus and feline leukemia virus using SNAP FIV/FeLV Combo Test (IDEXX, Westbrook, US), and feline calicivirus and feline parvovirus by ELISA KIT (NuoYuan, Shanghai, China) prior to the experiment. Also, cats tested seronegative for the presence of specific anti-*T. gondii* antibodies using indirect fluorescent antibody test (IFAT). Cats were supplied with a commercial diet (Royal Canine Inc., St. Charles, MO, USA) and water ad libitum during the 3 weeks prior to experimentation. During the experiment cats were fed a maintenance diet, based on their daily energy requirement.

Parasite Strain, Infection and Sample Collection

T. gondii Pru strain (genotype II) was maintained by passage through Kunming mice (26). The number of *T. gondii* cysts (determined using an optical microscope) was adjusted to 100 cysts per 1ml phosphate buffered saline (PBS, pH 7.4). Each experimental animal was infected with 100 cysts in 1 ml PBS by intragrastric inoculation. The enteroepithelial sexual cycle of *T. gondii* is completed within 3-10 days post ingestion of *T. gondii* cysts. This period can be extended to >18 days if cats are infected by oocysts. Control cats were sham-infected with 1 ml PBS only. Six different tissues (brain, heart, liver, lung, small intestine, and spleen) were collected from cats seven days after infection, in order to allow sufficient time for infection to establish. Tissue collection was performed as a terminal procedure from cats under deep isoflurane anesthesia, and unresponsiveness to all stimuli. Collected tissue samples were rinsed in saline, flash frozen in liquid nitrogen and stored at −80°C until processing.

Confirmation of Infection

Total genomic DNA was extracted from all harvested tissues using TIANamp Genomic DNA kit (TianGen™, Beijing, China). A PCR assay targeting *T. gondii* B1 gene was used to detect *T. gondii* infection in all cat tissues (27, 28). The PCR products were subjected to electrophoresis on ethidium bromide-stained 2% agarose–Tris-acetate-EDTA gels, and the banding pattern was visualized by UV transillumination. All of the electrophoresed PCR products were run with positive and negative control. *T. gondii* genotype was confirmed by PCR-restriction fragment length polymorphism (RFLP) analysis of the positive amplicons (29).

RNA Extraction and Qualification

Total RNA was extracted individually from the six tissues of the cats using TRIzol Reagent according to the manufacturer's protocol (Invitrogen, CA, USA). The RNA was checked for degradation and contamination using 1% agarose gels. RNA purity was evaluated with a NanoPhotometer® spectrophotometer (IMPLEN, CA, USA) and RNA concentration was measured using the Qubit® RNA Assay Kit in Qubit® 2.0 Fluorometer (Life Technologies, CA, USA). RNA integrity was assessed using the RNA Nano 6000 Assay Kit of the Agilent Bioanalyzer 2100 system (Agilent Technologies, CA, USA).

cDNA Library Preparation and Illumina Deep Sequencing

RNA samples that conformed with Quality Control checks (QC) were used in the transcriptome-sequencing (RNA-seq) analysis. Samples were run in duplicate, and each RNA template consisted of three pooled biological replicates from the same group. 3 μg RNA per sample was used as input material for RNA-seq library preparation using NEBNext® Ultra™ RNA Library Prep Kit for Illumina® (NEB, USA). Index codes were added to correlate sequences to their respective samples. The mRNA was purified from total RNA using poly-T oligo-attached magnetic beads. Fragmentation was carried out using divalent cations under elevated temperature in NEBNext First Strand Synthesis Reaction Buffer (5X). First strand cDNA was synthesized using a random hexamer primer and M-MuLV Reverse Transcriptase (RNase H-). Second strand cDNA was synthesized using DNA Polymerase I and RNase H. Remaining overhangs were converted into blunt ends using exonuclease/polymerase. Following adenylation of the 3′ends of DNA fragments, NEBNext Adaptor with hairpin loop structures were ligated to prepare for hybridization. In order to select cDNA fragments of 150~200 bp in length, library fragments were purified using the AMPure XP system (Beckman Coulter, Beverly, USA). Then, 3 μl USER Enzyme (NEB, USA) were used with size-selected, adaptor-ligated cDNA at 37°C for 15 min followed by 5 min at 95°C before PCR, which was performed with Phusion High-Fidelity DNA polymerase, Universal PCR primers and Index (X) Primer. PCR products were purified (AMPure XP system) and the library quality was assessed with the Agilent Bioanalyzer 2100 system. The clustering of index-coded samples was performed on a cBot Cluster Generation System using TruSeq PE Cluster Kit v3-cBot-HS (Illumia) according to the manufacturer's instructions. Following cluster generation, library preparations were sequenced on an Illumina Hiseq 2500 platform and 125 bp paired-end reads were generated.

Quality Trimming of Illumina Paired-End Reads
Before read alignment, all the data files (Fastq) were adaptor trimmed using "scythe" (v0.994 BETA) (https://github.com/vsbuffalo/scythe) and quality trimmed using the library "sickle" (v1.33) (https://github.com/najoshi/sickle).

Read Alignment and Transcript Assembly
Index of the reference genome was built using Hisat2 (v2.1.0) (30). Trimmed paired-end reads were aligned to the reference genome using Hisat2 for expression estimation. StringTie (v1.3.3) was then used to assemble the read alignments into known transcripts for each sample (31). In addition, StringTie also produces a gene abundance table (FPKM and TPM), which was used for clustering analysis.

Tissue-Specific Differential Expression Analysis
A combined read count table at the gene level for all the samples was generated using a python script available from StringTie. The Bioconductor package edgeR (v3.18.1) (32) was used to identify the differentially expressed (DE) genes per-tissue condition (infected vs. uninfected; two biological replicates per condition). Genes with a 5% false discovery rate (FDR < 0.05) and log fold change (logFC) ≥ 1 were considered differentially expressed.

Gene Ontology (GO) and Pathway Analyses
The Bioconductor package GOstats (v2.42.0) (33) was used to test for over-representation of GO terms using a hypergeometric test (hyperGTest). Orthologues for cat gene-sets were found using Ensembl BioMart against human data; then the cat gene orthologues were used for gene ontology analysis. GO terms with a corrected $P < 0.05$ were considered significantly enriched. Pathway analysis was performed using bioconductor package "pathview" (v1.16.5), which implements Kyoto Encyclopedia of Genes and Genomes (KEGG) pathways. The significance level of enrichment of KEGG pathways was identified using FDR < 0.05 and a corrected $P < 0.05$.

K-Means Clustering
The 21,890 genes identified through HiSat2 and StringTie were subjected to clustering analysis. In detail: the FPKM values of the genes from both replicates of each tissue and each treatment (e.g., rep 1 and rep 2 of infected brain tissues) were averaged; the log of the ratio between infected and non-infected conditions for each tissue was calculated; then, two subsequent k-means clustering analyses were performed [MeV_4_8 v10.2 (Multi Experiment viewer)] using Euclidean distance and k = 10 number of clusters. A stringent expression cutoff was applied to each sub-group of genes to discard background noise. Specifically, in each of the six generated clusters where genes showed increased expression

levels concentrated on a single infected tissue, only those genes with FPKM values >1 in the specific infected condition were considered as expressed and selected for further analysis. To visualize gene expression in each cluster, bean plots (which represent the actual distribution of the individual data sets) were produced using BoxPlotR: a web-tool for generation of box plots.

Quantitative Real Time (RT)-PCR
Total RNA was extracted from various cat tissues using the TRIzol method (Invitrogen) and reverse-transcribed to single strand cDNA using the GoScript™ Reverse Transcription System (Promega, MI, USA). GoTaq® qPCR Master Mix (Promega, MI, USA) was used to perform RT-PCR reactions in a QIAGEN's real-time PCR cycler (Rotor-Gene Q). Amplification reactions were performed under the following conditions: 2 min at 95°C, 40 cycles of 95°C for 15s, 55°C for 30s, and 72°C for 30s. All quantitative measurements were carried out in triplicate and normalized to the housekeeping gene glyceraldehyde-3-phosphatedehydrogenase (*GAPDH*) for every reaction (34). Twelve significant DEGs were selected to validate the sequencing data. Primers used for RT-PCR are listed in **Table 1**. The mRNA fold change was calculated using the following equations (35):

$$^\Delta C_T = {}^\Delta C_{T(target)} - {}^\Delta C_{T(GAPDH)};$$
$$^{\Delta\Delta} C_T = {}^\Delta C_{T(infected)} - {}^\Delta C_{T(control)}; \text{mRNA fold change} = 2^{-\Delta\Delta C_T}$$

RESULTS

Presence of *T. Gondii* Infection in Cats
Parasite dissemination from the intestine to other tissues, both close to the inoculation site (small intestine, liver, and spleen) and to distantly placed organs (brain, heart, and lungs) was confirmed seven days post infection. *T. gondii* B1 gene-based PCR analysis detected the parasite DNA in the brain, heart, liver, lung, small intestine, and spleen of all infected cats (**Figure S1**). The parasite load did not seem to vary across the cat tissues. However, it is possible that the parasite load may vary over the course of infection. *T. gondii* DNA was not detected in any tissue of the control cats. All positive amplicons that were characterized by RFLP produced a restriction fragment pattern that correlated with *T. gondii* genotype II.

General Features of the Transcriptome Data
Transcriptome-sequencing analysis generated ~143 million sequence reads (125 bp in length) from 24 libraries. After quality control analysis and the removal of low quality reads, ~170 Gb clean reads were obtained, with an average of 7 Gb clean reads/tissue. Less than 95% of the clean reads had Phred-like quality scores at the Q20 level and GC content of about 50% (**Table S1**). The clean reads were mapped to the genome of *Felis catus*. The majority of the clean reads were distributed in the exon region, with fewer in the intergenic region and the intron region. Approximately 80% of the clean reads were unique (**Table S2**); and subsequent analyses were based on these uniquely mapped reads.

TABLE 1 | Gene names and primers used in qRT-PCR analysis.

Gene	Primer name*	Primer sequence (5′ to 3′)
ADAM11	ADAM11-F	5′-CTGTGGCTTCCTCCTCTGTGT–3′
	ADAM11-R	5′-TTGCCCTGGTGGTAGAAGGT–3′
APOA2	APOA2-F	5′-CGGTGACTGACTACGGCAAG-3′
	APOA2-R	5′-TAACTGCTCCTGGGTCTTCTCAA–3′
MEP1A	MEP1A-F	5′-CACCATCATCAACATCCTGTCTC–3′
	MEP1A-R	5′-AAGGAAGGTCTGAAGTAGCAAAGGT-3′
ENO4	ENO4-F	5′-TGCATCTCTGTGTTGGTTATGCT–3′
	ENO4-R	5′- CGAAGGGCTACATACCGATTTTAC-3′
IGFI	IGFI-F	5′-GAGAGGAGTGGAAAACGCAGA–3′
	IGFI-R	5′-AGCGGTGAGTCCAAGACAGAG–3′
GKN2	GKN2-F	5′-CATGCTCCTCTACCACGGTTT–3′
	GKN2-R	5′-GCAGGGATGGCTTTATGTTTC–3′
GBP5	GBP5-F	5′-GCTAAAGGAAGGCACCGATAAA–3′
	GBP5-R	5′-AGTGAGCAGGAGAGTCGAAGATAAA–3′
OAS1	OAS1-F	5′-AGCCATCCACATCATCTCCAC–3′
	OAS1-R	5′- AGAGCCACCCTTGACCACTTT–3′
IDO1	IDO1-F	5′-GAACCAAGGCGGTGAAGATG–3′
	IDO1-R	5′-GCATAAACCAGAATAGGAGGCAGA–3′
PI16	PI16-F	5′-CTGCCAGAACTGTCTGCCTCT–3′
	PI16-R	5′-GTCCTTCATCTGCCCCTCAC–3′
ACTG2	ACTG2-F	5′-AACAGGGAGAAGATGACCCAGA–3′
	ACTG2-R	5′-CCAGAAGCATAGAGAGAGAGCACA–3′
ANKFN1	ANKFN1-F	5′-ATACCTCTACACCAGGCAAGGAAC–3′
	ANKFN1-R	5′-GCAGGGAGCAGGAGAAGAAA–3′
GAPDH	GAPDH(CAT)-F	5′-AAGCCCATCACCATCTTCCA–3′
	GAPDH(CAT)-R	5′-TTCACGCCCATCACAAACA–3′

Forward (F) and reverse (R) primers.
ADAM11, ADAM metallopeptidase domain 11; APOA2, apolipoprotein A2; MEP1A, Meprin A Subunit Alpha; ENO4, enolase family member 4; IGFI, Insulin-like growth factor 1 level; GKN2, gastrokine 2; GBP5, Guanylate Binding Protein 5; OAS1, 2'-5'-Oligoadenylate Synthetase 1; IDO1, indoleamine 2,3-dioxygenase 1; PI16, Peptidase Inhibitor 16; ACTG2, actin, gamma 2; ANKFN1, ankyrin repeat and fibronectin type III domain containing 1; GAPDH, glyceraldehyde-3-phosphate dehydrogenase.

Infection Induced Significant Alterations in Gene Expression

We investigated the distribution of gene expression values across the six tissues by fragment Per Kilobase of exon per Million mapped reads (FPKM) (**Table S3**). ~47% of the expressed genes had low expression values ($0 < \text{FPKM} \leq 1$). The number of genes with moderate expression values ($1 < \text{FPKM} \leq 60$) and high expression values ($\text{FPKM} > 60$) accounted for ~53% of the total annotated genes. Genes with $\text{FPKM} \geq 1$ [ranging from 12,195 (43.80%) to 16,734 (60.10%)] in the six tissues were considered expressed genes. We used the Bioconductor package edgeR (v3.18.1) to identify DEGs in each body tissue of the infected and uninfected cats. A total of 737 genes were differentially expressed in infected vs. uninfected cats, of which 410 were up-regulated and 327 were down-regulated. Large differences in gene expression were observed between cat tissues, indicating heterogenities in the response of cat tissues to *T. gondii* infection. Liver exhibited the highest number of DEGs

(151 genes) compared to lung (149 genes), small intestine (130 genes), heart (123 genes), brain (104 genes), and spleen (80 genes) (**Figure 1**). DEGs of each tissue are listed in **Table S4**. We also used quantitative real-time PCR to validate the expression levels of representative genes, across cat tissues, detected by RNA-sequencing analysis (**Figure 2**).

Gene Ontology (GO) Enrichment and Functional Annotation Analyses

GO enrichment analysis was used to identify the significantly enriched GO terms in all DEGs using the GOseq R package. The enriched GO terms of each tissue are shown in **Table S5**. All DEGs were mapped to terms in the KEGG database. DEGs and KEGG pathways related to immune response were highly represented and are summarized in **Table S6**.

Signatures of Gene Co-expression

Differences were detected between the transcriptomes of cat tissues, with significant variations in gene expression between infected and uninfected tissues (**Table S4**). Gene co-expression analysis of DEGs indicated that phosphatase and indoleamine 2,3-dioxygenase (IDO) were co-expressed in five tissues (brain, heart, liver, small intestine, and spleen); while the HES1 (Hes Family BHLH Transcription Factor 1) was co-expressed in brain, heart, liver, and small intestine. Guanylate-binding protein 5 was detected in heart, liver, lung, and spleen (**Figure 3**, **Table S7**). Expression patterns and pathways associated with co-expressed DEGs across the various cat tissues are shown (**Figure S2**).

Global Gene Regulation During *T. Gondii* Infection

We employed cluster analysis, which was based on the partition of genes into clusters according to the log-ratios of gene expression between infected and uninfected tissues using a two-tier K-means algorithm. This analysis identified a set of 10 gene groups each characterized by a unique pattern. The patterns corresponding to individual clusters are visualized as line plots (**Figure 4**). Seven of these 10 clusters showed significant expression levels: spleen (cluster 2); brain (cluster 3); lung (cluster 7); liver (cluster 8), and heart (cluster 9), included up-regulated genes. Small intestine tissue produced two clusters with opposite regulation: cluster 4 (up-regulated genes) and cluster 10 (down-regulated genes). Two clusters (5 and 6) did not exhibit gene expression patterns specific to any tissue. To isolate the most representative genes in each cluster, a second clustering analysis was performed, focusing on genes contained in each of the seven clusters identified by the initial cluster analysis. Ultimately, seven groups of tissue-specific genes were identified, and are shown in heat maps and graphical formats, based on patterns of expression of individual genes across various tissues (**Figures 5A,B**).

Refined Gene Clusters After FPKM Filtering

Here, a stringent expression cutoff was applied to each sub-group of genes to remove background noise. In each of the six clusters where genes showed increased expression concentrated on a single infected tissue, only those genes with FPKM values >1 in the infected condition were selected for further analysis. Five

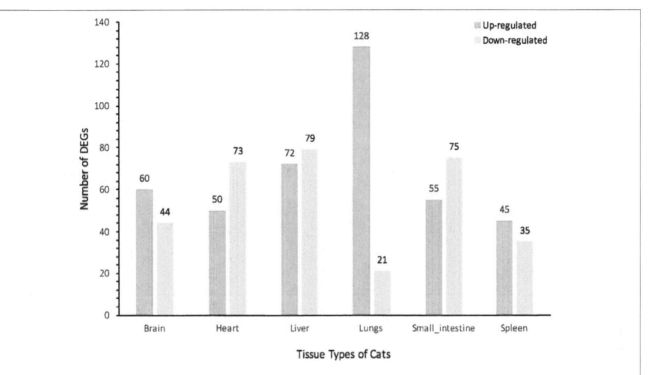

FIGURE 1 | Bar plot representation of the differentially Expressed Genes (DEGs) across the cat tissues after acute *T. gondii* infection. The numbers of up-regulated and down-regulated DEGs assigned to each cat tissue are indicated above the bars. The greatest changes in DEGs between infected and uninfected tissues were observed in the liver and lung.

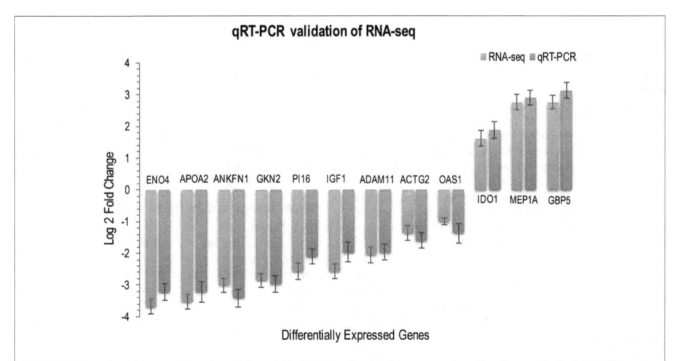

FIGURE 2 | RNA-seq transcriptome analysis and quantitative, real-time RT–PCR produced similar gene expression profiles. The expression levels of 12 DEGs across various cat tissues were determined by qRT-PCR for validation of RNA-seq data. Relative expression levels were calculated using the the $\Delta\Delta CT$ threshold cycle (CT) method and *GAPDH* as the reference gene. RNA-seq data are mean of two biological replicates + standard deviation (SD) of normalized read counts. qRT–PCR data are mean of three biological replicates + SD. *P* values are calculated with unpaired, two-tailed *t*-test. The height of the bars represents the log-transformed median fold changes in gene expression between infected and uninfected cats.

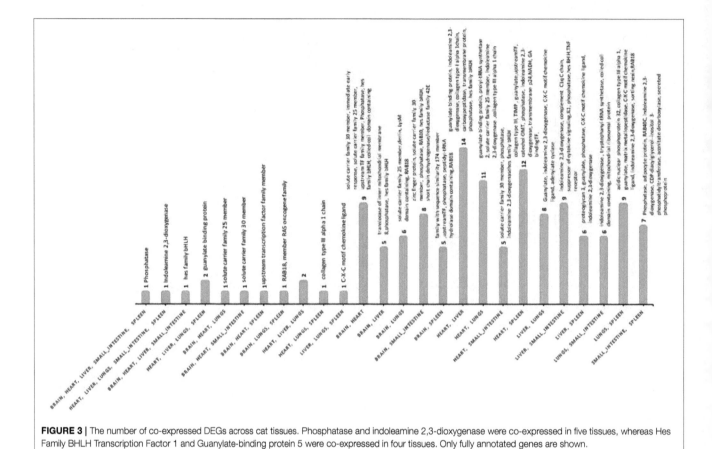

FIGURE 3 | The number of co-expressed DEGs across cat tissues. Phosphatase and indoleamine 2,3-dioxygenase were co-expressed in five tissues, whereas Hes Family BHLH Transcription Factor 1 and Guanylate-binding protein 5 were co-expressed in four tissues. Only fully annotated genes are shown.

of these clusters contained up-regulated genes in the spleen (6 genes), brain (13 genes), lung (75 genes), liver (1 gene), and heart (6 genes). However, the small intestine produced one cluster of 19 up-regulated genes and one cluster of 21 down-regulated genes. GO analysis of genes within these seven clusters provided new insights into biological processes, cellular processes and molecular functions regulated in cats during *T. gondii* infection. The five most highly associated biological process terms with the enrichment *P*-values of each cluster are shown (**Figure 5C**).

KEGG analysis of the DEGs within these seven final clusters was performed to gain more insight into the biological processes influenced during infection. We found no similarity in gene annotation in any cluster in any of the tissues examined. In small intestine cluster, KEGG analysis identified networks associated with hematopoietic cell lineage, metabolism of xenobiotics by cytochrome-P, chemical carcinogenesis and cytokine-cytokine receptor interaction. Lung cluster showed high expression levels of genes involved in nicotine addiction, biosynthesis of unsaturated fatty acids, long-term potentiation, glycosaminoglycan biosynthesis - heparan sulfate/heparin, cell adhesion molecules, insulin secretion, GABAergic synapse, fatty acid metabolism, amyotrophic lateral sclerosis, and adrenergic signaling in cardiomyocytes. The heart cluster showed high expression levels in complement and coagulation cascades and platelet activation. Small intestine cluster showed high expression levels of genes involved in metabolic metabolism, drug metabolism and fatty acid and amino acid metabolism.

Genes with different expression patterns across the seven clusters are shown in **Table S8**. All of the analyzed clusters contained genes annotated to GO terms from the three ontologies at roughly equivalent levels. However, we found considerable bias in some tissues in regards to the representation of clustered genes among the three ontologies (**Figure S3**). The high proportion of genes annotated to biological process, reflects a trend toward clustering of metabolic and immune pathways. The most striking example was in the lung cluster, where 253 terms were found in the biological process.

Tissue-Specific Changes in Gene Expression

Even though the number of genes in each cluster was small, large-magnitude gene expression changes between infected and uninfected was observed in most of the tissues (**Figure 6**). The liver gene cluster had the highest magnitude (7.68 fold), followed by lung (5.44 fold), brain (3.58 fold), small intestine cluster 4 (3.55 fold), spleen (3.09 fold), and heart (2.98 fold); whereas small intestine tissue cluster 10 had a magnitude of −3.22 fold. Apart from the liver with only on gene, lung, brain, small intestine, and heart showed large magnitude transcriptional changes occurring in a small number of genes. This suggests that changes induced by *T. gondii* infection seem to rely on a small number of genes, but with large transcriptional changes. The lung was the tissue showing the greatest number of genes with the largest magnitude of transcriptional change. Among all highly expressed genes, the

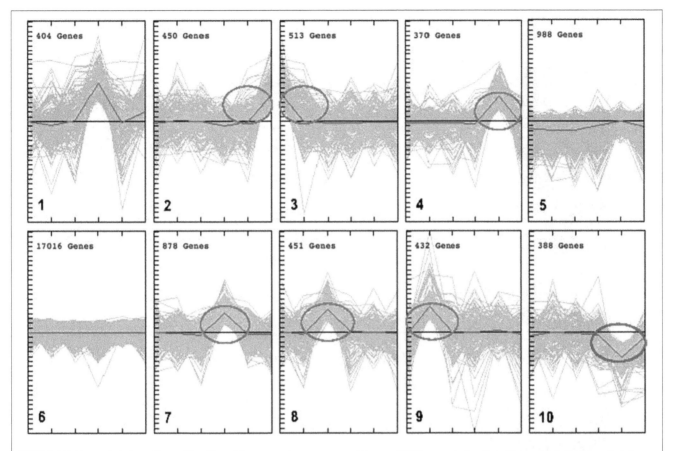

FIGURE 4 | k-Means clustering patterns of the differentially expressed genes across cat tissues. All DEGs were clustered into 10 groups using k-means clustering method and visualized with TM4 software. The pink line shows average expression z-scores to visualize the dominant expression trend of each cluster. Each line in the figure represents an expression value of the corresponding gene. The horizontal axis indicates the type of cat tissues and the vertical axis is the log2 expression ratio. Fold expression changes between various tissues from infected and uninfected cats were calculated using the log2 ratios. The numbers of genes for each cluster are indicated. The clusters included DEGs whose expression was either up regulated (clusters 2, 3, 4, 7, 8, and 9) or down regulated (cluster 10). There were no changes in gene expression observed in clusters 5 and 6. DEGs in cluster 1 was not considered due to lack of specificity to a single tissue.

metallothionein 3 (MT3) gene showed the highest expression in the infected lung, and it was also one of the genes with the highest log ratio between infected and uninfected tissues. Metallothionein-3 protein encoded by MT3 gene binds metals both in natural (such as Zn, Cu, Se) and xenobiotic (such as Ag, Cd) conditions, conferring a protective role against metal toxicity and oxidative stress.

DISCUSSION

The influence of *T. gondii* infection on the transcriptome of different tissue of cats is largely unknown. In this study, we examined the transcriptomes of liver, lung, small intestine, heart, brain, and spleen tissues of cats, seven days post infection. Inter-tissue transcriptome comparison revealed that the levels of DEGs were highest in the liver (151 genes) and lungs (149 genes), indicating a significant gene transcriptional response to infection in the liver and lung compared to other feline tissues. This result supports previous reports, wherein liver and lung seemed to be the most likely tissues to be involved in clinical cases of toxoplasmosis with a rapid fatal outcome (11–13, 34, 36).

It is plausible that the timing and duration of infection can influence host tissue transcriptional response to the parasite, as previously indicated by the difference in the transcriptomes of mouse brain between acute and chronic *T. gondii* infection (17), and this could alter cytokine responses of the host to infection.

The transcriptional landscape of infected cat tissues was dominated by an immune gene expression signature, wherein, cytokine-cytokine receptor interaction, Jak-STAT signaling pathway, NOD-like receptor signaling pathway, NF-kappa B signaling pathway, MAPK signaling pathway, T cell receptor signaling pathway and the cytosolic DNA sensing pathway, were amongst the up-regulated immune pathways in almost all tissues. The importance of Toll-like receptor signaling in controlling *T. gondii* infection has been established (37). Many of the upregulated genes (e.g., CXCL10, SOCS3, MAPK13, CXCL9, CD2, CSF2RA, PI4K2B, IGF1, PFKFB1, MMP7, FZD8, TNFSF10, and RelB) identified in the livers are involved in immune-related pathways. Some of these genes are involved in the development of Natural Killer (NK) and adaptive T cell responses, leading to the production of Interferon gamma (IFN-γ) and resistance to infection (38). *T. gondii* is very

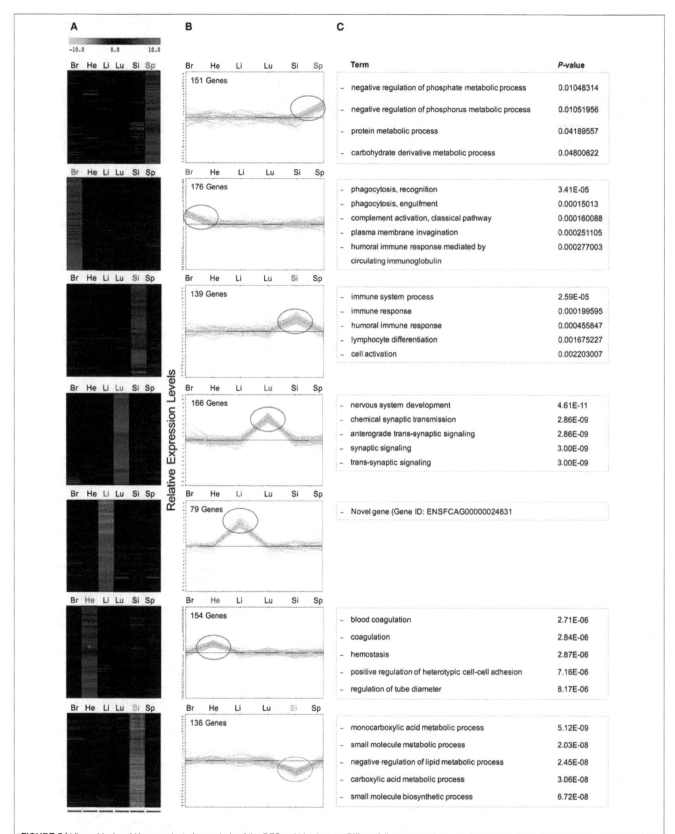

FIGURE 5 | Hierarchical and K-mean clustering analysis of the DEGs within clusters. Differentially expressed, co-regulated genes in each cluster were grouped using k-means clustering. Average cluster size varied considerably among tissues with lung containing the largest cluster with 75 genes. The smallest cluster was found in

(Continued)

FIGURE 5 | the liver, averaging 1 gene per cluster. The DEGs clustered into 7 major groups, demonstrated in **(A)** heat map and **(B)** graphical format, based on patterns of gene expression across the differing cat tissues. Red and green circles indicate the tissue-specific up- and down regulated genes, respectively. Negative values indicate decreased expression, and positive values indicate increased expression. **(C)** GO analysis of DEGs within clusters after FPKM filtering identified the top associated enriched GO terms with corresponding enrichment *P*-values, shown on right.

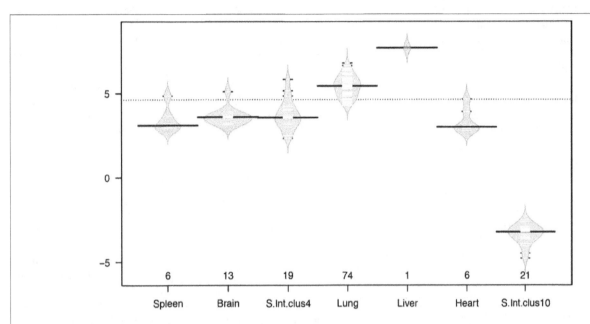

FIGURE 6 | Beanplots showing variation in the magnitude of gene expression within clusters in infected vs. uninfected tissues. The x-axis shows the number of genes of each cluster in the corresponding tissue. The y-axis indicates the average log2 fold change in gene expression. The width of the plot represents the distribution of data, short lines inside the shapes depict individual data points and heavy horizontal lines show the medians within each cluster, while the dotted line indicates the overall average. Plots were drawn using the R beanplot package.

efficient in manipulating the host's immune defense (39, 40); and previous studies have indicated that host immune response is a key determinant of clinical outcome following infection with *T. gondii* (16–20, 41, 42).

Although spleen had the lowest number of DEGs (80 genes) compared to other tissues, KEGG analysis identified multiple immune signaling pathways that were influenced by infection. Most of the immune pathways were up-regulated in spleen of infected cats; such as Toll-like receptor signaling pathway, cytosolic DNA-sensing pathway, RIG-I-like receptor signaling, TNF signaling pathway, FoxO signaling pathway, chemokine signaling pathway, and PI3K/Akt signaling pathway. Of note, C-X-C motif chemokine 10 (CXCL10) was involved in most of the immune-related pathways. Our previous study demonstrated that CXCL10 was up-regulated in pig peripheral blood mononuclear cells during early *T. gondii* infection (20, 21). CXCL10 is a chemokine secreted from cells stimulated with IFN-γ, and plays an important role in chemo-attraction of immune cells (43). This result indicates that *T. gondii* influences chemokine gene expression in spleen during early *T. gondii* infection.

T. gondii is a food-borne pathogen and infection is initially established in the small intestine by consuming prey containing parasite cysts or oocyst-contaminated water (44); leading to enteropathy (45). Therefore, successful infection of the host intestine is essential for subsequent parasite dissemination to different tissues. Others have showed that *in vitro* infection of rat intestinal epithelial cells can trigger an inflammatory response characterized by Tumor Necrosis Factor alpha (TNFα) signaling via NF-κB (46). However, feline host factors that are influenced by intestinal infection remain largely unknown. In our study, the global transcriptomic changes in the intestine of the definitive feline host, have been investigated. A total of 130 DEGs in the small intestine of infected cats were identified; of which 75 were down-regulated and 55 up-regulated. Some of the DEGs were involved in immune processes and signaling pathways, including LOC100302541, TNFSF18, CCL20, TNFRSF6B, IFNG, SOCS3, ICAM1, CD36, and FGF19. Other immune pathways up-regulated in liver and spleen tissues were also up-regulated in the small intestine.

An earlier study investigating the transcriptome of mouse brain during *T. gondii* infection reported an increased expression of genes involved in immune responses and cell activation (16). Also, host immune and inflammatory response was the major feature of genes affected by *T. gondii* infection of mouse peritoneal cells at five days post infection (47). We also showed that the expression of genes and signaling pathways involved in host immune response and cell fate, such as PI3K-Akt signaling pathway, Hippo signaling pathway and MAPK signaling pathway, was altered in the cat brain. Transcriptional signatures observed in the cat brain tissue showed also that Notch signaling pathway is involved in *T. gondii* neuro-pathogenesis. Previous *T. gondii* host/pathogen KEGG pathway interactome analysis suggested the involvement of six genes of the Notch pathway in psychiatric/neurological disorders (45, 48). Notch signaling interacts with other signaling pathways, including phosphatidylinositol-3-kinase (PI3K)/serine/threonine kinase (Akt) and NF-κB to regulate cell fate. PI3K/Akt signaling pathway regulates diverse cellular activities related to cell growth, metabolism, migration, and apoptosis (49). Notch signaling plays an important role in various facets of *T. gondii* pathogenesis (50). The possibility that PI3K/Akt signaling pathway participates in promoting *T. gondii* survival and proliferation (51) and in mediating cell survival and blockage of apoptotic responses during *T. gondii* infection (50), suggests a link between *T. gondii* and this signal pathway. This finding supports an earlier observation wherein many *T. gondii* strains were found able to regulate genes enriched for processes involved in cell cycle regulation in murine macrophages (15).

    T. gondii exploits heterotrimeric Gi-protein-mediated signaling to activate PI3K, leading to phosphorylation of downstream serine/threonine kinase AKT and extracellular signal-regulated protein kinases 1/2 (ERK1/2), and the inhibition of apoptosis (52). In our study, down-regulation of PI3K/AKT signaling in all tissues, except spleen, was detected and this can enhance apoptosis of host tissue and limits parasite growth. Phosphatase (a negative regulator of PI3K/Akt signaling, by converting PIP3 to PIP2, an opposite action to PI3K) can interfere with a number of cellular functions, such as cell proliferation and cell-cycle progression (53), was co-expressed in five cat tissues. These results indicate diverse roles played by PI3K/Akt signaling in *T. gondii*-host interaction. Further investigation into how the PI3K/Akt pathway interacts with other signaling mediators is required. NF-κB and mitogen-activated protein kinase (MAPK) signaling pathways are involved in the innate immune response to *T. gondii* (54). Altered MAPK signaling has been also implicated in toxoplasmosis of mice (55, 56) and humans (57). Considering that NF-κB and MAPK are downstream effectors of Akt, it is of significance to clarify whether this pathway influences the fate of infected cells via the regulation of NF-κB and MAPK.

Gene co-association Across Tissues

Co-expression analysis of DEGs indicated that phosphatase gene expression overlapped in five tissues; including brain, heart, liver, small intestine, and spleen. Transcripts for the inner-membrane complex (IMC) protein phosphatase have been involved in gene expression and cell division (46). Indoleamine 2,3-dioxygenase (IDO) was also co-expressed in five tissues: heart, liver, lung, small intestine, and spleen, but not in the brain tissue. IDO, the rate limiting catabolic enzyme in the degradation pathway of tryptophan, initiates the production of tryptophan degradation products, which exert important immuno-regulatory functions. IDO, through T-cell functions and other mechanisms (58), modulates pathophysiological processes, such as antimicrobial and antioxidant activities, and

immune-regulation. IFNγ produced in response to *T. gondii* infection induces IDO enzyme to degrade L-tryptophan, an amino acid for which *T. gondii* is auxotrophic (59, 60). IFNγ-induced L-tryptophan starvation was believed to trigger *T. gondii* clearance via noncanonical, ubiquitin-mediated autophagy (61). Guanylate-binding protein (GBP) was detected in the heart, liver, lung, and spleen. GBP, IFN-γ-inducible effector, is a member of the GTPase family, and plays an essential role in mediating host defense against *T. gondii* (62). Human guanylate-binding protein 1 (hGBP1) functions against *T. gondii* infection in human MSCs (hMSCs). *T. gondii* replication can be significantly inhibited by the recruitment of hGBP1 to the parasitophorous vacuole (PV) membrane in IFN-γ-stimulated hMSCs (63). In mice, the recruitment of mGBP2 to *T. gondii*-containing PV was essential for controlling *T. gondii* replication (64).

Patterns of Gene Clusters

Genes clustered according to their pattern of expressions across the six tissues examined, led to the identification of seven clusters featuring expressions differentiated across tissues and infected/non-infected conditions. We also detected tissue-specific variations in the percentage of clustered genes, and in the properties of gene clusters including functional annotation and magnitude of gene expression. The differences in each tissue's response to infection may imply that some tissue-specific defense mechanisms exist in order to maintain the balance between enhancing the host's response to infection and promoting the parasite's survival. The genes within these clusters after a further processing step imposing a stringent expression cutoff to avoid any background expression noise were analyzed for differential transcriptional changes between infected and uninfected samples (magnitude). Interestingly, the lung besides showing the greater number of genes showed also the largest magnitude of transcriptional changes between infected and non-infected conditions, suggesting that changes induced by infection in lungs seem to rely on genes, which had large transcriptional changes.

CONCLUSION

We used two complementary approaches to characterize alterations in tissue-specific gene expression in cats infected with *T. gondii*. Our results revealed considerable transcriptional differences between cat body tissues, and between infected and healthy cats. We identified significant tissue-specific differences in gene expression, and in gene cluster content and functional annotations. The differences in gene expression and gene clusters may result from tissue-specific differences in the defense processes that shape the host-pathogen interaction. Our data also underlined the importance of immune and inflammatory response to *T. gondii* infection, regardless of tissue types. Genes and pathways discovered in this study, should serve as a basis for further understanding the cellular and molecular basis of cat response to *T. gondii*. These results may assist the selection of biomarkers useful for developing new diagnostic tools or therapeutic interventions to control toxoplasmosis in cats.

Acute Toxoplasma Gondii Infection in Cats Induced Tissue-Specific Transcriptional Response...

191

ACCESSION NUMBER(S)

The RNA-seq data reported in this study have been deposited in GenBank's Short Read Archive (SRA) database under BioProject number PRJNA296557.

AUTHOR CONTRIBUTIONS

X-QZ, HE, and WC designed the experiment. WC supervised the experimental infection. WC, F-KZ, C-XZ, J-JH, and X-XZ performed the experiments. WC, HE, TD, FK, and RE contributed reagents, materials, and analysis tools. TD, FK, and RE developed computational algorithms and performed the bioinformatics analysis. WC, HE, and X-QZ wrote the paper. All authors commented on the manuscript.

FUNDING

Project support was kindly provided by the International Science and Technology Cooperation Project of Gansu Provincial Key Research and Development Program (Grant No. 17JR7WA031), the National Natural Science Foundation of China (Grant Nos. 31230073 and 31702383), the Elite Program of Chinese Academy of Agricultural Sciences, and the Agricultural Science and Technology Innovation Program (ASTIP) (Grant No. CAAS-ASTIP-2016-LVRI-03).

ACKNOWLEDGMENTS

We thank Hind Mamdowh Saad for excellent drawing of the **Graphical Abstract**.

REFERENCES

1. Montoya JG, Liesenfeld O. Toxoplasmosis. *Lancet* (2004) 363:1965–76. doi: 10.1016/S0140-6736(04)16412-X
2. Elsheikha HM. Congenital toxoplasmosis: priorities for further health promotion action. *Public Health* (2008) 122:335–53. doi: 10.1016/j.puhe.2007.08.009
3. Hill DE, Dubey JP. *Toxoplasma gondii* prevalence in farm animals in the United States. *Int J Parasitol.* (2013) 43:107–13. doi: 10.1016/j.ijpara.2012.09.012
4. Doliwa C, Escotte-Binet S, Aubert D, Sauvage V, Velard F, Schmid A, et al. Sulfadiazine resistance in *Toxoplasma gondii*: no involvement of overexpression or polymorphisms in genes of therapeutic targets and ABC transporters. *Parasite* (2013) 20:19. doi: 10.1051/parasite/2013020
5. Katlama C, De Wit S, O'Doherty E, Van Glabeke M, Clumeck N. Pyrimethamine-clindamycin versus pyrimethamine-sulfadiazine as acute and long-term therapy for toxoplasmic encephalitis in patients with aids. *Clin Infect Dis.* (1996) 22:268–75.
6. Dubey JP, Jones JL. *Toxoplasma gondii* infection in humans and animals in the United States. *Int J Parasitol.* (2008) 38:1257–78. doi: 10.1016/j.ijpara.2008.03.007
7. Hill DE, Dubey JP. *Toxoplasma gondii*: transmission, diagnosis and prevention. *Clin Microbiol Infect.* (2002) 8:634–40. doi: 10.1046/j.1469-0691.2002.00485.x
8. Dubey JP, Zajac SAA, Osofsky TobiasL. Acute primary toxoplasmic hepatitis in an adult cat shedding *Toxoplasma gondii* oocysts. *J Am Vet Med Assoc.* (1990) 197:1616–8.

9. Anfray P, Bonetti C, Fabbrini F, Magnino S, Mancianti F, Abramo F. Feline cutaneous toxoplasmosis: a case report. *Vet Dermatol.* (2005) 16:131–6. doi: 10.1111/j.1365-3164.2005.00434.x
10. Spycher A, Geigy C, Howard J, Posthaus H, Gendron K, Gottstein B, et al. Isolation and genotyping of *Toxoplasma gondii* causing fatal systemic toxoplasmosis in an immunocompetent 10-year-old cat. *J Vet Diagn Invest.* (2011) 23:104–8. doi: 10.1177/104063871102300117
11. Nagel SS, Williams JH, Schoeman JP. Fatal disseminated toxoplasmosis in an immunocompetent cat. *J S Afr Vet Assoc.* (2013) 84: E1–6. doi: 10.4102/jsava.v84i1.299
12. Foster SF, Charles JA, Canfield PJ, Beatty JA, Martin P. Reactivated toxoplasmosis in a FIV-positive cat. *Aus Vet Pract.* (1998) 28:159–63.
13. Atmaca HT, Dincel GC, Macun HC, Terzi OS, Uzunalioglu T, Kalender H, et al. A rare case of feline congenital *Toxoplasma gondii* infection: fatal outcome of systemic toxoplasmosis for the mother and its kitten. *Berl Munch Tierarztl Wochenschr* (2013) 126:216–9.
14. Dubey JP, Prowell M. Ante-mortem diagnosis, diarrhea, oocyst shedding, treatment, isolation, and genetic typing of *Toxoplasma gondii* associated with clinical toxoplasmosis in a naturally infected cat. *J Parasitol.* (2013) 99:158–60. doi: 10.1645/GE-3257.1
15. Melo MB, Nguyen QP, Cordeiro C, Hassan MA, Yang N, McKell R, et al. Transcriptional analysis of murine macrophages infected with different *Toxoplasma* strains identifies novel regulation of host signaling pathways. *PLoS Pathog.* (2013) 9:e1003779. doi: 10.1371/journal.ppat.1003779
16. Tanaka S, Nishimura M, Ihara F, Yamagishi J, Suzuki Y, Nishikawa Y. Transcriptome analysis of mouse brain infected with *Toxoplasma gondii. Infect Immun.* (2013) 81:3609–19. doi: 10.1128/IAI.00439-13

SUPPLEMENTARY MATERIAL

Figure S1 | Agarose gel electrophoresis of PCR amplicons after nested amplification of *Toxoplasma gondii B1* gene-specific fragment from cat tissue DNA. ~96-bp products of *B1* gene were amplified from ~193-bp *B1* PCR products, originally generated from genomic DNA extracted from different cat tissues, using the nested primers 5′-TGCATAGGTTGCAGTCACTG-3′ and 5′-GGCGACCAATCTGCGAATACACC-3′. Samples were analyzed by electrophoresis through 2% (wt/vol) agarose gels. Gels were stained with ethidium bromide and DNA was visualized under UV. Lanes: M, DNA ladder marker (TAKARA, China); 1, positive control; 2, negative control without DNA template; 3–8, positive PCR products from brain, heart, liver, lung, spleen and small intestine of infected cats; 9–14, negative results of samples obtained from the equivalent tissues of uninfected cats. The numbers to the left refer to the size (bp) of marker DNA fragments.

Figure S2 | Differential gene expression patterns across tissues and GO terms of the overlapping DEGs. **(A)** A heatmap of the genes expressed in all six tissues. **(B)** Gene Ontology terms associated with the co-expressed DEGs.

Figure S3 | Gene Ontology terms and KEGG pathways distribution per gene cluster.

Table S1 | Summary of RNA-Sequencing data obtained by Illumina HiSeq 2500 platform.

Table S2 | Summary of read mapping.

Table S3 | The number of gene in different expression level intervals.

Table S4 | Differentially expressed genes in various cat tissues.

Table S5 | Functional enrichment analysis of DEGs in various cat tissues.

Table S6 | DEGs involved in immune-related pathways in cat tissues.

Table S7 | Differentially co-expressed genes across various cat tissues.

Table S8 | Gene Ontology analysis of seven gene clusters.

17. Pittman KJ, Aliota MT, Knoll LJ. Dual transcriptional profiling of mice and *Toxoplasma gondii* during acute and chronic infection. *BMC Genomics* (2014) 15:806. doi: 10.1186/1471-2164-15-806

18. He JJ, Ma J, Li FC, Song HQ, Xu MJ, Zhu XQ. Transcriptional changes of mouse splenocyte organelle components following acute infection with *Toxoplasma gondii*. *Exp Parasitol*. (2016) 167:7–16. doi: 10.1016/j.exppara.2016.04.019

19. He JJ, Ma J, Song HQ, Zhou DH, Wang JL, Huang SY, et al. Transcriptomic analysis of global changes in cytokine expression in mouse spleens following acute *Toxoplasma gondii* infection. *Parasitol Res*. (2016) 115:703–12. doi: 10.1007/s00436-015-4792-5

20. Zhou CX, Elsheikha HM, Zhou DH, Liu Q, Zhu XQ, Suo X. Dual identification and analysis of differentially expressed transcripts of Porcine PK-15 cells and *Toxoplasma gondii* during *in vitro* infection. *Front Microbiol*. (2016) 7:721. doi: 10.3389/fmicb.2016.00721

21. Zhou CX, Zhou DH, Liu GX, Suo X, Zhu XQ. Transcriptomic analysis of porcine PBMCs infected with *Toxoplasma gondii* RH strain. *Acta Trop*. (2016) 154:82–8. doi: 10.1016/j.actatropica.2015.11.009

22. Emrich SJ, Barbazuk WB, Li L, Schnable PS. Gene discovery and annotation using LCM-454 transcriptome sequencing. *Genome Res*. (2007) 17:69–73. doi: 10.1101/gr.5145806

23. Huang Y, Huang X, Yan Y, Cai J, Ouyang Z, Cui H, et al. Transcriptome analysis of orange-spotted grouper (*Epinephelus coioides*) spleen in response to Singapore grouper iridovirus. *BMC Genomics* (2011) 12:556. doi: 10.1186/1471-2164-12-556

24. Videvall E, Cornwallis CK, Palinauskas V, Valkiunas G, Hellgren O. The avian transcriptome response to *Malaria* infection. *Mol Biol Evol*. (2015) 32:1255–67. doi: 10.1093/molbev/msv016

25. Hehl AB, Basso WU, Lippuner C, Ramakrishnan C, Okoniewski M, Walker RA, et al. Asexual expansion of *Toxoplasma gondii* merozoites is distinct from tachyzoites and entails expression of non-overlapping gene families to attach, invade, and replicate within feline enterocytes. *BMC Genomics* (2015) 16:66. doi: 10.1186/s12864-015-1225-x

26. Yan HK, Yuan ZG, Song HQ, Petersen E, Zhou Y, Ren D, et al. Vaccination with a DNA vaccine coding for perforin-like protein 1 and MIC6 induces significant protective immunity against *Toxoplasma gondii*. *Clin Vaccine Immunol*. (2012) 19:684–9. doi: 10.1128/CVI.05578-11

27. Cong W, Liu GH, Meng QF, Dong W, Qin SY, Zhang FK, et al. *Toxoplasma gondii* infection in cancer patients: prevalence, risk factors, genotypes and association with clinical diagnosis. *Cancer Lett*. (2015) 359:307–13. doi: 10.1016/j.canlet.2015.01.036

28. Jones CD, Okhravi N, Adamson P, Tasker S, Lightman S. Comparison of PCR detection methods for B1, P30, and 18S rDNA genes of *T. gondii* in aqueous humor. *Invest Ophthalmol Vis Sci*. (2000) 41:634–44.

29. Cong W, Meng QF, Song HQ, Zhou DH, Huang SY, Qian AD, et al. Seroprevalence and genetic characterization of *Toxoplasma gondii* in three species of pet birds in China. *Parasit Vectors* (2014) 7:152. doi: 10.1186/1756-3305-7-152

30. Kim D, Langmead B, Salzberg SL. HISAT: a fast spliced aligner with low memory requirements. *Nat Methods* (2015) 12:357-360. doi: 10.1038/nmeth.3317

31. Pertea M, Pertea GM, Antonescu CM, Chang TC, Mendell JT, Salzberg SL. StringTie enables improved reconstruction of a transcriptome from RNA-seq reads. *Nat Biotechnol*. (2015) 33:290–5. doi: 10.1038/nbt.3122

32. Robinson MD, McCarthy DJ, Smyth GK. edgeR: a Bioconductor package for differential expression analysis of digital gene expression data. *Bioinformatics* (2010) 26:139–40. doi: 10.1093/bioinformatics/btp616

33. Falcon S, Gentleman R. Using GOstats to test gene lists for GO term association. *Bioinformatics* (2007) 23:257–8. doi: 10.1093/bioinformatics/btl567

34. Schmittgen TD, Livak KJ. Analyzing real-time PCR data by the comparative CT method. *Nat Protoc*. (2008) 3:1101–8. doi: 10.1038/nprot.2008.73

35. Livak KJ, Schmittgen TD. Analysis of relative gene expression data using realtime quantitative PCR and the $2^{-\Delta\Delta}$ CT method. *Methods* (2001) 25:402–8. doi: 10.1006/meth.2001.1262

36. Tobias S. Acute primary toxoplasmic hepatitis in an adult cat shedding *Toxoplasma gondii* oocysts. *J Am Vet Med Asso*. (1990) 197:1616–8.

37. Yarovinsky F. Innate immunity to *Toxoplasma gondii* infection. *Nat Rev Immunol*. (2014) 14:109–21. doi: 10.1038/nri3598

38. Caamaño J, Alexander J, Craig L, Bravo R, Hunter CA. The NF-kappa B family member RelB is required for innate and adaptive immunity to *Toxoplasma gondii*. *J Immunol*. (1999) 163:4453–61.

39. Butcher BA, Fox BA, Rommereim LM, Kim SG, Maurer KJ, Yarovinsky F, et al. *Toxoplasma gondii* rhoptry kinase ROP16 activates STAT3 and STAT6 resulting in cytokine inhibition and arginase-1-dependent growth control. *PLoS Pathog*. (2011) 7:e1002236. doi: 10.1371/journal.ppat.1002236

40. Hunter CA, Sibley LD. Modulation of innate immunity by *Toxoplasma gondii* virulence effectors. *Nat Rev Microbiol*. (2012) 10:766–78. doi: 10.1038/nrmicro2858

41. Yarovinsky F. Toll-like receptors and their role in host resistance to *Toxoplasma gondii*. *Immunol Lett* (2008) 119:17-21. doi: 10.1016/j.imlet.2008.05.007

42. Pifer R, Yarovinsky F. Innate responses to *Toxoplasma gondii* in mice and humans. *Trends Parasitol*. (2011) 27:388–93. doi: 10.1016/j.pt.2011.03.009

43. Dufour JH, Dziejman M, Liu MT, Leung JH, Lane TE, Luster AD. IFN-γ-inducible protein 10 (IP-10; CXCL10)-deficient mice reveal a role for IP-10 in effector T cell generation and trafficking. *J Immunol*. (2002) 168:3195–204. doi: 10.4049/jimmunol.168.7.3195

44. Dubey JP. Toxoplasmosis - a waterborne zoonosis. *Vet Parasitol*. (2004) 126:57–72. doi: 10.1016/j.vetpar.2004.09.005

45. Schreiner M, Liesenfeld O. Small intestinal inflammation following oral infection with *Toxoplasma gondii* does not occur exclusively in C57BL/6 mice: Review of 70 reports from the literature. *Mem Inst Oswaldo Cruz*. (2009) 104:221–33. doi: 10.1590/S0074-02762009000200015

46. Guiton PS, Sagawa JM, Fritz HM, Boothroyd JC. An *in vitro* model of intestinal infection reveals a developmentally regulated transcriptome of *Toxoplasma* sporozoites and a NF-κB-like signature in infected host cells. *PLoS ONE* (2017) 12:e0173018. doi: 10.1371/journal.pone.0173018

47. Hill RD, Gouffon JS, Saxton AM, Su C. Differential gene expression in mice infected with distinct *Toxoplasma* strains. *Infect Immun*. (2012) 80:968–74. doi: 10.1128/IAI.05421-11

48. Carter CJ. Toxoplasmosis and polygenic disease susceptibility genes: extensive *Toxoplasma gondii* host/pathogen interactome enrichment in nine psychiatric or neurological disorders. *J Pathog*. (2013) 2013:965046. doi: 10.1155/2013/965046

49. Franke TF. Intracellular signaling by Akt: bound to be specific. *Sci Signal*. (2008) 1:pe29. doi: 10.1126/scisignal.124pe29

50. Quan JH, Cha GH, Zhou W, Chu JQ, Nishikawa Y, Lee YH. Involvement of PI 3 kinase/Akt-dependent Bad phosphorylation in *Toxoplasma gondii*-mediated inhibition of host cell apoptosis. *Exp Parasitol*. (2013) 133:462–71. doi: 10.1016/j.exppara.2013.01.005

51. Zhou W, Quan JH, Lee YH, Shin DW, Cha GH. *Toxoplasma gondii* proliferation require down-regulation of host Nox4 expression via activation of PI3 Kinase/Akt signaling pathway. *PLoS ONE* (2013) 8:e66306. doi: 10.1371/journal.pone.0066306

52. Kim L, Denkers EY. *Toxoplasma gondii* triggers Gi-dependent PI 3-kinase signaling required for inhibition of host cell apoptosis. *J Cell Sci*. (2006) 119 (Pt 10):2119–26. doi: 10.1242/jcs.02934

53. Jiang BH, Liu LZ. PI3K/PTEN signaling in angiogenesis and tumorigenesis. *Adv Cancer Res*. (2009) 102:19–65. doi: 10.1016/S0065-230X(09)02002-8

54. Yang CS, Yuk JM, Lee YH, Jo EK. *Toxoplasma gondii* GRA7-induced TRAF6 activation contributes to host protective immunity. *Infect Immun*. (2015) 84:339–50. doi: 10.1128/IAI.00734-15

55. Kim L, Butcher BA, Denkers EY. *Toxoplasma gondii* interferes with lipopolysaccharide-induced mitogen-activated protein kinase activation by mechanisms distinct from endotoxin tolerance. *J Immunol*. (2004) 172:3003–10. doi: 10.4049/jimmunol.172.5.3003

56. Valère A, Garnotel R, Villena I, Guenounou M, Pinon JM, Aubert D. Activation of the cellular mitogen-activated protein kinase pathways ERK, P38 and JNK during *Toxoplasma gondii* invasion. *Parasite* (2003)10:59–64. doi: 10.1051/parasite/2003101p59

57. Braun L, Brenier-Pinchart MP, Yogavel M, Curt-Varesano A, Curt-Bertini RL, Hussain T, et al. A *Toxoplasma* dense granule protein, GRA24, modulates the early immune response to infection by promoting a direct

and sustained host p38 MAPK activation. *J Exp Med.* (2013) 210:2071–86. doi: 10.1084/jem.20130103

58. Mbongue JC, Nicholas DA, Torrez TW, Kim NS, Firek AF, Langridge WH. The Role of Indoleamine 2, 3-Dioxygenase in immune suppression and autoimmunity. Vaccines (Basel) (2015) 3:703-729. doi: 10.3390/vaccines3030703

59. Pfefferkorn ER. Interferon gamma blocks the growth of *Toxoplasma gondii* in human fibroblasts by inducing the host cells to degrade tryptophan. *Proc Natl Acad Sci USA.* (1984) 81:908–12. doi: 10.1073/pnas.81.3.908

60. Hunt NH, Too LK, Khaw LT, Guo J, Hee L, Mitchell AJ, et al. The kynurenine pathway and parasitic infections that affect CNS function. *Neuropharmacology* (2017) 112(Pt B):389–98. doi: 10.1016/j.neuropharm.2016.02.029

61. Krishnamurthy S, Konstantinou EK, Young LH, Gold DA, Saeij JPJ. The human immune response to *Toxoplasma*: Autophagy versus cell death. *PLoS Pathog.* (2017) 13:e1006176. doi: 10.1371/journal.ppat.1006176

62. Kravets E, Degrandi D, Ma Q, Peulen TO, Klümpers V, Felekyan S, et al. Guanylate binding proteins directly attack *Toxoplasma gondii* via supramolecular complexes. *Elife* (2016) 5:e11479. doi: 10.7554/eLife.11479

63. Qin A, Lai DH, Liu Q, Huang W, Wu YP, Chen X, et al. Guanylate-binding protein 1 (GBP1) contributes to the immunity of human mesenchymal stromal cells against *Toxoplasma gondii*. *Proc Natl Acad Sci USA.* (2017) 114:1365–70. doi: 10.1073/pnas.1619665114

64. Degrandi D, Kravets E, Konermann C, Beuter-Gunia C, Klümpers V, Lahme S, et al. Murine guanylate binding protein 2 (mGBP2) controls *Toxoplasma gondii* replication. *Proc Natl Acad Sci USA.* (2013) 110:294–9. doi: 10.1073/pnas.1205635110

15

Sticking for a Cause: The Falciparum Malaria Parasites Cytoadherence Paradigm

Wenn-Chyau Lee[1], Bruce Russell[2] and Laurent Rénia[1]*

[1] Singapore Immunology Network (SIgN), Agency for Science, Technology and Research (A*STAR), Singapore, Singapore,
[2] Department of Microbiology and Immunology, University of Otago, Dunedin, New Zealand

*Correspondence:
Laurent Rénia
renia_laurent@immunol.a-star.edu.sg

After a successful invasion, malaria parasite *Plasmodium falciparum* extensively remodels the infected erythrocyte cellular architecture, conferring cytoadhesive properties to the infected erythrocytes. Cytoadherence plays a central role in the parasite's immune-escape mechanism, at the same time contributing to the pathogenesis of severe falciparum malaria. In this review, we discuss the cytoadhesive interactions between *P. falciparum* infected erythrocytes and various host cell types, and how these events are linked to malaria pathogenesis. We also highlight the limitations faced by studies attempting to correlate diversity in parasite ligands and host receptors with the development of severe malaria.

Keywords: malaria, *Plasmodium*, cytoadherence, pathogenesis, host immune responses

INTRODUCTION

Malaria continues to be a significant healthcare problem to many human populations, despite efforts to eliminate this debilitating and potentially fatal tropical disease. While the malaria mortality did not significantly change between 2015 and 2016, the number of malaria cases increased by five millions within the same period (1). Among the medically important malaria parasites (2, 3), *Plasmodium falciparum* is the primary cause of severe disease and death (4, 5).

As with other malaria parasites, *P. falciparum* has a complex life cycle involving humans as the intermediate host and *Anopheles* mosquitoes as the definitive host (where sexual reproductive forms of the parasites establish) (**Figure 1**). During its blood meal, the infected female *Anopheles* mosquito releases *Plasmodium* sporozoites from its salivary glands into the dermis of human host. A proportion of sporozoites migrate rapidly to the blood capillaries, then to the liver and invade the parenchymal hepatocytes after traversing the Kupffer cells (6). Inside the invaded parenchymal cells, parasites asexually multiply, producing numerous (~20,000–40,000) liver merozoites. Subsequently, these merozoites are released into the blood circulation, where they target and invade the erythrocytes (RBCs). It is the erythrocytic life cycle that is responsible for the manifestation of signs and symptoms in malaria. Within the infected erythrocytes (IRBCs), the blood stage-parasites develop from the early ring forms into trophozoites, subsequently form schizonts, which upon maturation will rupture and release blood stage merozoites to invade other uninfected erythrocytes (URBCs). Meanwhile, a fraction of the parasites are driven into the formation of sexual forms (gametocytes), which will be taken up by mosquitoes during feeding. Inside the mosquito, fertilization of male and female gametocytes leads to zygote formation. Subsequent developments lead to formation of salivary gland sporozoites, which are infective to the human host.

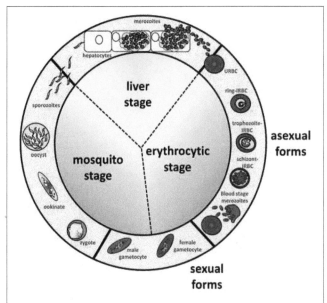

FIGURE 1 | Schematic diagram depicting life cycles of *Plasmodium falciparum*, involving *Anopheles* mosquito and human hosts, where the stages in humans can be furthered divided into liver (exoerythrocytic) and erythrocytic stages.

One fascinating aspect of *P. falciparum* infection is the cytoadherence phenomenon associated with the late stage-IRBC (7), which is considered to be a major contributor to the pathogenesis of falciparum malaria (8). As the parasite develops and matures within the host RBC, it causes substantial alteration to the IRBC membrane architecture, which changes various rheological properties of the IRBC, including its cytoadhesive characteristics (9–11). Here, we review the different types of cytoadhesive interactions of the IRBCs, how they are linked to each other, the molecular and cellular mechanisms behind these phenomena and their proposed involvement in malaria pathology. We also discuss knowledge gap, controversies and diverging views on the role of cytoadherence in *P. falciparum* immunopathogenesis.

COMPLEX PROFILE OF *P. falciparum*-IRBC CYTOADHERENCE

The cytoadherence of IRBCs to host cells in falciparum malaria is highly complex, involving at least three distinct groups of parasite-derived variant surface antigens (VSAs) encoded by multigene families, namely; *P. falciparum* Erythrocyte Membrane Protein 1 (PfEMP1) (12, 13), Subtelomeric Variable Open Reading frame (STEVOR) proteins (14), and repetitive interspersed family (RIFIN) proteins (15). The temporal expression of these ligands also differs, with PfEMP1 being expressed the earliest (transcription starts at ring forms and protein surface expression happens when parasites mature into trophozoites) (16, 17), followed by RIFIN (17, 18), then STEVOR (17, 19–21). In addition, only few members of VSA are expressed by a single IRBC. Members of these VSA families bind to a

wide range of different host-derived proteins, proteoglycans, and glycosaminoglycans (as summarized in **Table 1**). The role of RIFINs and STEVORs in the cytoadhesion of *P. falciparum* IRBCs is undoubtedly of significance. Apart from forming rosettes (a cytoadherence phenomenon by the late stage-IRBCs, which is elaborated in latter section) via interactions with the A antigens on the URBCs (15), some RIFINs can interact with leukocyte immunoglobulin-like receptor B1 (LILRB1), which inhibits the activation of B cells and natural killer (NK) cells expressing LILRB1 (51). This discovery suggests the involvement of RIFIN in the parasite's immune-evasion mechanisms. STEVOR proteins interact with the RBCs, and current evidence suggests their involvement in immune evasion, rosette formation and merozoite invasion (14, 21). By comparison, PfEMP1 binds to diverse array of host receptors on different host cells, leading to suggestions of its involvement in immune evasion (52) and immune modulation (53). Hence, it is generally accepted that the PfEMP1 is the most important of the VSAs. A detailed description of PfEMP1 variant domains and their binding targets, as well as the switching of expressions, have been elegantly reviewed elsewhere (54–56). In general, the extracellular domain of PfEMP1 can be classified into four major regions, which are the N-terminal segment (NTS), the C2 region, the Cysteine-rich inter-domain region (CIDR), and the Duffy binding-like region (DBL). These regions are responsible for the diverse cytoadherence phenomena attributed to PfEMP1, and difference in these regions gives rise to different cytoadherence properties, hence different tissue tropism for different strains of parasites (57, 58). Importantly, the various parasite-derived antigens that are expressed on IRBC surface make IRBCs an obvious target for host's immune system (59).

The IRBC-cytoadherence events are usually classified based on their binding sites, i.e., endothelial cytoadhesion, cytoadhesion to placental syncytiotrophoblasts, platelets, URBCs (rosetting phenomenon) and leukocytes (monocytes, macrophages, and dendritic cells) (23, 60–62). *P. falciparum* IRBCs can adhere to each other through platelet bridges, forming aggregates of IRBCs, a mechanism defined as autoagglutination (63–65). This phenomenon has been shown to be uncorrelated to rosetting and parasitemia, but significantly associated with severe malaria (63). These different interactions between the parasites and the host described above have been proposed to shape the immunopathobiology of malaria.

WHY DO *P. falciparum* IRBC CYTOADHERE?

Within hours after the *P. falciparum* merozoite invading the RBCs, the relatively low intra-erythrocytic viscosity of liquid hemoglobin is transformed into viscous gel-like cytoplasm of a developing IRBC (66). Besides, the parasite also remodels the IRBC by building a trafficking network with its parasite-derived proteins and organelles (such as Maurer's cleft) to bring in nutrients essential for its survival (67). The net consequence of these modifications (~10 h post-invasion) is a host cell with a compromised rheological profile (68). Such biomechanical

TABLE 1 | Host-derived receptors for *P. falciparum* cytoadherence ligands.

Ligands	Receptors	Expression sites	References
PfEMP1	Complement receptor 1 (CR1/CD35)	RBCs, leukocytes, splenic follicular dendritic cells	(22)
	Chondroitin sulfate A (CSA)	Endothelial cells, placental syncytiotrophoblasts	(23, 24)
	Hyaluronic acid (HA)	Placenta, and other connective, epithelial and neural tissues	(25)
	Heparan sulfate (HS)	All tissues	(26, 27)
	Platelet glycoprotein 4 (CD36)	Platelets, RBCs, monocytes, differentiated adipocytes, microdermal endothelial cells, skeletal muscles	(28–33)
	Intercellular adhesion molecule 1 (ICAM1/CD54)	Endothelial cells, leukocytes	(29, 31, 33–36)
	Vascular cell adhesion protein molecule 1 (VCAM1/CD106)	Endothelial cells	(31, 33, 35)
	RBC group A/B antigens	RBCs	(37, 38)
	Platelet endothelial cell adhesion molecule 1 (PECAM-1/CD31)	Platelets, monocytes, neutrophils, T-cells, endothelial cell (intercellular junctions)	(39, 40)
	Ig M	Circulation	(41–43)
	P-selectin (CD62P)	Activated platelets, activated endothelial cells	(31, 33, 44)
	E-selectin (CD62E)	Activated endothelial cells	(29, 35)
	Endothelial protein C receptor (EPCR/CD201)	Endothelial cells	(45–47)
	Hyaluronan-binding protein 1 (HABP1/gC1qR/P32)	Extracellular matrix, endothelial cells, platelets	(48, 49)
	Neural cell adhesion molecule (NCAM)	Endothelial cells	(50)
STEVOR	Glycophorin C (Gly C)	RBC	(14)
RIFIN	RBC group A antigen	RBC, B cells, NK cells	(15, 51)

changes render the IRBCs highly susceptible to splenic filtration. Within a spleen, the sinusoids of the red pulps act as a mechanical filter of the circulation. All entities in circulation have to move through the narrow (4 μm at its widest point) inter-endothelial slits (IES) of the red pulps (69). These are the smallest passage space for the blood circulation (69, 70). Healthy erythrocytes with normal morphology and rheology will be able to move through these IES whereas the abnormal cells will be retained and engulfed by the macrophages. As the red pulp of spleen is very effective in destroying rheologically impaired and less deformable erythrocytes, the developing malaria parasite has developed mechanisms that alters the host cell in some ways to escape splenic clearance (71). To this end, *P. falciparum* IRBCs avoid splenic clearance by cytoadhering to the vascular endothelium and sequestering in capillary beds of organs that are less dangerous than the spleen (72).

The central role of the spleen as a selective pressure for the evolution of cytoadhesive IRBCs is supported by the fact that in falciparum malaria patients and *P. falciparum*-infected monkeys whose spleens were removed prior to the infection, late stage-IRBCs that do not sequester are readily detected in peripheral blood (73–75). These circulating late-stage IRBCs have lost the capacity to cytoadhere to endothelial cells (74). These observations form the basis for the development of an anti-sequestration vaccine against *P. falciparum* (76). Theoretically, under spleen-intact conditions, the blockade of late stage-IRBCs to cytoadhere to endothelial cells will render these forms highly susceptible to splenic filtration. Thus, IRBC-cytoadherence plays critical roles in the immune-escape strategies by *P. falciparum*.

Besides endothelial cells, late stage-IRBCs can also adhere to URBC, forming flower-like structures known as "rosettes" (61). To date, *P. falciparum* rosetting has been attributed to three ligands, namely PfEMP1, STEVOR, and RIFIN (11, 13–15). Various host-derived receptors on RBCs have been found to be rosetting receptors (**Table 1**), the majority of these interact with the variant extracellular domains of PfEMP1. The binding affinity of these variants to the various receptors depends on the sequences coded for these regions, which has been described in detail elsewhere (55, 57, 77). Various roles have been proposed for rosetting; firstly, to facilitate merozoite invasion by bringing URBCs closer to the intracellular parasite. However, this "invasion facilitation" hypothesis for rosettes has been ruled out (78). The second proposed role for rosetting is that URBCs mask parasite-derived antigens (VSAs) expressed on the surface of IRBCs, allowing them to escape immune-recognition by antibodies or phagocytes. Practically, this masking strategy is similar to those applied by other parasites such as the blood flukes *Schistosoma* spp., where the flukes adsorb host-derived antigens (such as the blood surface A, B, H, Lewis b+ antigens) onto its surface (79–81). During the course of malaria infection, phagocytosis of IRBC plays a critical role in the clearance of parasites, especially in the spleen as mentioned earlier (82, 83). Opsonization of IRBCs leads to phagocytosis by the host phagocytes. The opsonization of IRBCs happens via antibody-mediated recognition and complement deposition (84–87). For instance, complement-decorated IRBCs are opsonized through the complement receptor 1 (CR1/CD35) (86, 88). Interestingly, CR1 on URBC is a receptor used by PfEMP1 on the surface of *P.*

falciparum-IRBC in rosetting (22). Formation of rosette via CR1 may block this phagocytosis pathway. Meanwhile, phagocytosis can also be mediated in a complement-independent, CD36-dependent manner (89, 90). Likewise, CD36 is also one of the receptors that bind with PfEMP1 for rosette formation (28) (**Table 1**). Although direct evidence of rosette hampering phagocytosis has yet to be reported, a previous study has demonstrated an inverse relationship between the amount of group A antigens (another rosetting receptor) being expressed on IRBC and its susceptibility to phagocytosis (91), and this may be linked to the better ability of blood group A-IRBCs to form rosettes (92). In addition, the larger size of a rosette relative to individual IRBCs may be more difficult to be engulfed by individual phagocytes as well. Previously, it has been demonstrated that opsonized targets larger than 3 μm and non-opsonized targets larger than 2 μm negatively affect the attachment step of phagocytosis (93). Of note, the thickest point of a RBC is 2–2.5 μm whereas the thinnest point of this cell is ~1 μm. Thus, size wise, a rosette will affect at least this critical step of phagocytosis. Furthermore, adherence of an IRBC to a URBC significantly reduces the deformability of the whole rosetting structure further, as compared to a non-rosetting IRBC harboring parasite of similar stage (68, 94). Such larger, more rigid yet stable structures are likely to be "mechanically" sequestered in microvasculature and may not even be able to reach the spleen.

Apart from endothelial cytoadhesion and rosetting as described above, some strains of *P. falciparum* can sequester within the placental intervillous space of pregnant patients (95), particularly the first-time-pregnant mothers (96). This enables the parasite to escape maternal immune responses (97). Interestingly, parasites that can sequester in placenta usually do not form rosettes well (98). On top of these evasion mechanisms, there are reports showing ability of PfEMP1 and RIFIN to modulate or suppress the host's immune responses as mentioned earlier (51, 53). Thus, it seems that *P. falciparum* uses various cytoadherence phenomena as an immune-escape mechanism.

HOST IMMUNE RESPONSES AND ANTIGENIC VARIATION OF THE CYTOADHERENCE LIGANDS

Since the cytoadherence of IRBCs relies on the IRBC-surface expression of parasite-derived cytoadherence ligands, these ligands would be easily recognized and hence destroyed by the host's immune system (59, 99). For instance, antibodies against PfEMP1 have been shown to inhibit rosette formation and induce phagocytosis in experiments using a laboratory-adapted *P. falciparum* strain (100). Antibodies raised against STEVOR expressed by different stages of *P. falciparum* can also inhibit either rosetting or merozoite reinvasion (14). Furthermore, the level of antibodies specific for RIFINs in pediatric malaria patients was reported to be positively correlated with the speed of parasite clearance (101). In fact, antibodies targeting the VSA have been shown to confer protection against malaria (101–106). For an extra level of survival advantage to the parasites,

these critical cytoadhesion ligands are VSA coded by multigene families as mentioned earlier (107). During multiplication, VSA expression changes, with a fraction of the progeny expressing a different set of VSAs. Such switching of VSA expression hampers the successful development of an immune response against all IRBCs (108–110). Taking PfEMP1 as an example, DBL and CIDR are the two regions of its extracellular domain responsible for the most of its cytoadherence activities (55, 111). Following the expression switching, the extracellular domains of PfEMP1, hence the binding receptors (targets) are different (112). Nevertheless, many binding receptors targeted by various PfEMP1 extracellular domains are available on endothelial cells. This also partly explains the diverse cytoadhesion receptors for PfEMP1, where the sequestration of IRBCs continues even with altered PfEMP1 variant expression.

SIDE EFFECTS OF THE PARASITE SEQUESTRATION ESCAPE STRATEGY

While the evolution of cytoadhesive IRBCs by *P. falciparum* has proven to be a potent immune-evasion strategy, the sequestration of IRBCs has an important side effect, which is the development of severe malaria (113). The manifestation of severe malaria largely depends on the site of sequestration. For instance, cytoadhesion of the IRBCs to syncytiotrophoblasts causes placental malaria, which is characterized by the inflammation of placental tissues, occlusion of nutrient supply to the fetus by the mother, resulting in higher risk of premature delivery, low birth weight of the neonates and subsequent negative impacts on future growth and development (114, 115).

Cytoadhesion of IRBCs to endothelial cells directly activates the endothelial cells, as shown *in vivo* (116) and *in vitro* (117), which in part may lead to endothelial injuries and vascular leakage (118). Various studies have implicated PfEMP1 [particularly its interaction with endothelial protein C receptor (EPCR)] in the pathogenesis of cerebral malaria, one of the most important forms of malaria-induced complications (45, 119–121). Nevertheless, the definitive *in vivo* demonstration of its involvement remains to be performed. There are apparent differences between the *in vitro* and *in vivo* conditions, encompassing content of nutrients, waste products, hormones, cytokines, oxygen level and shear force to name a few, as highlighted elsewhere (122). These differences may become the confounding factors in *in vitro* studies. However, the advancement of technology in the *in vivo* vascular imaging may provide a platform for the relevant *in vivo* works in future (123).

Based on the available information, a simplified sequential development of PfEMP1-mediated cerebral malaria has been suggested (7). The series of parasite-host interactive events start with the IRBCs binding to the endothelial cells via EPCR (119). EPCR plays protective role in maintaining the integrity of circulation through its ability to activate protein C, which is anti-coagulative and anti-inflammatory. The binding of IRBC-PfEMP1 to EPCR may hamper the protein C activation by EPCR, hence reducing the level of activated protein C in the microvasculature affected, which facilitates thrombin formation

(112). Such pro-coagulative environment further contributes to compromising microvasculature integrity. Following this, endothelial activation and inflammation may happen (124). The early onset of endothelial inflammation is characterized by the release of Weibel-Palade bodies and subsequent endothelial surface expression of P-selectin and von Willebrand factor (vWF) (113, 125, 126), which in turn mediate leukocyte and platelet rolling on inflamed endothelial cells (127).

Weibel-Palade bodies are the storage granules of endothelial cells (128). This structure contains of a number of components (P-selectin, VWF, angiopoietin 2, IL-8) that have been associated with endothelial injuries and vasculature leakage in malaria pathogenesis (113, 125, 126, 129–134). Other reported components of Weibel-Palade bodies include eotaxin 3, CD63, tissue plasminogen activator (TPA), factor VIII, endothelin 1, osteoprotegerin (OPG), alpha-(1,3)-fucosyltransferase (FUT6), endothelin-converting enzyme, calcitonin gene-related peptide, and insulin-like growth factor-binding protein 7 (IGFBP7). These components are involved in various homeostasis and inflammation related functions encompassing vasculature toning, inflammation and repair, regulating blood coagulation and angiogenesis (135–143). Remarkably, the release of different components within Weibel-Palade bodies is tightly regulated according to the microenvironment of the vasculature (140, 144, 145). This enables the endothelial cells to respond to changes of its microenvironment such as injuries, inflammation or shear stress changes. For instance, the release of VWF from Weibel-Palade bodies by endothelial cells can be triggered by interruption of blood flow (146). In such pro-coagulation environment, platelets can also serve as the bridge between IRBCs and endothelial cells, allowing cytoadhesion to happen even on endothelial cells devoid of principal cytoadhesion receptors (147). Additionally, platelet-mediated autoagglutination of IRBCs may happen in parallel (63), which further disrupts blood flow and activates the endothelial cells (148). Furthermore, angiopoietin-2 released from Weibel-Palade bodies can disrupt the integrity of endothelial junctions, which drives vasculature leakage (149). Following the "first bout" of endothelial inflammation, the expression of EPCR and thrombomodulin by host endothelial cells is downregulated (150), aggravating the pro-coagulation situation. The subsequent release of cytokines triggers expression upregulation of endothelial cell adhesion molecules (CAMs) such as ICAM1, E-selectin, and VCAM (151, 152). ICAM1 is used by other IRBCs to remain sequestering in the microvasculature, possibly with an expression switch of PfEMP1 variants (7). Notably, the disrupted blood flow can cause metabolic acidosis, which further facilitates the acidic pH-dependent binding of IRBCs to receptors like ICAM1 and CD36 (153). The vicious cycle continues, and the integrity of blood brain barrier is altered, leading to hemorrhages and possibly death if left without proper medical intervention.

The hypothesized sequences of pathological events described above remain to be validated fully. Of note, the dual EPCR/ICAM1 binding ability by certain PfEMP1 variants has been demonstrated (154), which may confound the hypothesized sequences of vascular pathogenesis events. Nevertheless, the critical role of EPCR in severe malaria pathogenesis has been highlighted by recent studies. The EPCR-binding *P. falciparum* isolates have been shown to be associated with severe malaria in both adults and children, with different clinical presentations including cerebral malaria, retinopathy and severe malaria-induced anemia (45–47, 155–159). On the other hand, falciparum malaria cases with predominantly CD36-binding parasites have been correlated with uncomplicated clinical presentations (159). Succinctly, the complex IRBC cytoadherence events trigger biological cascade reactions that lead to severe malaria pathologies.

P. falciparum ROSETTING AND SEVERE DISEASE

Rosetting was first reported in the simian malaria parasite *P. fragile,* and subsequently in *P. falciparum* and all other human malaria parasites (61, 160, 161). While it has been suggested that rosetting may aggravate the vasculature occlusion initiated by endothelial-cytoadhered IRBCs (162–164), its importance to pathogenesis of falciparum malaria is still debated. Associations between rosetting rates and malaria severity have been confounded with locality. African cohorts showed positive correlation between rosetting and malaria severity, where association of rosetting rates with parasitemia and different clinical parameters of severe malaria, as well as correlation between malaria severity and impairment of rosette formation due to availability of anti-rosette antibodies in serum and genetic blood disorders with abnormal erythrocytes have been reported (165–169). On the other hand, those conducted in Asia could not find such correlation (170, 171). Although correlation-based findings help to generate hypotheses, it is also important not to overlook the availability of confounding factors in many correlation studies, and the difference between a correlation and a causation.

As mentioned earlier, PfEMP1 is one of the key rosetting ligands for *P. falciparum*. The PfEMP1-mediated rosetting and endothelial cytoadhesion are two distinct biological phenomena, as demonstrated by previous studies (61, 162, 163). Nevertheless, dual cytoadhesion of rosetting IRBCs to endothelial cells have been demonstrated (164, 172), and distinct domain of PfEMP1 variant that possesses dual cytoadhesive (to endothelial cells and URBCs) properties has been described, albeit with very weak affinity to endothelia (the rosetting IRBCs were seen rolling instead of stably adhering to endothelial cells) under flow conditions mimicking microvasculature shear stress (164). Therefore, it remains to be investigated if such dual-binding phenomenon by IRBCs exists *in vivo*.

Importantly, all rosetting studies have been conducted under *in vitro* or *ex vivo* conditions using blood samples collected from peripheral circulation of patients, or clones of parasites derived from such sampling methods. The conundrum lies in the fact that the IRBCs that stably cytoadhere to microvasculature endothelium are responsible for parasite sequestration and may be the major contributor to the manifestation of severe malaria. However, the subpopulation of IRBCs collected from peripheral blood may be phenotypically different from those sequestering in the microvasculature when it comes to propensity of the IRBCs to cytoadhere. From another viewpoint, if the cytoadhesive phenotypes of IRBCs (usually the early stages) collected from the peripheral circulation are essentially similar to the sequestering late stage-IRBCs, the findings from *in vitro* rosetting studies (conducted on these parasites after *ex vivo* maturation) may not imply the actual situation *in vivo* since the recruited IRBCs are not given an equal exposure to URBCs and endothelial cells in rosetting assays, which raises doubts if rosetting ever happens *in vivo*. If this were the case, the rosetting phenomenon seen *in vitro* is merely an indication of "IRBC's stickiness," where the IRBCs would probably adhere to the microvasculature wall *in vivo*. Such situation makes it difficult to extrapolate the importance of rosetting in contributing to pathogenesis of severe malaria.

Malaria pathogenesis develops with time and often takes days to occur. One of the important shortcomings of studies correlating severe malaria with cytoadhesive IRBCs is that these studies are essentially snapshots of a multi-step process, which may be difficult to capture the complete chronology of an infection's pathogenesis. For cases with low parasite density, IRBCs have plenty of endothelial cells to cytoadhere to, leaving the non-endothelial cytoadhering IRBCs available in peripheral circulation. To avoid splenic clearance, these IRBCs may default to form rosettes over IRBC-endothelial cytoadhesion. Hence, it would be difficult to draw any correlation between rosetting phenomenon by this IRBC subpopulation and the pathology development that is happening in the deep microvasculature. On the other hand, parasite density in certain patients from certain localities may become too high (depending on parasite's virulence, genetic background and immunity status of the host, or lack of accessibility to timely treatment) and over-saturated relative to the total surface area of deep vasculature endothelial cells available for IRBC cytoadhesion. Thus, the IRBCs that do not get to cytoadhere to endothelia will be available in peripheral circulation. Of note, the availability of late stage *P. falciparum*-IRBCs in peripheral blood of a patient suffering hyperparasitemia has been reported (173). When these IRBCs are collected for rosetting assay, they are provided with only URBCs. Without their preferred cytoadhesive target (endothelial cells), these IRBCs may form rosette with the URBCs. Such alternative binding may happen as host-derived receptors like heparan sulfate (HS) (26, 164, 174–176), and CD36 (28, 177) have been reported as the receptor for endothelial cytoadhesion and rosette formation by the IRBCs. Rosetting rates obtained from such samples may reflect the relative endothelial cytoadhesion propensity of the IRBCs, which is associated with the severe malaria development. This may explain the positive correlation between rosetting and parasitemia in African clinical isolates previously reported (168). This hypothesis may also partly explain the discrepancies in correlation studies of rosetting rates and malaria severity conducted in different parts of the world. Notably, earlier studies have shown that the parasite clones in peripheral circulation and those sequestering in deep vasculature are similar (178, 179). Nevertheless, these molecular findings were based only on MSP-1 and MSP-2 alleles, and the tissue tropisms of the parasite subpopulations in a patient may not be revealed without specifically analyzing genes related to cytoadherence, as highlighted by the study (179).

So, the question remains: does the rosetting phenomenon contribute to severe malaria apart from its role as an immune-evasion strategy? To date, there is still a lack of solid evidence demonstrating stable, direct binding of rosetting IRBCs to endothelial cells under flow conditions. Nevertheless, such event may still be possible if the site of occurrence (microvasculature) has its blood flow hampered significantly in advance by the IRBC-endothelial cytoadhesion. Alternately, the rosetting IRBCs may be adhered securely to the endothelial cells via platelet as elaborated earlier (147). Regardless of how the rosette-endothelial binding interactions are, the contribution by rosetting to vasculature occlusion may not even require direct cytoadherence of rosetting IRBC to the endothelial cells. As mentioned earlier, it was shown that rosettes are less deformable and takes longer time to flow through a capillary-mimicking micropipette (68). In addition, Kaul et al. (180) demonstrated in an *ex vivo* system using rat isolated mesocecum that rosetting IRBCs contributed to microvasculature occlusion under flow condition. In this system, rosette-forming *P. falciparum* IRBC formed aggregates at venule junction, which restricted the flow. These aggregates were eventually dissociated slowly by the induced upstream force mimicking blood flow, leaving some IRBCs still attached to the endothelial cells afterwards. Here, rosetting was seen as an event that "widens the zone of vasculature occlusion." With merely IRBC-endothelial cytoadhesion, blockade may only happen at fine capillaries with lumen size ($\sim$5–10 μm) close to the size of a normal RBC. However, sites of IRBC sequestration encompass capillaries and venules (lumen size of $\sim$ 7 μm to 1 mm) (73, 181). As pointed out by Nash et al. (68), even with a monolayer of IRBCs cytoadhering to its endothelial wall, venules should has lumen wide enough to allow circulation flow, albeit with higher resistance. Following this theory, rosetting may occlude microvasculature distal to the endothelial-cytoadhered IRBC-obstructed fine capillaries. Nevertheless, it is important to note that another species of human malaria parasite, *P. vivax*, also readily forms rosettes (182, 183). Besides, the rigidity of *P. vivax* rosettes also increases (94). However, *P. vivax*-related cerebral malaria cases are not as common, with majority of such cases being reported from India (184–190), suggesting involvement of the human host-derived factors in this relatively geography-restricted pathology. Importantly, the endothelial cytoadhesion phenomenon by *P. vivax* IRBCs has been demonstrated, which is of similar binding strength but ten times lower in frequency than that of *P. falciparum* IRBCs (191). Therefore, this suggests that the key player that drives vasculature occlusion is IRBC-endothelial cytoadhesion. In this context, rosette formation is likely to play a subsidiary role.

Genetic polymorphisms influencing rosetting receptor expression is another factor to consider when assessing the roles of rosetting in malaria pathogenesis. For example, low level expression of CR1 on the surface of URBC (receptor for both rosette formation and IRBC clearance by the host) was reported to be a risk factor for severe malaria in Thai population (192). Another polymorphism that increases RBC surface expression of CR1 was reported to confer protection against cerebral malaria development in Thai population (193). On the other hand, studies conducted in India yielded complex picture, where low CR1 expression was found to be correlated with severe malaria susceptibility in non-endemic regions whereas high CR1 levels were associated with disease development in the malaria-endemic areas (194). Another study conducted in eastern part of India reported that extremely high and extremely low expression level of CR1 can lead to the higher risk of cerebral malaria development (195). Likewise, studies from Africa and Papua New Guinea yielded conflicting outcomes (196–198). Recently, two distinct CR1 polymorphisms commonly seen in African populations were found to demonstrate opposing correlation with the development of cerebral malaria in Kenya (199). The *Sl2* allele was reported to confer protection against cerebral malaria, possibly due partly to its reduced rosetting phenomenon in addition to other factors, as suggested by the authors; whereas *McC^b* allele served as a risk factor to develop cerebral malaria, but arises from selection probably due to survival advantage against other infections (199). Based on the example above, it is not easy to draw clear conclusions based on the correlations between genetic polymorphisms in a population and the outcome of a *P. falciparum* infection. More downstream experiments with carefully controlled longitudinal studies are needed to validate the significance of these findings.

ROSETTING AGAINST ENDOTHELIAL CYTOADHESION?

Parasitism is a relationship between two organisms where one party (the parasite) causes harms to the other party (the host) while living in/on the host. Evolution, through selection process, tends to drive this relationship toward a relatively "peaceful" one, where the selected parasites cause as little harm as possible to the host while the host is evolved and adapted to accommodate the parasite, without eliciting much immune response against the parasites. Following this evolutionary point of view, it would make more sense that *P. falciparum* that do not kill its human host while trying to survive within its host would be selected over time. As elaborated earlier, the *P. falciparum* late stage-IRBCs require sequestration to escape host's immune system. However, the endothelial cytoadhesion-mediated sequestration causes potentially fatal outcomes to the host, which is disadvantageous to the parasite as well.

Importantly, in areas with seasonal malaria transmission, asymptomatic carriers of *P. falciparum* serve as the parasite reservoirs during dry seasons, when the *Anopheline* mosquito number is low (200–203). Parasites persist within the hosts for months without causing clinical symptoms. In addition, the severity of clinical presentations for falciparum malaria covers a broad spectrum. This suggests that sequestration of late stage-IRBCs away from peripheral circulation can still happen without inducing grave outcomes to the host. Is endothelial cytoadhesion the only way for the parasites to sequester and escape splenic clearance?

Interestingly, cytoadhesive events such as rosetting, autoagglutination, and endothelial cytoadhesion use PfEMP1 as their ligand. Is there any form of competition between these events *in vivo*? In fact, the whorl of URBCs around a rosetting IRBCs can serve as a mechanical barrier against IRBC-endothelial cytoadhesion (164, 204, 205) and autoagglutination (206). Does rosetting carry any merit in reducing or preventing the endothelial injuries? Such theory has been raised no long after the discovery of rosetting phenomenon, where the role of rosetting either as a friend or foe to human host relies on the location or timing of rosette formation (68). IRBC-endothelial cytoadhesion occurs at capillaries and venules. If rosettes are formed ahead of these sites, rosettes can prevent IRBC-endothelial cytoadhesion. If rosettes can only be formed at similar vasculature sites as the IRBC-endothelial cytoadhesion, rosettes formed by the already endothelial-cytoadhered IRBCs can worsen the vasculature occlusion.

The manifestation of rosetting relies on the stability of rosetting complex under flow conditions. Rosettes are stable under sheared conditions, from very low shear forces to shear stress of about 1.5 Pa (68, 207), which is applicable to shear stress generated by blood flowing through arteries (208). This suggests that rosettes are available throughout the systemic circulation and that the *in vivo* rosettes may prevent IRBC-endothelial cytoadhesion. One concern was raised by an earlier study based on observation from its micropipette assay (68), where a rosetting IRBC that is forced into a capillary by blood flow will eventually have direct contact with the capillary wall (endothelial cells), hence IRBC-endothelial cytoadhesion may still happen even with rosetting. It is important to note that the force applied by that study to maneuver the rosetting IRBC into the micropipette was much higher (30 Pa) than the *in vivo* arterial shear force. Assuming that rosettes cannot move into capillaries *in vivo*, they may block the flow of blood into the capillary bed. If this were the case, the brain tissues covered by the affected capillary bed would suffer hypoxia and irreversible damages. However, cerebral malaria cases with irreversible hypoxia-induced brain tissue damages (as in stroke patients) following microvasculature occlusion by the IRBCs are rarely seen (209). Interestingly, via microvasculature-mimicking microfluidics channels, it was observed that the more rigid *P. vivax* rosettes that blocked the channel openings did not occlude the flow of normal URBCs through the channels (94). Although the experiment was conducted with *P. vivax*, we believe that it is applicable to *P. falciparum* as well, since both species preferably rosette with normocytes (matured RBCs) with similar binding strength (94, 183), and the rosettes formed by both species show enhanced rigidity (68, 94).

Another interesting evidence that suggests rosetting as "counter-endothelial cytoadhesion" stems from studies that investigated effects of sulfated glycoconjugates on rosetting and IRBC-endothelial adhesion. A number of sulfated glycoconjugates such as fucoidan, dextran sulfate, and heparin can disrupt rosettes (174, 210, 211). However, these molecules were found to enhance cytoadherence of IRBCs to CD36-bearing endothelial cells (177). An earlier study also reported the need of rosette disruption to allow IRBC adherence to CD36

(205). These findings suggest the need of cautious approach in considering heparin-derived molecules as malaria adjunctive treatment on the ground that they can disrupt rosette formation, as such adjunctive therapy may worsen the clinical situation by promoting IRBC-endothelial cytoadhesion (177). Is rosetting by the IRBCs purely a risk factor to human host, or an attempt by the parasites to minimize damages to the host without compromising its own survival? Various host- and parasite-derived confounding factors complicate the role characterization of rosetting.

INVOLVEMENT OF HUMAN-DERIVED FACTORS IN SHAPING THE DIRECTION OF IRBC-CYTOADHERENCE?

To date, most of the studies on human host-malaria parasite interactions in the context of IRBC cytoadherence focus on injuries sustained by the host from the parasites. Whether there is any "damage control" approach by either party in this parasitism relationship remains unknown. This is rather bizarre for a parasitism relationship with such a long evolutionary history. Importantly, as mentioned earlier, the parasites can persist in some human hosts for a very long time without causing signs and symptoms. This suggests that the survival-essential phenomena of the parasites, such as deep vasculature sequestration to avoid splenic clearance, can be tolerated by the host, and these phenomena may be the result of host-parasite interactions. Interestingly, the host-derived complement factor D, albumin, and anti-band 3 IgG have been reported as the rosette-promoting factors for P. falciparum (212). On top of that, a recent study reported "something" other than IgG from pooled human sera inhibited cytoadhesion of PfEMP1 to EPCR (213). Such serum-mediated IRBC-cytoadherence inhibition suggests intervention attempts by the host to control damages. According to this study, the inhibitors are available in circulation even under non-malaria infected conditions (usage of pooled donor sera) (213). Nevertheless, it is not known if there is any underlying medical condition among the donors. This is important since the serum component profiles of individual with cardiovascular problems, diabetes or chronic subclinical inflammation may be different from those of optimal health condition (214, 215). In addition, the components of serum from peripheral blood maybe different from that of the microenvironment within deep vasculature suffering endothelial injuries following IRBC-endothelial cytoadhesion. Nevertheless, this study sheds lights on potential host-parasite interactions in malaria pathogenesis.

As stated earlier, the adherence of IRBCs to endothelial cells trigger endothelial activation and inflammation. Subsequently, the level of various cytokines at the inflamed site is increased. Weibel-Palade body is one of the components being released by endothelial cells upon the onset of endothelial activation. As elaborated earlier, of the various components found within Weibel-Palade bodies, some have been associated with severe malaria pathogenesis and some have important role in regulating homeostasis in vasculature. It would be interesting to examine the effects of all key components in Weibel-Palade bodies on

the dynamics of IRBC cytoadherence, as well as other interplays between the host and the parasite.

Based on the currently available literature, it is likely that the malaria-related cytoadherence phenomena may give rise to

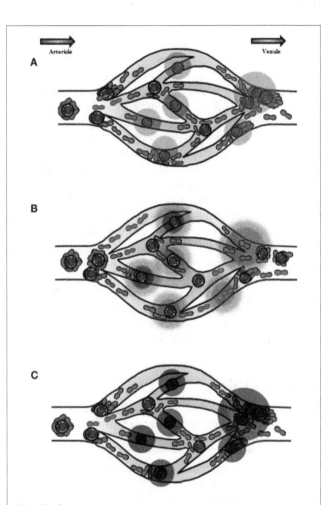

FIGURE 2 | Schematic diagram to illustrate the postulated chronology and mechanism of P. falciparum sequestration and pathogenesis in deep vasculature. The blue arrows on top of the diagram represent the direction of blood flow from arteriole to venule. **(A)** Cytoadhesion of IRBCs on endothelial cells causes endothelial inflammation. In addition, rosette formation at the capillary junctions opening into venules also contributes to the hampering of blood flow within the vasculature. The endothelial inflammation by direct IRBC-cytoadherence, coupled with hampering of blood flood stimulate the affected endothelial cells (pink halo) to release various substances in response to the changes in its environment. **(B)** Some of the components released by the endothelial cells (blue halo) may reverse and prevent IRBC-endothelial cytoadhesion, at the same time stimulate rosette formation. Rosetting mechanically prevents IRBCs from binding to endothelial cells while enabling the IRBCs to sequester in larger microvasculature. This will enable the parasite to escape splenic clearance. This switch of cytoadhesive characteristics also prevents complete occlusion of blood flow, thus minimizing, if not preventing irreversible tissue damages from tissue hypoxia. **(C)** However, for hosts with endothelial cells that are not as well-responsive to IRBC-endothelial cytoadhesion and slowing down of blood flow, the components that can reverse and prevent IRBC-endothelial cytoadhesion may be inadequate to exert such effect. As a result, vasculature occlusion ensures. At the same time, endothelial injury and vasculature leakage worsen (black halo), which may lead to fatal outcome.

homeostasis in vasculature. It would be interesting to examine the effects of all key components in Weibel-Palade bodies on complex host-parasite immunopathological interactions, starting from IRBC-endothelial cytoadhesion at the microvasculature (**Figure 2**). This results in endothelial activation and vasculature inflammation. Blood flow slows down due to the IRBC sequestration, which enables some immediately reformed rosettes with dual cytoadhesive capability to adhere at the venular junction. In fact, vasculature areas subjected to complex shear stresses such as the vascular branching junctions have abundant VWF-containing Weibel-Palade bodies (144), which may facilitate IRBC-endothelial binding. This further aggravates vasculature occlusion. On the other hand, stable rosettes that are formed before entering capillary bed will stay at the arteriole due to the higher rigidity of the whole rosetting structure. This form of rosettes prevents the rosetting IRBCs from having direct contact with the capillary endothelial, hence preventing endothelial cytoadhesion. Meanwhile, the reduction in shear stress of the microvasculature (capillaries and venules), coupled with endothelial inflammation trigger the affected endothelial cells to alter their expression, releasing unknown factors that may reverse IRBC-endothelial cytoadhesion. The endothelial cells may also secrete some other components to shield the endothelia from cytoadherence by incoming IRBCs, or the aforementioned unknown factors may be capable of reversing and preventing IRBC-endothelial cytoadhesion. The IRBCs detached from endothelial cells will flow out of the capillary bed

into the venule, and form rosettes. The rigid structure of rosettes enables the IRBCs to escape splenic clearance by mechanically sequester in larger-size microvasculature. This may avoid further damaging of host's vasculature, minimize complete occlusion of blood flow hence hypoxia and tissue necrosis. Finally, the ability of the host to respond to IRBC-induced endothelial activation by secreting and releasing these anti-endothelial cytoadhesion mediators will determine his survival in battling malaria.

CONCLUDING REMARKS

Undeniably, IRBC cytoadhesion is an important aspect in the pathogenesis of malaria, and a key interplay between the malaria parasite and its host. However, there are many "unresolved issues," such as the role of rosetting and feedback responses by the host following malaria-induced vascular injury, which deserve further research attention. A better understanding on these issues will enable us to understand malaria pathogenesis better, and design a reliable and safe clinical intervention strategies to improve the clinical management of malaria patients.

AUTHOR CONTRIBUTIONS

All authors listed have made a substantial, direct and intellectual contribution to the work, and approved it for publication.

REFERENCES

1. Alonso P, Noor AM. The global fight against malaria is at crossroads. *Lancet.* (2017) 390:2532–4. doi: 10.1016/S0140-6736(17)33080-5
2. White NJ. *Plasmodium knowlesi*: the fifth human malaria parasite. *Clin Infect Dis.* (2008) 46:172–3. doi: 10.1086/524889
3. Ta TH, Hisam S, Lanza M, Jiram AI, Ismail N, Rubio JM. First case of a naturally acquired human infection with *Plasmodium cynomolgi*. *Malar J.* (2014) 13:68. doi: 10.1186/1475-2875-13-68
4. Olliaro P. Editorial commentary: mortality associated with severe *Plasmodium falciparum* malaria increases with age. *Clin Infect Dis.* (2008) 47:158–60. doi: 10.1086/589288
5. Baird JK. Evidence and implications of mortality associated with acute *Plasmodium vivax* malaria. *Clin Microbiol Rev.* (2013) 26:36–57. doi: 10.1128/CMR.00074-12
6. Frevert U. Sneaking in through the back entrance: the biology of malaria liver stages. *Trends Parasitol.* (2004) 20:417–24. doi: 10.1016/j.pt.2004.07.007
7. Hviid L, Jensen AT. PfEMP1—A parasite protein family of key importance in *Plasmodium falciparum* malaria immunity and pathogenesis. *Adv Parasitol.* (2015) 88:51–84. doi: 10.1016/bs.apar.2015.02.004
8. Smith JD, Rowe JA, Higgins MK, Lavstsen T. Malaria's deadly grip: cytoadhesion of *Plasmodium falciparum*-infected erythrocytes. *Cell Microbiol.* (2013) 15:1976–83. doi: 10.1111/cmi.12183
9. Boddey JA, Cowman AF. *Plasmodium* nesting: remaking the erythrocyte from the inside out. *Annu Rev Microbiol.* (2013) 67:243–69. doi: 10.1146/annurev-micro-092412-155730
10. Elsworth B, Crabb BS, Gilson PR. Protein export in malaria parasites: an update. *Cell Microbiol.* (2014) 16:355–63. doi: 10.1111/cmi.12261

11. Yam XY, Niang M, Madnani KG, Preiser PR. Three is a crowd—new insights into rosetting in *Plasmodium falciparum*. *Trends Parasitol.* (2017) 33:309–20. doi: 10.1016/j.pt.2016.12.012
12. Howard RJ, Barnwell JW, Rock EP, Neequaye J, Ofori-Adjei D, Maloy WL, et al. Two approximately 300 kilodalton *Plasmodium falciparum* proteins at the surface membrane of infected erythrocytes. *Mol Biochem Parasitol.* (1988) 27:207–23. doi: 10.1016/0166-6851(88)90040-0
13. Chen Q, Barragan A, Fernandez V, Sundstrom A, Schlichtherle M, Sahlen A, et al. Identification of *Plasmodium falciparum* erythrocyte membrane protein 1 (PfEMP1) as the rosetting ligand of the malaria parasite *P. falciparum*. *J Exp Med.* (1998) 187:15–23. doi: 10.1084/jem.187.1.15
14. Niang M, Bei AK, Madnani KG, Pelly S, Dankwa S, Kanjee U, et al. STEVOR is a *Plasmodium falciparum* erythrocyte binding protein that mediates merozoite invasion and rosetting. *Cell Host Microbe.* (2014) 16:81–93. doi: 10.1016/j.chom.2014.06.004
15. Goel S, Palmkvist M, Moll K, Joannin N, Lara P, Akhouri RR, et al. RIFINs are adhesins implicated in severe *Plasmodium falciparum* malaria. *Nat Med.* (2015) 21:314–7. doi: 10.1038/nm.3812
16. Kyes S, Pinches R, Newbold C. A simple RNA analysis method shows var and rif multigene family expression patterns in *Plasmodium falciparum*. *Mol Biochem Parasitol.* (2000) 105:311–5. doi: 10.1016/S0166-6851(99)00193-0
17. Bachmann A, Petter M, Tilly AK, Biller L, Uliczka KA, Duffy MF, et al. Temporal expression and localization patterns of variant surface antigens in clinical *Plasmodium falciparum* isolates during erythrocyte schizogony. *PLoS ONE.* (2012) 7:e49540. doi: 10.1371/journal.pone.0049540
18. Kyes SA, Rowe JA, Kriek N, Newbold CI. Rifins: a second family of clonally variant proteins expressed on the surface of red cells infected with *Plasmodium falciparum*. *Proc Natl Acad Sci USA.* (1999) 96:9333–8. doi: 10.1073/pnas.96.16.9333

19. Kaviratne M, Khan SM, Jarra W, Preiser PR. Small variant STEVOR antigen is uniquely located within Maurer's clefts in *Plasmodium falciparum*-infected red blood cells. *Eukaryot Cell.* (2002) 1:926–35. doi: 10.1128/EC.1.6.926-935.2002

20. Lavazec C, Sanyal S, Templeton TJ. Expression switching in the stevor and Pfmc-2TM superfamilies in *Plasmodium falciparum*. *Mol Microbiol.* (2007) 64:1621–34. doi: 10.1111/j.1365-2958.2007.05767.x

21. Niang M, Yan Yam X, Preiser PR. The *Plasmodium falciparum* STEVOR multigene family mediates antigenic variation of the infected erythrocyte. *PLoS Pathog.* (2009) 5:e1000307. doi: 10.1371/journal.ppat.1000307

22. Rowe JA, Moulds JM, Newbold CI, Miller LH. *P. falciparum* rosetting mediated by a parasite-variant erythrocyte membrane protein and complement-receptor 1. *Nature.* (1997) 388:292–5. doi: 10.1038/40888

23. Fried M, Duffy PE. Adherence of *Plasmodium falciparum* to chondroitin sulfate A in the human placenta. *Science.* (1996) 272:1502–4. doi: 10.1126/science.272.5267.1502

24. Khattab A, Kun J, Deloron P, Kremsner PG, Klinkert MQ. Variants of *Plasmodium falciparum* erythrocyte membrane protein 1 expressed by different placental parasites are closely related and adhere to chondroitin sulfate A. *J Infect Dis.* (2001) 183:1165–9. doi: 10.1086/319288

25. Beeson JG, Rogerson SJ, Cooke BM, Reeder JC, Chai W, Lawson AM, et al. Adhesion of *Plasmodium falciparum*-infected erythrocytes to hyaluronic acid in placental malaria. *Nat Med.* (2000) 6:86–90. doi: 10.1038/71582

26. Vogt AM, Barragan A, Chen Q, Kironde F, Spillmann D, Wahlgren M. Heparan sulfate on endothelial cells mediates the binding of *Plasmodium falciparum*-infected erythrocytes via the DBL1alpha domain of PfEMP1. *Blood.* (2003) 101:2405–11. doi: 10.1182/blood-2002-07-2016

27. Barragan A, Fernandez V, Chen Q, Von Euler A, Wahlgren M, Spillmann D. The duffy-binding-like domain 1 of *Plasmodium falciparum* erythrocyte membrane protein 1 (PfEMP1) is a heparan sulfate ligand that requires 12 mers for binding. *Blood.* (2000) 95:3594–9.

28. Handunnetti SM, Van Schravendijk MR, Hasler T, Barnwell JW, Greenwalt DE, Howard RJ. Involvement of CD36 on erythrocytes as a rosetting receptor for *Plasmodium falciparum*-infected erythrocytes. *Blood.* (1992) 80:2097–104.

29. Turner GD, Morrison H, Jones M, Davis TM, Looareesuwan S, Buley ID, et al. An immunohistochemical study of the pathology of fatal malaria. Evidence for widespread endothelial activation and a potential role for intercellular adhesion molecule-1 in cerebral sequestration. *Am J Pathol.* (1994) 145:1057–69.

30. Baruch DI, Ma XC, Singh HB, Bi X, Pasloske BL, Howard RJ. Identification of a region of PfEMP1 that mediates adherence of Plasmodium falciparum infected erythrocytes to CD36: conserved function with variant sequence. *Blood.* (1997) 90:3766–75.

31. Udomsangpetch R, Reinhardt PH, Schollaardt T, Elliott JF, Kubes P, Ho M. Promiscuity of clinical *Plasmodium falciparum* isolates for multiple adhesion molecules under flow conditions. *J Immunol.* (1997) 158:4358–64.

32. Baruch DI, Ma XC, Pasloske B, Howard RJ, Miller LH. CD36 peptides that block cytoadherence define the CD36 binding region for *Plasmodium falciparum*-infected erythrocytes. *Blood.* (1999) 94:2121–7.

33. Yipp BG, Anand S, Schollaardt T, Patel KD, Looareesuwan S, Ho M. Synergism of multiple adhesion molecules in mediating cytoadherence of *Plasmodium falciparum*-infected erythrocytes to microvascular endothelial cells under flow. *Blood.* (2000) 96:2292–8.

34. Smith JD, Craig AG, Kriek N, Hudson-Taylor D, Kyes S, Fagan T, et al. Identification of a *Plasmodium falciparum* intercellular adhesion molecule-1 binding domain: a parasite adhesion trait implicated in cerebral malaria. *Proc Natl Acad Sci USA.* (2000) 97:1766–71. doi: 10.1073/pnas.040545897

35. Armah H, Dodoo AK, Wiredu EK, Stiles JK, Adjei AA, Gyasi RK, et al. High-level cerebellar expression of cytokines and adhesion molecules in fatal, paediatric, cerebral malaria. *Ann Trop Med Parasitol.* (2005) 99:629–47. doi: 10.1179/136485905X51508

36. Gullingsrud J, Saveria T, Amos E, Duffy PE, Oleinikov AV. Structure-function-immunogenicity studies of PfEMP1 domain DBL2betaPF11_0521, a malaria parasite ligand for ICAM-1. *PLoS ONE.* (2013) 8:e61323. doi: 10.1371/journal.pone.0061323

37. Barragan A, Kremsner PG, Wahlgren M, Carlson J. Blood group A antigen is a coreceptor in *Plasmodium falciparum* rosetting. *Infect Immun.* (2000) 68:2971–5. doi: 10.1128/IAI.68.5.2971-2975.2000

38. Vigan-Womas I, Guillotte M, Juillerat A, Hessel A, Raynal B, England P, et al. Structural basis for the ABO blood-group dependence of *Plasmodium falciparum* rosetting. *PLoS Pathog.* (2012) 8:e1002781. doi: 10.1371/journal.ppat.1002781

39. Treutiger CJ, Heddini A, Fernandez V, Muller WA, Wahlgren M. PECAM-1/CD31, an endothelial receptor for binding *Plasmodium falciparum*-infected erythrocytes. *Nat Med.* (1997) 3:1405–8. doi: 10.1038/nm1297-1405

40. Berger SS, Turner L, Wang CW, Petersen JE, Kraft M, Lusingu JP, et al. *Plasmodium falciparum* expressing domain cassette 5 type PfEMP1 (DC5-PfEMP1) bind PECAM1. *PLoS ONE.* (2013) 8:e69117. doi: 10.1371/journal.pone.0069117

41. Rowe JA, Shafi J, Kai OK, Marsh K, Raza A. Nonimmune IgM, but not IgG binds to the surface of Plasmodium falciparum-infected erythrocytes and correlates with rosetting and severe malaria. *Am J Trop Med Hyg.* (2002) 66:692–9. doi: 10.4269/ajtmh.2002.66.692

42. Creasey AM, Staalsoe T, Raza A, Arnot DE, Rowe JA. Nonspecific immunoglobulin M binding and chondroitin sulfate A binding are linked phenotypes of *Plasmodium falciparum* isolates implicated in malaria during pregnancy. *Infect Immun.* (2003) 71:4767–71. doi: 10.1128/IAI.71.8.4767-4771.2003

43. Akhouri RR, Goel S, Furusho H, Skoglund U, Wahlgren M. Architecture of human IgM in complex with *P. falciparum* erythrocyte membrane protein 1. *Cell Rep.* (2016) 14:723–36. doi: 10.1016/j.celrep.2015.12.067

44. Senczuk AM, Reeder JC, Kosmala MM, Ho M. *Plasmodium falciparum* erythrocyte membrane protein 1 functions as a ligand for P-selectin. *Blood.* (2001) 98:3132–5. doi: 10.1182/blood.V98.10.3132

45. Kessler A, Dankwa S, Bernabeu M, Harawa V, Danziger SA, Duffy F, et al. Linking EPCR-binding PfEMP1 to brain swelling in pediatric cerebral malaria. *Cell Host Microbe.* (2017) 22:601–14.e605. doi: 10.1016/j.chom.2017.09.009

46. Bernabeu M, Danziger SA, Avril M, Vaz M, Babar PH, Brazier AJ, et al. Severe adult malaria is associated with specific PfEMP1 adhesion types and high parasite biomass. *Proc Natl Acad Sci USA.* (2016) 113:E3270–9. doi: 10.1073/pnas.1524294113

47. Shabani E, Hanisch B, Opoka RO, Lavstsen T, John CC. *Plasmodium falciparum* EPCR-binding PfEMP1 expression increases with malaria disease severity and is elevated in retinopathy negative cerebral malaria. *BMC Med.* (2017) 15:183. doi: 10.1186/s12916-017-0945-y

48. Biswas AK, Hafiz A, Banerjee B, Kim KS, Datta K, Chitnis CE. *Plasmodium falciparum* uses gC1qR/HABP1/p32 as a receptor to bind to vascular endothelium and for platelet-mediated clumping. *PLoS Pathog.* (2007) 3:1271–80. doi: 10.1371/journal.ppat.0030130

49. Magallon-Tejada A, Machevo S, Cistero P, Lavstsen T, Aide P, Rubio M, et al. Cytoadhesion to gC1qR through *Plasmodium falciparum* erythrocyte membrane protein 1 in severe malaria. *PLoS Pathog.* (2016) 12:e1006011. doi: 10.1371/journal.ppat.1006011

50. Pouvelle B, Matarazzo V, Jurzynski C, Nemeth J, Ramharter M, Rougon G, et al. Neural cell adhesion molecule, a new cytoadhesion receptor for *Plasmodium falciparum*-infected erythrocytes capable of aggregation. *Infect Immun.* (2007) 75:3516–22. doi: 10.1128/IAI.01852-06

51. Saito F, Hirayasu K, Satoh T, Wang CW, Lusingu J, Arimori T, et al. Immune evasion of *Plasmodium falciparum* by RIFIN via inhibitory receptors. *Nature.* (2017) 552:101–5. doi: 10.1038/nature24994

52. Gomes PS, Bhardwaj J, Rivera-Correa J, Freire-De-Lima CG, Morrot A. Immune escape strategies of malaria parasites. *Front Microbiol.* (2016) 7:1617. doi: 10.3389/fmicb.2016.01617

53. Sampaio NG, Eriksson EM, Schofield L. *Plasmodium falciparum* PfEMP1 modulates monocyte/macrophage transcription factor activation and cytokine and chemokine responses. *Infect Immun.* (2018) 86:e00447–17. doi: 10.1128/IAI.00447-17

54. Flick K, Chen Q. var genes, PfEMP1 and the human host. *Mol Biochem Parasitol.* (2004) 134:3–9. doi: 10.1016/j.molbiopara.2003.09.010

55. Kraemer SM, Smith JD. A family affair: var genes, PfEMP1 binding, and malaria disease. *Curr Opin Microbiol.* (2006) 9:374–80. doi: 10.1016/j.mib.2006.06.006

56. Smith JD. The role of PfEMP1 adhesion domain classification in *Plasmodium falciparum* pathogenesis research. *Mol Biochem Parasitol.* (2014) 195:82–7. doi: 10.1016/j.molbiopara.2014.07.006

57. Smith JD, Subramanian G, Gamain B, Baruch DI, Miller LH. Classification of adhesive domains in the *Plasmodium falciparum* erythrocyte membrane protein 1 family. *Mol Biochem Parasitol.* (2000) 110:293–310. doi: 10.1016/S0166-6851(00)00279-6

58. Juillerat A, Lewit-Bentley A, Guillotte M, Gangnard S, Hessel A, Baron B, et al. Structure of a *Plasmodium falciparum* PfEMP1 rosetting domain reveals a role for the N-terminal segment in heparin-mediated rosette inhibition. *Proc Natl Acad Sci USA.* (2011) 108:5243–8. doi: 10.1073/pnas.1018692108

59. Beeson JG, Chan JA, Fowkes FJ. PfEMP1 as a target of human immunity and a vaccine candidate against malaria. *Expert Rev Vaccines.* (2013) 12:105–8. doi: 10.1586/erv.12.144

60. Barnwell JW, Ockenhouse CF, Knowles DM II. Monoclonal antibody OKM5 inhibits the *in vitro* binding of *Plasmodium falciparum*-infected erythrocytes to monocytes, endothelial, and C32 melanoma cells. *J Immunol.* (1985) 135:3494–7.

61. Udomsangpetch R, Wahlin B, Carlson J, Berzins K, Torii M, Aikawa M, et al. *Plasmodium falciparum*-infected erythrocytes form spontaneous erythrocyte rosettes. *J Exp Med.* (1989) 169:1835–40. doi: 10.1084/jem.169.5.1835

62. Wassmer SC, Lepolard C, Traore B, Pouvelle B, Gysin J, Grau GE. Platelets reorient *Plasmodium falciparum*-infected erythrocyte cytoadhesion to activated endothelial cells. *J Infect Dis.* (2004) 189:180–9. doi: 10.1086/380761

63. Roberts DJ, Pain A, Kai O, Kortok M, Marsh K. Autoagglutination of malaria-infected red blood cells and malaria severity. *Lancet.* (2000) 355:1427–8. doi: 10.1016/S0140-6736(00)02143-7

64. Pain A, Ferguson DJ, Kai O, Urban BC, Lowe B, Marsh K, et al. Platelet-mediated clumping of *Plasmodium falciparum*-infected erythrocytes is a common adhesive phenotype and is associated with severe malaria. *Proc Natl Acad Sci USA.* (2001) 98:1805–10. doi: 10.1073/pnas.98.4.1805

65. Chotivanich K, Sritabal J, Udomsangpetch R, Newton P, Stepniewska KA, Ruangveerayuth R, et al. Platelet-induced autoagglutination of *Plasmodium falciparum*-infected red blood cells and disease severity in Thailand. *J Infect Dis.* (2004) 189:1052–5. doi: 10.1086/381900

66. Russell BM, Cooke BM. The rheopathobiology of *Plasmodium vivax* and other important primate malaria parasites. *Trends Parasitol.* (2017) 33:321–34. doi: 10.1016/j.pt.2016.11.009

67. Mbengue A, Yam XY, Braun-Breton C. Human erythrocyte remodelling during *Plasmodium falciparum* malaria parasite growth and egress. *Br J Haematol.* (2012) 157:171–9. doi: 10.1111/j.1365-2141.2012.09044.x

68. Nash GB, Cooke BM, Carlson J, Wahlgren M. Rheological properties of rosettes formed by red cells parasitized by *Plasmodium falciparum. Br J Haematol.* (1992) 82:757–63. doi: 10.1111/j.1365-2141.1992.tb06955.x

69. Pivkin IV, Peng Z, Karniadakis GE, Buffet PA, Dao M, Suresh S. Biomechanics of red blood cells in human spleen and consequences for physiology and disease. *Proc Natl Acad Sci USA.* (2016) 113:7804–9. doi: 10.1073/pnas.1606751113

70. Mebius RE, Kraal G. Structure and function of the spleen. *Nat Rev Immunol.* (2005) 5:606–16. doi: 10.1038/nri1669

71. Sosale NG, Rouhiparkouhi T, Bradshaw AM, Dimova R, Lipowsky R, Discher DE. Cell rigidity and shape override CD47's "self"-signaling in phagocytosis by hyperactivating myosin-II. *Blood.* (2015) 125:542–52. doi: 10.1182/blood-2014-06-585299

72. Suwanarusk R, Cooke BM, Dondorp AM, Silamut K, Sattabongkot J, White NJ, et al. The deformability of red blood cells parasitized by *Plasmodium falciparum* and *P. vivax J Infect Dis.* (2004) 189:190–4. doi: 10.1086/380468

73. David PH, Hommel M, Miller LH, Udeinya IJ, Oligino LD. Parasite sequestration in Plasmodium falciparum malaria: spleen and antibody modulation of cytoadherence of infected erythrocytes. *Proc Natl Acad Sci USA.* (1983) 80:5075–9. doi: 10.1073/pnas.80.16.5075

74. Bachmann A, Esser C, Petter M, Predehl S, Von Kalckreuth V, Schmiedel S, et al. Absence of erythrocyte sequestration and lack of multicopy gene family expression in *Plasmodium falciparum* from a splenectomized malaria patient. *PLoS ONE.* (2009) 4:e7459. doi: 10.1371/journal.pone.0007459

75. Buffet PA, Safeukui I, Deplaine G, Brousse V, Prendki V, Thellier M, et al. The pathogenesis of *Plasmodium falciparum* malaria in humans: insights from splenic physiology. *Blood.* (2011) 117:381–92. doi: 10.1182/blood-2010-04-202911

76. Franke-Fayard B, Fonager J, Braks A, Khan SM, Janse CJ. Sequestration and tissue accumulation of human malaria parasites: can we learn anything from rodent models of malaria? *PLoS Pathog.* (2010) 6:e1001032. doi: 10.1371/journal.ppat.1001032

77. Rowe JA, Claessens A, Corrigan RA, Arman M. Adhesion of *Plasmodium falciparum*-infected erythrocytes to human cells: molecular mechanisms and therapeutic implications. *Expert Rev Mol Med.* (2009) 11:e16. doi: 10.1017/S1462399409001082

78. Clough B, Atilola FA, Pasvoi G. The role of rosetting in the multiplication of *Plasmodium falciparum*: rosette formation neither enhances nor targets parasite invasion into uninfected red cells. *Br J Haematol.* (1998) 100:99–104. doi: 10.1046/j.1365-2141.1998.00534.x

79. Smithers SR, Terry RJ, Hockley DJ. Host antigens in schistosomiasis. *Proc R Soc Lond B Biol Sci.* (1969) 171:483–94. doi: 10.1098/rspb.1969.0007

80. Goldring OL, Clegg JA, Smithers SR, Terry RJ. Acquisition of human blood group antigens by *Schistosoma mansoni. Clin Exp Immunol.* (1976) 26:181–7.

81. Loukas A, Jones MK, King LT, Brindley PJ, Mcmanus DP. Receptor for Fc on the surfaces of schistosomes. *Infect Immun.* (2001) 69:3646–51. doi: 10.1128/IAI.69.6.3646-3651.2001

82. Chotivanich K, Udomsangpetch R, Mcgready R, Proux S, Newton P, Pukrittayakamee S, et al. Central role of the spleen in malaria parasite clearance. *J Infect Dis.* (2002) 185:1538–41. doi: 10.1086/340213

83. Chua CL, Brown G, Hamilton JA, Rogerson S, Boeuf P. Monocytes and macrophages in malaria: protection or pathology? *Trends Parasitol.* (2013) 29:26–34. doi: 10.1016/j.pt.2012.10.002

84. Groux H, Gysin J. Opsonization as an effector mechanism in human protection against asexual blood stages of *Plasmodium falciparum*: functional role of IgG subclasses. *Res Immunol.* (1990) 141:529–42. doi: 10.1016/0923-2494(90)90021-P

85. Mota MM, Brown KN, Holder AA, Jarra W. Acute *Plasmodium chabaudi chabaudi* malaria infection induces antibodies which bind to the surfaces of parasitized erythrocytes and promote their phagocytosis by macrophages *in vitro. Infect Immun.* (1998) 66:4080–6.

86. Turrini F, Giribaldi G, Carta F, Mannu F, Arese P. Mechanisms of band 3 oxidation and clustering in the phagocytosis of *Plasmodium falciparum*-infected erythrocytes. *Redox Rep.* (2003) 8:300–3. doi: 10.1179/135100003225002943

87. Dasari P, Fries A, Heber SD, Salama A, Blau IW, Lingelbach K, et al. Malarial anemia: digestive vacuole of *Plasmodium falciparum* mediates complement deposition on bystander cells to provoke hemophagocytosis. *Med Microbiol Immunol.* (2014) 203:383–93. doi: 10.1007/s00430-014-0347-0

88. Silver KL, Higgins SJ, Mcdonald CR, Kain KC. Complement driven innate immune response to malaria: fuelling severe malarial diseases. *Cell Microbiol.* (2010) 12:1036–45. doi: 10.1111/j.1462-5822.2010.01492.x

89. Smith TG, Serghides L, Patel SN, Febbraio M, Silverstein RL, Kain KC. CD36-mediated nonopsonic phagocytosis of erythrocytes infected with stage I and IIA gametocytes of *Plasmodium falciparum. Infect Immun.* (2003) 71:393–400. doi: 10.1128/IAI.71.1.393-400.2003

90. Patel SN, Serghides L, Smith TG, Febbraio M, Silverstein RL, Kurtz TW, et al. CD36 mediates the phagocytosis of *Plasmodium falciparum*-infected erythrocytes by rodent macrophages. *J Infect Dis.* (2004) 189:204–13. doi: 10.1086/380764

91. Wolofsky KT, Ayi K, Branch DR, Hult AK, Olsson ML, Liles WC, et al. ABO blood groups influence macrophage-mediated phagocytosis of *Plasmodium falciparum*-infected erythrocytes. *PLoS Pathog.* (2012) 8:e1002942. doi: 10.1371/journal.ppat.1002942

92. Moll K, Palmkvist M, Ch'ng J, Kiwuwa MS, Wahlgren M. Evasion of immunity to *Plasmodium falciparum*: rosettes of blood group A impair recognition of PfEMP1. *PLoS ONE.* (2015) 10:e0145120. doi: 10.1371/journal.pone.0145120

93. Champion JA, Walker A, Mitragotri S. Role of particle size in phagocytosis of polymeric microspheres. *Pharm Res.* (2008) 25:1815–21. doi: 10.1007/s11095-008-9562-y

94. Zhang R, Lee WC, Lau YL, Albrecht L, Lopes SC, Costa FT, et al. Rheopathologic consequence of *Plasmodium vivax* rosette formation. *PLoS Negl Trop Dis.* (2016) 10:e0004912. doi: 10.1371/journal.pntd.0004912

95. Sharma L, Shukla G. Placental malaria: a new insight into the pathophysiology. *Front Med.* (2017) 4:117. doi: 10.3389/fmed.2017.00117

96. Rogerson SJ, Hviid L, Duffy PE, Leke RF, Taylor DW. Malaria in pregnancy: pathogenesis and immunity. *Lancet Infect Dis.* (2007) 7:105–17. doi: 10.1016/S1473-3099(07)70022-1

97. Reeder JC. Malaria in pregnancy: getting to grips with a sticky problem. *P N G Med J.* (1999) 42:73–6.

98. Maubert B, Fievet N, Tami G, Boudin C, Deloron P. *Plasmodium falciparum*-isolates from Cameroonian pregnant women do not rosette. *Parasite.* (1998) 5:281–3. doi: 10.1051/parasite/1998053281

99. Bull PC, Abdi AI. The role of PfEMP1 as targets of naturally acquired immunity to childhood malaria: prospects for a vaccine. *Parasitology.* (2016) 143:171–86. doi: 10.1017/S0031182015001274

100. Ghumra A, Khunrae P, Ataide R, Raza A, Rogerson SJ, Higgins MK, et al. Immunisation with recombinant PfEMP1 domains elicits functional rosette-inhibiting and phagocytosis-inducing antibodies to *Plasmodium falciparum*. *PLoS ONE.* (2011) 6:e16414. doi: 10.1371/journal.pone.0016414

101. Abdel-Latif MS, Dietz K, Issifou S, Kremsner PG, Klinkert MQ. Antibodies to *Plasmodium falciparum* rifin proteins are associated with rapid parasite clearance and asymptomatic infections. *Infect Immun.* (2003) 71:6229–33. doi: 10.1128/IAI.71.11.6229-6233.2003

102. Marsh K, Howard RJ. Antigens induced on erythrocytes by *P. falciparum*: expression of diverse and conserved determinants. *Science.* (1986) 231:150–3. doi: 10.1126/science.2417315

103. Marsh K, Otoo L, Hayes RJ, Carson DC, Greenwood BM. Antibodies to blood stage antigens of *Plasmodium falciparum* in rural Gambians and their relation to protection against infection. *Trans R Soc Trop Med Hyg.* (1989) 83:293–303. doi: 10.1016/0035-9203(89)90478-1

104. Bull PC, Lowe BS, Kortok M, Molyneux CS, Newbold CI, Marsh K. Parasite antigens on the infected red cell surface are targets for naturally acquired immunity to malaria. *Nat Med.* (1998) 4:358–60. doi: 10.1038/nm0398-358

105. Fried M, Nosten F, Brockman A, Brabin BJ, Duffy PE. Maternal antibodies block malaria. *Nature.* (1998) 395:851–2. doi: 10.1038/27570

106. Baruch DI, Gamain B, Barnwell JW, Sullivan JS, Stowers A, Galland GG, et al. Immunization of *Aotus* monkeys with a functional domain of the *Plasmodium falciparum* variant antigen induces protection against a lethal parasite line. *Proc Natl Acad Sci USA.* (2002) 99:3860–5. doi: 10.1073/pnas.022018399

107. Wahlgren M, Goel S, Akhouri RR. Variant surface antigens of *Plasmodium falciparum* and their roles in severe malaria. *Nat Rev Microbiol.* (2017) 15:479–91. doi: 10.1038/nrmicro.2017.47

108. Hommel M, David PH, Oligino LD. Surface alterations of erythrocytes in *Plasmodium falciparum* malaria. *Antigenic variation, antigenic diversity, and the role of the spleen J Exp Med.* (1983) 157:1137–48. doi: 10.1084/jem.157.4.1137

109. Fandeur T, Le Scanf C, Bonnemains B, Slomianny C, Mercereau-Puijalon O. Immune pressure selects for *Plasmodium falciparum* parasites presenting distinct red blood cell surface antigens and inducing strain-specific protection in *Saimiri sciureus* monkeys. *J Exp Med.* (1995) 181:283–95. doi: 10.1084/jem.181.1.283

110. Scherf A, Lopez-Rubio JJ, Riviere L. Antigenic variation in *Plasmodium falciparum*. *Annu Rev Microbiol.* (2008) 62:445–70. doi: 10.1146/annurev.micro.61.080706.093134

111. Smith JD, Gamain B, Baruch DI, Kyes S. Decoding the language of var genes and *Plasmodium falciparum* sequestration. *Trends Parasitol.* (2001) 17:538–45. doi: 10.1016/S1471-4922(01)02079-7

112. Bernabeu M, Smith JD. EPCR and malaria severity: the center of a perfect storm. *Trends Parasitol.* (2017) 33:295–308. doi: 10.1016/j.pt.2016.11.004

113. Craig AG, Khairul MF, Patil PR. Cytoadherence and severe malaria. *Malays J Med Sci.* (2012) 19:5–18.

114. Menendez C, Ordi J, Ismail MR, Ventura PJ, Aponte JJ, Kahigwa E, et al. The impact of placental malaria on gestational age and birth weight. *J Infect Dis.* (2000) 181:1740–5. doi: 10.1086/315449

115. Walther B, Miles DJ, Crozier S, Waight P, Palmero MS, Ojuola O, et al. Placental malaria is associated with reduced early life weight development of affected children independent of low birth weight. *Malar J.* (2010) 9:16. doi: 10.1186/1475-2875-9-16

116. Elhassan IM, Hviid L, Satti G, Akerstrom B, Jakobsen PH, Jensen JB, et al. Evidence of endothelial inflammation, T cell activation, and T cell reallocation in uncomplicated *Plasmodium falciparum* malaria. *Am J Trop Med Hyg.* (1994) 51:372–9. doi: 10.4269/ajtmh.1994.51.372

117. Tripathi AK, Sha W, Shulaev V, Stins MF, Sullivan DJ Jr. *Plasmodium falciparum*-infected erythrocytes induce NF-kappaB regulated inflammatory pathways in human cerebral endothelium. *Blood.* (2009) 114:4243–52. doi: 10.1182/blood-2009-06-226415

118. Gillrie MR, Ho M. Dynamic interactions of *Plasmodium* spp. with vascular endothelium. *Tissue Barriers.* (2017) 5:e1268667. doi: 10.1080/21688370.2016.1268667

119. Turner L, Lavstsen T, Berger SS, Wang CW, Petersen JE, Avril M, et al. Severe malaria is associated with parasite binding to endothelial protein C receptor. *Nature.* (2013) 498:502–5. doi: 10.1038/nature12216

120. Mosnier LO, Lavstsen T. The role of EPCR in the pathogenesis of severe malaria. *Thromb Res.* (2016) 141(Suppl. 2):S46–9. doi: 10.1016/S0049-3848(16)30364-4

121. Mkumbaye SI, Wang CW, Lyimo E, Jespersen JS, Manjurano A, Mosha J, et al. The severity of *Plasmodium falciparum* infection Is associated with transcript levels of var genes encoding endothelial protein C receptor-binding *P. falciparum* erythrocyte membrane protein 1. *Infect Immun.* (2017) 85:e00841-16. doi: 10.1128/IAI.00841-16

122. Leroux M, Lakshmanan V, Daily JP. *Plasmodium falciparum* biology: analysis of *in vitro* versus *in vivo* growth conditions. *Trends Parasitol.* (2009) 25:474–81. doi: 10.1016/j.pt.2009.07.005

123. Hong G, Lee JC, Robinson JT, Raaz U, Xie L, Huang NF, et al. Multifunctional *in vivo* vascular imaging using near-infrared II fluorescence. *Nat Med.* (2012) 18:1841–6. doi: 10.1038/nm.2995

124. Viebig NK, Wulbrand U, Forster R, Andrews KT, Lanzer M, Knolle PA. Direct activation of human endothelial cells by *Plasmodium falciparum*-infected erythrocytes. *Infect Immun.* (2005) 73:3271–7. doi: 10.1128/IAI.73.6.3271-3277.2005

125. Van Mourik JA, Romani De Wit T, Voorberg J. Biogenesis and exocytosis of Weibel-Palade bodies. *Histochem Cell Biol.* (2002) 117:113–22. doi: 10.1007/s00418-001-0368-9

126. Dole VS, Bergmeier W, Mitchell HA, Eichenberger SC, Wagner DD. Activated platelets induce Weibel-Palade-body secretion and leukocyte rolling *in vivo*: role of P-selectin. *Blood.* (2005) 106:2334–9. doi: 10.1182/blood-2005-04-1530

127. Cambien B, Wagner DD. A new role in hemostasis for the adhesion receptor P-selectin. *Trends Mol Med.* (2004) 10:179–86. doi: 10.1016/j.molmed.2004.02.007

128. Valentijn KM, Sadler JE, Valentijn JA, Voorberg J, Eikenboom J. Functional architecture of Weibel-Palade bodies. *Blood.* (2011) 117:5033–43. doi: 10.1182/blood-2010-09-267492

129. Hermsen CC, Konijnenberg Y, Mulder L, Loe C, Van Deuren M, Van Der Meer JW, et al. Circulating concentrations of soluble granzyme A and B increase during natural and experimental *Plasmodium falciparum* infections. *Clin Exp Immunol.* (2003) 132:467–72. doi: 10.1046/j.1365-2249.2003.02160.x

130. Yeo TW, Lampah DA, Gitawati R, Tjitra E, Kenangalem E, Piera K, et al. Angiopoietin-2 is associated with decreased endothelial nitric oxide and poor clinical outcome in severe falciparum malaria. *Proc Natl Acad Sci USA.* (2008) 105:17097–102. doi: 10.1073/pnas.0805782105

131. Lovegrove FE, Tangpukdee N, Opoka RO, Lafferty EI, Rajwans N, Hawkes M, et al. Serum angiopoietin-1 and−2 levels discriminate cerebral malaria from uncomplicated malaria and predict clinical outcome in African children. *PLoS ONE.* (2009) 4:e4912. doi: 10.1371/journal.pone.0004912

132. Conroy AL, Phiri H, Hawkes M, Glover S, Mallewa M, Seydel KB, et al. Endothelium-based biomarkers are associated with cerebral malaria in Malawian children: a retrospective case-control study. *PLoS ONE.* (2010) 5:e15291. doi: 10.1371/journal.pone.0015291

133. Conroy AL, Glover SJ, Hawkes M, Erdman LK, Seydel KB, Taylor TE, et al. Angiopoietin-2 levels are associated with retinopathy and predict mortality in Malawian children with cerebral malaria: a retrospective case-control study. *Crit Care Med.* (2012) 40:952–9. doi: 10.1097/CCM.0b013e3182373157

134. O'Regan N, Gegenbauer K, O'sullivan JM, Maleki S, Brophy TM, Dalton N, et al. A novel role for von Willebrand factor in the pathogenesis of experimental cerebral malaria. *Blood.* (2016) 127:1192–201. doi: 10.1182/blood-2015-07-654921

135. Vischer UM, Wagner DD. CD63 is a component of Weibel-Palade bodies of human endothelial cells. *Blood.* (1993) 82:1184–91.

136. Galbusera M, Zoja C, Donadelli R, Paris S, Morigi M, Benigni A, et al. Fluid shear stress modulates von Willebrand factor release from human vascular endothelium. *Blood.* (1997) 90:1558–64.

137. Rosnoblet C, Vischer UM, Gerard RD, Irminger JC, Halban PA, Kruithof EK. Storage of tissue-type plasminogen activator in Weibel-Palade bodies of human endothelial cells. *Arterioscler Thromb Vasc Biol.* (1999) 19:1796–803. doi: 10.1161/01.ATV.19.7.1796

138. Schnyder-Candrian S, Borsig L, Moser R, Berger EG. Localization of α1,3-fucosyltransferase VI in Weibel-Palade bodies of human endothelial cells. *Proc Natl Acad Sci USA.* (2000) 97:8369–74. doi: 10.1073/pnas.97.15.8369

139. Zannettino AC, Holding CA, Diamond P, Atkins GJ, Kostakis P, Farrugia A, et al. Osteoprotegerin (OPG) is localized to the Weibel-Palade bodies of human vascular endothelial cells and is physically associated with von Willebrand factor. *J Cell Physiol.* (2005) 204:714–23. doi: 10.1002/jcp.20354

140. Rondaij MG, Bierings R, Kragt A, Van Mourik JA, Voorberg J. Dynamics and plasticity of Weibel-Palade bodies in endothelial cells. *Arterioscler Thromb Vasc Biol.* (2006) 26:1002–7. doi: 10.1161/01.ATV.0000209501.56852.6c

141. Van Breevoort D, Van Agtmaal EL, Dragt BS, Gebbinck JK, Dienava-Verdoold I, Kragt A, et al. Proteomic screen identifies IGFBP7 as a novel component of endothelial cell-specific Weibel-Palade bodies. *J Proteome Res.* (2012) 11:2925–36. doi: 10.1021/pr300010r

142. Turner NA, Moake JL. Factor VIII Is synthesized in human endothelial cells, packaged in Weibel-Palade bodies and secreted bound to ULVWF strings. *PLoS ONE.* (2015) 10:e0140740. doi: 10.1371/journal.pone.0140740

143. Maleszewski JJ, Lai CK, Veinot JP. Chapter 1—anatomic considerations and examination of cardiovascular specimens (excluding devices) A2 - Buja, L. Maximilian. In: Butany J, editor. *Cardiovascular Pathology, 4th ed.* San Diego: Academic Press (2016). p. 1–56. doi: 10.1016/B978-0-12-420219-1.00001-X

144. Babich V, Meli A, Knipe L, Dempster JE, Skehel P, Hannah MJ, et al. Selective release of molecules from Weibel-Palade bodies during a lingering kiss. *Blood.* (2008) 111:5282–90. doi: 10.1182/blood-2007-09-113746

145. Kiskin NI, Babich V, Knipe L, Hannah MJ, Carter T. Differential cargo mobilisation within Weibel-Palade bodies after transient fusion with the plasma membrane. *PLoS ONE.* (2014) 9:e108093. doi: 10.1371/journal.pone.0108093

146. Dekker RJ, Boon RA, Rondaij MG, Kragt A, Volger OL, Elderkamp YW, et al. KLF2 provokes a gene expression pattern that establishes functional quiescent differentiation of the endothelium. *Blood.* (2006) 107:4354–63. doi: 10.1182/blood-2005-08-3465

147. Combes V, Coltel N, Faille D, Wassmer SC, Grau GE. Cerebral malaria: role of microparticles and platelets in alterations of the blood-brain barrier. *Int J Parasitol.* (2006) 36:541–6. doi: 10.1016/j.ijpara.2006.02.005

148. Jenkins NT, Padilla J, Boyle LJ, Credeur DP, Laughlin MH, Fadel PJ. Disturbed blood flow acutely induces activation and apoptosis of the human vascular endothelium. *Hypertension.* (2013) 61:615–21. doi: 10.1161/HYPERTENSIONAHA.111.00561

149. Scholz A, Plate KH, Reiss Y. Angiopoietin-2: a multifaceted cytokine that functions in both angiogenesis and inflammation. *Ann N Y Acad Sci.* (2015) 1347:45–51. doi: 10.1111/nyas.12726

150. Moxon CA, Wassmer SC, Milner DA Jr, Chisala NV, Taylor TE, Seydel KB, et al. Loss of endothelial protein C receptors links coagulation and inflammation to parasite sequestration in cerebral malaria in African children. *Blood.* (2013) 122:842–51. doi: 10.1182/blood-2013-03-490219

151. Turner GD, Ly VC, Nguyen TH, Tran TH, Nguyen HP, Bethell D, et al. Systemic endothelial activation occurs in both mild and severe malaria. Correlating dermal microvascular endothelial cell phenotype and soluble cell adhesion molecules with disease severity. *Am J Pathol.* (1998) 152:1477–87.

152. Tripathi AK, Sullivan DJ, Stins MF. *Plasmodium falciparum*-infected erythrocytes increase intercellular adhesion molecule 1 expression on brain endothelium through NF-κB. *Infect Immun.* (2006) 74:3262–70. doi: 10.1128/IAI.01625-05

153. Pouvelle B, Fusai T, Lepolard C, Gysin J. Biological and biochemical characteristics of cytoadhesion of *Plasmodium falciparum*-infected erythrocytes to chondroitin-4-sulfate. *Infect Immun.* (1998) 66:4950–6.

154. Avril M, Bernabeu M, Benjamin M, Brazier AJ, Smith JD. Interaction between endothelial protein C receptor and intercellular adhesion molecule 1 to mediate binding of *Plasmodium falciparum*-infected erythrocytes to endothelial cells. *mBio.* (2016) 7:e00615–16. doi: 10.1128/mBio.00615-16

155. Lavstsen T, Turner L, Saguti F, Magistrado P, Rask TS, Jespersen JS, et al. *Plasmodium falciparum* erythrocyte membrane protein 1 domain cassettes 8 and 13 are associated with severe malaria in children. *Proc Natl Acad Sci USA.* (2012) 109:E1791–800. doi: 10.1073/pnas.1120455109

156. Bertin GI, Lavstsen T, Guillonneau F, Doritchamou J, Wang CW, Jespersen JS, et al. Expression of the domain cassette 8 *Plasmodium falciparum* erythrocyte membrane protein 1 is associated with cerebral malaria in Benin. *PLoS ONE.* (2013) 8:e68368. doi: 10.1371/journal.pone.0068368

157. Abdi AI, Kariuki SM, Muthui MK, Kivisi CA, Fegan G, Gitau E, et al. Differential *Plasmodium falciparum* surface antigen expression among children with Malarial Retinopathy. *Sci Rep.* (2015) 5:18034. doi: 10.1038/srep18034

158. Seydel KB, Kampondeni SD, Valim C, Potchen MJ, Milner DA, Muwalo FW, et al. Brain swelling and death in children with cerebral malaria. *N Engl J Med.* (2015) 372:1126–37. doi: 10.1056/NEJMoa1400116

159. Jespersen JS, Wang CW, Mkumbaye SI, Minja DT, Petersen B, Turner L, et al. *Plasmodium falciparum* var genes expressed in children with severe malaria encode CIDRalpha1 domains. *EMBO Mol Med.* (2016) 8:839–50. doi: 10.15252/emmm.201606188

160. David PH, Handunnetti SM, Leech JH, Gamage P, Mendis KN. Rosetting: a new cytoadherence property of malaria-infected erythrocytes. *Am J Trop Med Hyg.* (1988) 38:289–97. doi: 10.4269/ajtmh.1988.38.289

161. Lowe BS, Mosobo M, Bull PC. All four species of human malaria parasites form rosettes. *Trans R Soc Trop Med Hyg.* (1998) 92:526. doi: 10.1016/S0035-9203(98)90901-4

162. Wahlgren M, Carlson J, Udomsangpetch R, Perlmann P. Why do *Plasmodium falciparumm*-infected erythrocytes form spontaneous erythrocyte rosettes? *Parasitol Today.* (1989) 5:183–5. doi: 10.1016/0169-4758(89)90141-5

163. Carlson J, Holmquist G, Taylor DW, Perlmann P, Wahlgren M. Antibodies to a histidine-rich protein (PfHRP1) disrupt spontaneously formed *Plasmodium falciparum* erythrocyte rosettes. *Proc Natl Acad Sci USA.* (1990) 87:2511–5. doi: 10.1073/pnas.87.7.2511

164. Adams Y, Kuhnrae P, Higgins MK, Ghumra A, Rowe JA. Rosetting *Plasmodium falciparum*-infected erythrocytes bind to human brain microvascular endothelial cells in vitro, demonstrating a dual adhesion phenotype mediated by distinct P. falciparum erythrocyte membrane protein 1 domains. *Infect Immun.* (2014) 82:949–59. doi: 10.1128/IAI.01233-13

165. Treutiger CJ, Hedlund I, Helmby H, Carlson J, Jepson A, Twumasi P, et al. Rosette formation in *Plasmodium falciparum* isolates and anti-rosette activity of sera from Gambians with cerebral or uncomplicated malaria. *Am J Trop Med Hyg.* (1992) 46:503–10. doi: 10.4269/ajtmh.1992.46.503

166. Carlson J, Nash GB, Gabutti V, Al-Yaman F, Wahlgren M. Natural protection against severe *Plasmodium falciparum* malaria due to impaired rosette formation. *Blood.* (1994) 84:3909–14.

167. Rowe A, Obeiro J, Newbold CI, Marsh K. *Plasmodium falciparum* rosetting is associated with malaria severity in Kenya. *Infect Immun.* (1995) 63:2323–6.

168. Rowe JA, Obiero J, Marsh K, Raza A. Short report: positive correlation between rosetting and parasitemia in Plasmodium falciparum clinical isolates. *Am J Trop Med Hyg.* (2002) 66:458–60. doi: 10.4269/ajtmh.2002.66.458

169. Doumbo OK, Thera MA, Kone AK, Raza A, Tempest LJ, Lyke KE, et al. High levels of *Plasmodium falciparum* rosetting in all clinical forms of severe malaria in African children. *Am J Trop Med Hyg.* (2009) 81:987–93. doi: 10.4269/ajtmh.2009.09-0406

170. Ho M, Davis TM, Silamut K, Bunnag D, White NJ. Rosette formation of *Plasmodium falciparum*-infected erythrocytes from patients with acute malaria. *Infect Immun.* (1991) 59:2135–9.

171. Al-Yaman F, Genton B, Mokela D, Raiko A, Kati S, Rogerson S, et al. Human cerebral malaria: lack of significant association between erythrocyte

rosetting and disease severity. *Trans R Soc Trop Med Hyg.* (1995) 89:55–8. doi: 10.1016/0035-9203(95)90658-4

172. Udomsangpetch R, Webster HK, Pattanapanyasat K, Pitchayangkul S, Thaithong S. Cytoadherence characteristics of rosette-forming *Plasmodium falciparum*. *Infect Immun.* (1992) 60:4483–90.

173. Branco A, Melo-Cristino J. Extreme parasitemia in *P. falciparum malaria Blood.* (2018) 132:868. doi: 10.1182/blood-2018-07-861880

174. Carlson J, Ekre HP, Helmby H, Gysin J, Greenwood BM, Wahlgren M. Disruption of *Plasmodium falciparum* erythrocyte rosettes by standard heparin and heparin devoid of anticoagulant activity. *Am J Trop Med Hyg.* (1992) 46:595–602. doi: 10.4269/ajtmh.1992.46.595

175. Vogt AM, Winter G, Wahlgren M, Spillmann D. Heparan sulphate identified on human erythrocytes: a *Plasmodium falciparum* receptor. *Biochem J.* (2004) 381:593–7. doi: 10.1042/BJ20040762

176. Angeletti D, Sandalova T, Wahlgren M, Achour A. Binding of subdomains 1/2 of PfEMP1-DBL1alpha to heparan sulfate or heparin mediates *Plasmodium falciparum* rosetting. *PLoS ONE.* (2015) 10:e0118898. doi: 10.1371/journal.pone.0118898

177. McCormick CJ, Newbold CI, Berendt AR. Sulfated glycoconjugates enhance CD36-dependent adhesion of *Plasmodium falciparum*-infected erythrocytes to human microvascular endothelial cells. *Blood.* (2000) 96:327–33.

178. Dembo EG, Phiri HT, Montgomery J, Molyneux ME, Rogerson SJ. Are *Plasmodium falciparum* parasites present in peripheral blood genetically the same as those sequestered in the tissues? *Am J Trop Med Hyg.* (2006) 74:730–2. doi: 10.4269/ajtmh.2006.74.730

179. Montgomery J, Milner DA Jr, Tse MT, Njobvu A, Kayira K, Dzamalala CP, et al. Genetic analysis of circulating and sequestered populations of *Plasmodium falciparum* in fatal pediatric malaria. *J Infect Dis.* (2006) 194:115–22. doi: 10.1086/504689

180. Kaul DK, Roth EF Jr, Nagel RL, Howard RJ, Handunnetti SM. Rosetting of *Plasmodium falciparum*-infected red blood cells with uninfected red blood cells enhances microvascular obstruction under flow conditions. *Blood.* (1991) 78:812–9.

181. Berendt AR, Ferguson DJ, Newbold CI. Sequestration in *Plasmodium falciparum* malaria: sticky cells and sticky problems. *Parasitol Today.* (1990) 6:247–54. doi: 10.1016/0169-4758(90)90184-6

182. Chotivanich KT, Pukrittayakamee S, Simpson JA, White NJ, Udomsangpetch R. Characteristics of *Plasmodium vivax*-infected erythrocyte rosettes. *Am J Trop Med Hyg.* (1998) 59:73–6. doi: 10.4269/ajtmh.1998.59.73

183. Lee WC, Malleret B, Lau YL, Mauduit M, Fong MY, Cho JS, et al. Glycophorin C (CD236R) mediates vivax malaria parasite rosetting to normocytes. *Blood.* (2014) 123:e100–9. doi: 10.1182/blood-2013-12-541698

184. Ozen M, Gungor S, Atambay M, Daldal N. Cerebral malaria owing to *Plasmodium vivax*: case report. *Ann Trop Paediatr.* (2006) 26:141–4. doi: 10.1179/146532806X107494

185. Thapa R, Patra V, Kundu R. *Plasmodium vivax* cerebral malaria. *Indian Pediatr.* (2007) 44:433–4.

186. Sarkar S, Bhattacharya P. Cerebral malaria caused by *Plasmodium vivax* in adult subjects. *Indian J Crit Care Med.* (2008) 12:204–5. doi: 10.4103/0972-5229.45084

187. Mahgoub H, Gasim GI, Musa IR, Adam I. Severe *Plasmodium vivax* malaria among sudanese children at New Halfa Hospital, Eastern Sudan. *Parasit Vectors.* (2012) 5:154. doi: 10.1186/1756-3305-5-154

188. Pinzon MA, Pineda JC, Rosso F, Shinchi M, Bonilla-Abadia F. *Plasmodium vivax* cerebral malaria complicated with venous sinus thrombosis in Colombia. *Asian Pac J Trop Med.* (2013) 6:413–5. doi: 10.1016/S1995-7645(13)60050-4

189. Karanth SS, Marupudi KC, Gupta A. Intracerebral bleed, right haemiparesis and seizures: an atypical presentation of vivax malaria. *BMJ Case Rep.* (2014) 2014:bcr2014204833. doi: 10.1136/bcr-2014-204833

190. Gupta H, Dhunputh P, Bhatt AN, Satyamoorthy K, Umakanth S. Cerebral malaria in a man with *Plasmodium vivax* mono-infection: a case report. *Trop Doct.* (2016) 46:241–5. doi: 10.1177/0049475515624857

191. Carvalho BO, Lopes SC, Nogueira PA, Orlandi PP, Bargieri DY, Blanco YC, et al. On the cytoadhesion of *Plasmodium vivax*-infected erythrocytes. *J Infect Dis.* (2010) 202:638–47. doi: 10.1086/654815

192. Nagayasu E, Ito M, Akaki M, Nakano Y, Kimura M, Looareesuwan S, et al. CR1 density polymorphism on erythrocytes of falciparum

malaria patients in Thailand. *Am J Trop Med Hyg.* (2001) 64:1–5. doi: 10.4269/ajtmh.2001.64.1.11425154

193. Teeranaipong P, Ohashi J, Patarapotikul J, Kimura R, Nuchnoi P, Hananantachai H, et al. A functional single-nucleotide polymorphism in the CR1 promoter region contributes to protection against cerebral malaria. *J Infect Dis.* (2008) 198:1880–91. doi: 10.1086/593338

194. Sinha S, Jha GN, Anand P, Qidwai T, Pati SS, Mohanty S, et al. CR1 levels and gene polymorphisms exhibit differential association with falciparum malaria in regions of varying disease endemicity. *Hum Immunol.* (2009) 70:244–50. doi: 10.1016/j.humimm.2009.02.001

195. Rout R, Dhangadamajhi G, Mohapatra BN, Kar SK, Ranjit M. High CR1 level and related polymorphic variants are associated with cerebral malaria in eastern-India. *Infect Genet Evol.* (2011) 11:139–44. doi: 10.1016/j.meegid.2010.09.009

196. Zimmerman PA, Fitness J, Moulds JM, Mcnamara DT, Kasehagen LJ, Rowe JA, et al. CR1 Knops blood group alleles are not associated with severe malaria in the Gambia. *Genes Immun.* (2003) 4:368–73. doi: 10.1038/sj.gene.6363980

197. Cockburn IA, Mackinnon MJ, O'donnell A, Allen SJ, Moulds JM, Baisor M, et al. A human complement receptor 1 polymorphism that reduces *Plasmodium falciparum* rosetting confers protection against severe malaria. *Proc Natl Acad Sci USA.* (2004) 101:272–7. doi: 10.1073/pnas.0305306101

198. Thathy V, Moulds JM, Guyah B, Otieno W, Stoute JA. Complement receptor 1 polymorphisms associated with resistance to severe malaria in Kenya. *Malar J.* (2005) 4:54. doi: 10.1186/1475-2875-4-54

199. Opi DH, Swann O, Macharia A, Uyoga S, Band G, Ndila CM, et al. Two complement receptor one alleles have opposing associations with cerebral malaria and interact with alpha(+)thalassaemia. *Elife.* (2018) 7:e31579. doi: 10.7554/eLife.31579

200. Babiker HA, Abdel-Muhsin AM, Ranford-Cartwright LC, Satti G, Walliker D. Characteristics of *Plasmodium falciparum* parasites that survive the lengthy dry season in eastern Sudan where malaria transmission is markedly seasonal. *Am J Trop Med Hyg.* (1998) 59:582–90. doi: 10.4269/ajtmh.1998.59.582

201. Zwetyenga J, Rogier C, Spiegel A, Fontenille D, Trape JF, Mercereau-Puijalon O. A cohort study of *Plasmodium falciparum* diversity during the dry season in Ndiop, a Senegalese village with seasonal, mesoendemic malaria. *Trans R Soc Trop Med Hyg.* (1999) 93:375–80. doi: 10.1016/S0035-9203(99)90122-0

202. Baliraine FN, Afrane YA, Amenya DA, Bonizzoni M, Menge DM, Zhou G, et al. High prevalence of asymptomatic Plasmodium falciparum infections in a highland area of western Kenya: a cohort study. *J Infect Dis.* (2009) 200:66–74. doi: 10.1086/599317

203. Sagna AB, Gaayeb L, Sarr JB, Senghor S, Poinsignon A, Boutouaba-Combe S, et al. *Plasmodium falciparum* infection during dry season: IgG responses to *Anopheles gambiae* salivary gSG6-P1 peptide as sensitive biomarker for malaria risk in Northern Senegal. *Malar J.* (2013) 12:301. doi: 10.1186/1475-2875-12-301

204. Howard RJ, Gilladoga AD. Molecular studies related to the pathogenesis of cerebral malaria. *Blood.* (1989) 74:2603–18.

205. Handunnetti SM, Hasler TH, Howard RJ. *Plasmodium falciparum*-infected erythrocytes do not adhere well to C32 melanoma cells or CD36 unless rosettes with uninfected erythrocytes are first disrupted. *Infect Immun.* (1992) 60:928–32.

206. Rogerson SJ, Beck HP, Al-Yaman F, Currie B, Alpers MP, Brown GV. Disruption of erythrocyte rosettes and agglutination of erythrocytes infected with *Plasmodium falciparum* by the sera of Papua New Guineans. *Trans R Soc Trop Med Hyg.* (1996) 90:80–4. doi: 10.1016/S0035-9203(96)90487-3

207. Chotivanich KT, Dondorp AM, White NJ, Peters K, Vreeken J, Kager PA, et al. The resistance to physiological shear stresses of the erythrocytic rosettes formed by cells infected with *Plasmodium falciparum*. *Ann Trop Med Parasitol.* (2000) 94:219–26. doi: 10.1080/00034983.2000.11813532

208. Saxer T, Zumbuehl A, Muller B. The use of shear stress for targeted drug delivery. *Cardiovasc Res.* (2013) 99:328–33. doi: 10.1093/cvr/cvt102

209. Idro R, Marsh K, John CC, Newton CR. Cerebral malaria: mechanisms of brain injury and strategies for improved neurocognitive outcome. *Pediatr Res.* (2010) 68:267–74. doi: 10.1203/PDR.0b013e3181eee738

210. Rogerson SJ, Reeder JC, Al-Yaman F, Brown GV. Sulfated glycoconjugates as disrupters of *Plasmodium falciparum* erythrocyte rosettes. *Am J Trop Med Hyg.* (1994) 51:198–203. doi: 10.4269/ajtmh.1994.51.198

211. Rowe A, Berendt AR, Marsh K, Newbold CI. *Plasmodium falciparum*: a family of sulphated glycoconjugates disrupts erythrocyte rosettes. *Exp Parasitol.* (1994) 79:506–16. doi: 10.1006/expr.1994.1111

212. Luginbuhl A, Nikolic M, Beck HP, Wahlgren M, Lutz HU. Complement factor D, albumin, and immunoglobulin G anti-band 3 protein antibodies mimic serum in promoting rosetting of malaria-infected red blood cells. *Infect Immun.* (2007) 75:1771–7. doi: 10.1128/IAI.01514-06

213. Azasi Y, Lindergard G, Ghumra A, Mu J, Miller LH, Rowe JA. Infected erythrocytes expressing DC13 PfEMP1 differ from recombinant proteins in EPCR-binding function. *Proc Natl Acad Sci USA.* (2018) 115:1063–8. doi: 10.1073/pnas.1712879115

214. Haffner SM. Pre-diabetes, insulin resistance, inflammation and CVD risk. *Diabetes Res Clin Pract.* (2003) 61(Suppl. 1):S9–18. doi: 10.1016/S0168-8227(03)00122-0

215. Movva LR, Ho DKL, Corbet EF, Leung WK. Type-2 diabetes mellitus, metabolic control, serum inflammatory factors, lifestyle, and periodontal status. *J Dent Sci.* (2014) 9:1–9. doi: 10.1016/j.jds.2013.10.006

16

Diet-Microbe-Host Interactions that Affect Gut Mucosal Integrity and Infection Resistance

*Andrew J. Forgie, Janelle M. Fouhse and Benjamin P. Willing**

Department of Agricultural, Food and Nutritional Science, University of Alberta, Edmonton, AB, Canada

Correspondence:
Benjamin P. Willing
willing@ualberta.ca

The gastrointestinal tract microbiome plays a critical role in regulating host innate and adaptive immune responses against pathogenic bacteria. Disease associated dysbiosis and environmental induced insults, such as antibiotic treatments can lead to increased susceptibility to infection, particularly in a hospital setting. Dietary intervention is the greatest tool available to modify the microbiome and support pathogen resistance. Some dietary components can maintain a healthy disease resistant microbiome, whereas others can contribute to an imbalanced microbial population, impairing intestinal barrier function and immunity. Characterizing the effects of dietary components through the host-microbe axis as it relates to gastrointestinal health is vital to provide evidence-based dietary interventions to mitigate infections. This review will cover the effect of dietary components (carbohydrates, fiber, proteins, fats, polyphenolic compounds, vitamins, and minerals) on intestinal integrity and highlight their ability to modulate host-microbe interactions as to improve pathogen resistance.

Keywords: microbiota, diet, infection resistance, gastrointestinal integrity, disease susceptibility

INTRODUCTION

Infectious enteric diseases are a major cause of morbidity and mortality worldwide and are of particular concern in hospital settings and developing countries. According to the World Health Organization, infectious enteric diseases are one of the top 10 causes of death leading to over two billion cases and one million deaths worldwide in 2010 (1). Host resistance toward invading pathogens requires tight regulation of the gastrointestinal environment, maintained through a synergistic relationship between the host immune system and microbiome. Disruption to a host's intestinal homeostasis, including insults from diet, stress, antibiotic and drug treatment, allergies, cancer, and related illnesses can leave the host vulnerable to enteric pathogens (2). It is well-understood that diet can play a major role on health by positively and negatively shaping gastrointestinal ecology (3, 4), and therefore should be a major focus in mitigating the severity of infection.

Although humans have successfully reduced pathogen exposure through effective sanitation practices, the adoption of a "Western diet," over-sanitation and lack of physical exercise are hypothesized to have contributed to the rise in autoimmune disorders (5). The "Western diet" is characterized by the excessive consumption of fats, proteins, refined sugar, and low intake of dietary fiber. Other dietary patterns such as the Mediterranean, Vegetarian-based, Japanese-based, and Ketogenic type diets can positively regulate immune responsiveness to reduce immune activity and support health (6). However, human epidemiology studies on diet tend to exclude important interindividual variations that govern the gastrointestinal microbiota and may explain the diverse claims to which foods are known as "protective" and "harmful" (7). Establishing a mechanistic link between individual diet components using microbe-host interactions will aid to provide evidence driven recommendations to help control an overactive immune response.

An overactive immune system is associated with autoimmune disorders such as irritable bowel disease (IBD) that affects host immune activity and leads to increased incidence of infection (8, 9). Likewise, "westernized diets" have shown to enhance *Escherichia coli* colonization and associated inflammation in mice by altering the host mucus layer, increasing intestinal permeability, and impairing immune function (10). Dietary fiber and other microbiota-accessible carbohydrates (MACs) are a key component missing from the "westernized diet" that when re-introduced provides a beneficial balance to host health and microbiome (11). Fiber is exhaustively studied as a microbial fermentation substrate that produces short chain fatty acids (SCFAs) with known benefits to host intestinal homeostasis and health (12). However, we fear that this focus on the beneficial effects of fiber-associated SCFA production has led researchers to overlook other common dietary components that may positively or negatively influence the host gastrointestinal environment and health.

Diet intervention should be considered a valuable tool to manipulate the host-microbe axis to help sustain intestinal homeostasis and infection resistance. Dietary components such as carbohydrates, lipids, proteins, phytochemicals, minerals, and vitamins all have unique structural and chemical (physicochemical) properties that influence host pathogen resistance directly and indirectly through the microbiome. Bridging the gap between diet, host, and microbiome as they relate to immunity and disease resistance is a multifaceted field that requires an understanding of their combined effects on intestinal homeostasis (**Figure 1**). This review explores the role of common dietary components on host-microbe interactions that modulate host resistance and tolerance toward common infectious diseases. We highlight the opportunity to improve outcomes, yet recognize the current knowledge limits the ability to provide concrete dietary advice. This is partially limited by the fact that diet focused infection resistance research is scarce and difficult to translate to humans.

GALT AND MICROBIOME REGULATE HOST DEFENSES

The gut associated lymphoid tissue (GALT) plays a crucial role in regulating intestinal homeostasis and is composed of lymph nodes, lamina propria, and epithelial cells that together provide the host with a protective barrier and immune defense against invading pathogens (13). On the other hand, the microbiota provides a physical presence that can directly prevent pathogen colonization by competing for attachment sites or nutrient resources. Indirectly, the microbiota helps to improve host resistance by modulating intestinal integrity through the mucus layer, tight junction proteins, and antimicrobial peptides (AMPs: cathelicidins, C-type lectins, and defensins) (14, 15). Mucins

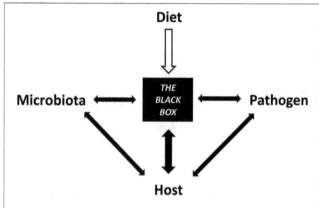

FIGURE 1 | Diet contributes to a black box of intertwined mechanisms between the microbiota, host, and pathogen that have yet to be elucidated.

secreted by goblet cells provide the first line of defense by forming a physical barrier composed of highly glycosylated and interlinked proteins between luminal bacteria and host epithelial cells (16). The mucus layer provides lubricant and is metabolized by mucin-degrading (mucolytic) bacteria forming the loosely attached layer (17), whereas the adherent layer, when properly formed, secures a balance of host AMPs and immune factors that maintain intestinal homeostasis (18).

Disruptions to the balanced microbial ecosystem greatly increase a host's vulnerability to infection (19). In particular, antibiotic exposure can cause major shifts in microbial communities leading to mucus layer thinning, predisposing, and exacerbating infections, as shown with antibiotic accompanied *Citrobacter rodentium* infections in mice (20). Antibiotic-induced microbiota imbalances are well-documented to alter the production of AMPs, tight junction proteins, and immune factors that normally contribute to intestinal homeostasis and infection resistance (21, 22). Secretory immunoglobulin A (SIgA) antibodies are abundant immune factors of the intestinal lumen that protect epithelial cells from enteric pathogens and toxins by blocking their access to epithelial receptors and entrapping them in mucus to promote clearance (23). Although SIgA targets and disrupts pathogens and antigens, commensal microbes such as *Bacteroides fragilis* alter their surface proteins to attract SIgA to enhance mucosal colonization (24). Intestinal epithelial cells (IECs) produce reactive oxygen species (ROS) (25) and Resistin-like molecules (e.g., RELMβ) (26) that hinder commensal and pathogenic bacteria colonization, further maintaining intestinal hemostasis. IECs apical surface fucosylation is another useful host strategy that controls commensal microbes and inhibits pathogens. Secreted fucose is metabolized by bacteria to produce bioactive metabolites, reduce virulence factors, and enrich beneficial gut microbes to strengthen colonization exclusion (27). Alternatively, fucose can be fermented by commensal microbes into 1,2-propanediol and utilized by *Salmonella* during inflammation to drive their fitness in the colon (28).

The host has significant control over microbial communities of the small and large intestine; however, this relationship is complex and is managed in part through gastric acid secretions, intestinal motility, bile secretions, oxygen gradients, and regulation of pattern recognition receptors (PPRs), such as Toll-like receptors (TLRs) (4). The host recognizes commensal bacteria through activation of TLRs and relays an appropriate response in accordance to the specific microbial derived ligands [e.g., peptidoglycan, lipoprotein, lipopolysaccharide (LPS), and flagellin] (29). Innate lymphoid cells (ILCs) have been identified as key immune regulatory cells of the GALT controlling pathogen resistance, inflammation, and metabolic homeostasis (30). ILCs concentrate within mucosal surfaces and relay signals sent between the microbiota, epithelia, immune cells, and metabolites in the intestine to maintain epithelial barrier function. Transcriptomic analysis of 15 ILC subtypes revealed their regulatory functions depend on the presence of the microbiome, nutrients, and xenobiotics (31). Ultimately, it is the combined relationship between the gut microbiota, host, and diet that help improve or worsen a host's ability to tolerate and resist pathogenic bacteria (**Figure 2**). The remainder of this review will focus on specific dietary components and how they stimulate some of these and other host-microbe interactions resulting in impaired or improved host disease resistance.

CARBOHYDRATES

Dietary carbohydrates are often classified by their degree of polymerization into mono-, di-, oligo-, or poly-saccharides and composition of their monosaccharides: glucose, fructose, galactose, and xylose. Typically, carbohydrates are categorized as either digestible or indigestible (fiber). Binding and structural properties of carbohydrates dictate the glucosidase enzymes required to break bonds into their basic units for absorption (32). The digestible carbohydrates escaping host small intestinal digestion, along with dietary fiber, become available as microbial energy substrates and are able to substantially alter the intestinal ecosystem and community structure (33).

Increasing intake of digestible carbohydrates has been scrutinized for contributing to the worldwide obesity and diabetes epidemics. However, carbohydrates are essential energy substrates for the central nervous system and red blood cells, are required to maintain cellular energy balance after sustained increases in metabolic activity, and to restore energy levels and glycogen stores (34). Humans and animals are able to regulate blood glucose levels; however, excessive dietary carbohydrate consumption can worsen acute hyperglycemia, particularly during times of an illness (35, 36) and stress (37, 38). A medical illness can enhance the negative effects of acute hyperglycemia, which include inhibition of neutrophil migration, phagocytosis, superoxide production, and microbial killing, compromising host innate immunity against bacterial and fungal infections (39). Diets high in simple and refined carbohydrates are shown to negatively impact gastrointestinal microbial communities leading to intestinal barrier dysfunction and greater risk for enteric infection (36). Whereas, balanced diets containing resistant starch and fiber stimulate microbial fermentation leading to a stable diverse microbiome and production of beneficial SCFAs (40). Understanding both negative and positive effects of carbohydrate consumption

on gastrointestinal immunity and microbial populations will provide vital insight toward dietary strategies to help maintain pathogen resistance.

Dietary trehalose, a food component used to improve a product's texture, flavor, glycemic index and shelf life, was introduced in the early 2000's and has since been proposed to have contributed to the global *Clostridioides difficile* epidemic (41). Trehalose is a disaccharide composed of two glucose molecules linked by a resistant α,α−1,1-glucosidic bond found in plants, algae, fungi, yeast, bacteria, insects, and other invertebrates (42). Mammals and other vertebrates lack the ability to synthesize trehalose, and the dietary fate of trehalose depends on the capacity of the small intestinal trehalase enzyme to hydrolyze it into glucose (43). Trehalase deficiency is rare in humans but excessive consumption of trehalose can lead to negative intestinal imbalances similar to those associated with lactose and fructose intolerances. Researchers believe the increased use of trehalose in food production has naturally selected for *C. difficile* with the capacity to metabolize trehalose more efficiently, thus increasing pathogen fitness and contributing to their hypervirulent outbreaks in the human population (41). To combat reoccurring *C. difficile* infections a fecal microbial transplant (FMT) from a healthy donor has become a helpful treatment option, however the mechanism of remission remains unclear (44). The success of FMTs to treat *C. difficile* infections highlights the importance of a "healthy" gut microbiome to promote infection resistance. Additional research is needed to confirm the impact of specific carbohydrates and their malabsorption on immune and microbial networks in the gut as it relates to pathogen fitness. Interestingly, studies in mice comparing fiber-rich and fiber-deprived diets support the detrimental effect of a simple carbohydrate dominated diet and the importance of fiber on infection resistance (11, 33).

DIETARY FIBER

Health benefits associated with foods rich in non-digestible dietary fiber depend on their type, source, and proportion of water soluble and insoluble carbohydrate components (45). Fruits, vegetables, and grains are excellent sources of numerous fiber types, however, not all fiber sources and types are created equal. The food source, glycosylated chain structures, and their fermentability, along with other inherent components are key parameters for their functional quality within the gastrointestinal tract (12). Non-digestible carbohydrates are composed of monosaccharide units (glucose, fructose, galactose, xylose, fucose, and sialic acid) found naturally in plants, algae, fungi, bacteria, and mammalian milk, or produced by chemical or enzymatic processes (46, 47). Short chain fructo-oligosaccharides (FOS) have received a great deal of attention due to their prebiotic effects (48) and fact that they occur naturally (mostly as inulin) with different degrees of polymerization in foods (47). The consumption of prebiotic fibers have helped with diarrhea and constipation (49–51), however, not everyone benefits from their consumption, and can even lead to excessive gas production, bloating, and discomfort (50, 52). In cases of gastrointestinal

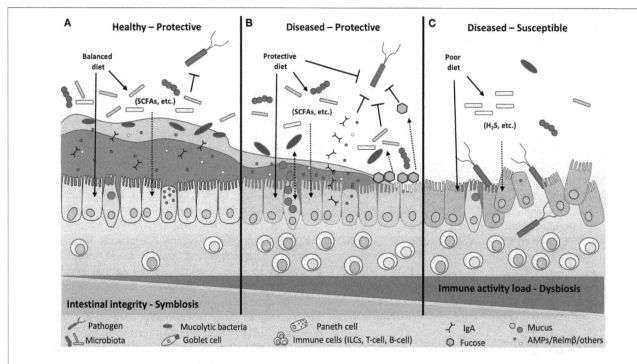

FIGURE 2 | Diet and immune activity load (allergies, cancer, other illness, etc.) determine host intestinal integrity toward invading pathogens. Diet affects intestinal integrity directly by stimulating IECs, ILCs, and microbial communities, and indirectly through microbial fermentation by-products (SCFAs, H₂S, etc.). A healthy individual following a balanced diet to maintain symbiosis between host and microbial populations has enhanced intestinal integrity with a thick inner and outer mucus layer that retains AMPs and other compounds to protect the host against pathogen colonization **(A)**. A diseased host with heightened immune activity maintains symbiosis by consuming dietary components that protect and boost host innate defenses (IgA, AMPs, mucus, fucosylation) and adaptive immune responses to prevent pathogen colonization **(B)**. Whereas, diseased individuals with heightened immune activity consuming a poor diet are more susceptible to enteric infections due to impaired host defenses that cannot control the dysbiotic intestinal environment **(C)**.

discomfort, a diet low in fructans (FODMAP-restricted diet) or reducing dietary fiber is often effective but remains controversial, and individualized (53–55).

The effects of various non-digestible fiber on health and microbiota is thoroughly reviewed (12, 45, 46). In general, dietary fiber can modify gastrointestinal function directly through fecal bulking and indirectly through the modification of microbial community structure, and by increasing microbial biomass and fermentation products (45). Fiber fermentation leads to beneficial SCFAs (mainly acetate, propionate, and butyrate) but also undesired gases such as carbon dioxide, hydrogen, and methane (56). Increased gas production, fecal bulking and delayed gastric emptying can lead to discomfort, bloating, and flatus in many individuals (45). Microbial fermentation products such as SCFAs interact with the intestinal epithelium to promote certain defense mechanisms. In particular, microbial production of butyrate provides an energy substrate to epithelial cells (57), maintains the hypoxic environment (58), and promotes improved barrier function through hypoxia inducible factor (HIF) (59). Induction of HIF transcription factor subsequently stimulates downstream signaling to increase mucus production (60) and expression of AMPs (61) ultimately helping to minimize facultative pathogen growth.

According to the Global Burden of Diseases, Injuries, and Risk Factors Study of 2015 infectious diarrhea is a leading cause

of death globally among all ages (1.3 million deaths); with a large proportion of those occurring in infants under 5 years of age (499,000 deaths) (62). Providing children with MACs is an important strategy to mitigate infection burden by stabilizing the microbiota and by bolstering intestinal immunity. Infants that are exclusively breast fed have reduced risk of developing diarrheal disease (63), partially due to the naturally occurring human milk oligosaccharides (HMOs) present in breast milk. HMOs are soluble complex carbohydrates that act as prebiotics, providing a substrate for the intestinal microbiota and can prevent pathogenic bacterial adhesion through a variety of mechanisms (64). *In vitro* studies determined that HMOs act as pathogen decoy receptors to prevent infections and their activities depend on the location and degree of fucosylation (65). Human breast milk contains a multitude of other bioactive factors, immunoglobulins, cytokines, chemokines, growth factors, hormones, and lactoferrin which all likely contribute to the improved disease resistance of breast fed infants and is reviewed elsewhere (66). Human milk has shown the ability to directly inhibit the adherence of *Streptococcus pneumonia* and *Haemophilus influenza* to human mucosal cells *ex vivo* (67). When HMOs were fractioned, it was found that the acidic fraction had greater anti-adhesive properties toward enteropathogenic *E. coli* (EPEC), *Vibrio cholera*, and *Salmonella fyris* compared to the neutral high and low molecular weight fractions (68). Similarly, HMOs blocked EPEC adherence to epithelial cells *in vitro* and reduced EPEC colonization in newborn mice, further implying the essential role HMO play in the prevention of infectious disease in human infants (69). Experimentally, it was shown that supplementing formula with HMO reduced the duration of diarrhea in rotavirus-infected pigs and promoted IFNγ and IL-10 expression in the ileum, suggesting HMOs may also protect infants against rotavirus infection (70). Therefore, research efforts have focused on HMO substitutes that can be added to formula fed to infants that are unable to breastfeed. Human and animal studies suggest supplementing formula with fermentable fiber (e.g., soy polysaccharides, fructo- & galacto- oligosaccharide) reduces infection-associated diarrhea burden by improving intestinal homeostasis (71) and increasing beneficial *Bifidobacterium* species (72–74).

Minimizing infectious diarrheal disease with dietary tools has become the focus of recent research efforts. The importance of non-digestible fermentable fiber or MACs intake in adults has clearly been shown where a greater intake (comparing top vs. bottom quartiles) reduced risk of death from cardiovascular, infectious, and respiratory disease by 24–56% in men and 34–59% in women (75). Galacto-oligosaccharides (GOS) have shown to increase bifidobacteria and beneficially modulate immune function when supplemented to elderly volunteers. Along with improving phagocytosis and natural killer cell activity, the GOS supplemented volunteers had an anti-inflammatory cytokine profiles with increased IL-10 and reduced IL-1B, IL-6, and TNFα (76). In a double blind placebo controlled trial, those supplemented with GOS had reduced diarrhea incidence, duration, and severity (77). *Clostridioides difficile* is the leading cause of health care-associated diarrheal infections, commonly affecting the elderly and antibiotic treated hospitalized patients (78). Significant evidence suggests that the inclusion of soluble fiber to the diet, specifically MACs that increase SCFA production, may be a useful strategy to enhance infection resistance (79). In a mouse model, dietary inclusion of MACs or inulin alone was shown to suppress *C. difficile* infection; whereas diets devoid of MACs exacerbated the infection (11). The mechanisms by which MACs help to mitigate *C. difficile* infection is through the expansion of fiber fermenting microbiota (via competitive exclusion) and subsequent increases in their immune-stimulatory metabolites (promote host defenses), which limit a pathogen's fitness (11).

β-glucans are one type of fermentable fiber that is frequently studied due to its common occurrence in the cell walls of yeast, fungi, and cereals such as barley and oats. Aside from acting as a microbial fermentation substrate, β-glucans are also of great interest for their direct effect on host immune activities and functions that alter immunity toward infections. In humans, the immune modulating property is due to the binding of β-glucans with host receptor dectin-1 (80), which contributes to macrophages activation, and induce phagocytosis (81). Studies in mice found that oat derived β-glucans supplemented at 3 mg every other day stimulated a systemic immune response that reduced fecal oocyst shedding of *Eimeria vermiformis* by 39.6% post-challenge by increasing

specific antibodies against the parasite (81). Oral administration of β-glucan from a fungal source (*Sclerotinia sclerotiorum* at 80 mg/kg every 2 or 3 days) was shown to directly stimulate proliferative responses of Peyer's patches to both T and B-cell mitogens, suggesting β-glucans may also stimulate a mucosal immune activation (82). Intraperitoneal injection of β-glucans has also shown to work as a potent adjuvant to enhance host resistance to both bacterial (81) and parasitic (Leishmania) infections (83). The use of immunostimulants derived from naturally occurring polysaccharides (e.g., β-glucan or chitosan) has become somewhat commonplace in the aquaculture industry as an alternative strategy for disease prevention. Inclusion of oligo-β-glucans (100–200 mg/kg) to striped catfish has shown to improve growth performance and reduce mortality post *Edwardsiella ictaluri* challenge via heightened phagocytic and lysozyme activity (84). The inclusion of dietary β-glucans (200 mg/kg) in poultry has also been used effectively to reduce the severity of necrotic enteritis when challenged with *Eimeria* and *C. perfringens* (85) and inhibited growth depression when challenged with *Salmonella enteritidis* (86) by increasing specific antibody levels. In both cases, inclusion of dietary β-glucans reduced pathogen colonization (*C. perfringens* and *S. enteritidis*).

Generally, increasing fiber will change the microbiome and improve gastrointestinal heath. As stated previously, the benefits associated from consuming food sources or supplements high in fiber is individualized and should be carefully monitored for side-effects.

FATS

Fats are an essential dietary macronutrient that have been criticized and are commonly avoided in developed countries with the objective of reducing weight, cholesterol levels, and cardiovascular disease risk. Fat avoidance and subsequent reliance on simple carbohydrates for caloric intake with reduced energy expenditure is believed to have contributed to the unintended rise of obesity worldwide (87). In healthy individuals most fats are emulsified and absorbed in the small intestine; however, in excess and during intestinal stress fats can travel toward the colon as a substrate for the microbiota (88). Human and animal studies have shown that intestinal microbes have the capacity to alter host homeostasis through a variety of metabolites, including carcinogenic and cytotoxic secondary bile acids (89). The effects of the microbiota on host homeostasis is through alteration to hepatic lipid and bile metabolism, reverse cholesterol transport, energy expenditure, and insulin sensitivity in peripheral tissue (90). In this respect, dietary lipids are capable of directly affecting the host and microbiome, while indirectly altering host homeostasis through the microbiome and their metabolites.

The direct effect of microbial fat metabolism on intestinal health has yet to be established but studies have shown that dietary lipid profiles can alter the outcome of enteric infections. Fat consumption with regards to infection have been thoroughly reviewed elsewhere (91), and provides a bases to establish the connection between microbe and host on enteric pathogen resistance. A study comparing dietary saturated (SFA, milk), monounsaturated (MUFA, olive oil), and polyunsaturated (PUFA, omega-6 corn oil) fatty acids uncovered distinct lipid mediated immune responses in mice after an acute *C. rodentium* challenge (92). SFA and MUFA dominated diets induced protective T-regulatory cells, interleukin (IL)-10, IL-33, and SCFAs that helped mitigate inflammation during enteric infection (92). Interestingly, in a dextran sodium sulfate (DSS) model, IL-10 knockout mice fed a diet containing milk SFAs, but not lard fat SFAs, resulted in a pro-inflammatory T_H1 immune response associated with a bloom of *Bilophila wadsworthia* and its metabolites, hydrogen sulfide and secondary bile acids (93). Diets high in medium-chain SFAs like coconut oil have antifungal action toward *Candida albicans* (94) and antibacterial properties against enteric pathogens (95). Moreover, the addition of fish oil, high in omega-3 (n-3) fatty acids to a SFA dominated diet activated intestinal alkaline phosphatase (IAP), an enzyme that detoxifies proinflammatory lipopolysaccharide (LPS) endotoxins from gram-negative bacteria that accumulates during infection; whereas supplementing n-3 to an n-6 rich diet did not enhance IAP activity (92). Previously it has been observed that high levels of dietary n-6 PUFAs in fact reduce IAP activity leading to LPS endotoxemia in mice (96). Transgenic *Fat-1* mice, which genetically retain a higher concentration of n-3 in their tissues, demonstrated elevated serum IL-10 and IAP activity (96). In mice, safflower and canola oil based diets (high in n-6) heighten mucosal T_H1/T_H17 responses and inflammation, whereas a fish oil based diet has shown to have a protective anti-inflammatory effect following a *C. rodentium* infection (97). Diets rich in n-3 PUFAs have proven protective against many extracellular pathogens (*Mycobacterium tuberculosis, Salmonella typhimurium, S. pneumoniae, Pseudomonas aeruginosa, E. coli, Staphylococcus aureus, C. rodentium, Helicobacter hepaticus, H. pylori,* and *Listeria monocytogene*); however, potentially damaging effects were observed during intracellular viral infections (98, 99). Dose and timing of n-3 PUFAs is critical for intestinal immune homeostasis. Sustained high doses alter microbial communities and host immune system toward an anti-inflammatory state that could exacerbate infections, especially when proinflammatory responses are essential for infection clearance (98). Interestingly, lipid composition affects host-microbial interactions even when administered via a non-enteral route. The inclusion of mixed lipids containing soybean oil, medium-chain triglycerides, olive oil, and fish oil in parenteral formula was shown to reduce intestinal inflammation and alter microbial composition in a piglet model of infant total parenteral nutrition as compared to soybean oil alone (100).

PROTEIN

Protein homeostasis is crucial for host health, physiology, and immune development that together foster a fast-acting immune response toward pathogens. The role of dietary protein and amino acids on host immune function related to diet malnutrition and pathogen interactions has been thoroughly reviewed (101, 102). Amino acids play a major role in regulating immune cell activation, cellular redox homeostasis, lymphocyte proliferation, and production of cytokines, cytotoxins, and antibodies (101). Protein deficiency is well-known to impair immunity and infection resistance, especially during stress and illness due to protein malabsorption and protein consuming processes such as tissue repair (103). Protein deficits have been shown to exacerbate parasitic *Cryptosporidium* infections in mice through disruption of baseline (primary) Th1-type mucosal immunity (104). Furthermore, protein-deprived diets decreased small intestinal macrophage proliferation and IL-10 production independently of the microbiota (105).

In contrast, researchers propose that protein-rich diets can be just as harmful since they lead to an increase in undigested proteins that encourage protein-fermenting bacteria and disease susceptibility (106). Resistant and undigested proteins can interfere with host functions directly as biologically active proteins (BAP) like trypsin and chymotrypsin inhibitors, and indirectly through microbial proteolytic fermentation by-products [H_2, CO_2, CH_4, H_2S, SCFA, branched chain amino acids (BCAA), nitrogenous compounds, phenols, and indoles] with poorly understood health outcomes (107). It is important to note that dietary crude protein can contain a high concentration of BAPs whose activities can be reduced upon hydrolysis digestion (heating, chemical, or enzymatic). A study replacing crude protein (wheat and casein) with purified amino acids to diets fed to weaned pigs reduced proteolytic fermentation before and after an enterotoxigenic *E. coli* (ETEC) K88 challenge (108). Three days post-infection, ETEC K88 colonized the small intestine of pigs fed the crude protein diet whereas no colonization was observed in the small intestine of pigs receiving the purified amino acid diet. In this context, undigested protein or other components associated with crude protein diets promoted ETEC growth and colonization in the small intestine.

Furthermore, the source of proteins can impact microbial communities depending on the digestibility and total amino acids in the diet (106). For instance, animal proteins tend to be highly digestible in the proximal intestine compared to plant-based proteins (109). Processing proteins with heat can impact their digestibility, for example rats fed thermolyzed (heated to 180°C for 1–2 h) casein, soy, or egg white protein had reduced proximal intestinal digestibility, leading to a greater degree of protein fermentation in the cecum (110). The number of aberrant crypts were measured after azoxymethane challenge to assess the carcinogenic promoting properties of casein, soy, and egg proteins. For the heat-treated proteins, the number of aberrant crypts increased with casein, remained unchanged with soy, and decreased with egg white compared to untreated protein diets. In agreement, a DSS mouse model study using multiple custom diets demonstrated that casein and soy proteins worsened DSS associated weight loss, whereas no effect was seen in mice fed the egg white protein diets (111). In contrast, a human trial compared high- and low-fat diets with non-meat protein (legumes, nuts, grains, soy), red meat protein (beef) or white meat protein (chicken and turkey) on the gut microbiome and found only a modest impact of protein source on the microbiome (112). For cardiovascular health, the plant-based proteins outperformed meat protein diets but white meat was no better than red meat for reducing disease risk (113). However, animal protein dominated diets tend to include higher amounts of fats, which ultimately may be more impactful on health than the proteins themselves. Plant-based protein diets may inherently contain detrimental components. For example, soybean isoflavones are suggested to contribute to greater parasitic oocyst fecal output and reduce immune responsiveness in mice fed a soy-based diet compared to casein and whey protein fed groups (114). For this reason, crude protein diet studies make it difficult to identify the bioactive component responsible for the observed phenotype. A study in rats comparing protein from soy, casein, pork, beef, chicken, and fish indicates that protein source alters microbial composition (115). Specifically, white meat (chicken and fish) increased beneficial *Lactobacillus* species. Blood levels of lipopolysaccharide-binding protein (LBP), a marker for lipopolysaccharide (LPS) endotoxemia, was found to be significantly higher in the soy protein diet group compared to fish, chicken, pork, beef, and casein protein fed groups. Further research is needed in controlled animal models to investigate isolated protein types and processing techniques on host digestion, microbiome, and fermentation products to mechanistically link the impact of protein on infection resistance.

Dietary glutamine supplementation has proven to be an effective therapy to help restore intestinal integrity in patients with post-infectious associated irritable bowel syndrome (116). Although glutamine significantly improved IBS scores compared to a placebo supplemented group, a larger cohort and mechanistic studies are warranted. The effect of glutamine supplementation may be associated with glutamines ability to enhance intestinal cell proliferation (117), decrease the Firmicute population, and activate innate immunity through NF-κB, MAPK, and PI3K-Akt signaling pathways (118). Similar effects have been observed with arginine supplementation (119). Over a 14-day study, daily supplementation of 30 g of L-glutamine to overweight individuals led to a significant decrease in Firmicute populations, including species from the genus *Dialister*, *Dorea*, *Pseudobutyrivibrio*, and *Veillonella* (120). Since overweight individuals typically have a higher Firmicute/Bacteroidetes ratio than lean individuals (121), a decrease in Firmicutes with glutamine supplementation suggests that dietary glutamine may play a beneficial role in restoring microbiota balance. In accordance, glutamine and arginine supplementation promoted the activation of innate immunity and lowered intestinal pathogen load in ETEC-infected mice (122). In humans, enteral glutamine administration in critically ill patients with severe trauma, burns, and sepsis significantly reduced the number of isolated enteric bacteria such as *Pseudomonas* sp., *Klebsiella* sp., *E. coli*, and *Acinetobacter* sp., all of which can contribute to pneumonia if transmitted to the lungs (123, 124). Enteral glutamine administration reduced bacterial overgrowth within the gastrointestinal tract, which may have reduced the chance of bacterial exposure to the lungs and explain the reduced incidence of pneumonia in patients. Moreover, a systematic review and meta-analysis concluded that glutamine-enriched enteral formulae can significantly reduce gut permeability in critically ill patients (125). The requirement and importance of enteric glutamine has been extensively reviewed (126), but

requires further research in healthy subjects and animals models to understand the impact on the microbiome and enteric infection resistance.

Further emerging evidence suggests that numerous microbially-derived indoles from tryptophan catabolism can promote intestinal homeostasis by activating regulatory T cells (Tregs) through their interaction with the aryl hydrocarbon receptor (AhR) (127). Roager and Licht summarize known microbes responsible for producing tryptophan-derivatives that positively act on tight junctions, gastrointestinal motility, host metabolism, AhR to activate IL-22, along with their systemic anti-oxidative and anti-inflammatory properties (128). In this respect, dietary tryptophan likely contributes to infection resistance by priming host defense strategies. The importance of tryptophan is further supported by the ability of host dendritic cells to metabolize tryptophan into kynurenine using indoleamine 2,3-dioxygenase-1 (IDO1) in order to control host inflammation during a *C. difficile* infection (129). Kynurenine production during *C. difficile* infection is proposed to be beneficial as it reduces excessive interferon-γ (IFNγ) cytokine production by limiting neutrophil populations in the lamina propria (129). Clinically, these findings provide important insight into the use of IDO1 inhibitors for cancer treatment which would prevent kynurenine production, and increase the severity of *C. difficile* infection (129). Like tryptophan, threonine is another essential amino acid that must be obtained from diet with deficiencies leading to immune and barrier dysfunctions (130). Dietary threonine is essential for the production of mucin with deficient diets leading to altered mucosal integrity and persistent diarrhea in neonatal piglets (131). The importance of dietary threonine for mucus production and structure may not only provide protection for host IECs but also could stimulate mucolytic bacteria with unknown functions (**Figure 3**).

Dietary protein source, amount, and processing can alter their impact and effects within gastrointestinal environment. Clearly host protein digestion shares an intimate relationship with the gut microbiome and their fermentation products (132). A balanced macronutrient or low indigestible protein diet is recommended to discourage proteolytic bacteria from overproducing cytotoxic, genotoxic, and carcinogenic by-products that disrupt intestinal integrity and increase the risk of infection (106).

PHYTOCHEMICALS

Plants synthesize a large pool of compounds known as phytochemicals to protect themselves from stress, predation, and infection. Complex mixtures of phytochemicals are found in the roots, seeds, leaves, bark, flowers, and fruit of plants and have been intensively studied for their antimicrobial, anti-inflammatory, and antioxidants activities (133). The physicochemical properties of phytochemicals give plants their unique color, smell, and flavor profiles, and dictates their bioactivities and bioavailability within the gastrointestinal tract (134). Condensed tannins, mainly polymeric flavanols can act as antinutritional factors that reduce host digestion

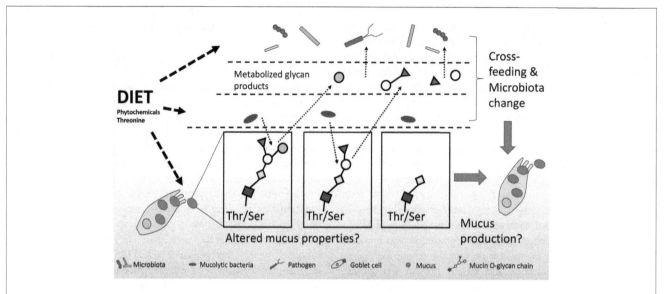

FIGURE 3 | Diet alters host-microbiota-pathogen mechanisms of mucus production and consumption. Mucolytic specialists that digest the mucus O-glycans and subsequently cross-feed with other bacteria and pathogens can lead to further microbiota changes and alterations to mucosal integrity.

through enzyme inhibition and protein precipitation (135). However, the consumption of phytochemicals is typically associated with beneficial health outcomes from their activities on the resident microbial population and host metabolism (14, 136, 137). Phytochemicals are treated as xenobiotics by the host and because of this, the liver can reintroduce phytochemical derivatives to microbes through enterohepatic circulation, further complicating their effects on host health. Many studies fail to demonstrate and characterize absorbed phytochemical derivatives to investigate whether their impact on host are direct or indirect through the microbiota.

Research has focused on the use of phytochemicals as an alternative to antibiotics and as a dietary supplement to strengthen host pathogen resistance (138). For instance, chickens fed a mixture of pepper (*Capsicum*) and turmeric oleoresin had less weight loss and reduced intestinal lesions scores in a necrotic enteritis disease model (139). The phytochemical mixture lowered intestinal but increased splenic proinflammatory cytokines/chemokines (IL-8, lipopolysaccharide-induced TNF-a factor, IL-17) levels altering host immunity through immune cell differentiation, proliferation, apoptosis and NO production (139). Reactive nitrogen and oxygen species produced by peripheral leucocytes is an essential defense strategy against pathogens. In fish, dietary supplementation of a grass extract (*Cynodon dactylon*) to infected *Catla catla* carp stimulated reactive oxygen and nitrogen species production and decreased mortality in a dose depend manner (140). Screening multiple phytonutrients revealed that the dietary flavonoid naringenin can act as an agonist on the AhR to induce regulatory T cells (Treg) that suppress allergy and autoimmune disease (141). Interestingly, phytochemicals such as indole-3-carbinol (I3C) present in cruciferous vegetables (e.g., broccoli, cabbage) act as ligands for AhR leading to the expansion of the

anti-inflammatory IL-22 producing ILCs (142). Functioning AhR has proven to be crucial for immunity because AhR-deficient mice failed to control *C. rodentium* infections (143). Moreover, mice fed a phytochemical-free diet had a reduced formation of lymphocyte aggregates and follicles, a similar phenotype as seen in AhR-deficient mice (142). Dietary I3C supplementation protected against *C. difficile* infection through activation of AhR but also through unknown AhR-independent mechanisms likely caused by changes to microbial populations (144).

Anti-adhesion properties are well sought after when studying the direct effects of phytochemicals on pathogen fitness. Cranberry extracts are documented to inhibit pathogenic *E. coli* adhesins (e.g., fimbriae) limiting their ability to attach to host cells (145, 146). The anti-adhesion activity of cranberry extract is attributed to the polyphenolic flavan-3-ol compounds known as A-type proanthocyanidins (PACs) (147). Cranberry A-type PACs reduced adherence of multiple strains uropathogenic *E. coli* and *Proteus mirabilis in vitro* (145). However, *in vivo*, intestinal and microbial PACs metabolites are found at higher concentrations in urine than the intact PACs and thus may be the bioactive metabolites responsible for the anti-adhesive properties (148). Interestingly, an analysis of urine phytochemical metabolites indicated that they change over-time due to multiple rounds of enterohepatic circulation modifications (148) with poorly understood activities (149). Moreover, cranberry PACs are thought to inhibit host and microbial enzymes (e.g., lipase, glycosidases) protecting against diet-induced obesity (150). PACs are associated with increased *Akkermansia* sp. abundance; however, it is unknown whether microbiota changes are a direct action of PACs or an indirect result of their effects on host metabolism (151). B-type PACs are known to be less inhibitory to both bacteria and host metabolism (150). Work from our group demonstrates that pea seed coats rich in B-type PACs lead to a significant decrease in the Firmicutes population, increased fecal mucin content, and caused greater pathogen colonization in mice compared to a PAC-poor diet (152). B-type PACs may have led to improper mucus formation leading to a greater concentration of mucin excreted in feces. Phytonutrient supplementation is associated with increases in beneficial Clostridia species and can strengthen mucosal barrier function by increasing mucus production and thickness (153), protecting epithelial cells from invading pathogens and disease. Interestingly, a positive feedback loop may be established between mucolytic bacteria such as *Akkermansia* sp. that can degrade mucus O-linked glycans, thereby producing SCFAs that could stimulate goblet cells to secrete more mucus (14). Polyphenolic compounds may stimulate the microbiota directly or indirectly through modulation of mucus production, however further research is needed to establish direct links between diet and infection resistance (**Figure 3**).

VITAMINS AND MINERALS

Micronutrients are essential for proper metabolic and immune function. Nutrient and mineral deficiencies, typical in those that are critically-ill and in developing countries, can lead to metabolic changes, oxidative damage, immunological defects, weakness, and death (154). The effects of essential minerals, including iron, zinc, copper, selenium, silver, sulfur, calcium, phosphorus, and magnesium have been shown to affect resident microbial populations and health outcomes in both animal and human studies (155). Phagocytes have been shown to utilize the bactericidal actions of copper and zinc to enhance intracellular killing of pathogens (156). For instance, mice fed a zinc-deficient diet and challenged with Enteroaggregative *E. coli* (EAEC) had reduced leukocyte infiltration and increased virulence factors in luminal content, indicating an impaired immune response and increased infection severity (157). Regular supplementation of vitamin C (1–2 g/day) and zinc (<100 mg/day) reduced the duration of the common cold by 8–14 and 33%, respectively (158, 159). For vitamin C, prophylactic doses >0.2 g/day alleviated respiratory associated problems, particularly in physically strained and stressed individuals, however, its use as a therapy to treat the common cold remains controversial (160). In contrast, zinc supplementation studies support its use as a treatment option to reduce the duration and severity of the common cold (159). Vitamin D had the best overall protection against the common cold, however baseline vitamin D levels and dose must be considered since lower doses and deficient individuals experienced the most benefit (158). More mechanistic research is required to understand the impact of vitamins on immune responsiveness, especially with respect to the microbe-host gut axis in deficient and in excess conditions. Experiments in germ-free, conventionalized and infectious *C. rodentium* mice models confirm that the microbiota influences vitamin D metabolism by lowering fibroblast growth factor (FGF) 23 through increased activation of TNF-α in the colon (161). The fact that the presence of the microbial community or mono-colonization with *C. rodentium* increases serum vitamin

D levels highlights their role on host homeostasis, especially since vitamin D levels control calcium homeostasis and bone formation (161). Research suggests that proper regulation of vitamins and minerals is key for establishing a proper immune response and intestinal barrier function. Similar to vitamin and mineral deficiencies, excessive supplementation can impair a host ability to resist enteric infections by altering intestinal integrity or enhancing pathogen fitness.

Recently, oral iron and vitamin B12 supplementation are suggested to impair microbiota dependent infection resistance. A systematic review and meta-analysis comprising 6831 adult participants concluded that oral ferrous sulfate (iron) supplementation is associated with a significant increase in gastrointestinal side-effects compared to placebo and intravenous iron delivery (162). This reveals that the effects of iron supplementation are possibly initiated through the microbe-gut axis with unknown consequences and should be used cautiously. For instance, excessive luminal iron affects intestinal integrity through oxygen radical production, encourages pathogen virulence, and alters microbial populations leading to pathogen overgrowth (163, 164). In a dose dependent manner, iron increased epithelial invasion and translocation of *S. typhimurium* in Caco-2 cells *in vitro* and reduced the survival of the nematode *Caenorhabditis elegans* infected with *S. typhimuriumi* (163, 165). Regulation of luminal iron is extremely important for maintaining intestinal integrity and controlling pathogen expansion (166). Furthermore, lipocalin-2 is a protein produced by neutrophils and epithelial cells during inflammation that directly limits bacterial iron uptake, reducing pathogen overgrowth and severity (167). Unlike iron, vitamin B12 is directly regulated in the gut by intrinsic factors for absorption and in excess, it can escape host absorption and affect microbial competition. The gut commensal bacteria *Bacteroides thetaiotaomicron* may compete against enterohemorrhagic *E. coli* (EHEC) to sequester dietary vitamin B12 (168). *In vitro* competition assays show that *B. thetaiotaomicron* reduced EHEC shiga toxins but when co-cultured with a mutant *B. thetaiotaomicron* lacking a vitamin B12 transporter, EHEC had normal shiga toxin production (168). Microbial vitamin B12 transporters have different affinities toward vitamin B12 allowing them to compete with host cells and other microbes to take up exogenous vitamin B12 (169, 170). More research is needed into micronutrient supplementation on host-microbe interactions toward pathogens, especially in the context of over-supplementation, which may be detrimental depending on the micronutrient balance and host intestinal homeostasis. Limiting the expansion of enteric pathogens can be accomplished by reducing their access to vitamin or minerals either through diet or stimulation of gut commensals to compete with pathogen for vital nutrients.

CONCLUSION

Pathogen resistance and tolerance requires tight host regulation of dietary components and subsequent microbial actions that together influence each other and host immunity. Undigested and unabsorbed dietary components are able to influence microbial populations and their fermentation by-products can indirectly contribute to infection resistance by modulating host intestinal integrity. Dietary intervention studies are difficult to control and compare due to seasonal variations in diets sources. We suggest that dietary intervention studies should include diet backgrounds designed with macro- and micro- nutrients that stress and protect the gastrointestinal environment, as to give a proper assessment of that dietary component on host. In general, a balanced diet of SFA, MUFA, MACs, protein, phytochemicals, vitamins, and minerals with limited sources of n-6 PUFAs, simple carbohydrates, BAPs, and iron may help restore intestinal homeostasis in compromised individuals. Dietary individuality makes it difficult to make general diet recommendations as each individual may have genetic, microbiota, and unforeseen environmental factors that influence diet digestibility and utilization. Together, these factors ultimately provide the context to which dietary components may influence intestinal integrity and homeostasis.

AUTHOR CONTRIBUTIONS

The concept of this review was developed by BW and AF. This review was written by AF and JF, and was edited by BW, AF, and JF.

FUNDING

BW was supported by the Canada Research Chair program. JF was supported by a Natural Sciences and Engineering Research Council Postdoctoral Fellowship.

REFERENCES

1. Kirk MD, Pires SM, Black RE, Caipo M, Crump JA, Devleesschauwer B, et al. World Health Organization estimates of the global and regional disease burden of 22 foodborne bacterial, protozoal, and viral diseases, 2010: a data synthesis. *PLoS Med.* (2015) 12:e1001921. doi: 10.1371/journal.pmed.1001921
2. Stecher B. The roles of inflammation, nutrient availability and the commensal microbiota in enteric pathogen infection. *Microbiol Spectr.* (2015) 3:297–320. doi: 10.1128/microbiolspec.MBP-0008-2014
3. Singh RK, Chang H-W, Yan D, Lee KM, Ucmak D, Wong K, et al. Influence of diet on the gut microbiome and implications for human health. *J Transl Med.* (2017) 15:73. doi: 10.1186/s12967-017-1175-y
4. Byndloss MX, Pernitzsch SR, Bäumler AJ. Healthy hosts rule within: ecological forces shaping the gut microbiota. *Mucosal Immunol.* (2018) 11:1299–305. doi: 10.1038/s41385-018-0010-y
5. Manzel A, Muller DN, Hafler DA, Erdman SE, Linker RA, Kleinewietfeld M. Role of "Western diet" in inflammatory autoimmune diseases. *Curr Allergy Asthma Rep.* (2014) 14:404. doi: 10.1007/s11882-013-0404-6
6. Soldati L, Di Renzo L, Jirillo E, Ascierto PA, Marincola FM, De Lorenzo A. The influence of diet on anti-cancer immune responsiveness. *J Transl Med.* (2018) 16:75. doi: 10.1186/s12967-018-1448-0
7. Ananthakrishnan AN. Epidemiology and risk factors for IBD. *Nat Rev Gastroenterol Hepatol.* (2015) 12:205–17. doi: 10.1038/nrgastro.2015.34
8. Singh H, Nugent Z, Yu BN, Lix LM, Targownik LE, Bernstein CN. Higher incidence of *Clostridium difficile* infection among individuals with inflammatory bowel disease. *Gastroenterology.* (2017) 153:430–8.e2. doi: 10.1053/j.gastro.2017.04.044
9. Hong SN, Kim HJ, Kim KH, Han SJ, Ahn IM, Ahn HS. Risk of incident *Mycobacterium tuberculosis* infection in patients with inflammatory bowel disease: a nationwide population-based study in South Korea. *Aliment Pharmacol Ther.* (2017) 45:253–63. doi: 10.1111/apt.13851
10. Martinez-Medina M, Denizot J, Dreux N, Robin F, Billard E, Bonnet R, et al. Western diet induces dysbiosis with increased e coli in CEABAC10 mice, alters host barrier function favouring AIEC colonisation. *Gut.* (2014) 63:116–24. doi: 10.1136/gutjnl-2012-304119
11. Hryckowian AJ, Van Treuren W, Smits SA, Davis NM, Gardner JO, Bouley DM, et al. Microbiota-accessible carbohydrates suppress *Clostridium difficile* infection in a murine model. *Nat Microbiol.* (2018) 3:662–9. doi: 10.1038/s41564-018-0150-6
12. Makki K, Deehan EC, Walter J, Bäckhed F. The impact of dietary fiber on gut microbiota in host health and disease. *Cell Host Microbe.* (2018) 23:705–15. doi: 10.1016/j.chom.2018.05.012
13. Forchielli ML, Walker WA. The role of gut-associated lymphoid tissues and mucosal defence. *Br J Nutr.* (2005) 93:S41. doi: 10.1079/BJN20041356
14. Anhê FF, Varin TV, Le Barz M, Desjardins Y, Levy E, Roy D, et al. Gut microbiota dysbiosis in obesity-linked metabolic diseases and prebiotic potential of polyphenol-rich extracts. *Curr Obes Rep.* (2015) 4:389–400. doi: 10.1007/s13679-015-0172-9
15. Dudek-Wicher RK, Junka A, Bartoszewicz M. The influence of antibiotics and dietary components on gut microbiota. *Prz Gastroenterol.* (2018) 13:85–92. doi: 10.5114/pg.2018.76005
16. Dupont A, Heinbockel L, Brandenburg K, Hornef MW. Antimicrobial peptides and the enteric mucus layer act in concert to protect the intestinal mucosa. *Gut Microbes.* (2014) 5:761–5. doi: 10.4161/19490976.2014.972238
17. Sicard J-F, Le Bihan G, Vogeleer P, Jacques M, Harel J. Interactions of intestinal bacteria with components of the intestinal mucus. *Front Cell Infect Microbiol.* (2017) 7:387. doi: 10.3389/fcimb.2017.00387
18. Antoni L, Nuding S, Weller D, Gersemann M, Ott G, Wehkamp J, et al. Human colonic mucus is a reservoir for antimicrobial peptides. *J Crohn's Colitis.* (2013) 7:e652–64. doi: 10.1016/j.crohns.2013.05.006
19. Willing BP, Russell SL, Finlay BB. Shifting the balance: antibiotic effects on host-microbiota mutualism. *Nat Rev Microbiol.* (2011) 9:233–43. doi: 10.1038/nrmicro2536
20. Wlodarska M, Willing B, Keeney KM, Menendez A, Bergstrom KS, Gill N, et al. Antibiotic treatment alters the colonic mucus layer and predisposes the host to exacerbated *Citrobacter rodentium*-induced colitis. *Infect Immun.* (2011) 79:1536–45. doi: 10.1128/IAI.01104-10
21. Menendez A, Willing BP, Montero M, Wlodarska M, So CC, Bhinder G, et al. Bacterial stimulation of the TLR-MyD88 pathway modulates the homeostatic expression of ileal paneth cell α-defensins. *J Innate Immun.* (2013) 5:39–49. doi: 10.1159/000341630
22. Cash HL. Symbiotic bacteria direct expression of an intestinal bactericidal lectin. *Science.* (2006) 313:1126–30. doi: 10.1126/science.1127119
23. Mantis NJ, Rol N, Corthésy B. Secretory IgA's complex roles in immunity and mucosal homeostasis in the gut. *Mucosal Immunol.* (2011) 4:603–11. doi: 10.1038/mi.2011.41
24. Donaldson GP, Ladinsky MS, Yu KB, Sanders JG, Yoo BB, Chou WC, et al. Gut microbiota utilize immunoglobulin a for mucosal colonization. *Science.* (2018) 360:795–800. doi: 10.1126/science.aaq0926
25. Knaus UG, Hertzberger R, Pircalabioru GG, Yousefi SPM, Branco Dos Santos F. Pathogen control at the intestinal mucosa - H2O2 to the rescue. *Gut Microbes.* (2017) 8:67–74. doi: 10.1080/19490976.2017.1279378
26. Pine GM, Batugedara HM, Nair MG. Here, there and everywhere: resistin-like molecules in infection, inflammation, and metabolic disorders. *Cytokine.* (2018) 110:442–51. doi: 10.1016/j.cyto.2018.05.014
27. Pickard JM, Chervonsky AV. Intestinal fucose as a mediator of host-microbe symbiosis. *J Immunol.* (2015) 194:5588–93. doi: 10.4049/jimmunol.1500395
28. Faber F, Thiennimitr P, Spiga L, Byndloss MX, Litvak Y, Lawhon S, et al. Respiration of microbiota-derived 1,2-propanediol

drives salmonella expansion during colitis. *PLoS Pathog.* (2017) 13:e1006129. doi: 10.1371/journal.ppat.1006129

29. Hug H, Mohajeri MH, La Fata G. Toll-like receptors: regulators of the immune response in the human gut. *Nutrients.* (2018) 10:11–3. doi: 10.3390/nu10020203

30. Klose CSN, Artis D. Innate lymphoid cells as regulators of immunity, inflammation and tissue homeostasis. *Nat Immunol.* (2016) 17:765–74. doi: 10.1038/ni.3489

31. Gury-BenAri M, Thaiss CA, Serafini N, Winter DR, Giladi A, Lara-Astiaso D, et al. The spectrum and regulatory landscape of intestinal innate lymphoid cells are shaped by the microbiome. *Cell.* (2016) 166:1231–46.e13. doi: 10.1016/j.cell.2016.07.043

32. Goodman BE. Insights into digestion and absorption of major nutrients in humans. *Adv Physiol Educ.* (2010) 34:44–53. doi: 10.1152/advan.00094.2009

33. Desai MS, Seekatz AM, Koropatkin NM, Kamada N, Hickey CA, Wolter M, et al. A dietary fiber-deprived gut microbiota degrades the colonic mucus barrier and enhances pathogen susceptibility. *Cell.* (2016) 167:1339–53.e21. doi: 10.1016/j.cell.2016.10.043

34. Mergenthaler P, Lindauer U, Dienel GA, Meisel A. Sugar for the brain: the role of glucose in physiological and pathological brain function. *Trends Neurosci.* (2013) 36:587–97. doi: 10.1016/j.tins.2013.07.001

35. Ingels C, Vanhorebeek I, Van den Berghe G. Glucose homeostasis, nutrition and infections during critical illness. *Clin Microbiol Infect.* (2018) 24:10–5. doi: 10.1016/j.cmi.2016.12.033

36. Thaiss CA, Levy M, Grosheva I, Zheng D, Soffer E, Blacher E, et al. Hyperglycemia drives intestinal barrier dysfunction and risk for enteric infection. *Science.* (2018) 1383:eaar3318. doi: 10.1126/science.aar3318

37. Marfella R, Quagliaro L, Nappo F, Ceriello A, Giugliano D, Pennathur S, et al. Acute hyperglycemia induces an oxidative stress in healthy subjects. *J Clin Invest.* (2001) 108:635–6. doi: 10.1172/JCI13727

38. van der Kooij MA, Jene T, Treccani G, Miederer I, Hasch A, Voelxen N, et al. Chronic social stress-induced hyperglycemia in mice couples individual stress susceptibility to impaired spatial memory. *Proc Natl Acad Sci USA.* (2018) 115:E10187–96. doi: 10.1073/pnas.1804412115

39. Jafar N, Edriss H, Nugent K. The effect of short-term hyperglycemia on the innate immune system. *Am J Med Sci.* (2016) 351:201–11. doi: 10.1016/j.amjms.2015.11.011

40. Martens EC, Neumann M, Desai MS. Interactions of commensal and pathogenic microorganisms with the intestinal mucosal barrier. *Nat Rev Microbiol.* (2018) 16:457–70. doi: 10.1038/s41579-018-0036-x

41. Collins J, Robinson C, Danhof H, Knetsch CW, Van Leeuwen HC, Lawley TD, et al. Dietary trehalose enhances virulence of epidemic *Clostridium difficile*. *Nature.* (2018) 553:291–4. doi: 10.1038/nature25178

42. Richards AB, Krakowka S, Dexter LB, Schmid H, Wolterbeek APM, Waalkens-Berendsen DH, et al. Trehalose: a review of properties, history of use and human tolerance, and results of multiple safety studies. *Food Chem Toxicol.* (2002) 40:871–98. doi: 10.1016/S0278-6915(02)00011-X

43. Argüelles JC. Why can't vertebrates synthesize trehalose? *J Mol Evol.* (2014) 79:111–6. doi: 10.1007/s00239-014-9645-9

44. Baktash A, Terveer EM, Zwittink RD, Hornung BVH, Corver J, Kuijper EJ, et al. Mechanistic insights in the success of fecal microbiota transplants for the treatment of *Clostridium difficile* infections. *Front Microbiol.* (2018) 9:1242. doi: 10.3389/fmicb.2018.01242

45. Eswaran S, Muir J, Chey WD. Fiber and functional gastrointestinal disorders. *Am J Gastroenterol.* (2013) 108:718–27. doi: 10.1038/ajg.2013.63

46. Mussatto SI, Mancilha IM. Non-digestible oligosaccharides: a review. *Carbohydr Polym.* (2007) 68:587–97. doi: 10.1016/j.carbpol.2006.12.011

47. Belorkar SA, Gupta AK. Oligosaccharides: a boon from nature's desk. *AMB Express.* (2016) 6:82 doi: 10.1186/s13568-016-0253-5

48. Singh SP, Jadaun JS, Narnoliya LK, Pandey A. Prebiotic oligosaccharides: special focus on fructooligosaccharides, its biosynthesis and bioactivity. *Appl Biochem Biotechnol.* (2017) 183:613–35. doi: 10.1007/s12010-017-2605-2

49. Suares NC, Ford AC. Systematic review: the effects of fibre in the management of chronic idiopathic constipation. *Aliment Pharmacol Ther.* (2011) 33:895–901. doi: 10.1111/j.1365-2036.2011.04602.x

50. Souza D da S, Tahan S, Weber TK, de Araujo-Filho HB, de Morais MB. Randomized, double-blind, placebo-controlled parallel clinical trial assessing the effect of fructooligosaccharides in infants with constipation. *Nutrients.* (2018) 10:E1602. doi: 10.3390/nu10111602

51. Beleli CAV, Antonio MARGM, Dos Santos R, Pastore GM, Lomazi EA. Effect of 4′ galactooligosaccharide on constipation symptoms. *J Pediatr.* (2015) 91:567–73. doi: 10.1016/j.jped.2015.01.010

52. Yang J, Wang HP, Zhou L, Xu CF. Effect of dietary fiber on constipation: a meta-analysis. *World J Gastroenterol.* (2012) 18:7378–83. doi: 10.3748/wjg.v18.i48.7378

53. Ho KS, Tan CYM, Daud MAM, Seow-Choen F. Stopping or reducing dietary fiber intake reduces constipation and its associated symptoms. *World J Gastroenterol.* (2012) 18:4593–6. doi: 10.3748/wjg.v18.i33.4593

54. Eswaran S, Farida JP, Green J, Miller JD, Chey WD. Nutrition in the management of gastrointestinal diseases and disorders: the evidence for the low FODMAP diet. *Curr Opin Pharmacol.* (2017) 37:151–7. doi: 10.1016/j.coph.2017.10.008

55. Rao SSC, Yu S, Fedewa A. Systematic review: dietary fibre and FODMAP-restricted diet in the management of constipation and irritable bowel syndrome. *Aliment Pharmacol Ther.* (2015) 41:1256–70. doi: 10.1111/apt.13167

56. Krompiewski S. Graphene nanoribbons with end- and side-contacted electrodes. *Acta Phys Pol A.* (2012) 121:1216–8. doi: 10.12693/APhysPolA.121.1216

57. Hamer HM, Jonkers D, Venema K, Vanhoutvin S, Troost FJ, Brummer RJ. Review article: the role of butyrate on colonic function. *Aliment Pharmacol Ther.* (2008) 27:104–9. doi: 10.1111/j.1365-2036.2007.03562.x

58. Litvak Y, Byndloss MX, Bäumler AJ. Colonocyte metabolism shapes the gut microbiota. *Science.* (2018) 362:eaat9076. doi: 10.1126/science.aat9076

59. Kelly CJ, Zheng L, Campbell EL, Saeedi B, Scholz CC, Bayless AJ, et al. Crosstalk between microbiota-derived short-chain fatty acids and intestinal epithelial HIF augments tissue barrier function. *Cell Host Microbe.* (2015) 17:662–71. doi: 10.1016/j.chom.2015.03.005

60. Louis NA, Hamilton KE, Canny G, Shekels LL, Ho SB, Colgan SP. Selective induction of mucin-3 by hypoxia in intestinal epithelia. *J Cell Biochem.* (2006) 99:1616–27. doi: 10.1002/jcb.20947

61. Kelly CJ, Glover LE, Campbell EL, Kominsky DJ, Ehrentraut SF, Bowers BE, et al. Fundamental role for HIF-1α in constitutive expression of human β defensin-1. *Mucosal Immunol.* (2013) 6:1110–8. doi: 10.1038/mi.2013.6

62. Troeger C, Forouzanfar M, Rao PC, Khalil I, Brown A, Reiner RC, et al. Estimates of global, regional, and national morbidity, mortality, and aetiologies of diarrhoeal diseases: a systematic analysis for the Global Burden of Disease Study 2015. *Lancet Infect Dis.* (2017) 17:909–48. doi: 10.1016/S1473-3099(17)30276-1

63. Popkin BM, Adair L, Akin JS, Black R, Briscoe J, Flieger W. Breast-feeding and diarrheal morbidity. *Pediatrics.* (1990) 86:874–82.

64. Le Doare K, Holder B, Bassett A, Pannaraj PS. Mother's milk: a purposeful contribution to the development of the infant microbiota and immunity. *Front Immunol.* (2018) 9:361. doi: 10.3389/fimmu.2018.00361

65. Craft KM, Thomas HC, Townsend SD. Interrogation of human milk oligosaccharide fucosylation patterns for antimicrobial and antibiofilm trends in group B streptococcus. *ACS Infect Dis.* (2018) 4:1755–65. doi: 10.1021/acsinfecdis.8b00234

66. Andreas NJ, Kampmann B, Mehring Le-Doare K. Human breast milk: a review on its composition and bioactivity. *Early Hum Dev.* (2015) 91:629–35. doi: 10.1016/j.earlhumdev.2015.08.013

67. Andersson B, Porras O, Hanson L, Lagergård T, Svanborg-Eden C. Inhibition of attachment of streptococcus pneumoniae and haemophilus influenza by human milk and receptor oligosaccharides. *J Infect Dis.* (1986) 153:368–70. doi: 10.1093/infdis/153.2.232

68. Coppa GV, Zampini L, Galeazzi T, Facinelli B, Ferrante L, Capretti R, et al. Human milk oligosaccharides inhibit the adhesion to Caco-2 cells of diarrheal pathogens: *Escherichia coli, Vibrio cholerae,* and *Salmonella fyris. Pediatr Res.* (2006) 59:377–82. doi: 10.1203/01.pdr.0000200805.45593.17

69. Manthey CF, Autran CA, Eckmann L, Bode L. Human milk oligosaccharides reduce EPEC attachment *in vitro* and EPEC colonization in mice. *J Pediatr Gastroenterol Nutr.* (2014) 58:165–8. doi: 10.1097/MPG.0000000000000172

70. Li M, Monaco MH, Wang M, Comstock SS, Kuhlenschmidt TB, Fahey GC, et al. Human milk oligosaccharides shorten rotavirus-induced diarrhea and

modulate piglet mucosal immunity and colonic microbiota. *ISME J.* (2014) 8:1609–20. doi: 10.1038/ismej.2014.10

71. Correa-Matos NJ, Donovan SM, Isaacson RE, Gaskins HR, White BA, Tappenden KA. Fermentable fiber reduces recovery time and improves intestinal function in piglets following *Salmonella typhimurium* infection. *J Nutr.* (2003) 133:1845–52. doi: 10.1093/jn/133.6.1845

72. Giovannini M, Verduci E, Gregori D, Ballali S, Soldi S, Ghisleni D, et al. Prebiotic effect of an infant formula supplemented with galacto-oligosaccharides: randomized multicenter trial. *J Am Coll Nutr.* (2014) 33:385–93. doi: 10.1080/07315724.2013.878232

73. Brown KH, Perez F, Peerson JM, Fadel J, Brunsgaard G, Ostrom KM, et al. Effect of dietary fiber (soy polysaccharide) on the severity, duration, and nutritional outcome of acute, watery diarrhea in children. *Pediatrics.* (1993) 92:241–7.

74. Vanderhoof JA, Murray ND, Paule CL, Ostrom KM. Use of soy fiber in acute diarrhea in infants and toddlers. *Clin Pediatr.* (1997) 36:135–9. doi: 10.1177/000992289703600303

75. Park Y, Subar AF, Hollenbeck A, Schatzkin A. Dietary fiber intake and mortality in the NIH-AARP diet and health study. *Arch Intern Med.* (2011) 171:1061–8. doi: 10.1001/archinternmed.2011.18

76. Vulevic J, Drakoularakou A, Yaqoob P, Tzortzis G, Gibson GR. Modulation of the fecal microflora profile and immune function by a novel trans-galactooligosaccharide mixture (B-GOS) in healthy elderly volunteers. *Am J Clin Nutr.* (2008) 88:1438–46. doi: 10.3945/ajcn.2008.26242

77. Drakoularakou A, Tzortzis G, Rastall RA, Gibson GR. A double-blind, placebo-controlled, randomized human study assessing the capacity of a novel galacto-oligosaccharide mixture in reducing travellers' diarrhoea. *Eur J Clin Nutr.* (2010) 64:146–52. doi: 10.1038/ejcn.2009.120

78. Leffler DA, Lamont JT. *Clostridium difficile* infection. *N Engl J Med.* (2015) 372:1539–48. doi: 10.1056/NEJMra1403772

79. Verspreet J, Damen B, Broekaert WF, Verbeke K, Delcour JA, Courtin CM. A critical look at prebiotics within the dietary fiber concept. *Annu Rev Food Sci Technol.* (2016) 7:167–90. doi: 10.1146/annurev-food-081315-032749

80. Brown GD, Gordon S. Immune recognition: a new receptor for β-glucans. *Nature.* (2001) 413:36–7. doi: 10.1038/35092620

81. Yun CH, Estrada A, Van Kessel A, Park BC, Laarveld B. β-Glucan, extracted from oat, enhances disease resistance against bacterial and parasitic infections. *FEMS Immunol Med Microbiol.* (2003) 35:67–75. doi: 10.1016/S0928-8244(02)00460-1

82. Hashimoto K, Suzuki I, Yadomae T. Oral administration of SSG, a β-glucan obtained from *Sclerotinia sclerotiorum*, affects the function of Peyer's patch cells. *Int J Immunopharmacol.* (1991) 13:437–42. doi: 10.1016/0192-0561(91)90014-X

83. Abid Obaid K, Ahmad S, Manzoor Khan H, Ali Mahdi A, Khanna R. Protective effect of L. donovani antigens using glucan as an adjuvant. *Int J Immunopharmacol.* (1989) 11:229–35. doi: 10.1016/0192-0561(89)90159-8

84. Nguyen ND, Van Dang P, Le AQ, Nguyen TKL, Pham DH, Van Nguyen N, et al. Effect of oligochitosan and oligo-β-glucan supplementation on growth, innate immunity, and disease resistance of striped catfish (*Pangasianodon hypophthalmus*). *Biotechnol Appl Biochem.* (2017) 64:564–71. doi: 10.1002/bab.1513

85. Tian X, Shao Y, Wang Z, Guo Y. Effects of dietary yeast β-glucans supplementation on growth performance, gut morphology, intestinal *Clostridium perfringens* population and immune response of broiler chickens challenged with necrotic enteritis. *Anim Feed Sci Technol.* (2016) 215:144–55. doi: 10.1016/j.anifeedsci.2016.03.009

86. Shao Y, Wang Z, Tian X, Guo Y, Zhang H. Yeast β-d-glucans induced antimicrobial peptide expressions against Salmonella infection in broiler chickens. *Int J Biol Macromol.* (2016) 85:573–84. doi: 10.1016/j.ijbiomac.2016.01.031

87. Liu AG, Ford NA, Hu FB, Zelman KM, Mozaffarian D, Kris-Etherton PM. A healthy approach to dietary fats: understanding the science and taking action to reduce consumer confusion. *Nutr J.* (2017) 16:1–15. doi: 10.1186/s12937-017-0271-4

88. Agans R, Gordon A, Kramer DL, Perez-Burillo S, Rufián-Henares JA, Paliy O. Dietary fatty acids sustain growth of human gut microbiota. *Appl Environ Microbiol.* (2018) 84:e01525-18. doi: 10.1128/AEM.01525-18

89. Ridlon JM, Wolf PG, Gaskins HR. Taurocholic acid metabolism by gut microbes and colon cancer. *Gut Microbes.* (2016) 7:201–15. doi: 10.1080/19490976.2016.1150414

90. Ghazalpour A, Cespedes I, Bennett BJ, Allayee H. Expanding role of gut microbiota in lipid metabolism. *Curr Opin Lipidol.* (2016) 27:141–7. doi: 10.1097/MOL.0000000000000278

91. Quin C, Gibson DL. Dietary lipids and enteric infection in rodent models. In: Patel VB, editor. *The Molecular Nutrition of Fats.* Elsevier (2019). p. 49–64. doi: 10.1016/B978-0-12-811297-7.00004-4

92. DeCoffe D, Quin C, Gill SK, Tasnim N, Brown K, Godovannyi A, et al. Dietary lipid type, rather than total number of calories, alters outcomes of enteric infection in mice. *J Infect Dis.* (2016) 213:1846–56. doi: 10.1093/infdis/jiw084

93. Devkota S, Wang Y, Musch M. 43 dietary fat-induced taurocholic acid production promotes pathobiont and colitis in IL-10$^{-/-}$ mice. *Gastroenterology.* (2012) 142:S–12. doi: 10.1016/S0016-5085(12)60043-2

94. Gunsalus KTW, Tornberg-Belanger SN, Matthan NR, Lichtenstein AH, Kumamoto CA. Manipulation of host diet to reduce gastrointestinal colonization by the opportunistic pathogen candida albicans. *mSphere.* (2016) 1:e00020–15. doi: 10.1128/mSphere.00020-15

95. Shilling M, Matt L, Rubin E, Visitacion MP, Haller NA, Grey SF, et al. Antimicrobial effects of virgin coconut oil and its medium-chain fatty acids on *Clostridium difficile*. *J Med Food.* (2013) 16:1079–85. doi: 10.1089/jmf.2012.0303

96. Kaliannan K, Wang B, Li XY, Kim KJ, Kang JX. A host-microbiome interaction mediates the opposing effects of omega-6 and omega-3 fatty acids on metabolic endotoxemia. *Sci Rep.* (2015) 5:11276. doi: 10.1038/srep11276

97. Hekmatdoost A, Wu X, Morampudi V, Innis SM, Jacobson K. Dietary oils modify the host immune response and colonic tissue damage following *Citrobacter rodentium* infection in mice. *AJP Gastrointest Liver Physiol.* (2013) 304:G917–28. doi: 10.1152/ajpgi.00292.2012

98. Husson MO, Ley D, Portal C, Gottrand M, Hueso T, Desseyn JL, et al. Modulation of host defence against bacterial and viral infections by omega-3 polyunsaturated fatty acids. *J Infect.* (2016) 73:523–35. doi: 10.1016/j.jinf.2016.10.001

99. Jones GJB, Roper RL. The effects of diets enriched in omega-3 polyunsaturated fatty acids on systemic vaccinia virus infection. *Sci Rep.* (2017) 7:15999. doi: 10.1038/s41598-017-16098-7

100. Lavallee CM, Lim DW, Wizzard PR, Mazurak VC, Mi S, Curtis JM, et al. Impact of clinical use of parenteral lipid emulsions on bile acid metabolism and composition in neonatal piglets. *JPEN J Parenter Enter Nutr.* (2018) 43:668–76. doi: 10.1002/jpen.1437

101. Li P, Yin Y, Li D, Woo Kim S, Wu G. Amino acids and immune function. *Br J Nutr.* (2007) 98:237. doi: 10.1017/S000711450769936X

102. Ren W, Rajendran R, Zhao Y, Tan B, Wu G, Bazer FW, et al. Amino acids as mediators of metabolic cross talk between host and pathogen. *Front Immunol.* (2018) 9:319. doi: 10.3389/fimmu.2018.00319

103. Jonker R, Engelen MPKJ, Deutz NEP. Role of specific dietary amino acids in clinical conditions. *Br J Nutr.* (2012) 108(Suppl.):S139–48. doi: 10.1017/S0007114512002358

104. Bartelt LA, Bolick DT, Kolling GL, Roche JK, Zaenker EI, Lara AM, et al. Cryptosporidium priming is more effective than vaccine for protection against cryptosporidiosis in a murine protein malnutrition model. *PLoS Negl Trop Dis.* (2016) 10:e0004820. doi: 10.1371/journal.pntd.0004820

105. Ochi T, Feng Y, Kitamoto S, Nagao-Kitamoto H, Kuffa P, Atarashi K, et al. Diet-dependent, microbiota-independent regulation of IL-10-producing lamina propria macrophages in the small intestine. *Sci Rep.* (2016) 6:27634. doi: 10.1038/srep27634

106. Ma N, Tian Y, Wu Y, Ma X. Contributions of the interaction between dietary protein and gut microbiota to intestinal health. *Curr Protein Pept Sci.* (2017) 18:795–808. doi: 10.2174/1389203718666170216153505

107. Yao CK, Muir JG, Gibson PR. Review article: insights into colonic protein fermentation, its modulation and potential health implications. *Aliment Pharmacol Ther.* (2016) 43:181–96. doi: 10.1111/apt.13456

108. Opapeju FO, Krause DO, Payne RL, Rademacher M, Nyachoti CM. Effect of dietary protein level on growth performance, indicators of enteric health, and gastrointestinal microbial ecology of weaned pigs induced with postweaning colibacillosis. *J Anim Sci.* (2009) 87:2635–43. doi: 10.2527/jas.2008-1310

109. Windey K, de Preter V, Verbeke K. Relevance of protein fermentation to gut health. *Mol Nutr Food Res.* (2012) 56:184–96. doi: 10.1002/mnfr.201100542

110. Corpet DE, Yin Y, Zhang XM, Rémésy C, Stamp D, Medline A, et al. Colonic protein fermentation and promotion of colon carcinogenesis by thermolyzed casein. *Nutr Cancer.* (1995) 23:271–81. doi: 10.1080/01635589509514381

111. Llewellyn SR, Britton GJ, Contijoch EJ, Vennaro OH, Mortha A, Colombel JF, et al. Interactions between diet and the intestinal microbiota alter intestinal permeability and colitis severity in mice. *Gastroenterology.* (2018) 154:1037–46.e2. doi: 10.1053/j.gastro.2017.11.030

112. Lang JM, Pan C, Cantor RM, Tang WHW, Garcia-Garcia JC, Kurtz I, et al. Impact of individual traits, saturated fat, and protein source on the gut microbiome. *MBio.* (2018) 9:1–14. doi: 10.1128/mBio.01604-18

113. Bergeron N, Chiu S, Williams PT, King SM, Krauss RM. Effects of red meat, white meat, and nonmeat protein sources on atherogenic lipoprotein measures in the context of low compared with high saturated fat intake: a randomized controlled trial. *Am J Clin Nutr.* 110:24–33. (2019). doi: 10.1093/ajcn/nqz035

114. Ford JT, Wong CW, Colditz IG. Effects of dietary protein types on immune responses and levels of infection with *Eimeria vermiformis* in mice. *Immunol Cell Biol.* (2001) 79:23–8. doi: 10.1046/j.1440-1711.2001.00788.x

115. Zhu Y, Lin X, Zhao F, Shi X, Li H, Li Y, et al. Meat, dairy and plant proteins alter bacterial composition of rat gut bacteria. *Sci Rep.* (2015) 5:15220. doi: 10.1038/srep16546

116. Zhou Q, Verne ML, Fields JZ, Lefante JJ, Basra S, Salameh H, et al. Randomised placebo-controlled trial of dietary glutamine supplements for postinfectious irritable bowel syndrome. *Gut.* (2018) 68:996–1002. doi: 10.1136/gutjnl-2017-315136

117. Ren W, Duan J, Yin J, Liu G, Cao Z, Xiong X, et al. Dietary l-glutamine supplementation modulates microbial community and activates innate immunity in the mouse intestine. *Amino Acids.* (2014) 46:2403–13. doi: 10.1007/s00726-014-1793-0

118. Chen S, Xia Y, Zhu G, Yan J, Tan C, Deng B, et al. Glutamine supplementation improves intestinal cell proliferation and stem cell differentiation in weanling mice. *Food Nutr Res.* (2018) 62:2403–13. doi: 10.29219/fnr.v62.1439

119. Ren W, Chen S, Yin J, Duan J, Li T, Liu G, et al. Dietary arginine supplementation of mice alters the microbial population and activates intestinal innate immunity. *J Nutr.* (2014) 144:988–95. doi: 10.3945/jn.114.192120

120. Zambom de Souza AZ, Zambom AZ, Abboud KY, Reis SK, Tannihão F, Guadagnini D, et al. Oral supplementation with l-glutamine alters gut microbiota of obese and overweight adults: a pilot study. *Nutrition.* (2015) 31:884–9. doi: 10.1016/j.nut.2015.01.004

121. Koliada A, Syzenko G, Moseiko V, Budovska L, Puchkov K, Perederiy V, et al. Association between body mass index and Firmicutes/Bacteroidetes ratio in an adult Ukrainian population. *BMC Microbiol.* (2017) 17:120. doi: 10.1186/s12866-017-1027-1

122. Liu G, Ren W, Fang J, Hu CAA, Guan G, Al-Dhabi NA, et al. l-Glutamine and l-arginine protect against enterotoxigenic *Escherichia coli* infection via intestinal innate immunity in mice. *Amino Acids.* (2017) 49:1945–54. doi: 10.1007/s00726-017-2410-9

123. Conejero R, Bonet A, Grau T, Esteban A, Mesejo A, Montejo JC, et al. Effect of a glutamine-enriched enteral diet on intestinal permeability and infectious morbidity at 28 days in critically ill patients with systemic inflammatory response syndrome: a randomized, single-blind, prospective, multicenter study. *Nutrition.* (2002) 18:716–21. doi: 10.1016/S0899-9007(02)00847-X

124. Sader HS, Castanheira M, Mendes RE, Flamm RK. Frequency and antimicrobial susceptibility of Gram-negative bacteria isolated from patients with pneumonia hospitalized in ICUs of US medical centres (2015–17). *J Antimicrob Chemother.* (2018) 73:3053–9. doi: 10.1093/jac/dky279

125. Mottaghi A, Yeganeh MZ, Golzarand M, Jambarsang S, Mirmiran P. Efficacy of glutamine-enriched enteral feeding formulae in critically ill patients: a systematic review and meta-analysis of randomized controlled trials. *Asia Pac J Clin Nutr.* (2016) 25:504–12. doi: 10.6133/apjcn.092015.24

126. Biolo G. Protein metabolism and requirements. *World Rev Nutr Diet.* (2013) 105:12–20. doi: 10.1159/000341545

127. Mezrich JD, Fechner JH, Zhang X, Johnson BP, Burlingham WJ, Bradfield CA. An interaction between kynurenine and the aryl hydrocarbon receptor can generate regulatory T cells. *J Immunol.* (2010) 185:3190–8. doi: 10.4049/jimmunol.0903670

128. Roager HM, Licht TR. Microbial tryptophan catabolites in health and disease. *Nat Commun.* (2018) 9:1–10. doi: 10.1038/s41467-018-05470-4

129. El-Zaatari M, Chang Y-M, Zhang M, Franz M, Shreiner A, McDermott AJ, et al. Tryptophan catabolism restricts IFN-γ-expressing neutrophils and *Clostridium difficile* immunopathology. *J Immunol.* (2014) 193:807–16. doi: 10.4049/jimmunol.1302913

130. Dong YW, Feng L, Jiang WD, Liu Y, Wu P, Jiang J, et al. Dietary threonine deficiency depressed the disease resistance, immune and physical barriers in the gills of juvenile grass carp (*Ctenopharyngodon idella*) under infection of *Flavobacterium columnare*. *Fish Shellfish Immunol.* (2018) 72:161–73. doi: 10.1016/j.fsi.2017.10.048

131. Law GK, Bertolo RF, Adjiri-Awere A, Pencharz PB, Ball RO. Adequate oral threonine is critical for mucin production and gut function in neonatal piglets. *Am J Physiol Gastrointest Liver Physiol.* (2007) 292:G1293–301. doi: 10.1152/ajpgi.00221.2006

132. Diether N, Willing B. Microbial fermentation of dietary protein: an important factor in diet–microbe–host interaction. *Microorganisms.* (2019) 7:19. doi: 10.3390/microorganisms7010019

133. Ayseli MT, Ipek Ayseli Y. Flavors of the future: health benefits of flavor precursors and volatile compounds in plant foods. *Trends Food Sci Technol.* (2016) 48:69–77. doi: 10.1016/j.tifs.2015.11.005

134. Kemperman RA, Bolca S, Roger LC, Vaughan EE. Novel approaches for analysing gut microbes and dietary polyphenols: challenges and opportunities. *Microbiology.* (2010) 156:3224–31. doi: 10.1099/mic.0.042127-0

135. Gilani GS, Xiao CW, Cockell KA. Impact of antinutritional factors in food proteins on the digestibility of protein and the bioavailability of amino acids and on protein quality. *Br J Nutr.* (2012) 108(Suppl. 2):S315–32. doi: 10.1017/S0007114512002371

136. Pandey KB, Rizvi SI. Plant polyphenols as dietary antioxidants in human health and disease. *Oxid Med Cell Longev.* (2009) 2:270–8. doi: 10.4161/oxim.2.5.9498

137. Dueñas M, Muñoz-González I, Cueva C, Jiménez-Girón A, Sánchez-Patán F, Santos-Buelga C, et al. A survey of modulation of gut microbiota by dietary polyphenols. *Biomed Res Int.* (2015) 2015:850902. doi: 10.1155/2015/850902

138. Willing BP, Pepin DM, Marcolla CS, Forgie AJ, Diether NE, Bourrie BCT. Bacterial resistance to antibiotic alternatives: a wolf in sheep's clothing? *Anim Front.* (2018) 8:39–47. doi: 10.1093/af/vfy003

139. Lee SH, Lillehoj HS, Jang SI, Lillehoj EP, Min W, Bravo DM. Dietary supplementation of young broiler chickens with Capsicum and turmeric oleoresins increases resistance to necrotic enteritis. *Br J Nutr.* (2013) 110:840–7. doi: 10.1017/S0007114512006083

140. Kaleeswaran B, Ilavenil S, Ravikumar S. Dietary supplementation with *Cynodon dactylon* (L.) enhances innate immunity and disease resistance of Indian major carp, *Catla catla* (Ham.). *Fish Shellfish Immunol.* (2011) 31:953–62. doi: 10.1016/j.fsi.2011.08.013

141. Wang HK, Yeh CH, Iwamoto T, Satsu H, Shimizu M, Totsuka M. Dietary flavonoid naringenin induces regulatory T cells via an aryl hydrocarbon receptor mediated pathway. *J Agric Food Chem.* (2012) 60:2171–8. doi: 10.1021/jf204625y

142. Kiss EA, Vonarbourg C, Kopfmann S, Hobeika E, Finke D, Esser C, et al. Natural aryl hydrocarbon receptor ligands control organogenesis of intestinal lymphoid follicles. *Science.* (2011) 334:1561–5. doi: 10.1126/science.1214914

143. Qiu J, Heller JJ, Guo X, Chen ZE, Fish K, Fu Y-X, et al. The aryl hydrocarbon receptor regulates gut immunity through modulation of innate lymphoid cells. *Immunity.* (2012) 36:92–104. doi: 10.1016/j.immuni.2011.11.011

144. Julliard W, De Wolfe TJ, Fechner JH, Safdar N, Agni R, Mezrich JD. Amelioration of *Clostridium difficile* infection in mice by dietary supplementation with indole-3-carbinol. *Ann Surg.* (2017) 265:1183–91. doi: 10.1097/SLA.0000000000001830

145. Nicolosi D, Tempera G, Genovese C, Furneri P. Anti-adhesion activity of A2-type proanthocyanidins (a cranberry major component) on uropathogenic *E. coli* and *P. mirabilis* strains. *Antibiotics.* (2014) 3:143–54. doi: 10.3390/antibiotics3020143

146. Luís Â, Domingues F, Pereira L, Luís Â. Can cranberries contribute to reduce the incidence of urinary tract infections? A systematic review with meta-analysis and trial sequential analysis of clinical trials. *J Urol.* (2017) 198:614–21. doi: 10.1016/j.juro.2017.03.078

147. Howell AB. Bioactive compounds in cranberries and their role in prevention of urinary tract infections. *Mol Nutr Food Res.* (2007) 51:732–7. doi: 10.1002/mnfr.200700038

148. Peron G, Sut S, Pellizzaro A, Brun P, Voinovich D, Castagliuolo I, Dall'Acqua S. The antiadhesive activity of cranberry phytocomplex studied by metabolomics: intestinal PAC-A metabolites but not intact PAC-A are identified as markers in active urines against uropathogenic *Escherichia coli*. *Fitoterapia*. (2017) 122:67–75. doi: 10.1016/j.fitote.2017.08.014

149. Tian L, Tan Y, Chen G, Wang G, Sun J, Ou S, et al. Metabolism of anthocyanins and consequent effects on the gut microbiota. *Crit Rev Food Sci Nutr.* (2019) 59:982–91. doi: 10.1080/10408398.2018.1533517

150. Yokota K, Kimura H, Ogawa S, Akihiro T. Analysis of A-type and B-type highly polymeric proanthocyanidins and their biological activities as nutraceuticals. *J Chem.* (2013) 2013:352042. doi: 10.1155/2013/352042

151. Anhê FF, Roy D, Pilon G, Dudonné S, Matamoros S, Varin TV, et al. A polyphenol-rich cranberry extract protects from diet-induced obesity, insulin resistance and intestinal inflammation in association with increased *Akkermansia* spp. population in the gut microbiota of mice. *Gut.* (2015) 64:872–83. doi: 10.1136/gutjnl-2014-307142

152. Forgie AJ, Gao Y, Ju T, Pepin DM, Yang K, Gänzle MG, et al. Pea polyphenolics and hydrolysis processing alter microbial community structure and early pathogen colonization in mice. *J Nutr Biochem.* (2019) 67:101–10. doi: 10.1016/j.jnutbio.2019.01.012

153. Wlodarska M, Willing BP, Bravo DM, Finlay BB. Phytonutrient diet supplementation promotes beneficial Clostridia species and intestinal mucus secretion resulting in protection against enteric infection. *Sci Rep.* (2015) 5:9253. doi: 10.1038/srep09253

154. Shenkin A. Micronutrients in health and disease. *Postgrad Med J.* (2006) 82:559–67. doi: 10.1136/pgmj.2006.047670

155. Skrypnik K, Suliburska J. Association between the gut microbiota and mineral metabolism. *J Sci Food Agric.* (2018) 98:2449–60. doi: 10.1002/jsfa.8724

156. Djoko KY, Ong Clynn Y, Walker MJ, McEwan AG. The role of copper and zinc toxicity in innate immune defense against bacterial pathogens. *J Biol Chem.* (2015) 290:18954–61. doi: 10.1074/jbc.R115.647099

157. Bolick DT, Kolling GL, Moore JH, de Oliveira LA, Tung K, Philipson C, et al. Zinc deficiency alters host response and pathogen virulence in a mouse model of enteroaggregative escherichia coli-induced diarrhea. *Gut Microbes.* (2015) 5:618–27. doi: 10.4161/19490976.2014.969642

158. Rondanelli M, Miccono A, Lamburghini S, Avanzato I, Riva A, Allegrini P, et al. Self-care for common colds: the pivotal role of vitamin D, vitamin C, zinc, and echinacea in three main immune interactive clusters (physical barriers, innate and adaptive immunity) involved during an episode of common colds - practical advice on dosages. *Evid Based Complement Altern Med.* (2018) 2018:5813095. doi: 10.1155/2018/5813095

159. Hemilä H. Zinc lozenges and the common cold: a meta-analysis comparing zinc acetate and zinc gluconate, and the role of zinc dosage. *JRSM Open.* (2017) 8:205427041769429. doi: 10.1177/2054270417694291

160. Douglas R, Hemilä H, Chalker E, Treacy B. Cochrane review: vitamin C for preventing and treating the common cold. *Evid Based Child Heal A Cochrane Rev J.* (2008) 3:672–720. doi: 10.1002/ebch.266

161. Bora SA, Kennett MJ, Smith PB, Patterson AD, Cantorna MT. The gut microbiota regulates endocrine vitamin D metabolism through fibroblast growth factor 23. *Front Immunol.* (2018) 9:408. doi: 10.3389/fimmu.2018.00408

162. Tolkien Z, Stecher L, Mander AP, Pereira DIA, Powell JJ. Ferrous sulfate supplementation causes significant gastrointestinal side-effects in adults: a systematic review and meta-analysis. *PLoS ONE.* (2015) 10:e0117383. doi: 10.1371/journal.pone.0117383

163. Kortman GAM, Boleij A, Swinkels DW, Tjalsma H. Iron availability increases the pathogenic potential of *Salmonella typhimurium* and other enteric pathogens at the intestinal epithelial interface. *PLoS ONE.* (2012) 7:e29968. doi: 10.1371/journal.pone.0029968

164. Natoli M, Felsani A, Ferruzza S, Sambuy Y, Canali R, Scarino ML. Mechanisms of defence from Fe(II) toxicity in human intestinal Caco-2 cells. *Toxicol Vitr.* (2009) 23:1510–5. doi: 10.1016/j.tiv.2009.06.016

165. Kortman GAM, Mulder MLM, Richters TJW, Shanmugam NKN, Trebicka E, Boekhorst J, et al. Low dietary iron intake restrains the intestinal inflammatory response and pathology of enteric infection by food-borne bacterial pathogens. *Eur J Immunol.* (2015) 45:2553–67. doi: 10.1002/eji.201545642

166. Hurrell R, Egli I. Iron bioavailability and dietary reference values. *Am J Clin Nutr.* (2010) 91:1461S–7S. doi: 10.3945/ajcn.2010.28674F

167. Liu Z, Petersen R, Devireddy L. Impaired neutrophil function in 24p3 null mice contributes to enhanced susceptibility to bacterial infections. *J Immunol.* (2013) 190:4692–706. doi: 10.4049/jimmunol.1202411

168. Cordonnier C, Le Bihan G, Emond-Rheault JG, Garrivier A, Harel J, Jubelin G. Vitamin B12 uptake by the gut commensal bacteria bacteroides thetaiotaomicron limits the production of shiga toxin by enterohemorrhagic *Escherichia coli*. *Toxins.* (2016) 8:E14. doi: 10.3390/toxins8 010014

169. Wexler AG, Schofield WB, Degnan PH, Folta-Stogniew E, Barry NA, Goodman AL. Human gut Bacteroides capture vitamin B12 via cell surface-exposed lipoproteins. *Elife.* (2018) 7:e37138. doi: 10.7554/eLife.37138

170. Degnan PH, Barry NA, Mok KC, Taga ME, Goodman AL. Human gut microbes use multiple transporters to distinguish vitamin B12 analogs and compete in the gut. *Cell Host Microbe.* (2014) 15:47–57. doi: 10.1016/j.chom.2013.12.007

17

Transcriptional Immunoprofiling at the Tick-Virus-Host Interface During Early Stages of Tick-Borne Encephalitis Virus Transmission

Saravanan Thangamani[1,2,3*], Meghan E. Hermance[1], Rodrigo I. Santos[1], Mirko Slovak[4], Dar Heinze[5], Steven G. Widen[6] and Maria Kazimirova[4]

[1] Department of Pathology, The University of Texas Medical Branch, Galveston, TX, United States, [2] Institute for Human Infections and Immunity, The University of Texas Medical Branch, Galveston, TX, United States, [3] Center for Tropical Diseases, The University of Texas Medical Branch, Galveston, TX, United States, [4] Institute of Zoology, Slovak Academy of Sciences, Bratislava, Slovakia, [5] Department of Surgery, Center for Regenerative Medicine, Boston University and Boston Medical Center, Boston, MA, United States, [6] Department of Biochemistry and Molecular Biology, The University of Texas Medical Branch, Galveston, TX, United States

*Correspondence:
Saravanan Thangamani
sathanga@utmb.edu

Emerging and re-emerging diseases transmitted by blood feeding arthropods are significant global public health problems. Ticks transmit the greatest variety of pathogenic microorganisms of any blood feeding arthropod. Infectious agents transmitted by ticks are delivered to the vertebrate host together with saliva at the bite site. Tick salivary glands produce complex cocktails of bioactive molecules that facilitate blood feeding and pathogen transmission by modulating host hemostasis, pain/itch responses, wound healing, and both innate and adaptive immunity. In this study, we utilized Illumina Next Generation Sequencing to characterize the transcriptional immunoprofile of cutaneous immune responses to *Ixodes ricinus* transmitted tick-borne encephalitis virus (TBEV). A comparative immune gene expression analysis of TBEV-infected and uninfected tick feeding sites was performed. Our analysis reveals that ticks create an inflammatory environment at the bite site during the first 3 h of feeding, and significant differences in host responses were observed between TBEV-infected and uninfected tick feeding. Gene-expression analysis reveals modulation of inflammatory genes after 1 and 3 h of TBEV-infected tick feeding. Transcriptional levels of genes specific to chemokines and cytokines indicated a neutrophil-dominated immune response. Immunohistochemistry of the tick feeding site revealed that mononuclear phagocytes and fibroblasts are the primary target cells for TBEV infection and did not detect TBEV antigens in neutrophils. Together, the transcriptional and immunohistochemistry results suggest that early cutaneous host responses to TBEV-infected tick feeding are more inflammatory than expected and highlight the importance of inflammatory chemokine and cytokine pathways in tick-borne flavivirus transmission.

Keywords: TBEV, flavivirus, tick, *Ixodes ricinus*, cutaneous, immune response

INTRODUCTION

Tick-borne encephalitis virus (TBEV) is a zoonotic tick-borne virus in the *Flaviviridae* family (genus *Flavivirus*). It is the causative agent of tick-borne encephalitis (TBE), a serious neurological disease in humans. During the last few decades, TBE has become a widespread public health concern in Eurasia with endemic regions extending from Western and Central Europe to Siberia and parts of Asia (Süss, 2011). The various strains of TBEV are subdivided into three main subtypes that are closely related genetically and antigenically: European (Eu), Siberian (Sib), and Far-Eastern (FE) (Gritsun et al., 2003a; Mansfield et al., 2009). TBEV-Eu is widely distributed in Europe, including the European regions of Russia, while TBEV-Sib is mainly found in Russia, the Baltic countries and Finland (Mansfield et al., 2009; Kovalev and Mukhacheva, 2014). TBEV-FE is present in Far-Eastern Russia and parts of China, Japan, and the Republic of Korea (Mansfield et al., 2009). Human infections with TBEV can range from mild flu-like symptoms to severe or fatal neuroinvasive disease, often with long-term neurological symptoms. There is a correlation between the TBEV subtype and severity of disease. TBEV-FE is associated with severe neurological disease and a case fatality rate of approximately 30–40%, while the case fatality rates for TBEV-Sib and TBEV-Eu are approximately 6–8% and 1–2%, respectively (Gritsun et al., 2003a; Tonteri et al., 2013). Although the incidence rates vary from year to year and between subtypes, several thousand human TBE cases are reported annually (CDC Tick-borne Encephalitis, 2017).

In nature, the *Ixodes ricinus* tick is the primary vector for TBEV-Eu while the *Ixodes persulcatus* tick is the main vector for the TBEV-Sib and TBEV-FE (Gritsun et al., 2003b). *I. ricinus* is widely distributed throughout Europe, extending to Turkey, and northern Iran, while *I. persulcatus* is distributed across the Urals, Siberia, Far-Eastern Russia, and parts of China and Japan (Gritsun et al., 2003a; Lindquist and Vapalahti, 2008). A sympatric zone exists in northern Baltics, western Finland and northwestern Russia where the habitats for *I. ricinus* and *I. persulcatus* overlap and multiple TBEV subtypes have been recorded (Lindquist and Vapalahti, 2008; Süss, 2011; Kovalev and Mukhacheva, 2014). TBEV is maintained in natural transmission cycles involving ixodid ticks and wild-living mammalian hosts. When infected with TBEV, a tick is supposed to remain infected throughout its life cycle (Gritsun et al., 2003a). Transovarial transmission of TBEV from an infected female tick to the egg mass can occur, but this route of tick infection is not entirely efficient at maintaining TBEV within the natural tick population (Danielová et al., 2002). During the tick feeding process, TBEV-infected ticks can transmit the virus to susceptible vertebrate hosts, but they can also transmit TBEV to uninfected ticks that are co-feeding on the same host (Mansfield et al., 2009; Randolph, 2011). During co-feeding, TBEV can be transmitted even non-viremically i.e., when the ticks feed on a non-viremic or virus-immune host (Labuda et al., 1993, 1997). The local skin site of tick feeding is understood to be an important focus for early TBEV replication, and immune cell infiltrates to this feeding site are believed to serve as vehicles for TBEV transmission between co-feeding ticks (Labuda et al., 1996).

Infectious agents transmitted by ticks are delivered to the vertebrate host together with saliva at the tick feeding site. Tick-borne viruses are transmitted to the host very early during the tick feeding process. TBEV can be transmitted from the saliva of an *I. ricinus* tick to the cement cone in the skin of a host as early as 1 h after the tick attaches and initiates feeding (Alekseev et al., 1996). As *I. ricinus* and *I. persulcatus* ticks feed, TBEV replicates to higher viral titers than in unfed ticks (Alekseev and Chunikhin, 1990; Belova et al., 2012; Slovák et al., 2014). The dynamic nature of TBEV replication in ticks has also been demonstrated in field-collected ticks. In partially engorged *I. ricinus* nymphs removed from humans, TBEV prevalence was higher than in questing, unfed nymphs collected in the same region (Süss et al., 2004). Experimental data suggest that in nature, ticks secrete repeated "pulses" of a few infectious virus particles over the course of feeding (Kaufman and Nuttall, 1996). Thus, virus transmission from an infected tick to a host is a very dynamic process that begins soon after the tick initiates feeding.

Ixodid ticks must remain attached to their hosts for several days to successfully acquire a bloodmeal and complete development, and have evolved salivary countermeasures directed against the host's immune and hemostatic defenses. Tick salivary glands produce complex cocktails of biologically active molecules that facilitate blood feeding and pathogen transmission by modulating host hemostasis, pain/itch responses, wound healing, and both innate and adaptive immunity. Bioactive tick salivary molecules include those with anti-pain/itch, antiplatelet, anticoagulation, vasodilatory, immunomodulatory, and anti-inflammatory activities (Ribeiro et al., 2006, Francischetti et al., 2009; Kazimírová and Štibrániová, 2013; Wikel, 2013; Šimo et al., 2017). As the course of tick feeding progresses, salivary gland genes are differentially expressed, reflecting the dynamic and complex composition of tick saliva (Ribeiro et al., 2006; Šimo et al., 2017).

The skin is the first host organ that tick saliva and a tick-borne pathogen contact during the tick feeding process. The cutaneous interface between the tick, pathogen, and host is crucial for influencing the initial host response to tick infestation and pathogen transmission (Kazimírová et al., 2017; Šimo et al., 2017). A prior study examined the tick-induced changes in cutaneous gene expression and histopathology during the early stages of uninfected *Ixodes scapularis* feeding. Early transcriptional and histopathological changes at the feeding site of uninfected *I. scapularis* nymphs are initially characterized by modulation of host responses in resident cells, followed by progression to a neutrophil-dominated immune response after 12 h of tick feeding (Heinze et al., 2012). Similarly, a complex proinflammatory environment was observed at the Powassan virus (POWV), a North American tick-borne flavivirus, infected tick feeding site. Together these findings from the cutaneous interface provide evidence of an immunologically privileged micro-environment at the tick feeding site that is established during the early stages of POWV-infected tick feeding (Hermance and Thangamani, 2014; Hermance et al., 2016).

In the present study, Illumina Next Generation Sequencing (NGS) and immunohistochemistry are utilized to understand host immunomodulation induced by TBEV-infected *I. ricinus* feeding at the earliest stages of TBEV transmission. By studying the interactions between the host immune response and tick-mediated immunomodulation during the early hours of infected tick feeding, we can begin to understand the immunologic processes that facilitate transmission of a tick-borne flavivirus to a host.

MATERIALS AND METHODS

Ethics Statement

All experiments involving mice were performed in accordance with the animal use protocol approved by the State Veterinary and Food Administration of the Slovak Republic (permit number 1335/12-221).

Animals

Five-week-old female BALB/c mice were purchased from Dobra Voda Breeding Station, Institute of Experimental Pharmacology and Toxicology, Slovak Academy of Sciences (SAS). The animals were housed at the Institute of Virology, Biomedical Research Center, SAS (Bratislava, Slovakia) under standard conditions. Food and water were provided *ad libitum*. Upon arrival, mice were allowed to adapt to the local environment before being incorporated into the study. Mice were 6 weeks old at the start of the study. At the end of the experiment animals were euthanized by cervical dislocation under anesthesia induced by carbon dioxide.

Virus and Tick Infection

I. ricinus ticks were obtained from a laboratory colony maintained at the Institute of Zoology SAS (Bratislava, Slovakia). The F1 generation of laboratory-bred *I. ricinus* females was used for virus inoculation. TBEV (Hypr strain prepared as a 10% mouse brain suspension of 1.1×10^9 PFU/ml in Leibovitz's L-15 medium) was provided by the Institute of Virology, Biomedical Research Center, SAS. Fasting *I. ricinus* females were inoculated into the haemocoel with TBEV (5.5×10^4 PFU per tick) through the coxal plate of the second pair of legs using a digital microinjector TM system (MINJ-D-CE; Tritech Research, Inc., USA) (Kazimírová et al., 2012). By this procedure, ~100% of the ticks were found to acquire TBEV infection (Slovák et al., 2014). Inoculated ticks were incubated at room temperature and 85% relative humidity in a desiccator for 21 days prior to the infestation experiments.

Infestation of Mice by Ticks

Two groups of mice ($n = 6$ per group) were infested with either TBEV-infected or uninfected (control) *I. ricinus* females. Ticks were placed in small neoprene capsules glued on the shaved backs of the mice (two capsules per mouse, four tick females per capsule) (Kazimírová et al., 2012; Hermance and Thangamani, 2014). Ticks in each capsule were allowed to feed for either 1 or 3 h. After the allotted feeding time, skin biopsies were taken from euthanized mice, at each tick feeding site using a Premier

Uni-Punch (Premier Products Co., Plymouth Meeting, PA). For immunohistochemical analysis, skin biopsies ($n = 3$) were harvested with attached ticks and placed in 4% formaldehyde. For RNA extraction, the attached ticks were removed from the skin biopsies and the biopsies ($n = 3$) were placed in RNALater (Ambion, Life Technologies, Carlsbad, CA). Control biopsies were taken from the shaved skin of naïve tick-free mice and stored in either 4% formaldehyde or RNALater.

Cutaneous Immune Response

Total RNA was extracted as previously described (Heinze et al., 2012; Hermance and Thangamani, 2014) and RNAseq analysis (Illumina deep sequencing / NGS) was performed on these samples. Briefly, 1 μg of total RNA from mouse skin biopsies ($n = 3$) was poly A+ selected and fragmented using divalent cations and heat (94°C, 8 min). Illumina TruSeq v2 sample preparation kits (Illumina Inc., San Diego, CA) were used for the RNA-Seq library construction. Each sample library was uniquely indexed to allow combining libraries during sequencing and subsequent separation post-sequencing. NGS was performed at the NGS core facility, Sealy Center for Molecular Medicine, The University of Texas Medical Branch (UTMB). Sample libraries were analyzed by the Illumina HiSeq 1500 using a 2×50 base paired end run protocol, with TruSeq v3 sequencing-by-synthesis chemistry. Reads were aligned to the mouse mm10 reference genome using TopHat version v2.0.4. Cuffdiff version 2.0.2 was used to estimate differential gene expression between TBEV-infected and uninfected feeding sites after 1 or 3 h of tick feeding. The total dataset of 23,000 genes was filtered for p-values ≤ 0.05 and a fold change ≤ -1.5 or $\geq +1.5$. The Log_2(fold change) and p-value data for each gene expression comparison (Supplement Table 1) were then uploaded to Ingenuity Pathway Analysis (IPA) software (Ingenuity Systems, Redwood City, CA) for further transcriptional analysis of the early cutaneous immune response, as previously described (Heinze et al., 2012; Hermance and Thangamani, 2014).

Real-Time PCR Validation

Real-time PCR was used to validate the NGS data (Supplement Table 1). Skin biopsies were harvested from the feeding sites of TBEV-infected and uninfected ticks as described above. At each time point, biopsies from three mice were used for the real-time PCR validation. Fifteen gene targets were selected for real-time PCR analysis. We selected these genes based our previous studies with POWV where these genes were shown to be modulated genes of interest during the host anti-tick response to POWV infection (Hermance and Thangamani, 2014, 2015). This list also includes genes that were not differentially modulated as per RNASeq analysis. Primers were purchased from Integrated DNA Technologies and the primer sequences are provided in Supplement Table 2. Primers were mixed with IQ SYBR green supermix (Bio-Rad) and loaded into iCycler IQ PCR 96-well plates (Bio-Rad) to create customized PCR arrays where each gene was measured in triplicate. For each PCR plate, 1 μg of total RNA extracted from skin biopsies was converted into cDNA using the RT[2] First Strand kit (Qiagen). cDNA was loaded onto the 96-well PCR plates, which were run on an iCycler iQ5 real-time PCR instrument (Bio-Rad) with the following cycling protocol: 10 min at 95°C; 15 s at 95°C, 1 min 60°C for 40 cycles, and an 80-cycle (+0.5°C /cycle) 55–95°C melt curve. Every array included GAPDH as an endogenous control gene and a no-template control. The iCycler's software was used to calculate the threshold cycle (C_T) values for all analyzed genes. The delta-delta C_T method was used to calculate fold-changes in gene expression between TBEV-infected and uninfected tick feeding sites. Data normalization was achieved by correcting all C_T values to the average C_T values of the GAPDH housekeeping gene. Statistically significant differences in gene expression between the 1 vs. 3 h tick feeding time points were determined by the Student's t-test. P-values less than 0.05 were considered significant. SPSS statistical software was used.

Immunohistochemistry

The skin biopsies with attached ticks were formalin-fixed for a minimum of 48 h in 4% formaldehyde. These biopsy samples were treated with Decal (Decal Chemical Corp, Tallman, NY) for 2 h, and then paraffin-embedded (Heinze et al., 2012). Five micron paraffin sections were taken from each sample and adhered to glass slides. The slides were deparaffinized in xylene and then rehydrated in decreasing concentrations of ethanol (Hermance et al., 2016). For antigen retrieval, the slides were treated with 10 mM Tris Base + 0.05% Tween 20 (pH 10) for 20 min with microwave heating. Upon returning to room temperature, endogenous peroxidase quenching was performed by incubating the slides in 4% H_2O_2 for 30 min. The primary antibody for TBEV detection used in this study was a Hyper Mouse Immune Ascitic Fluid (HMIAF) antibody against TBEV; therefore, the Mouse-On-Mouse kit (MOM, Vector labs, Burlingame, CA) was used in order to reduce the endogenous mouse Ig background staining generated when mouse primary antibodies are used on mouse tissue (Santos et al., 2016). Slides were incubated for 1 h at room temperature with the MOM mouse Ig blocking reagent. The HMIAF primary antibody against TBEV was diluted 1:250 in the MOM diluent and incubated for 30 min at room temperature. Secondary antibody consisted of MOM biotinylated horse anti-mouse IgG reagent, which was incubated for 30 min at room temperature. The biotinylated secondary antibody was detected with a streptavidin-peroxidase ultrasensitive polymer (Sigma-Aldrich, St. Louis, MO) followed by staining with the NovaRED HRP substrate kit (Vector Laboratories Inc., Burlingame, CA). Slides were counterstained with Harris hematoxylin and coverslips were mounted using Permount (ThermoFisher Scientific, Waltham, MA). Uninfected skin and tick biopsy sections generated from uninfected tick feeding sites were used as negative controls to verify the specificity of the MIAF anti-TBEV primary antibody. Secondary antibody only (no primary antibody) controls were used to confirm that the MOM biotinylated anti-mouse IgG reagent did not bind non-specifically to cellular components.

RESULTS AND DISCUSSION

In the present study, the host cutaneous immune response to TBEV-infected *I. ricinus* feeding after 1 and 3 h of tick attachment

was investigated by Illumina NGS and immunohistochemistry. No prior studies have examined the early host immune response at the feeding site of a TBEV-infected tick. We also used the RNASeq data to check for the presence of TBEV at the infected tick feeding site by aligning the sequences against a TBEV reference genome (NM_001672). TBEV sequences were detected in the 3 hpi (hours post infection), but not in the 1 hpi samples (**Figure 1A**).

The differences in the total number of significantly up- and downregulated host genes ($p \leq 0.05$) between TBEV-infected and uninfected tick feeding sites as well as between TBEV-infected feeding sites 1 and 3 h post tick attachment are shown in **Figure 1B**. When the TBEV-infected and uninfected tick feeding sites were compared, the total number of significantly upregulated genes decreased from 1 to 3 h, while there was an overall increase in significantly downregulated genes from 1 to 3 h tick attachment. An online tool (Oliveros, 2007) was used to generate a Venn diagram showing the overlap of significantly modulated genes between the 1 and 3 h comparison of the TBEV-infected vs. uninfected tick feeding sites (**Figure 1C**). 10.2% of significantly modulated genes were shared between the three comparisons; however, the majority of significantly modulated genes were unique to either the 1 h TBEV-infected vs. 1 h uninfected tick feeding site (18.7%), the 3 h TBEV-infected vs. 3 h uninfected tick feeding site (25.7%), or the 3 h TBEV-infected vs. 1 h TBEV-infected tick feeding site (14%). Additionally, a list of all modulated genes at either time point in the study was used to generate a heat map (**Figure 1D**). This heat map suggests that after 1 h of TBEV-infected tick feeding, there was a pattern of mostly upregulated cutaneous genes; however, after 3 h, the pattern changed to downregulation. This pattern of gene expression was further validated by the real-time PCR data. Though we could not recapitulate the exact fold changes of the selected immune genes observed by RNASeq data, our data clearly concur with the expression pattern of the selected genes: upregulation at 1 hpi and downregulation at 3 hpi (**Figure 1E**). Together these data suggest that a distinctive cutaneous immune response profile exists after 1 h of TBEV-infected tick feeding, but it changes to reflect a new and unique profile after 3 h. This change in gene expression profile could be attributed to the dynamic salivary secretion and physical injury during tick attachment/feeding mechanisms.

Ingenuity Pathway Analysis

In total, 1,548 genes were analyzed by Ingenuity Pathway Analysis (IPA) software (Supplement Table 1). The focus of the present study is on the cutaneous immune response observed at the TBEV-infected vs. the uninfected tick feeding sites after 1 and 3 h of tick feeding. The networks generated from IPA analysis illustrate the interrelationships between genes and the temporal changes in gene modulation. The top IPA-generated networks are shown for the TBEV-infected vs. uninfected tick feeding sites after 1 h of tick feeding (**Figure 2A**), the TBEV-infected vs. uninfected tick feeding sites after 3 h of tick feeding (**Figure 2B**), and the TBEV-infected tick feeding site after 3 h of tick feeding vs. the TBEV-infected tick feeding site after 1 h of feeding (**Figure 2C**). The three bio-functions most associated

Transcriptional Immunoprofiling at the Tick-Virus-Host Interface During Early Stages...

227

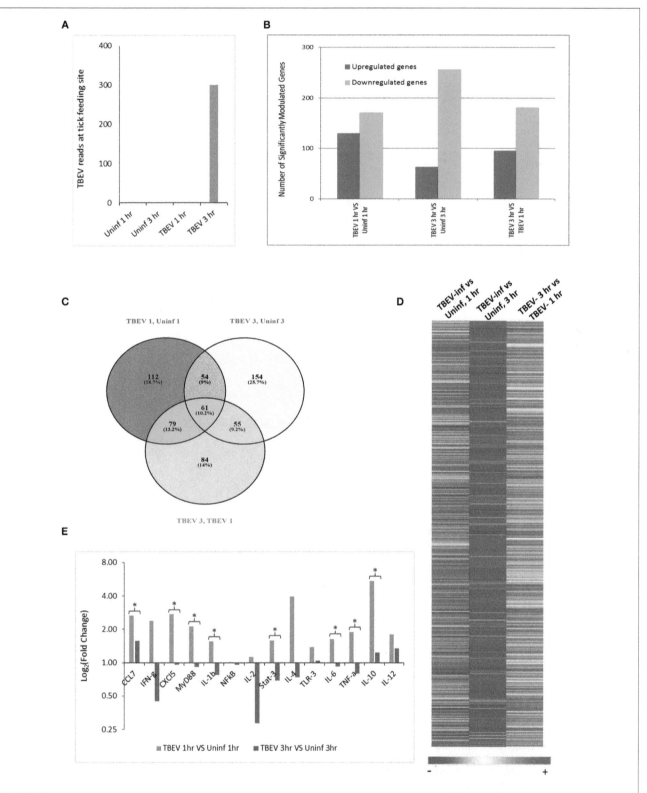

FIGURE 1 | Comparative transcriptional analysis of the TBEV-infected and uninfected *Ixodes ricinus* tick feeding loci. **(A)** The RNASeq data was screened for the presence of TBEV reads at the tick feeding site by aligning the sequences against a TBEV reference genome (MN_001672). The number of TBEV reads that match the TBEV reference genome is plotted for the uninfected tick feeding sites and the TBEV-infected tick feeding sites. **(B,C)** The following comparisons are depicted: TBEV-infected tick feeding loci at 1 h vs. uninfected tick feeding loci at 1 h, TBEV-infected tick feeding loci at 3 h vs. uninfected tick feeding loci at 3 h, TBEV-infected

(Continued)

FIGURE 1 | tick feeding loci at 3 h vs. TBEV-infected tick feeding loci at 1 h. **(B)** The total number of significantly up- or downregulated ($p \leq 0.05$) genes for each comparison. **(C)** Venn diagram showing overlap of significantly modulated genes for each of the three comparisons. **(D)** Heat map showing temporal changes in gene expression profiles. A list of all genes modulated at any time point in the study was used to generate a heatmap with Morpheus web server application (www. broadinstitute.org). **(E)** The immune genes selected for validation were shown to be modulated genes of interest during the host anti-tick response in previous studies. Pre-optimized primers were purchased from IDT and used for the real-time PCR validation. The delta-delta CT method was used to calculate fold-changes in gene expression between TBEV-infected and uninfected tick feeding sites as described in the methods section. GAPDH was used as an endogenous control gene. Statistically significant differences in gene expression between the 1 vs. 3 h tick feeding time points were determined by the Student's *t*-test. *P*-values less than 0.05 were considered significant. Significant differences are indicated by asterisks.

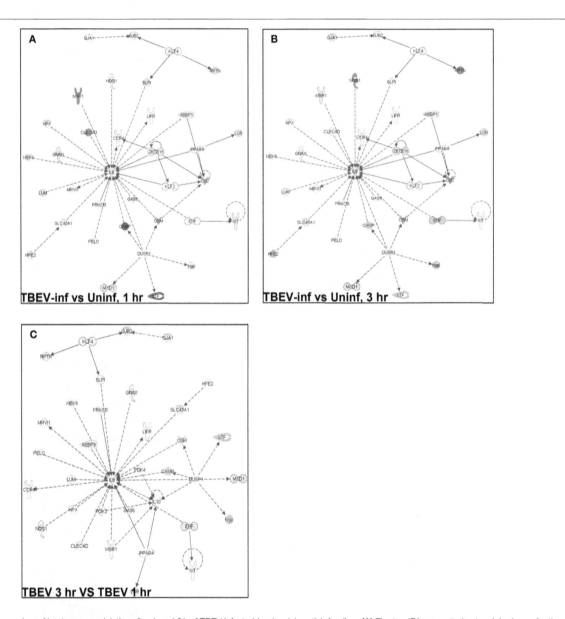

FIGURE 2 | An overview of host gene modulation after 1 and 3 h of TBEV-infected *Ixodes ricinus* tick feeding. **(A)** The top IPA-generated network is shown for the TBEV-infected tick feeding loci at 1 h vs. the uninfected tick feeding loci at 1 h **(B)** The top IPA-generated network is shown for the TBEV-infected tick feeding loci at 3 h vs. the uninfected tick feeding loci at 3 h. **(C)** The top-IPA-generated network is shown for the TBEV-infected tick feeding loci at 3 h vs. TBEV-infected tick feeding loci at 1 h. Note: Red/pink represents upregulated genes, green represents down-regulated genes, and gray represents unchanged or insignificant genes.

with the networks representing the TBEV-infected vs. uninfected comparisons (**Figures 2A,B**) are cellular movement, organismal injury and abnormalities, and hematological system development and function. After 1 h of TBEV-infected tick feeding, 19 host genes shown in the **Figure 2A** network were downregulated and 16 host genes were upregulated. After 3 h of TBEV-infected tick feeding, 22 host genes in the **Figure 2B** network were downregulated, 12 were upregulated, and one gene (Ngp) had a fold change of zero. Thus, as 1 h progressed to 3 h of TBEV-infected tick feeding, the network displayed a slight shift toward cutaneous gene downregulation (**Figure 2**). The IPA-generated network for the TBEV-infected 3 h vs. the TBEV-infected 1 h tick feeding site (**Figure 2C**) is unique from the **Figures 2A,B** networks, as it lacks Ccl2, KLF2, and ZBTB16, but instead includes 20 unique genes which contribute to this network's association with bio-functions such as molecular transport, organismal injury and abnormalities, and cellular movement.

In both the 1 and 3 h comparisons between TBEV-infected vs. uninfected tick feeding sites, inflammatory response was the primary predicted host response. Based on the IPA transcriptional immunoprofiling, the inflammatory response was

projected to be activated in the 1 h comparison of the TBEV-infected vs. uninfected tick feeding site (activation z-score = 1.549), and inhibited in the 3 h comparison (activation z-score = −1.26). Temporal changes in gene expression for all genes predicted to have direct correlative relationships with the inflammatory response were plotted after 1 or 3 h of TBEV-infected vs. uninfected tick feeding (**Figure 3**). Transcriptional levels of cytokines Ccl2, Ccl12, Cxcl1, Cxcl2, Cxcl5, IL6, and IL10 were all upregulated after 1 h of TBEV-infected tick feeding, thus contributing to the overall activation of the inflammatory response (**Figure 3**). At the 3 h time point, the majority of these cytokine transcriptional level were still upregulated, with the exception of Cxcl5 and IL10, which were both slightly downregulated. Real-time PCR validation of a few selected immune genes followed the general pattern observed in the

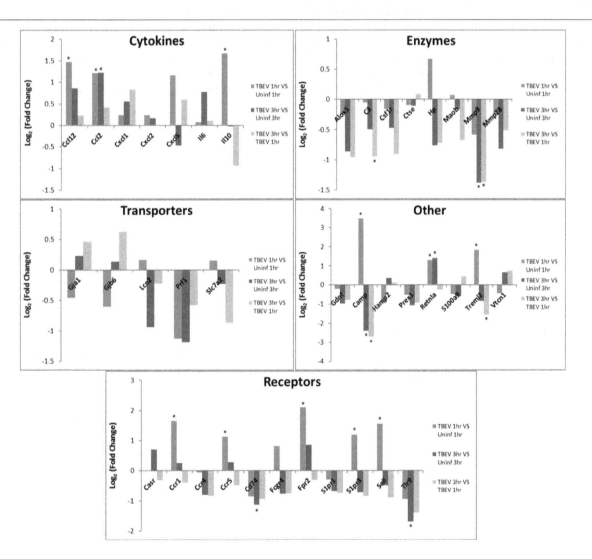

FIGURE 3 | Changes in gene expression related to the inflammatory response after 1 and 3 h of TBEV-infected *Ixodes ricinus* tick feeding. Temporal changes in gene expression data were analyzed by IPA software. Genes predicted to be directly involved in the "Inflammatory Response" were plotted to show temporal changes in gene expression for the following comparisons: TBEV-infected tick feeding loci at 1 h vs. uninfected tick feeding loci at 1 h, TBEV-infected tick feeding loci at 3 h vs. uninfected tick feeding loci at 3 h, TBEV-infected tick feeding loci at 3 h vs. TBEV-infected tick feeding loci at 1 h. Genes with significant modulation in expression (p ≤ 0.05) are marked with an asterisk.

Illumina NGS analysis (**Figure 1E**). All of the enzymes projected to have a direct, correlative relationship with the inflammatory response were downregulated at 3 h, further contributing to the predicted inhibition of the inflammatory response at the feeding site of a TBEV-infected tick (**Figure 3**). Additionally, transcript expression of several receptors (CCR1, CCR5, and Sell) were all significantly upregulated after 1 h of TBEV-infected tick feeding (**Figure 3**), likely contributing to the overall accumulation of immune cells to the tick attachment site. In summary, the cutaneous gene expression analysis indicates that the inflammatory response is activated after only 1 h of TBEV-infected tick feeding, and that increased recruitment and accumulation of immune cells is expected at the 1 h time point. However, after 3 h of TBEV-infected tick feeding, the cutaneous inflammatory response is predicted to undergo slight inhibition, as demonstrated by the downregulated expression of over half of the genes shown to have a correlative relationship with the inflammatory response (**Figure 3**).

An IPA core comparison analysis was used to analyze changes in host cutaneous gene expression in response to TBEV-infected tick feeding vs. uninfected tick feeding observed across the two experimental time points (1 and 3 h). **Figure 4** shows activation status prediction networks for the top five immune responses or bio-functions generated from the IPA core comparison analysis. "Maintenance of leukocytes" was the top predicted bio-function in the core comparison analysis (**Figure 4**). This IPA category moniker refers to bio-functions associated with the normal cellular activities that maintain cellular homeostasis, including engulfment, phagocytosis, regulation, and stasis of cells. The maintenance of leukocytes was predicted to be inhibited at both the 1 and 3 h comparisons of TBEV-infected vs. uninfected tick feeding (activation z-score $= -2$ for both time points). At both the 1 and 3 h time points, GATA3 transcription was downregulated (**Figure 4**). GATA3 is a transcription factor required for both the maintenance and development of Th2 cells (Pai et al., 2004). Furthermore, IL34, which is highly expressed by keratinocytes in the epidermis and plays an important role in the maintenance and development of Langerhans cells (Greter et al., 2012), was also downregulated after 1 and 3 h of TBEV-infected tick feeding (**Figure 4**). CCR4 knockout (CCR4$^{-/-}$) bone marrow-derived dendritic cells are less efficient in the maintenance of Th17 responses compared to wild type dendritic cells (Poppensieker et al., 2012); therefore, the downregulation of CCR4 transcription in the present study contributes to the

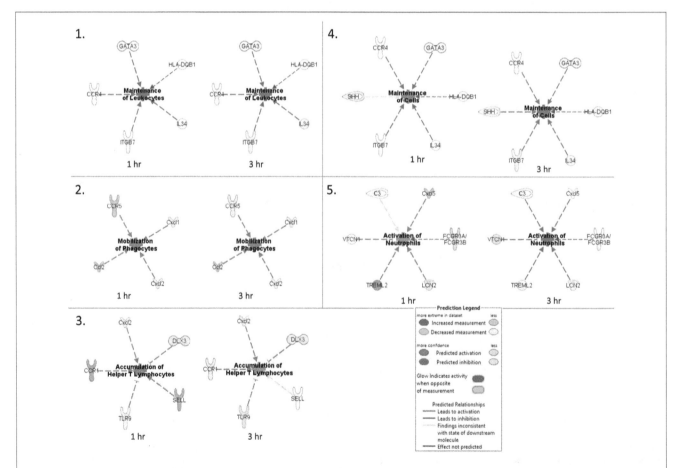

FIGURE 4 | Activation status prediction networks for the top five immune responses / bio-functions generated from the IPA core comparison analysis. An IPA core comparison analysis was used to analyze which biological processes are relevant at 1 and 3 h of TBEV-infected vs. uninfected tick feeding. The predicted activation status of each network is shown.

inhibition of leukocyte maintenance at the 1 and 3 h time points. Mouse integrin subunit beta 7 (ITGB7) is necessary for the maintenance of memory T lymphocytes expressing the CD4 protein (Yang et al., 2011). Since ITGB7 is downregulated in the present transcriptional immunoprofiling study, it likely contributes to the inhibited maintenance of memory CD4+ T cells after 1 and 3 h of TBEV-infected tick feeding.

"Mobilization of phagocytes" was the second predicted bio-function in the core comparison analysis. After 1 and 3 h of TBEV-infected vs. uninfected tick feeding, the mobilization of phagocytes was predicted to be activated (activation z-score = 1.982 for both time points) (**Figure 4**). Monocytes, macrophages, neutrophils, dendritic cells, and mast cells are several of the professional phagocytic cells. In mice, there are two Ccl2 homologs, Ccl2 and Ccl12, both of which are potent phagocyte chemoattractants. The transcript levels of these two chemokines are upregulated at both the 1 and 3 h time points, thereby increasing the mobilization and chemotaxis of phagocytes at the TBEV-infected tick feeding site (**Figures 3, 4**). CCR5 is known to regulate accumulation of activated macrophages in the West Nile virus-infected mouse brain (Glass et al., 2005), and upregulated transcription of this chemokine receptor in the present study likely contributes to the activated mobilization of phagocytes. Mast cells and tissue resident macrophages release the potent neutrophil chemoattractants, Cxcl1 and Cxcl2 (De Filippo et al., 2008, 2013). In response to tissue inflammation, mast cells positioned near the vasculature initiate neutrophil infiltration from the circulation by releasing Cxcl1 and Cxcl2, while tissue resident macrophages also release Cxcl1 and Cxcl2, recruiting neutrophils deeper into the inflamed tissue (De Filippo et al., 2013). In the present study transcript levels of both

these chemokines are both upregulated during TBEV-infected tick feeding, thus contributing to the activated mobilization of neutrophils that infiltrate the tick feeding site very early (**Figures 3, 4**).

The third predicted bio-function generated in the IPA core comparison analysis was "accumulation of helper T lymphocytes." The activation z-score for this bio-function decreased from 2.19 at 1 h post-TBEV-infected tick feeding to 1.452 at the 3 h time point. Transcript levels of CCR1 and Cxcl2 are upregulated at both time points in the present study and these genes are associated with the recruitment and accumulation of helper T lymphocytes at the cutaneous site of TBEV-infected tick feeding (**Figure 4**). Selectin L (SELL) is a cellular adhesion molecule found on the surface of most lymphocytes that mediates lymphocyte capture and rolling at sites of inflammation (Tedder et al., 1995). In the present study, SELL transcription was upregulated at the 1 h time point, contributing to the IPA prediction that helper T lymphocytes are accumulating, but the downregulated transcription of SELL at 3 h is inconsistent with the predicted activation pattern, as depicted by the yellow arrow in **Figure 4**. TLR9, a receptor that preferentially binds unmethylated CpG sequences in bacterial and viral DNA, was downregulated in the present study (**Figure 4**). Here, the downregulation of TLR9 transcription is predicted to activate the accumulation of T lymphocytes at the skin feeding site of a TBEV-infected tick. This prediction is supported by a recently developed mouse model of cutaneous lupus that is dependent on the expression of TLR7 and the loss of TLR9, which ultimately results in extensive accumulation of IFNγ-producing T lymphocytes (Mande et al., 2017). Distal-less 3 (DLX3) is a transcription factor involved in the terminal differentiation of keratinocytes. In a

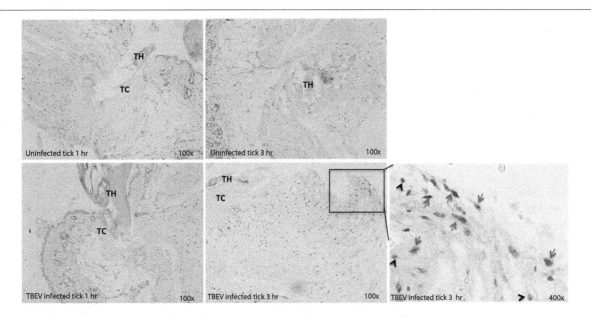

FIGURE 5 | Immunohistochemistry of the *Ixodes ricinus* feeding loci. Five micron sections from skin biopsies harvested at *I. ricinus* feeding sites were subjected to immunohistochemistry procedures to detect TBEV antigens. Red arrows point to TBEV infected fibroblasts; blue arrows point to TBEV infected mononuclear phagocytes, and black arrowheads point to uninfected neutrophils. TH, tick hypostome; TC, tick cement.

mouse model with epidermal ablation of DLX3, there was an increase of IL17-producing CD4$^+$ T cells, CD8$^+$ T cells, and γδ T cells in the skin and draining lymph nodes (Hwang et al., 2011); thus, the downregulated transcription of DLX3 in the skin biopsies from the present study likely contributes to the accumulation of helper T lymphocytes at the cutaneous feeding site of infected ticks (**Figure 4**).

"Maintenance of cells" was the fourth predicted bio-function in the IPA core comparison analysis. This bio-function was predicted to be inhibited at both experimental time points (1 h activation z-score = −1.342, 3 h activation z-score = −2.236). The "maintenance of cells" activation network is very similar to the top predicted network, "maintenance of leukocytes"; however, the only difference is that Sonic hedgehog (SHH) is present in the "maintenance of cells" network (**Figure 4**). The touch dome, a highly specialized mechanosensory epidermal structure composed of distinct keratinocytes in close association with innervated Merkel cells, is maintained by signaling with SHH to tissue-specific stem cells (Xiao et al., 2015). In the present study SHH transcription is upregulated after 1 h of TBEV-infected tick feeding, a finding that is inconsistent with the predicted pattern of inhibited cell maintenance (depicted by the yellow arrow in **Figure 4**); however, at the 3 h time point, SHH transcription was downregulated, contributing to the predicted inhibition of touch dome cell maintenance (**Figure 4**). Some damage to the perineural skin microenvironment is likely to occur because of the mechanical injury induced by tick feeding, and this could ultimately impact SHH signaling and the touch dome homeostasis.

The "activation of neutrophils" was the fifth predicted bio-function in the core comparison analysis. After 1 h of TBEV-infected vs. uninfected tick feeding, neutrophil activation was predicted to be activated (activation z-score = 1.342); however, after 3 h, neutrophils were predicted to be inhibited (activation z-score = −2.236) (**Figure 4**). The upregulated transcription of Cxcl5 and TREML2 at the 1 h time point, followed by the downregulation of these genes at the 3 h time point contribute to this phenomenon because Cxcl5 is a chemokine involved in the activation of neutrophils (Proost et al., 1993) and TREML2 potentiates neutrophil activation in response to G protein-coupled receptor signaling (Halpert et al., 2011). Likewise, Lipocalin-2 (LCN2) transcription was upregulated at 1 h post-TBEV-infected tick feeding and downregulated at 3 h. LCN2 is expressed in neutrophils and is a potent inducer of their chemotaxis and migration to sites of inflammation (Schroll et al., 2012); thus, its upregulation at the 1 h time point further contributes to the activation of neutrophils at the feeding site of TBEV-infected ticks. VTCN1 belongs to the B7 family of costimulatory proteins. VTCN1 inhibits the expansion of neutrophils from their progenitors, as demonstrated by VTCN1-deficient mice that display enhanced neutrophil-mediated innate immunity (Zhu et al., 2009); therefore, the downregulation of VTCN1 transcription after 1 h, and its upregulation after 3 h, contributes to the activation of neutrophils at the cutaneous feeding site of a TBEV-infected tick (**Figure 4**).

Immunohistochemistry

Immunohistochemical analysis was performed at the feeding sites of TBEV-infected and uninfected *I. ricinus* to determine if the gene expression data could be correlated to the tissue morphology and inflammation. The tick feeding site is characterized by extravasated erythrocytes and leucocytes, and with a steady influx of inflammatory cells. As early as 1 h post-TBEV-infected tick feeding, neutrophils were observed at both infected and uninfected tick feeding sites, with a marked increase at the infected tick feeding site. After 3 h of TBEV-infected tick feeding, increased recruitment of inflammatory cells was observed at the infected tick feeding site compared to the uninfected tick feeding site. Among these, TBEV antigens were localized in fibroblasts and mononuclear cells, but not in neutrophils (**Figure 5**). These immunohistochemistry observations support the cutaneous immune gene expression data, showing an inflammatory micro-environment at the feeding site of TBEV-infected ticks. The recruitment of inflammatory cells appears to be much more pronounced in the TBEV-infected tick feeding site than the uninfected tick feeding site.

CONCLUSIONS

The present study demonstrates that TBEV-infected *I. ricinus* adult ticks create an inflammatory environment at the murine cutaneous interface within 1 h of feeding. Significant differences in immune responses were observed between hosts infested with TBEV-infected vs. uninfected ticks. Furthermore, genes associated with neutrophil activation and mobilization were modulated in the presence of TBEV, suggesting that there is an influx of neutrophils and other phagocytic inflammatory cells to the tick feeding site after only 1 and 3 h of infected tick feeding. Immunohistochemistry further supported the cutaneous immune gene expression analysis, demonstrating pronounced recruitment of inflammatory cells, especially neutrophils, to the feeding site of TBEV-infected ticks. Taken together with our earlier study on POWV-infected tick feeding sites (Hermance and Thangamani, 2014), and the current study, it is clearly evident that during the earliest stages of flavivirus-infected tick feeding, a complex, inflammatory micro-environment is created in the host's skin. The present study serves to expand our understanding of the immunological events that occur at the cutaneous interface during the early stages of tick-borne flavivirus transmission to a host.

AUTHOR CONTRIBUTIONS

Conceived the idea: ST; Provided reagents and materials: ST and MK; Performed experiments: ST, MK, MH, RS, SW, MS, and DH; Data analysis: ST, MH, and SW; Wrote manuscript: ST and MH. All authors critically read and revised the manuscript.

FUNDING

ST is supported by NIH/NIAID grants R01AI127771 and R21AI113128. MK was supported by the Slovak Research and Development Agency (contract no. APVV-0737-12).

ACKNOWLEDGMENTS

The authors wish to thank Dr. Boris Klempa and Marta Siebenstichova from the Institute of Virology, Biomedical Research Center, Slovak Academy of Sciences (Bratislava, Slovakia) for providing TBEV MBS for tick inoculations.

REFERENCES

1. Alekseev, A. N., Burenkova, L. A., Vasilieva, I. S., Dubinina, H. V., and Chunikhin, S. P. (1996). Preliminary studies on virus and spirochete accumulation in the cement plug of ixodid ticks. *Exp. Appl. Acarol.* 20, 713–723. doi: 10.1007/BF00051556

2. Alekseev, A. N., and Chunikhin, S. P. (1990). The experimental transmission of the tick-borne encephalitis virus by ixodid ticks (the mechanisms, time periods, species and sex differences). *Parazitologiia* 24, 177–185.

3. Belova, O. A., Burenkova, L. A., and Karganova, G. G. (2012). Different tick-borne encephalitis virus (TBEV) prevalences in unfed versus partially engorged ixodid ticks -evidence of virus replication and changes in tick behavior. *Ticks Tick Borne Dis.* 3, 240–246. doi: 10.1016/j.ttbdis.2012.05.005

4. CDC Tick-borne Encephalitis (2017). *Tick-borne encephalitis (TBE). Risk of Exposure. 2017.* Available online at: https://www.cdc.gov/vhf/tbe/exposure/index.html

5. Danielová, V., Holubová, J., Pejcoch, M., and Daniel, M. (2002). Potential significance oftransovarial transmission in the circulation of tick-borne encephalitis virus. *Folia Parasitol.* 49, 323–325. doi: 10.14411/fp.2002.060

6. De Filippo, K., Dudeck, A., Hasenberg, M., Nye, E., van Rooijen, N., Hartmann, K., et al. (2013). Mast cell and macrophage chemokines CXCL1/CXCL2 control the early stage of neutrophil recruitment during tissue inflammation. *Blood* 121, 4930–4937. doi: 10.1182/blood-2013-02-486217

7. De Filippo, K., Henderson, R. B., Laschinger, M., and Hogg, N. (2008). Neutrophil chemokines KC and macrophage-inflammatory protein-2 are newly synthesized by tissue macrophages using distinct TLR signaling pathways. *J. Immunol.* 180, 4308–4315. doi: 10.4049/jimmunol.180.6.4308

8. Francischetti, I. M., Sa-Nunes, A., Mans, B. J., Santos, I. M., and Ribeiro, J. M. (2009). The role of saliva in tick feeding. *Front. Biosci.* 14:363. doi: 10.2741/3363

9. Glass, W. G., Lim, J. K., Cholera, R., Pletnev, A. G., Gao, J. L., and Murphy, P. M. (2005). Chemokine receptor CCR5 promotes leukocyte trafficking to the brain and survival in West Nile virus infection. *J. Exp. Med.* 202, 1087–1098. doi: 10.1084/jem.20042530

10. Greter, M., Lelios, I., Pelczar, P., Hoeffel, G., Price, J., Leboeuf, M., et al. (2012). Stroma-derived interleukin-34 controls the development and maintenance of Langerhans cells and the maintenance of microglia. *Immunity* 37, 1050–1060. doi: 10.1016/j.immuni.2012.11.001

11. Gritsun, T. S., Lashkevich, V. A., and Gould, E. A. (2003a). Tick-borne encephalitis. *Antiviral Res.* 57, 129–146. doi: 10.1016/S0166-3542(02)00206-1

12. Gritsun, T. S., Nuttall, P. A., and Gould, E. A. (2003b). Tick-borne flaviviruses. *Adv. Virus. Res.* 61, 317–371. doi: 10.1016/S0065-3527(03)61008-0

13. Halpert, M. M., Thomas, K. A., King, R. G., and Justement, L. B. (2011). TLT2 potentiates neutrophil antibacterial activity and chemotaxis in response to G protein-coupled receptor-mediated signaling. *J. Immunol.* 187, 2346–2355. doi: 10.4049/jimmunol.1100534

14. Heinze, D. M., Carmical, J. R., Aronson, J. F., and Thangamani, S. (2012). Early immunologic events at the tick-host interface. *PLoS ONE* 7:e47301. doi: 10.1371/journal.pone.0047301

15. Hermance, M. E., Santos, R. I., Kelly, B. C., Valbuena, G., and Thangamani, S. (2016). Immune cell targets of infection at the tick-skin interface during Powassan virus transmission. *PLoS ONE* 11:e0155889. doi: 10.1371/journal.pone.0155889

16. Hermance, M. E., and Thangamani, S. (2014). Proinflammatory cytokines and chemokines at theskin interface during Powassan virus transmission. *J. Invest. Dermatol.* 134, 2280–2283. doi: 10.1038/jid.2014.150

17. Hermance, M. E., and Thangamani, S. (2015). Tick saliva enhances Powassan virus transmission to the host, influencing its dissemination and the course of disease. *J. Virol.* 89, 7852–7860. doi: 10.1128/JVI.01056-15

18. Hwang, J., Kita, R., Kwon, H. S., Choi, E. H., Lee, S. H., Udey, M. C., et al. (2011). Epidermal ablation of Dlx3 is linked to IL-17-associated skin inflammation. *Proc. Natl. Acad. Sci. U.S.A.* 108, 11566–15671. doi: 10.1073/pnas.1019658108

19. Kaufman, W. R., and Nuttall, P. A. (1996). *Amblyomma variegatum* (Acari: Ixodidae): mechanism and control of arbovirus secretion in tick saliva. *Exp. Parasitol.* 82, 316–323. doi: 10.1006/expr.1996.0039

20. Kazimírová, M., and Štibrániová, I. (2013). Tick salivary compounds: their role in modulation of host defences and pathogen transmission. *Front. Cell. Infect. Microbiol.* 3:43. doi: 10.3389/fcimb.2013.00043

21. Kazimírová, M., Mantel, N., Raynaud, S., Slovák, M., Ustaniková, K., Lang, J., et al. (2012). Evaluation of chimeric yellow fever 17D/dengue viral replication in ticks. *Vector Borne Zoonot. Dis.* 12, 979–985. doi: 10.1089/vbz.2011.0947

22. Kazimírová, M., Thangamani, S., Bartíková, P., Hermance, M., Holíková, V., Štibrániová, I., et al. (2017). Tick-borne viruses and biological processes at the tick-host-virus interface. *Front. Cell. Infect. Microbiol.* 7:339. doi: 10.3389/fcimb.2017.00339

23. Kovalev, S. Y., and Mukhacheva, T. A. (2014). Tick-borne encephalitis virus subtypes emerged through rapid vector switches rather than gradual evolution. *Ecol. Evol.* 4, 4307–4316. doi: 10.1002/ece3.1301

24. Labuda, M., Austyn, J. M., Zuffova, E., Kozuch, O., Fuchsberger, N., Lysy, J., et al. (1996). Importance of localized skin infection in tick-borne encephalitis virus transmission. *Virology* 219, 357–366. doi: 10.1006/viro.1996.0261

25. Labuda, M., Jones, L. D., Williams, T., Danielova, V., and Nuttall, P. A. (1993). Efficient transmission of tick-borne encephalitis virus between cofeeding ticks. *J. Med. Entomol.* 30, 295–299. doi: 10.1093/jmedent/30.1.295

26. Labuda, M., Kozuch, O., Zuffová, E., Eleková, E., Hails, R. S., and Nuttall, P. A. (1997). Tick-borne encephalitis virus transmission between ticks cofeeding on specific immune natural rodent hosts. *Virology* 235, 138–143. doi: 10.1006/viro.1997.8622

27. Lindquist, L., and Vapalahti, O. (2008). Tick-borne encephalitis. *Lancet* 371, 1861–1871. doi: 10.1016/S0140-6736(08)60800-4

28. Mande, P., Taravati, K., Rosenblum, M., and Rothstein, A. M. (2017). Taking a 'Toll' on skin: a novel TLR9-deficient model of cutaneous lupus [Abstract]. *J. Immunol.* 198, 207.2.

29. Mansfield, K. L., Johnson, N., Phipps, L. P., Stephenson, J. R., Fooks, A. R., and Solomon, T. (2009). Tick-borne encephalitis virus - a review of an emerging zoonosis. *J. Gen. Virol.* 90, 1781–1794. doi: 10.1099/vir.0.011437-0

30. Oliveros, J. C. (2007). *Venny. An Interactive Tool for Comparing Lists with Venn Diagrams.* Available online at: http://bioinfogp.cnb.csic.es/tools/venny/index.html (Accessed February, 2017).

31. Pai, S. Y., Truitt, M. L., and Ho, I. C. (2004). GATA-3 deficiency abrogates the development and maintenance of T helper type 2 cells. *Proc. Natl. Acad. Sci. U.S.A.* 101, 1993–1998. doi: 10.1073/pnas.0308697100

32. Poppensieker, K., Otte, D. M., Schürmann, B., Limmer, A., Dresing, P., Drews, E., et al. (2012). CC chemokine receptor 4 is required for experimental autoimmune encephalomyelitis by regulating GM-CSF and IL-23

33. production in dendritic cells. *Proc. Natl. Acad. Sci. U.S.A.* 109, 3897–3902. doi: 10.1073/pnas.1114153109

34. Proost, P., Wuyts, A., Conings, R., Lenaerts, J. P., Billiau, A., Opdenakker, G., et al. (1993). Human and bovine granulocyte chemotactic protein-2: complete amino acid sequence and functional characterization as chemokines. *Biochemistry* 32, 10170–10177. doi: 10.1021/bi00089a037

35. Randolph, S. E. (2011). Transmission of tick-borne pathogens between co-feeding ticks: milan labuda's enduring paradigm. *Ticks Tick Borne Dis.* 2, 179–182. doi: 10.1016/j.ttbdis.2011.07.004

36. Ribeiro, J. M., Alarcon-Chaidez, F., Francischetti, I. M., Mans, B. J.,

Mather, T. N., Valenzuela, J. G., et al. (2006). An annotated catalog of salivary gland transcripts from *Ixodes scapularis* ticks. *Insect Biochem. Mol. Biol.* 36, 111–129. doi: 10.1016/j.ibmb.2005.11.005

37. Santos, R. I., Hermance, M. E., Gelman, B. B., and Thangamani, S. (2016). Spinal cord ventral horns and lymphoid organ involvement in *Powassan virus* infection in a mouse model. *Viruses* 8:220. doi: 10.3390/v8080220

38. Schroll, A., Eller, K., Feistritzer, C., Nairz, M., Sonnweber, T., Moser, P. A., et al. (2012). Lipocalin-2 ameliorates granulocyte functionality. *Eur. J. Immunol.* 42, 3346–3357. doi: 10.1002/eji.201142351

39. Slovák, M., Kazimírová, M., Siebenstichová, M., Ustaníková, K., Klempa, B., Gritsun, T., et al. (2014). Survival dynamics of tick-borne encephalitis virus in *Ixodes ricinus* ticks. *Ticks Tick Borne Dis.* 5, 962–969. doi: 10.1016/j.ttbdis.2014. 07.019

40. Süss, J. (2011). Tick-borne encephalitis 2010: epidemiology, risk areas, and virus strains in Europe and Asia-an overview. *Ticks Tick Borne Dis.* 2, 2–15. doi: 10.1016/j.ttbdis.2010.10.007

41. Süss, J., Schrader, C., Falk, U., and Wohanka, N. (2004). Tick-borne encephalitis (TBE) in Germany - epidemiological data, development of risk areas and virus prevalence in field-collected ticks and in ticks removed from humans. *Int. J. Med. Microbiol.* 293, 69–79. doi: 10.1016/S1433-1128(04)80011-1

42. Šimo, L., Kazimirova, M., Richardson, J., and Bonnet, S. I. (2017). The essential role of tick salivary glands and saliva in tick feeding and pathogen transmission. *Front. Cell. Infect. Microbiol.* 7:281. doi: 10.3389/fcimb.2017.00281

43. Tedder, T. F., Steeber, D. A., and Pizcueta, P. (1995). L-selectin-deficient mice have impaired leukocyte recruitment into inflammatory sites. *J. Exp. Med.* 181, 2259–2264. doi: 10.1084/jem.181.6.2259

44. Tonteri, E., Kipar, A., Voutilainen, L., Vene, S., Vaheri, A., Vapalahti, O., et al. (2013). The three subtypes of tick-borne encephalitis virus induce encephalitis in a natural host, the bank vole (*Myodes glareolus*). *PLoS ONE* 8:e81214. doi: 10.1371/journal.pone.0081214

45. Wikel, S. (2013). Ticks and tick-borne pathogens at the cutaneous interface: host defenses, tick countermeasures, and a suitable environment for pathogen establishment. *Front. Microbiol.* 4:337. doi: 10.3389/fmicb.2013.00337

46. Xiao, Y., Thoresen, D. T., Williams, J. S., Wang, C., Perna, J., Petrova, R., et al. (2015). Neural Hedgehog signaling maintains stem cell renewal in the sensory touch dome epithelium. *Proc. Natl. Acad. Sci. U.S.A.* 112, 7195–7200. doi: 10.1073/pnas.1504177112

47. Yang, L., Yu, Y., Kalwani, M., Tseng, T. W., and Baltimore, D. (2011). Homeostatic cytokines orchestrate the segregation of CD4 and CD8 memory T-cell reservoirs in mice. *Blood* 118, 3039–3050. doi: 10.1182/blood-2011-04-3 49746

48. Zhu, G., Augustine, M. M., Azuma, T., Luo, L., Yao, S., Anand, S., et al. (2009). B7- H4-deficient mice display augmented neutrophil-mediated innate immunity. *Blood* 113, 1759–1767. doi: 10.1182/blood-2008-01-133223

Permissions

The contributors of this book come from diverse backgrounds, making this book a truly international effort. This book will bring forth new frontiers with its revolutionizing research information and detailed analysis of the nascent developments around the world.

We would like to thank all the contributing authors for lending their expertise to make the book truly unique. They have played a crucial role in the development of this book. Without their invaluable contributions this book wouldn't have been possible. They have made vital efforts to compile up to date information on the varied aspects of this subject to make this book a valuable addition to the collection of many professionals and students.

This book was conceptualized with the vision of imparting up-to-date information and advanced data in this field. To ensure the same, a matchless editorial board was set up. Every individual on the board went through rigorous rounds of assessment to prove their worth. After which they invested a large part of their time researching and compiling the most relevant data for our readers.

The editorial board has been involved in producing this book since its inception. They have spent rigorous hours researching and exploring the diverse topics which have resulted in the successful publishing of this book. They have passed on their knowledge of decades through this book. To expedite this challenging task, the publisher supported the team at every step. A small team of assistant editors was also appointed to further simplify the editing procedure and attain best results for the readers.

Apart from the editorial board, the designing team has also invested a significant amount of their time in understanding the subject and creating the most relevant covers. They scrutinized every image to scout for the most suitable representation of the subject and create an appropriate cover for the book.

The publishing team has been an ardent support to the editorial, designing and production team. Their endless efforts to recruit the best for this project, has resulted in the accomplishment of this book. They are a veteran in the field of academics and their pool of knowledge is as vast as their experience in printing. Their expertise and guidance has proved useful at every step. Their uncompromising quality standards have made this book an exceptional effort. Their encouragement from time to time has been an inspiration for everyone.

The publisher and the editorial board hope that this book will prove to be a valuable piece of knowledge for researchers, students, practitioners and scholars across the globe.

List of Contributors

Jing Xia, Ling Kong, Li-Juan Zhou, Shui-Zhen Wu, Li-Jie Yao, Cheng He and Hong-Juan Peng
Department of Pathogen Biology, Guangdong Provincial Key Laboratory of Tropical Disease Research, School of Public Health, Southern Medical University, Guangzhou, China

Cynthia Y. He
Department of Biological Sciences, National University of Singapore, Singapore

Daniel Młocicki
Department of General Biology and Parasitology, Medical University of Warsaw, Warsaw, Poland
Witold Stefań ski Institute of Parasitology, Polish Academy of Sciences, Warsaw, Poland

Anna Sulima
Department of General Biology and Parasitology, Medical University of Warsaw, Warsaw, Poland

Justyna Bień, Anna Zawistowska-Deniziak and Katarzyna Basałaj
Witold Stefań ski Institute of Parasitology, Polish Academy of Sciences, Warsaw, Poland

Anu Näreaho
Department of Veterinary Biosciences, University of Helsinki, Helsinki, Finland

Rusłan Sałamatin
Department of General Biology and Parasitology, Medical University of Warsaw, Warsaw, Poland
Department of Parasitology and Vector-Borne Diseases, National Institute of Public Health National Institute of Hygiene, Warsaw, Poland

David Bruce Conn
Department of Invertebrate Zoology, Museum of Comparative Zoology, Harvard University, Cambridge, MA, United States
One Health Center, Berry College, Mount Berry, GA, United States

Kirsi Savijoki
Division of Pharmaceutical Biosciences, University of Helsinki, Helsinki, Finland

Taniya Mitra, Fana Alem Kidane and Dieter Liebhart
Clinic for Poultry and Fish Medicine, Department for Farm Animals and Veterinary Public Health, University of Veterinary Medicine Vienna, Vienna, Austria

Michael Hess
Clinic for Poultry and Fish Medicine, Department for Farm Animals and Veterinary Public Health, University of Veterinary Medicine Vienna, Vienna, Austria
Christian Doppler Laboratory for Innovative Poultry Vaccines (IPOV), University of Veterinary Medicine Vienna, Vienna, Austria

Sebastian Rausch, Ankur Midha, Nicole Affinass and Susanne Hartmann
Department of Veterinary Medicine, Institute of Immunology, Freie Universität Berlin, Berlin, Germany

Matthias Kuhring
Bioinformatics Unit (MF 1), Robert Koch Institute, Berlin, Germany
Core Unit Bioinformatics, Berlin Institute of Health (BIH), Berlin, Germany
Berlin Institute of Health Metabolomics Platform, Berlin Institute of Health (BIH), Berlin, Germany
Max Delbrück Center for Molecular Medicine, Berlin, Germany

Aleksandar Radonic
Centre for Biological Threats and Special Pathogens (ZBS 1), Robert Koch Institute, Berlin, Germany
Genome Sequencing Unit (MF 2), Robert Koch Institute, Berlin, Germany

Anja A. Kühl
iPATH.Berlin, Core Unit for Immunopathology for Experimental Models, Berlin Institute of Health, Charité - Universitätsmedizin Berlin, Corporate Member of Freie Universität Berlin, Humboldt-Universität zu Berlin, Berlin, Germany

André Bleich
Institute for Laboratory Animal Science, Hannover Medical School, Hannover, Germany

Bernhard Y. Renard
Bioinformatics Unit (MF 1), Robert Koch Institute, Berlin, Germany

Eduardo L. V. Silveira, Mariana R. Dominguez and Irene S. Soares
Department of Clinical and Toxicological Analyses, School of Pharmaceutical Sciences, University of São Paulo, São Paulo, Brazil

Vitomir Djokic, Shekerah Primus, Lavoisier Akoolo, Monideep Chakraborti and Nikhat Parveen
Department of Microbiology, Biochemistry and Molecular Genetics, Rutgers New Jersey Medical School, Newark, NJ, United States

Daria L. Ivanova, Stephen L. Denton, Kevin D. Fettel and Jason P. Gigley
Molecular Biology, University of Wyoming, Laramie, WY, United States

Kerry S. Sondgeroth and Berit Bangoura
Veterinary Sciences, University of Wyoming, Laramie, WY, United States

Juan Munoz Gutierrez
Microbiology, Immunology and Pathology, College of Veterinary Medicine and Biomedical Sciences, Colorado State University, Fort Collins, CO, United States

Ildiko R. Dunay
Institute of Inflammation and Neurodegeneration, Ottovon- Guericke Universität Magdeburg, Magdeburg, Germany

Mariana K. Galuppo, Eloiza de Rezende, Mauro Cortez and Beatriz S. Stolf
Department of Parasitology, Institute of Biomedical Sciences, University of São Paulo, São Paulo, Brazil

Andre A. Teixeira, Ricardo J. Giordano and Fabio L. Forti
Department of Biochemistry, Institute of Chemistry, University of São Paulo, São Paulo, Brazil

Mario C. Cruz
Department of Immunology, Institute of Biomedical Sciences, University of São Paulo, São Paulo, Brazil

Amin Zakeri, Sidsel D. Andersen and Peter Nejsum
Department of Clinical Medicine, Faculty of Health, Aarhus University, Aarhus, Denmark

Eline P. Hansen and Andrew R. Williams
Department of Veterinary and Animal Sciences, Faculty of Health and Medical Sciences, University of Copenhagen, Frederiksberg, Denmark

Magdalena Radwanska
Laboratory for Biomedical Research, Ghent University Global Campus, Incheon, South Korea

Nick Vereecke and Stefan Magez
Laboratory for Biomedical Research, Ghent University Global Campus, Incheon, South Korea
Laboratory of Cellular and Molecular Immunology, Vrije Universiteit Brussel, Brussels, Belgium

Violette Deleeuw and Joar Pinto
Laboratory of Cellular and Molecular Immunology, Vrije Universiteit Brussel, Brussels, Belgium

Woo H. Kim, Atul A. Chaudhari and Hyun S. Lillehoj
Animal Biosciences and Biotechnology Laboratory, U.S. Department of Agriculture, Beltsville Agricultural Research Center, ARS, Beltsville, MD, United States

Wongi Min
College of Veterinary Medicine and Institute of Animal Medicine, Gyeongsang National University, Jinju, South Korea

Neil A. Mabbott
The Roslin Institute & Royal (Dick) School of Veterinary Studies, University of Edinburgh, Edinburgh, United Kingdom

Wei Cong
State Key Laboratory of Veterinary Etiological Biology, Key Laboratory of Veterinary Parasitology of Gansu Province, Lanzhou Veterinary Research Institute, Chinese Academy of Agricultural Sciences, Lanzhou, China
Department of Marine Engineering, Marine College, Shandong University, Weihai, China

Tania Dottorini and Richard D. Emes
Faculty of Medicine and Health Sciences, School of Veterinary Medicine and Science, University of Nottingham, Loughborough, United Kingdom
Advanced Data Analysis Centre, University of Nottingham, Loughborough, United Kingdom

Faraz Khan
Advanced Data Analysis Centre, University of Nottingham, Loughborough, United Kingdom

Fu-Kai Zhang, Chun-Xue Zhou, Jun-Jun He, Xiao-Xuan Zhang and Xing-Quan Zhu
State Key Laboratory of Veterinary Etiological Biology, Key Laboratory of Veterinary Parasitology of Gansu Province, Lanzhou Veterinary Research Institute, Chinese Academy of Agricultural Sciences, Lanzhou, China

Hany M. Elsheikha
Faculty of Medicine and Health Sciences, School of Veterinary Medicine and Science, University of Nottingham, Loughborough, United Kingdom

Wenn-Chyau Lee and Laurent Rénia
Singapore Immunology Network (SIgN), Agency for Science, Technology and Research, Singapore

Bruce Russell
Department of Microbiology and Immunology, University of Otago, Dunedin, New Zealand

Andrew J. Forgie, Janelle M. Fouhse and Benjamin P. Willing
Department of Agricultural, Food and Nutritional Science, University of Alberta, Edmonton, AB, Canada

Saravanan Thangamani
Department of Pathology, The University of Texas Medical Branch, Galveston, TX, United States
Institute for Human Infections and Immunity, The University of Texas Medical Branch, Galveston, TX, United States
Center for Tropical Diseases, The University of Texas Medical Branch, Galveston, TX, United States

Meghan E. Hermance and Rodrigo I. Santos
Department of Pathology, The University of Texas Medical Branch, Galveston, TX, United States

Mirko Slovak and Maria Kazimirova
Institute of Zoology, Slovak Academy of Sciences, Bratislava, Slovakia

Dar Heinze
Department of Surgery, Center for Regenerative Medicine, Boston University and Boston Medical Center, Boston, MA, United States

Steven G. Widen
Department of Biochemistry and Molecular Biology, The University of Texas Medical Branch, Galveston, TX, United States

Index

Printed in the USA
CPSIA information can be obtained
at www.ICGtesting.com
JSHW051624061123
51533JS00005B/91